Infectious Complications in Biologic and Targeted Therapies

Carlos Cervera • Jose Maria Aguado
Editors

Infectious Complications in Biologic and Targeted Therapies

Springer

Editors
Carlos Cervera
Division of Infectious Diseases
University of Alberta
Edmonton, AB, Canada

Jose Maria Aguado
Complutense University of Madrid
University Hospital "October 12"
Madrid, Madrid, Spain

ISBN 978-3-031-11362-8 ISBN 978-3-031-11363-5 (eBook)
https://doi.org/10.1007/978-3-031-11363-5

This Springer imprint is published by the registered company Springer Nature Switzerland AG
The registered company address is: Gewerbestrasse 11, 6330 Cham, Switzerland

To Sonia, Laura, Carolina, and Carlos.

Preface

Biologic therapies include a wide range of products, from blood and blood products to gene therapies. These drugs represent a complete revolution in the therapy of many diseases. The common nexus of biologic therapy is their isolation from a variety of natural sources and their production from novel biotechnology methods. Commonly, these agents target key steps involved in the pathophysiological mechanisms of disease. This targeted approach leads to high efficacy and less toxicities than drugs with broad activity.

The expansion of the biologic therapy armamentarium has been exponential in the last decade. An increasing number of targets are constantly identified, and new biologic agents targeting the same protein but differing in activity, pharmacokinetics, and other characteristics are available for its use. In recent years, there is growing data on the use of combined biologic therapy or the incorporation of biologics to "classical" therapies for several diseases. It is not uncommon that malignancies combine classic chemotherapy with new biologics.

Despite the targeted approach of these treatments, some biologics can lead to unexpected side effects for which the increased risk of infections is certainly a major concern. The risk of infections can occur early after initiation of the biologic therapy but many times there is a delay in the occurrence of infections. Examples of this delay include the risk of tuberculosis with monoclonal antibodies against TNF-α or the risk of progressive multifocal leukoencephalopathy with the use of natalizumab. The concomitant use of different therapies and biologics, for example in the treatment of hematologic malignancies, can act synergistically increasing the risk of infections. Therefore, we should expect new infectious syndromes and risks with the incorporation of new biologics in the future.

This book is intended to offer an evidence-based guidance to understand the risk of infections associated with the use of biologics and it is divided in three parts. The first four chapters give a general view of the risks of infections and how to use vaccines for vaccine-preventable infections. Part II describes the risk of infections by specific agents in each major group of targets. This classical approach will allow to review specific biologics, their associated risk of infections, and how to prevent them. Finally, Part III analyzes the impact of biologic therapy in common infectious syndromes. For example, what would be the role of biologic therapies in patients with pulmonary infiltrates or CMV infection.

The most valuable aspect of the book is the extraordinary work of the contributing authors. Each chapter has been led by one or more international experts in the field. This book was developed during the COVID-19 pandemic, which reflects the unvaluable and resilient work of all contributing authors. The support of the European Group for the Study of Infections in the Immunocompromised Hosts (ESGICH) has been crucial for the development and completion of this extraordinary complex task. Finally, I must highlight the extraordinary work, excellent advice, and commitment of Prof. Jose Maria Aguado, coeditor of this book.

Edmonton, AB, Canada — Carlos Cervera
Madrid, Spain — Jose Maria Aguado
Rome, Italy — Paolo Grossi

Contents

Part I

Overview of the Epidemiology, Risk and Prevention of Infections

Overview of the Risk of Infection Associated with Biologic and Target Therapies

1

Mario Fernández-Ruiz

Overview of Targeted and Biological Therapies

A long journey has been traveled between the pioneer research carried out by Paul Ehrlich in the transition from nineteenth to twentieth centuries (Fig. 1.1) [1] and the approval of rituximab and imatinib for the treatment of hematological malignancies in 1997 and 2001, respectively [2, 3]. The number of biological therapies used in hematology, rheumatology, dermatology, or gastroenterology is a continuous increase, and there are more new molecules in the pipeline or at different stages of clinical development. The classification of these biological therapies can be made on the basis of their mode of action, targeted site, or structural properties. The two later classifications may not be useful in clinical practice, but they are still important for research purposes [4]. Three main categories can be established:

1. *Biological response modifiers,* which are agents that do not directly target cancer cells but rather exert a stimulating effect that boosts the immune system to fight against them. Biological response modifiers include exogenous interferons, interleukins (ILs) or colony-stimulating factors, as well as nonspecific immunomodulating agents (such as the *bacille Calmette-Guérin* [BCG]).
2. *Gene therapies,* which constitute a separate entity since genes can be manipulated through different ways [5]: replacing the defective gene with a normal gene (this approach mainly works against nonmalignant disorders with a single-gene aberration [6]), simulating the immune response against cancer cells [7], sensitizing cancer tissues to conventional chemotherapy and radiotherapy [8], delivering genes to cancer cells that change drugs from an inactive prodrug to the active form [9], blocking processes that protect cancer cells such as anti-apoptotic

M. Fernández-Ruiz (✉)
Unit of Infectious Diseases, Hospital Universitario "12 de Octubre", Instituto de Investigación Hospital "12 de Octubre" (imas12), Madrid, Spain

Department of Medicine, School of Medicine, Universidad Complutense, Madrid, Spain

C. Cervera, J. M. Aguado (eds.), *Infectious Complications in Biologic and Targeted Therapies*, https://doi.org/10.1007/978-3-031-11363-5_1

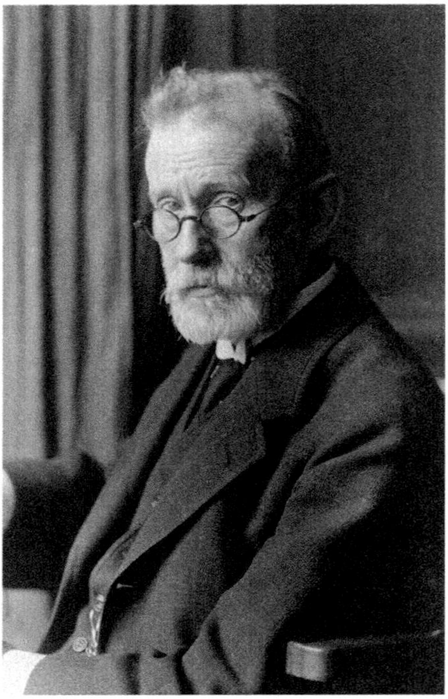

Fig. 1.1 Paul Ehrlich (1854–1915) and his "side-chain theory" constituted one of the foundations of modern immunology and paved the way for the design of targeted therapies. First formulated in 1897 and later developed as the "receptor-ligand concept," this theory postulated that cells expose on their surface a set of side-chains with distinct molecular structures and biological functions, which are uniquely recognized by different toxins (i.e., ligands) and inhibitory antagonists. In addition, these so-called chemoreceptors could serve as drug-binding sites, justifying the clinical use of specific antitoxins (i.e., therapeutic mAbs). Due to this and other major achievements, Paul Ehrlich was awarded in 1908 with the Nobel Prize in Physiology or Medicine together with Elie Metchnikoff. (Source: Wikimedia Commons, https://commons.wikimedia.org/w/index.php?curid=33752936)

mechanisms [10], using oncolytic viruses to kill cancer cells directly [11], or by means of DNA or RNA oligonucleotide therapies [12].

3. *Targeted therapies,* which are the most common biological approach not only for malignant diseases but also for inflammatory disorders. These agents have the advantage of directly targeting the cells or pathways involved in disease pathophysiology, thus minimizing the risk of treatment-related adverse events. There are a virtually endless number of potential therapeutic targets, from cell surface receptors to cytokines, immunoglobulins, intracellular enzymes, or bacterial toxins. The present book is mainly focused on these therapies.

Monoclonal Antibodies and Related Agents

Since more than three decades ago, monoclonal antibodies (mAbs) have become a standard component of the therapeutic approach for an increasing number of malignant, inflammatory, and rheumatological conditions [13]. The first agents within this class to be used in clinical practice were murine mAbs, although the inherent limitations associated with administering mouse immunoglobulins to humans—in particular the development of alloimmune responses leading to mAb clearance and the suboptimal induction of host's immunity against the targeted cells—were rapidly evident. The introduction of techniques of genetic engineering that allow for the sequential replacement of mouse-derived amino acids by human sequences

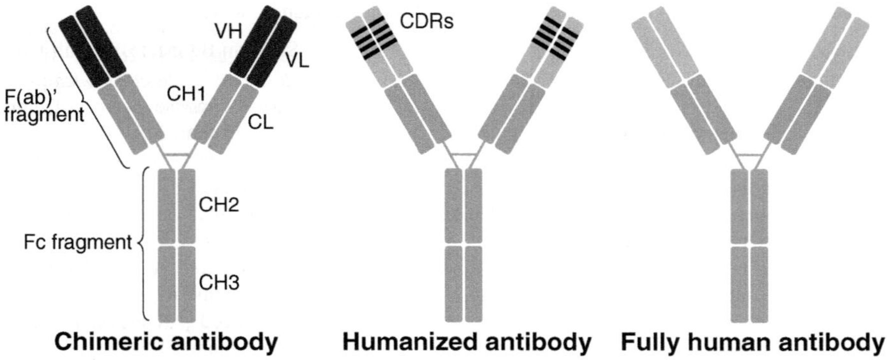

Fig. 1.2 Schematic representation of different types of therapeutic mAbs according to their progressive humanization. Regions of human and murine origin are shown in gray and black, respectively. *CDRs* complementarity-determining regions

constituted a crucial step forward. Chimerization process, in which the murine constant regions are replaced by human constant regions, were the first engineered improvement [14]. However, chimeric mouse-human mAbs still pose a meaningful risk of eliciting alloimmune responses since a significant portion of the antibody remains nonhuman. The humanization process—in which only the complementarity determining regions (CDRs) of the variable regions remain of mouse origin [15]—constituted the next achievement. In "fully human" mAbs the antigen specificity is selected either in vivo by the use of transgenic mice containing human immunoglobulin genes or through antibody engineering processes combined with screening in recombinant human antibody libraries (Fig. 1.2). Humanized and fully human mAbs exhibit a lower immunogenicity than mouse or chimeric antibodies [16].

A nomenclature scheme fixed by the WHO International Nonproprietary Names (INN) Programme has been consistently used for mAbs since the early 1990s (with the exception of the anti-CD3 agent muromonab-CD3). Each INN for a given mAb is composed of a random/fantasy prefix, a substem A indicating the target (molecule, cell or organ) class, a substem B indicating the species on which the immunoglobulin sequence is based (such as *-xi-* for chimeric or *-zu-* for humanized), and the stem *-mab* (Table 1.1) [17].

From a structural point of view, all these constructs mirror natural human IgG. The use of IgG-based agents has a number of advantages, since the half-lives of IgG1, IgG2, and IgG4 subclasses are considerably longer (about 23 days) than those of other immunoglobulin classes (ranging from 2 to 7 days), thus facilitating in most cases the administration in a weekly or monthly basis. The interaction between the IgG fragment crystallizable (Fc) region and immune cell receptors—Fcγ receptors (FcγRs) or complement protein C1q, among others—results in efficient cell lysis through complement-dependent cytotoxicity (CDC), antibody-dependent cell-mediated cytotoxicity (ADCC) and antibody-dependent cell-mediated phagocytosis (ADCP), as well as to enhanced antigen presentation to

Table 1.1 Revised WHO INN monoclonal antibody nomenclature scheme [17]

Prefix	Substem A (target class)	Substem B (species)	Substem
Random	*-ba-* bacterial *-ami-* serum amyloid protein (SAP)/amyloidosis (pre-substem) *-ci-* cardiovascular *-fung-* fungal *-gros-* skeletal muscle mass-related growth factors and receptors (pre-substem) *-ki-* interleukin *-li-* immunomodulating *-ne-* neural *-os-* bone *-toxa-* toxin *-tu-* or *-ta-* tumor *-vet-* veterinary use (pre-substem) *-vi-* viral	*-a-* rat *-axo-* rat-mouse (pre-substem) *-e-* hamster *-i-* primate *-o-* mouse *-u-* human *-xi-* chimeric *-xizu-* chimeric-humanized *-zu-* humanized	*-mab*

INN International Nonproprietary Names

dendritic cells [18]. The high diffusion coefficient of the IgG molecule allows for the rapid distribution to the extravascular compartment and the persistence within tumor environment for long periods of time. In opposition to the full-length mAbs, certolizumab (a new-generation tumor necrosis factor [TNF]-α-targeted agent) does not contain the IgG Fc region and, therefore, lacks in vitro CDC or ADCC effector activity (Fig. 1.3). A virtually unlimited quantity of recombinant human IgG with predetermined specificities and properties can be generated by means of modern mAb technology [19]. Since the development in 1981 of the anti-CD20 specific antibody B1 (renamed tositumomab) [20] and the Food and Drug Administration (FDA) approval in 1997 of rituximab for the treatment of indolent lymphoma [3], the clinical program of anti-CD20 agents exemplifies the improvements over the last decades in the engineering of therapeutic mAbs [21]. After binding to CD20, rituximab and ofatumumab—two type I anti-CD20 mAbs of first and second generation, respectively—induce the translocation of the antibody–antigen complex to lipid rafts in the cell membrane (membrane microdomains rich in cholesterol and sphingolipids). Lipid rafts serve as a setting for signal transduction, leading to strong CDC upon recruitment of C1q, but only to weak direct cytotoxicity. The second-generation mAb ofatumumab differs from rituximab in the binding site at the CD20 protein, resulting in higher affinity and enhanced CDC activity. Variations in lipid raft composition, however, contribute to the emergence of resistance to these type I mAbs. Type II anti-CD20 mAbs such as obinutuzumab or ocaratuzumab do not localize the antibody–antigen complex into lipid rafts and, therefore, induce a much weaker (10- to 100-fold) CDC activity than rituximab or ofatumumab. Nevertheless, reduced FcγR-mediated CD20 internalization increases the capacity to bind and activate natural killer (NK) and other FcγR-expressing cells (e.g., granulocytes or macrophages), which ultimately results in enhanced ADCC and ADCP [22].

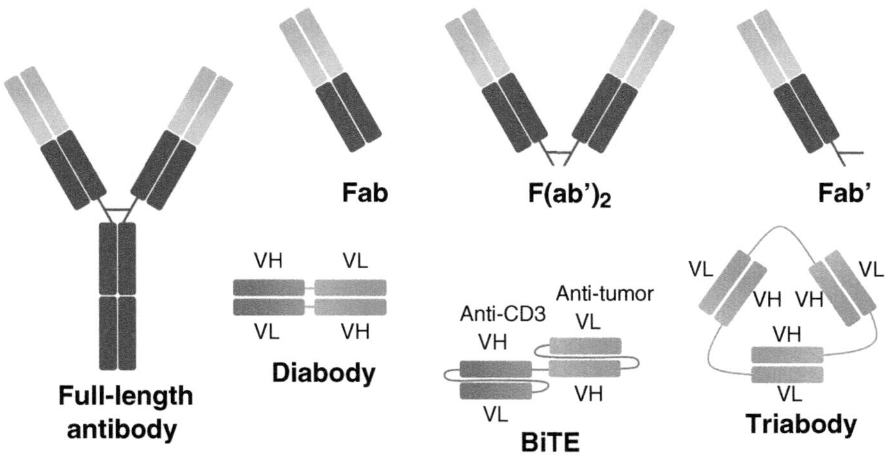

Fig. 1.3 Applications of engineered mAb technology. Fab fragment (50,000 Da) is a monovalent fragment consisting of the VH, CH1, VL, and CL domains linked by an intramolecular disulfide bond. Fab' fragment (55,000 Da), which may be obtained from a divalent $F(ab')_2$ fragment, contains a free sulfhydryl group that may be alkylated or utilized in conjugation with an enzyme, toxin, or other partner. Diabody is a noncovalent dimer formed by two single-chain variable regions (scFv), each consisting of the VH and VL domains connected by a small peptide linker. Triabody has three scFv heads, each consisting of the VH domain from one polypeptide paired with the VL domain from a neighboring polypeptide. Bispecific T-cell engagers (BiTEs) are composed of a single polypeptide chain that consists of two VL and VH pairs (i.e., two tandem scFv regions), each with a unique antigen specificity (one recognizes CD3 and the other recognizes an antigen on tumor cell surface). Constant regions (CH and CL) are shown in dark gray, variable regions (VH and VL) in clear gray

A pharmacokinetic refinement in the building of therapeutic mAbs is the covalent attachment of a polyethylene glycol (PEG) molecule, also termed PEGylation. The PEGylation process increases the hydrophilicity and serum half-life and reduces the glomerular filtration of the mAb, thus improving the therapeutic efficacy of the conjugate [23]. Such a strategy is particularly useful when the fragment antigen-binding (Fab) region of the mAb (which lacks the Fc region) is used as a therapeutic agent, since its clinical applicability would be limited by short serum half-life. Second-generation site-specific PEGylation techniques, which have been applied in the development of certolizumab, allow for well-defined and improved conjugated products compared to those obtained by nonspecific random conjugations [24].

Antibody–drug conjugates (ADCs), which are mAbs covalently attached to biologically active drugs by means of specialized chemical linkers, constitute a recent achievement in the development of targeted agents [25]. This approach allows for delivering and releasing potent cytotoxic agents at the precise tumor site due to the specific affinity of the mAb for the targeted antigen expressed on the surface of malignant cells. Surrounding nonmalignant tissues are spared, thus reducing the risk of systemic exposure and toxicity. The attached drug can be a bacterial toxin (i.e., *Pseudomonas* exotoxin A [PE]) or a cytotoxin that induces DNA or microtubule damage (i.e., auristatins or calicheamicins). Noncleavable linkers are the most commonly used since they require proteolytic degradation of the antibody part within the lysosome of the targeted cell to release the cytotoxic molecule, minimizing the amount of free circulating drug into the bloodstream. Examples of ADCs include CD22-targeted (moxetumomab pasudotox or inotuzumab ozogamicin), CD30-targeted (brentuximab vedotin), or CD33-targeted agents (gemtuzumab ozogamicin) [26].

In a similar way to ADCs, therapeutic MAbs also represents an excellent platform to deliver radioisotopes directly to tumor cells, minimizing the systemic toxicity of conventional radiotherapy. Due to the wide availability of specific target antigens and its relative radiosensitivity, lymphoma cells are particularly amenable for the use of radioimmunoconjugates. Two CD20-targeted agents, ibritumomab tiuxetan and tositumomab, which are conjugated to different isotopes (^{90}Y and ^{131}I respectively), have been FDA-approved for the treatment of patients with low-grade or follicular non-Hodgkin's lymphoma [26].

Bispecific T-cell engagers (BiTEs) are obtained through an innovative technology that fuses the antigen-binding variable regions of two different mAbs (Fig. 1.3). One of these arms targets a surface antigen expressed on cytotoxic T-cells, whereas the other binds to an antigen primarily found on malignant cells. The BiTE antibody forms a stable bridge between the immune and the tumor cell, enabling antigen recognition and the targeted deployment of cytotoxic mechanisms (i.e., degranulation of granzyme B and perforin) [27]. Blinatumomab, a CD19-targeted agent, is the first-in-class and so far the only approved BiTE antibody in clinical use [28]. Solitomab is a BiTE targeted to CD3 and the epithelial cell adhesion molecule (EpCAM), a transmembrane glycoprotein highly expressed in colon, gastric, prostate, ovarian, lung, and pancreatic cancer cells that is often correlated with poor outcomes.

Decoy receptors are also derived from the mAb technology and consist of the extracellular ligand-binding domains of naturally occurring receptors fused to the Fc region of a human immunoglobulin (usually IgG1). The resulting chimeric protein is able to trap the targeted soluble mediator (a cytokine or a growth factor), preventing its biological action. The Fc region partner contributes to improve the pharmacokinetic property of the recombinant fusion protein (prolonging its serum half-life) and facilitates large-scale production through processes similar to those applied for the production of therapeutic mAbs (expression in mammalian cells, secretion into culture supernatants and subsequent affinity-based purification). Etanercept, aflibercept, rilonacept, and olamkicept are examples of decoy receptors targeting TNF-α, vascular endothelium growth factor (VEGF), interleukin (IL)-1, and IL-6, respectively. Anakinra—the recombinant form of the native IL-1 receptor antagonist (IL-1Ra)—acts as a competitive inhibitor by binding to IL-1α and IL-1β and is based on an analogue therapeutic principle to decoy receptors. Due to the lack of the Fc region, anakinra must be administered daily following a loading dose due to its short half-life.

In addition to designing immunologically efficient and pharmacokinetically optimized mAbs, the choice of the targeted antigens is also critical. For cancer therapy, factors such as the density and consistency of expression on malignant cells of that targeted molecule, its limited expression on nontumor tissues, the lack of high-level soluble forms, and the limited tendency of antigen-negative escape tumor variants to emerge must be considered. For inflammatory diseases, the pathophysiological role displayed by certain cytokines, ILs, or soluble immune mediators in each specific condition guides the selection of targeted molecules.

Small-Molecule Enzyme Inhibitors

A completely different concept of targeted therapy is embodied by the so-called small-molecule inhibitors, whose development has been fueled by the continuous discovery of key oncogenic mutations involved in tumorigenesis and by the precise characterization of the critical role played by angiogenesis in tumor cell survival and metastatic dissemination. Since the approval in 2001 of imatinib for the treatment of Philadelphia chromosome (Ph)-positive chronic myeloid leukemia [29], a large number of kinase inhibitors have been designed over the past decades. In most cases, these agents block initial steps of intracellular downstream signaling cascades that are overexpressed in tumor cells due to point mutations (i.e., V600 mutations in the B-type Raf kinase *(BRAF)* oncogene in melanoma [30]) or chromosomal rearrangements (i.e., the BCR-ABL fusion tyrosine kinase resulting from the [9;22] translocation in Ph-positive leukemias [31]). The Ras/phosphatidylinositol-3-kinase (PI3K)/Akt/mTOR cascade and the Ras/Raf/MEK/ERK cascade (also known as MAPK/ERK) are two crucial pathways implied in the delicate control of cell survival, differentiation, and proliferation in response to extracellular stimuli. Thus, various drug classes are targeted to inhibit some steps of both that are overexpressed in tumor cells, including BRAF inhibitors (such as vemurafenib) [32], PI3K δ isoform inhibitors (idelalisib) [33], MEK inhibitors (trametinib or cobimetinib) [34], or mTOR inhibitors (everolimus or temsirolimus) [35]. While some small-molecule inhibitors exert a selective action on the tyrosine kinase domains integrated into the cytoplasmic tails of certain cell surface receptors (i.e., epidermal growth factor receptor [EGFR] or vascular endothelium growth factor receptor [VEGFR]), others indirectly block receptors that lack intrinsic enzymatic activity and rely on unspecific kinases to initiate the intracellular signaling pathway (i.e., type I and II cytokine receptors and the Janus family of tyrosine kinases) [36]. However, it should be noted that some degree of off-target inhibition results is unavoidable even with the more specific agents. As an example, imatinib has a large number of indications beyond Ph-positive leukemias, including c-Kit-positive gastrointestinal stromal tumor (GIST), myelodysplastic syndromes, systemic mastocytosis, or dermatofibrosarcoma protuberans. This concept is particularly evident for the multikinase inhibitors such as sorafenib or sunitinib, which in addition to VEGFR act on a large array of receptors (such as BRAF, c-Kit, platelet-derived growth factor receptor [PDGFR], or *fms*-like tyrosine kinase-3 [FLT3]) [37].

As compared to therapeutic mAbs and related agents, small-molecule inhibitors have pharmacokinetic advantages: good oral bioavailability, rapid absorption (reaching peak plasma levels within the first hours from administration), extensive tissue distribution (with good central nervous system penetration in some cases), and high protein bound [38]. However, they are not extent from drug-to-drug interactions since most of them are metabolized through the cytochrome P450 (CYP) 3A4 isoform (with other CYP-enzymes playing a secondary role) and are substrate of efflux transporters such as the ATP-binding cassette transporter family [39].

Assessment of the Risk of Infection

Targeted agents are directed towards cytokines, immune soluble mediators, cell surface molecules and receptors, and components of intracellular signaling cascades involved in the pathophysiology of cancer and autoimmune or inflammatory diseases. However, these targeted sites are often also key elements of physiological processes such as normal immune homeostasis or cell cycle control. The blockade of pathways controlling immune or inflammatory responses may result in an impaired immune function, with the consequent risk of infection [40]. Both innate and adaptive immunity may be targeted. Long-term immunological memory relies on CD4+ and CD8+ memory T-cells. Acquired immunity to extracellular and intracellular microorganisms depends on a network of Th17 and Th1 cells, cytotoxic CD8+ T-cells, and B-cells [41]. Targeted therapies may therefore affect responses to acute infection exposures as well as control of latent or chronic infections.

From a theoretical point of view, the potential of these agents to predispose to specific infectious complications or to overall increase infection risk mainly depend on their site of action (i.e., the targeted soluble immune mediator, cell surface antigen of intracellular signal transducer) and the subsequent impact on the functionality of the immune system [42]. Interestingly, the action some mAbs mirrors the immune defects that underlie the pathogenesis of well-defined primary immunodeficiencies, as is the case of CD40-targeted agents (lucatumumab or dacetuzumab) and the hyper-IgM syndrome [43, 44], or IL-17-targeted agents (secukinumab or brodalumab) and chronic mucocutaneous candidiasis [45].

However, in clinical practice such associations are far from deterministic, since they are modulated by a plethora of factors such as the nature and stage of the underlying condition, the prior or concurrent receipt of other immunosuppressive agents, the duration of therapy, or the cumulative exposure (Table 1.2). This notion is exemplified by the notable differences in the rates of infection observed with the

Table 1.2 Factors that modulate the risk of infectious complications in patients receiving biological agents

Clinical status and activity of the underlying malignancy or inflammatory disease
Prior or concomitant immunosuppressive therapies (i.e. corticosteroids)
Age and chronic comorbidities (i.e. diabetes mellitus)
Duration of therapy with the biological agent and mode of administration
Dose and cumulative exposure to the biological agent
Individual genetic susceptibility
Baseline incidence of infection in the overall population (i.e. latent tuberculosis)

use of the anti-CD52 mAb alemuzumb according to the indication of therapy, multiple sclerosis or B-cell malignancy (since the corresponding maximum annual doses vary from 36 to 1080 mg, respectively) [46, 47]. In the case of immune checkpoint inhibitors targeting inhibitory T-cell receptors, such as nivolumab or ipilimumab, the risk is not driven by the use of the agent itself, but by the subsequent requirement of additional immunosuppression therapy to manage the immune-related adverse effects emerging from the upregulation of immune response [48]. The underlying inflammatory state present in certain conditions may predispose to the activation of some pathogens (e.g., cytomegalovirus [CMV] via TNF-α). Thus, control of inflammation by targeted therapies would reduce the predisposition to infection intrinsically related to the disease [40]. In fact, a decline in the absolute risk of infection over time can be observed in some cohorts of patients under TNF-α-targeted agents due to the improvement in their clinical status and disease activity [49]. In addition, and despite its allegedly specific mode of action, some of these drugs do exert an off-target action on different cellular sites, further hampering the precise characterization of its impact on the host's susceptibility. As mentioned above, this should be anticipated when assessing the risk posed by the multikinase inhibitors like dasatinib, which has been recently associated to an increased incidence of CMV infection [50]. On the other hand, the abrupt discontinuation of therapy may lead to a paradoxical aggravation of the ongoing infection caused by the onset of immune reconstitution inflammatory syndrome (IRIS) or the aggravation of underlying disease, as observed in children with auto-inflammatory diseases receiving IL-1-targeted agents. Finally, immunosenescence, an emergent concept of immune degradation over time, is also a matter of concern because of its implications in the risk of infection. With chronic inflammation inducing continuous immune activation, accelerated T-cell senescence is unavoidable. The contraction of the immune repertoire may also determine the degree of susceptibility to new pathogens [51].

Moreover, the assessment of the infection risk associated to the use of targeted therapies is challenged by a number of methodological and practical difficulties. Pivotal RCTs that justify the approval by regulatory agencies are usually performed in patients with relapsed or refractory forms of disease, thus making it difficult to delineate the incremental risk of infection conferred by a certain agent from the background effect of previous lines of therapy. Caution must be exerted even if pivotal studies do not report an increased occurrence of infection, since most of the data on relatively uncommon complications has only emerged from the wide-scale use of a marketed agent, either in the form of case series or data from large post-marketing observational studies, such was the case of active tuberculosis with TNF-α-targeted agents [52] or progressive multifocal leukoencephalopathy (PML) with natalizumab or brentuximab vedotin [53, 54]. Unfortunately, post-marketing observational studies usually lack an adequate control group, leaving open to interpretation whether events are associated with the therapeutic agent or with the disease itself [55]. On the other hand, most RCTs do not provide detailed data on the clinical syndromes or causative agents in observed episodes of infection. The reported rates of infection for a given agent may substantially differ across different trials according to the geographic origin of the recruited patients (e.g., disparate incidence of active tuberculosis in low- or high-endemicity areas), the stringency of exclusion criteria (e.g., chronic infection with hepatitis virus), or the screening and prophylaxis strategies required per study protocol. Finally, since trials are usually designed to measure drug efficacy rather than detect rare adverse effects, the follow-up period may not be large enough to allow infections with protracted courses or long incubation periods (such as tuberculosis or certain endemic mycoses) to clinically emerge [55].

In view of the aforementioned limitations, the evaluation of the risk of infection for each targeted agent is far more complex than simply evaluating its efficacy or defining the expected safety profile within a given drug class. Although the majority of serious infections under these therapies are similar to those observed in the general population, it is clear that some specific events are much more likely to occur with certain agents or to evolve into a more severe course. While pathogens that exclusively cause disease among immunocompromised hosts can clearly be designated as "opportunistic," for most infections such concept is elusive. This is partly due to the lack of a formal definition in the context of targeted therapies, unlike other types of immunosuppression [56]. Prior attempts to define opportunistic infections associated with the use of targeted agents have been inconsistent, resulting in wide-ranging risk estimates across studies [57]. However, a multidisciplinary committee has recently reached an agreement upon a consensus definition for the reporting of each pathogen, recommending these criteria to be used in future studies to facilitate comparison between different agents [56].

References

1. Valent P, Groner B, Schumacher U, Superti-Furga G, Busslinger M, Kralovics R, et al. Paul Ehrlich (1854-1915) and his contributions to the foundation and birth of translational medicine. J Innate Immun. 2016;8:111–20.
2. Druker BJ, Talpaz M, Resta DJ, Peng B, Buchdunger E, Ford JM, et al. Efficacy and safety of a specific inhibitor of the BCR-ABL tyrosine kinase in chronic myeloid leukemia. N Engl J Med. 2001;344:1031–7.
3. Maloney DG, Grillo-Lopez AJ, White CA, Bodkin D, Schilder RJ, Neidhart JA, et al. IDEC-C2B8 (rituximab) anti-CD20 monoclonal antibody therapy in patients with relapsed low-grade non-Hodgkin's lymphoma. Blood. 1997;90:2188–95.
4. Santos R, Ursu O, Gaulton A, Bento AP, Donadi RS, Bologa CG, et al. A comprehensive map of molecular drug targets. Nat Rev Drug Discov. 2017;16:19–34.
5. Naldini L. Gene therapy returns to centre stage. Nature. 2015;526:351–60.
6. Ribeil JA, Hacein-Bey-Abina S, Payen E, Magnani A, Semeraro M, Magrin E, et al. Gene therapy in a patient with sickle cell disease. N Engl J Med. 2017;376:848–55.
7. Dahlberg CI, Sarhan D, Chrobok M, Duru AD, Alici E. Natural killer cell-based therapies targeting cancer: possible strategies to gain and sustain anti-tumor activity. Front Immunol. 2015;6:605.
8. Kim SS, Rait A, Kim E, Pirollo KF, Nishida M, Farkas N, et al. A nanoparticle carrying the p53 gene targets tumors including cancer stem cells, sensitizes glioblastoma to chemotherapy and improves survival. ACS Nano. 2014;8:5494–514.

9. Carruthers KH, Metzger G, During MJ, Muravlev A, Wang C, Kocak E. Gene-directed enzyme prodrug therapy for localized chemotherapeutics in allograft and xenograft tumor models. Cancer Gene Ther. 2014;21:434–40.
10. Albarakati N, Abdel-Fatah TM, Doherty R, Russell R, Agarwal D, Moseley P, et al. Targeting BRCA1-BER deficient breast cancer by ATM or DNA-PKcs blockade either alone or in combination with cisplatin for personalized therapy. Mol Oncol. 2015;9:204–17.
11. Foreman PM, Friedman GK, Cassady KA, Markert JM. Oncolytic virotherapy for the treatment of malignant glioma. Neurotherapeutics. 2017;14:333–44.
12. Amato RJ. Inhibition of DNA methylation by antisense oligonucleotide MG98 as cancer therapy. Clin Genitourin Cancer. 2007;5:422–6.
13. Nakamura RM. Monoclonal antibodies: methods and clinical laboratory applications. Clin Physiol Biochem. 1983;1:160–72.
14. Bruggemann M, Winter G, Waldmann H, Neuberger MS. The immunogenicity of chimeric antibodies. J Exp Med. 1989;170:2153–7.
15. Gussow D, Seemann G. Humanization of monoclonal antibodies. Methods Enzymol. 1991;203:99–121.
16. Presta LG. Engineering of therapeutic antibodies to minimize immunogenicity and optimize function. Adv Drug Deliv Rev. 2006;58:640–56.
17. World Health Organization. Programme on International Nonpropietary Names (INN). Revised monoclonal antibody nomenclature scheme. Geneva, May 2017. https://www.who.int/medicines/services/inn/Revised_mAb_nomenclature_scheme.pdf. Accesed 28 Mar 2021.
18. Glennie MJ, French RR, Cragg MS, Taylor RP. Mechanisms of killing by anti-CD20 monoclonal antibodies. Mol Immunol. 2007;44:3823–37.
19. Singh S, Kumar N, Dwiwedi P, Charan J, Kaur R, Sidhu P, et al. Monoclonal antibodies: a review. Curr Clin Pharmacol. 2018;13(2):85–99.
20. Nadler LM, Takvorian T, Botnick L, Bast RC, Finberg R, Hellman S, et al. Anti-B1 monoclonal antibody and complement treatment in autologous bone-marrow transplantation for relapsed B-cell non-Hodgkin's lymphoma. Lancet. 1984;2:427–31.
21. Oflazoglu E, Audoly LP. Evolution of anti-CD20 monoclonal antibody therapeutics in oncology. MAbs. 2010;2:14–9.
22. Lim SH, Beers SA, French RR, Johnson PW, Glennie MJ, Cragg MS. Anti-CD20 monoclonal antibodies: historical and future perspectives. Haematologica. 2010;95:135–43.
23. Zundorf I, Dingermann T. PEGylation—a well-proven strategy for the improvement of recombinant drugs. Pharmazie. 2014;69:323–6.
24. Pasut G. Pegylation of biological molecules and potential benefits: pharmacological properties of certolizumab pegol. BioDrugs. 2014;28(Suppl 1):S15–23.
25. Tolcher AW. Antibody drug conjugates: lessons from 20 years of clinical experience. Ann Oncol. 2016;27:2168–72.
26. Wolska-Washer A, Robak P, Smolewski P, Robak T. Emerging antibody-drug conjugates for treating lymphoid malignancies. Expert Opin Emerg Drugs. 2017;22:259–73.
27. Liu H, Saxena A, Sidhu SS, Wu D. Fc engineering for developing therapeutic bispecific antibodies and novel scaffolds. Front Immunol. 2017;8:38.
28. Wilke AC, Gokbuget N. Clinical applications and safety evaluation of the new CD19 specific T-cell engager antibody construct blinatumomab. Expert Opin Drug Saf. 2017;16:1191–202.
29. Buchdunger E, Zimmermann J, Mett H, Meyer T, Muller M, Druker BJ, et al. Inhibition of the Abl protein-tyrosine kinase in vitro and in vivo by a 2-phenylaminopyrimidine derivative. Cancer Res. 1996;56:100–4.
30. Dienstmann R, Tabernero J. BRAF as a target for cancer therapy. Anti Cancer Agents Med Chem. 2011;11:285–95.
31. Lin X, Qureshi MZ, Attar R, Khalid S, Tahir F, Yaqub A, et al. Targeting of BCR-ABL: lessons learned from BCR-ABL inhibition. Cell Mol Biol (Noisy-le-Grand). 2016;62:129–37.
32. Cosgarea I, Ritter C, Becker JC, Schadendorf D, Ugurel S. Update on the clinical use of kinase inhibitors in melanoma. J Dtsch Dermatol Ges. 2017;15:887–93.

33. Barrientos JC. Idelalisib for the treatment of indolent non-Hodgkin lymphoma: a review of its clinical potential. Onco Targets Ther. 2016;9:2945–53.
34. Cheng Y, Tian H. Current development status of MEK inhibitors. Molecules. 2017;22
35. Dancey JE. Clinical development of mammalian target of rapamycin inhibitors. Hematol Oncol Clin North Am. 2002;16:1101–14.
36. Gadina M, Hilton D, Johnston JA, Morinobu A, Lighvani A, Zhou YJ, et al. Signaling by type I and II cytokine receptors: ten years after. Curr Opin Immunol. 2001;13:363–73.
37. Rask-Andersen M, Zhang J, Fabbro D, Schioth HB. Advances in kinase targeting: current clinical use and clinical trials. Trends Pharmacol Sci. 2014;35:604–20.
38. van Erp NP, Gelderblom H, Guchelaar HJ. Clinical pharmacokinetics of tyrosine kinase inhibitors. Cancer Treat Rev. 2009;35:692–706.
39. Shao J, Markowitz JS, Bei D, An G. Enzyme- and transporter-mediated drug interactions with small molecule tyrosine kinase inhibitors. J Pharm Sci. 2014;103:3810–33.
40. Her M, Kavanaugh A. Alterations in immune function with biologic therapies for autoimmune disease. J Allergy Clin Immunol. 2016;137:19–27.
41. Boyman O, Comte D, Spertini F. Adverse reactions to biologic agents and their medical management. Nat Rev Rheumatol. 2014;10:612–27.
42. Salvana EM, Salata RA. Infectious complications associated with monoclonal antibodies and related small molecules. Clin Microbiol Rev. 2009;22:274–90, Table of Contents.
43. Qamar N, Fuleihan RL. The hyper IgM syndromes. Clin Rev Allergy Immunol. 2014;46:120–30.
44. Cabral-Marques O, Klaver S, Schimke LF, Ascendino EH, Khan TA, Pereira PV, et al. First report of the Hyper-IgM syndrome Registry of the Latin American Society for Immunodeficiencies: novel mutations, unique infections, and outcomes. J Clin Immunol. 2014;34:146–56.
45. Huppler AR, Bishu S, Gaffen SL. Mucocutaneous candidiasis: the IL-17 pathway and implications for targeted immunotherapy. Arthritis Res Ther. 2012;14:217.
46. Riera R, Porfirio GJ, Torloni MR. Alemtuzumab for multiple sclerosis. Cochrane Database Syst Rev. 2016;4:CD011203.
47. Warner JL, Arnason JE. Alemtuzumab use in relapsed and refractory chronic lymphocytic leukemia: a history and discussion of future rational use. Ther Adv Hematol. 2012;3:375–89.
48. Del Castillo M, Romero FA, Arguello E, Kyi C, Postow MA, Redelman-Sidi G. The spectrum of serious infections among patients receiving immune checkpoint blockade for the treatment of melanoma. Clin Infect Dis. 2016;63:1490–3.
49. Strangfeld A, Eveslage M, Schneider M, Bergerhausen HJ, Klopsch T, Zink A, et al. Treatment benefit or survival of the fittest: what drives the time-dependent decrease in serious infection rates under TNF inhibition and what does this imply for the individual patient? Ann Rheum Dis. 2011;70:1914–20.
50. Prestes DP, Arbona E, Nevett-Fernandez A, Woolley AE, Ho VT, Koo S, et al. Dasatinib use and risk of cytomegalovirus reactivation after allogeneic hematopoietic-cell transplantation. Clin Infect Dis. 2017;65:510–3.
51. Naylor K, Li G, Vallejo AN, Lee WW, Koetz K, Bryl E, et al. The influence of age on T cell generation and TCR diversity. J Immunol. 2005;174:7446–52.
52. Keane J, Gershon S, Wise RP, Mirabile-Levens E, Kasznica J, Schwieterman WD, et al. Tuberculosis associated with infliximab, a tumor necrosis factor alpha-neutralizing agent. N Engl J Med. 2001;345:1098–104.
53. Clifford DB, De Luca A, Simpson DM, Arendt G, Giovannoni G, Nath A. Natalizumab-associated progressive multifocal leukoencephalopathy in patients with multiple sclerosis: lessons from 28 cases. Lancet Neurol. 2010;9:438–46.
54. Carson KR, Newsome SD, Kim EJ, Wagner-Johnston ND, von Geldern G, Moskowitz CH, et al. Progressive multifocal leukoencephalopathy associated with brentuximab vedotin therapy: a report of 5 cases from the Southern Network on Adverse Reactions (SONAR) project. Cancer. 2014;120:2464–71.
55. Bongartz T, Sutton AJ, Sweeting MJ, Buchan I, Matteson EL, Montori V. Anti-TNF antibody therapy in rheumatoid arthritis and the risk of serious infections and malignancies:

systematic review and meta-analysis of rare harmful effects in randomized controlled trials. JAMA. 2006;295:2275–85.
56. Winthrop KL, Novosad SA, Baddley JW, Calabrese L, Chiller T, Polgreen P, et al. Opportunistic infections and biologic therapies in immune-mediated inflammatory diseases: consensus recommendations for infection reporting during clinical trials and postmarketing surveillance. Ann Rheum Dis. 2015;74:2107–16.
57. Bryant PA, Baddley JW. Opportunistic infections in biological therapy, risk and prevention. Rheum Dis Clin N Am. 2017;43:27–41.

Timeline and Infectious Disease Evaluation of Candidates to New Therapies

2

Francisco Lopez-Medrano and Jose Tiago Silva

Introduction

Biologic and targeted therapies, which have exponentially increased in the past years, have significantly changed the treatment of autoimmune, inflammatory, and onco-hematological life-threatening diseases, improving the prognosis and the quality of life for many patients. Nonetheless, this has been accompanied by an increase in the risk of developing opportunistic and agent-related infectious complications [1].

The prevention and management of these complications can be a challenge to the clinician. In some cases, there is a known cause–effect relationship between the agent and the infectious disease, which helps the physician in making a decision concerning the prophylactic treatment. Such is the case for tumor necrosis factor (TNF)-α inhibitor agents and the increased risk of latent tuberculous infection (LTBI) reactivation [2]. Unfortunately, in other cases, due to the lack of data, the risk of infection remains to be confirmed, e.g., novel drugs with insufficient data on uncommon complications due to small case series or postmarketing observational studies. Moreover, this risk is also determined by the patient's susceptibility (e.g., the patient's age, underlying disease, and prior and concurrent use of immunosuppressive drugs), the patient's environment (e.g., the local incidence of TB, which can differ greatly from country to country, or the possible existence of fungal and parasitic endemic diseases), and the patient's exposure to the drug (e.g., the duration of treatment). In these cases, deciding on the most adequate prophylactic treatment can be challenging for the physician.

F. Lopez-Medrano (✉) · J. T. Silva
Unit of Infectious Diseases, University Hospital 12 de Octubre, Instituto de Investigación del Hospital 12 de Octubre (imas12), School of Medicine, Universidad Complutense, Madrid, Spain

Centro de Investigación Biomédica en Red de Enfermedades Infecciosas (CIBERINFEC; CB21/13/00009), Instituto de Salud Carlos III, Madrid, Spain

C. Cervera, J. M. Aguado (eds.), *Infectious Complications in Biologic and Targeted Therapies*, https://doi.org/10.1007/978-3-031-11363-5_2

In this chapter, a review of the risk of developing an infectious complication is provided, according to the type and length of treatment. Recommendations of the evaluation and prevention of most of these complications is also provided.

Timeline of Infectious Complications in Patients on Biologic and Targeted Drugs

Determining the type and the moment that an infectious disease will arise for a patient receiving a biologic or targeted treatment is sometimes difficult, as it can even vary within different drugs of the same class. This is true for TB and TNF-α inhibitor agents, such as infliximab, adalimumab, and etanercept. A comparison between 13 selected studies published from 2001 to 2017, which examined the time to onset of TB in patients with inflammatory diseases on TNF-α inhibitor agents, disclosed that the median time to TB onset was significantly shorter in patients on infliximab and adalimumab than in patients on etanercept (3–6 months vs. more than 12 months, respectively) [2]. Although this finding could indicate a lower risk of developing TB with etanercept, it must be kept in mind that the risk of TB disease, and especially extrapulmonary and disseminated presentations of the disease, are increased regardless of the TNF-α inhibitor agent prescribed [3]. Active TB, which can result from acquisition of new infection or from reactivation of LTBI, must always be considered a serious possible complication in these patients.

Eculizumab is an example of a biological agent for which the risk of developing an infectious complication is immediate after the administration of the first dose. By preventing the formation of the terminal membrane attack complex (MAC) C5b-C9, which has a key effector role in killing bacteria belonging to the genus *Neisseria*, eculizumab is associated with a 10,000-fold increase in the risk of developing disseminated meningococcal infection [4], including strains that rarely cause diseases in healthy subjects [5]. The risk of disseminated infection by *Neisseria gonorrhoeae* is also increased [6].

JC polyomavirus (JCPyV) is a human polyomavirus, first identified in 1971 as the cause of progressive multifocal leukoencephalopathy (PML) [7]. Natalizumab is associated with a high risk of developing PML [7–9]. Contrary to eculizumab, natalizumab shows a long latency period from the drug initiation to the diagnosis of the infectious complication. A study that included 179 patients treated with natalizumab for relapsing-remitting multiple sclerosis reported an annualized seroconversion rate of 7.1% [10], with an incidence of 2 cases per 1000 treated patients beyond the 48th month of therapy and a swift increase after the 72nd month [11].

In some cases, infectious complications can be seen after the end of treatment. Approximately 5–15% of patients treated with rituximab develop a particular side effect, called late-onset neutropenia [12], a condition characterized by an otherwise unexplained grade III-IV neutropenia (an absolute neutrophil count under $0.5–1 \times 10^9$/L), beyond the fourth week of the last infusion of rituximab. Although its impact on the risk of infection is still unknown [12], cases of bacterial infections have been described [13]. Rituximab is also associated with reactivation of hepatitis

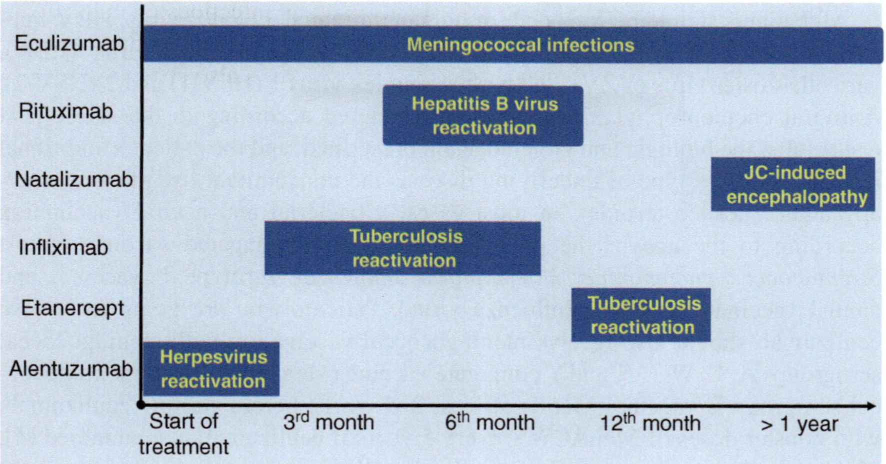

Fig. 2.1 Timeline of the onset of some of the most common infections associated to biologic and targeted therapies

B virus (HBV). Although HBV reactivation has been described to occur at a median of 23 weeks after the start of treatment [14], there have been cases described after the end of therapy [15]. As such, both hepatitis B surface antigen (HBsAg)-positive and HBsAg-negative/hepatitis B core antibody (anti-HBc)-positive patients should receive antiviral prophylaxis for at least 12–18 months after the last administration of rituximab [12]. Figure 2.1 shows a sensible approach to the most common infections according to the drug and the timeline in which the risk is maximum.

Evaluation and Prevention of Infectious Complications in Patients on Biologic and Targeted Treatment

A patient who is a candidate for a biologic and targeted treatment must be thoroughly evaluated for the presence of possible latent infections, should have their vaccines updated, and should be scheduled to receive chemoprophylaxis whenever necessary. Despite these recommendations, a multicenter study, performed among different Spanish medical societies that prescribe biologic treatments, reported that 43% of the surveyed physicians did not follow LTBI screening recommendations with an acceptable degree of adherence, that only 36.6% performed the appropriate diagnostic tests, and that only 63.9% started biologic therapy after the recommended length of LTBI treatment [16]. A similar cross-sectional survey, performed in 24 different countries of the European Union, which included 441 rheumatologists, 266 gastroenterologists, and 208 dermatologists who prescribed TNF-α inhibitor agents revealed that approximately 1 in every 10 physicians reported not following any guideline for pretreatment TB screening and that between 8% and 27% of physicians reported not screening their patients for TB [17].

All patients should be screened for human immunodeficiency virus, HBV, hepatitis C virus (HCV), cytomegalovirus (CMV), Epstein-Barr virus (EBV), varicella-zoster virus (VZV), and herpes simplex virus 1 (HSV-1) and 2 (HSV-2). Antiviral chemoprophylaxis should be considered according to the serological test results, the biologic and targeted agent prescribed, and the patient's additional risk-factors (e.g., type of underlying disease and concomitant use of chemotherapy and/or corticosteroids). In most cases, a bacterial and a viral vaccination according to the age of the patient is sufficient (conjugated vaccine against *Streptococcus pneumoniae*, *Haemophilus influenzae* serotype b vaccine, and annual vaccination against Influenza virus). Patients who are going to receive eculizumab should also receive meningococcal vaccination with meningococcal serogroups A, C, W-135, and Y conjugate vaccine (MenACWY) and meningococcal serogroup B vaccine (MenB) at least 2–4 weeks before starting eculizumab, with booster doses of MenACWY every 5 years if eculizumab is maintained [4]. Meningococcal chemoprophylaxis with penicillin V or ciprofloxacin for at least 4 weeks following completion of vaccination or until protective antibody titers are documented is also recommended [4]. Chemoprophylaxis for immunocompromised patients should be maintained, only to be discontinued after 4 weeks from the last dose of eculizumab [4, 18]. Screening for gonococcal infection in patients at high risk for sexually transmitted diseases and their sexual partners is also recommended in patients receiving eculizumab [4]. LTBI should be screened for all patients, especially those who are going to receive TNF-α inhibitor agents, and an appropriate prophylactic antibiotic treatment should be prescribed if needed. Conventional anti-*Pneumocystis* prophylaxis with cotrimoxazole should be used according to the agent prescribed (e.g., anti-*Pneumocystis* prophylaxis has been shown to be effective in patients with T-cell lymphomas treated with mogamulizumab) [19] and depending on the existence of additional risk factors, such as high-dose or prolonged corticosteroid treatment (steroids at the dose of 20 mg of prednisone daily [or equivalent] for at least 4 weeks). Finally, all patients should also be counselled on appropriate hygienic and food safety measures, such as avoiding raw meat or fish, undercooked eggs or unpasteurized milk, and thoroughly peeling or washing all fruits and vegetables before eating.

In order to plan the most adequate prophylactic regimen, it is extremely important to gather a detailed medical history, including the patient's place of birth and the countries where he or she has lived. As previously mentioned, the patient could have been exposed to diseases which are not endemic in the country where he or she is going to receive treatment, as these infections could reactivate while on therapy. Such is the case for *Leishmania* spp., which is endemic in Latin America, Africa, the Mediterranean Basin, the Indian subcontinent, and the Central-Southeast Asia Region [20]. Cases of *Leishmania* spp., including possible cases of reactivation, have been associated to TNF-α inhibitor agents [21, 22], rituximab [23], and alemtuzumab (a humanized IgG1 monoclonal antibody that binds to CD52 and produces a severe depletion of peripheral blood lymphocytes) [24]. Rare cases of submicroscopic *Plasmodium falciparum* [25] and Chagas disease reactivation [26], disseminated *Strongyloides stercoralis* infection [27], and adult T-cell leukemia associated to human T-cell leukemia virus type 1 (HTLV-1) [28] have also been described in patients originating of endemic countries that were being treated with TNF-α inhibitor agents. These patients could benefit from a specific microbiological study aimed at dismissing these endemic latent infections, with prophylactic treatment and close follow-up whenever indicated necessary. Table 2.1 includes the recommended measures for the prevention of viral infections in patients on biologic and targeted therapies.

Table 2.1 Measures for the prevention of viral infections in patients with biologic targeted agents (adapted from Noreña et al. [31])

Infective agent	Preventive recommendation
Influenza	– Seasonal vaccination
Hepatitis A virus	– Evaluate for HAV IgG in patients living in countries with intermediate to high rates of infection, and vaccinate whenever the serology is negative – Vaccinate patients travelling to these countries
Hepatitis B virus	– Serologic evaluation before beginning the biological treatment based on the detection of HBsAg and anti-HBc – Antiviral prophylaxis while on therapy should be offered to HBsAg-positive patients with moderate or high risk of reactivation and those with occult infection and high-risk of reactivation – Measure HBV DNA viral load before starting antiviral – Periodic liver and serologic tests (HBsAg and HBV-DNA) during and after the biological treatment, especially among anti-HBc-positive / HBsAg-negative patients
Hepatitis C virus	– Request HCV antibodies before initiating treatment
Cytomegalovirus	– Serologic evaluation before beginning the biological treatment – Patients receiving a biologic drug associated with a high risk of CMV reactivation[a] might benefit from a weekly or monthly monitoring of CMV viremia – Start preemptive antiviral therapy and stop the biologic treatment in case of CMV reactivation
Varicella zoster virus	– Serologic evaluation before beginning treatment and vaccination whenever negative[b] – Avoid vaccination in immunosuppressed patients[b] – Prophylaxis with (val)acyclovir in the case of VZV-seropositive patients receiving bortezomib-based regimens
Herpes simplex virus	– Serologic evaluation before beginning treatment – Prophylaxis with (val)acyclovir in bortezomib-based regimens
Epstein Barr virus	– Serologic evaluation before beginning treatment
JC polyomavirus[c]	– Serologic evaluation before beginning treatment – Periodic cerebral MR for early detection of PML in high-risk patients
Human papilloma virus	– HPV vaccination – Cervical cancer screening with periodic examination searching for pap smear abnormalities

Anti-HBc hepatitis B core antibody, *CMV* cytomegalovirus, *HAV* hepatitis A virus infection, *HBsAg* hepatitis B surface antigen, *HBV* hepatitis B virus infection, *HCV* hepatitis C virus, *HPV* human papilloma virus, *IgG* immunoglobulin G, *MR* magnetic resonance, *PML* progressive multifocal leukoencephalopathy, *VZV* varicella zoster virus

[a] Drugs associated with a high-risk of CMV reactivation include alemtuzumab, idelalisib, dasatinib

[b] Live-attenuated vaccines can only be administered up to 14 days before the initiation the biologic treatment or 1 month after stopping this therapy

[c] In the case of patients who will receive natalizumab

Table 2.2 Screening recommendations in patients coming from countries where these infections are endemic (adapted from Clemente et al. [32] and Pierrotti et al. [33])

Infective agent	Screening recommendation
Strongyloides stercoralis	Serological technique and parasitological stool testing
Leishmania spp.	Serological tests and a serum PCR[a]
Trypanosoma cruzi	Serological tests
Malaria	Detection of *Plasmodium* DNA or RNA by PCR
HTLV-1 and HTLV-2	Serological tests

DNA deoxyribonucleic acid, *HTLV* human T-cell leukemia virus, *PCR* polymerase chain reaction, *RNA* ribonucleic acid

[a] PCR should be performed in candidates with a positive serology

Lastly, patients on biologic treatment who are planning to travel to countries where these infections are endemic should seek proper pre-travel counsel and should have their prophylactic treatments adjusted. Severe cases of disseminated histoplasmosis [29] and *Plasmodium falciparum* infection [30], diagnosed within the first weeks after returning from their travel, have been described in patients on infliximab. In the latter, the refusal to take the recommended malaria chemoprophylaxis might have contributed to the infection. Table 2.2 shows the screening recommendations in patients coming from countries where parasitic infections are endemic.

Conclusion

Patients on biologic and targeted treatment have a higher risk of developing life-threatening infectious diseases. A thorough medical history before starting treatment is mandatory in order to plan the most adequate prophylactic approach and to schedule the follow-up. The physician should take into account the patient's underlying diseases and prior and concurrent immunosuppressive treatment, the patient's place of birth, and countries where he or she has lived. The physician must also take into consideration the mechanism of action of the agent and the scheduled duration of the treatment. A correct prophylactic strategy is extremely important, as it can avoid most infectious complications associated with biologic and targeted therapies.

References

1. Fernandez-Ruiz M, Meije Y, Manuel O, Akan H, Carratala J, Aguado JM, et al. ESCMID Study Group for Infections in Compromised Hosts (ESGICH) consensus document on the safety of targeted and biological therapies: an infectious diseases perspective (introduction). Clin Microbiol Infect. 2018;24(Suppl 2):S2–9.
2. Godfrey MS, Friedman LN. Tuberculosis and biologic therapies: anti-tumor necrosis factor-alpha and beyond. Clin Chest Med. 2019;40(4):721–39.

3. Cantini F, Niccoli L, Goletti D. Adalimumab, etanercept, infliximab, and the risk of tuberculosis: data from clinical trials, national registries, and postmarketing surveillance. J Rheumatol Suppl. 2014;91:47–55.
4. Winthrop KL, Mariette X, Silva JT, Benamu E, Calabrese LH, Dumusc A, et al. ESCMID Study Group for Infections in Compromised Hosts (ESGICH) consensus document on the safety of targeted and biological therapies: an infectious diseases perspective (soluble immune effector molecules [II]: agents targeting interleukins, immunoglobulins and complement factors). Clin Microbiol Infect. 2018;24(Suppl 2):S21–40.
5. Nolfi-Donegan D, Konar M, Vianzon V, MacNeil J, Cooper J, Lurie P, et al. Fatal nongroupable Neisseria meningitidis disease in vaccinated patient receiving eculizumab. Emerg Infect Dis. 2018;24(8)
6. Crew PE, Abara WE, McCulley L, Waldron PE, Kirkcaldy RD, Weston EJ, et al. Disseminated gonococcal infections in patients receiving eculizumab: a case series. Clin Infect Dis. 2019;69(4):596–600.
7. Multani A, Ho DY. JC polyomavirus infection potentiated by biologics. Infect Dis Clin N Am. 2020;34(2):359–88.
8. Mills EA, Mao-Draayer Y. Understanding progressive multifocal leukoencephalopathy risk in multiple sclerosis patients treated with immunomodulatory therapies: a bird's eye view. Front Immunol. 2018;9:138.
9. Grebenciucova E, Berger JR. Progressive multifocal leukoencephalopathy. Neurol Clin. 2018;36(4):739–50.
10. Vennegoor A, van Rossum JA, Leurs C, Wattjes MP, Rispens T, Murk JL, et al. High cumulative JC virus seroconversion rate during long-term use of natalizumab. Eur J Neurol. 2016;23(6):1079–85.
11. Redelman-Sidi G, Michielin O, Cervera C, Ribi C, Aguado JM, Fernandez-Ruiz M, et al. ESCMID Study Group for Infections in Compromised Hosts (ESGICH) consensus document on the safety of targeted and biological therapies: an infectious diseases perspective (immune checkpoint inhibitors, cell adhesion inhibitors, sphingosine-1-phosphate receptor modulators and proteasome inhibitors). Clin Microbiol Infect. 2018;24(Suppl 2):S95–S107.
12. Mikulska M, Lanini S, Gudiol C, Drgona L, Ippolito G, Fernandez-Ruiz M, et al. ESCMID Study Group for Infections in Compromised Hosts (ESGICH) consensus document on the safety of targeted and biological therapies: an infectious diseases perspective (agents targeting lymphoid cells surface antigens [I]: CD19, CD20 and CD52). Clin Microbiol Infect. 2018;24(Suppl 2):S71–82.
13. Wolach O, Bairey O, Lahav M. Late-onset neutropenia after rituximab treatment: case series and comprehensive review of the literature. Medicine (Baltimore). 2010;89(5):308–18.
14. Ogawa E, Wei MT, Nguyen MH. Hepatitis B virus reactivation potentiated by biologics. Infect Dis Clin N Am. 2020;34(2):341–58.
15. Cicculo A, Ponziani FR, Maiolo E, Pallavicini F, Pompili M. Late reactivation of hepatitis B virus after rituximab-containing chemotherapy for mantle cell lymphoma: a case report. Infection. 2019;47(2):313–6.
16. Quiros S, de la Rosa D, Uranga A, Madero R, Amaro R, Bruguera N, et al. Screening for latent tuberculosis infection in patients who are candidate for biological therapies in Spain? A multidisciplinary survey. Arch Bronconeumol. 2018;54(10):510–7.
17. Smith MY, Attig B, McNamee L, Eagle T. Tuberculosis screening in prescribers of anti-tumor necrosis factor therapy in the European Union. Int J Tuberc Lung Dis. 2012;16(9):1168–73.
18. Benamu E, Montoya JG. Infections associated with the use of eculizumab: recommendations for prevention and prophylaxis. Curr Opin Infect Dis. 2016;29(4):319–29.
19. Drgona L, Gudiol C, Lanini S, Salzberger B, Ippolito G, Mikulska M. ESCMID Study Group for Infections in Compromised Hosts (ESGICH) consensus document on the safety of targeted and biological therapies: an infectious diseases perspective (agents targeting lymphoid or myeloid cells surface antigens [II]: CD22, CD30, CD33, CD38, CD40, SLAMF-7 and CCR4). Clin Microbiol Infect. 2018;24(Suppl 2):S83–94.
20. Burza S, Croft SL, Boelaert M. Leishmaniasis. Lancet. 2018;392(10151):951–70.

21. Tektonidou MG, Skopouli FN. Visceral leishmaniasis in a patient with psoriatic arthritis treated with infliximab: reactivation of a latent infection? Clin Rheumatol. 2008;27(4):541–2.
22. Tung Chen Y, Perales C, Lacruz J, Senent L, Salavert M. Visceral leishmaniasis infection during adalimumab therapy: a case report and literature review. Int J Rheum Dis. 2014;17(7):822–4.
23. Casabianca A, Marchetti M, Zallio F, Feyles E, Concialdi E, Ferroglio E, et al. Seronegative visceral leishmaniasis with relapsing and fatal course following rituximab treatment. Infection. 2011;39(4):375–8.
24. Pitini V, Cascio A, Arrigo C, Altavilla G. Visceral leishmaniasis after alemtuzumab in a patient with chronic lymphocytic leukaemia. Br J Haematol. 2012;156(1):1.
25. Haeseleer C, Martiny D, Van Laethem Y, Cantinieaux B, Martin C. Reactivation of Plasmodium infection during a treatment with infliximab: a case report. Int J Infect Dis. 2020;91:101–3.
26. Vacas AS, Gomez-Santana LV, Torre AC, Galimberti RL. Reactivation of Chagas-Mazza disease during treatment with infliximab. An Bras Dermatol. 2017;92(6):899–900.
27. Krishnamurthy R, Dincer HE, Whittemore D. Strongyloides stercoralis hyperinfection in a patient with rheumatoid arthritis after anti-TNF-alpha therapy. J Clin Rheumatol. 2007;13(3):150–2.
28. Umekita K, Hashiba Y, Kariya Y, Kubo K, Miyauchi S, Aizawa A, et al. The time-sequential changes of risk factors for adult T-cell leukemia development in human T-cell leukemia virus-positive patients with rheumatoid arthritis: a retrospective cohort study. Mod Rheumatol. 2019;29(5):795–801.
29. Swaminathan N, Vinicius JM, Serrins J. Hemophagocytic lymphohistiocytosis (HLH) in a patient with disseminated histoplasmosis. Case Rep Hematol. 2020;2020:5638262.
30. Geraghty EM, Ristow B, Gordon SM, Aronowitz P. Overwhelming parasitemia with Plasmodium falciparum infection in a patient receiving infliximab therapy for rheumatoid arthritis. Clin Infect Dis. 2007;44(10):e82–4.
31. Norena I, Fernandez-Ruiz M, Aguado JM. Viral infections in the biologic therapy era. Expert Rev Anti-Infect Ther. 2018;16(10):781–91.
32. Clemente WT, Pierrotti LC, Abdala E, Morris MI, Azevedo LS, Lopez-Velez R, et al. Recommendations for management of endemic diseases and travel medicine in solid-organ transplant recipients and donors: Latin America. Transplantation. 2018;102(2):193–208.
33. Pierrotti LC, Levi ME, Di Santi SM, Segurado AC, Petersen E. Malaria disease recommendations for solid organ transplant recipients and donors. Transplantation. 2018;102(2S Suppl 2):S16–26.

Safety and Efficacy of Vaccines in Patients on Targeted and Biologic Therapies

3

Ashlesha Sonpar

Summary Table

	Inactivated vaccines	Live vaccines
TNF alpha inhibitors and abatacept		BCG, intranasal influenza, oral polio, rotavirus, yellow fever MMR, VZV
IL-1 inhibitors	For pneumococcal vaccine	Small number of cases
IL-6 inhibitors		
IL-12/23 inhibitors		
IL-17 inhibitors		
Eculizumab	Meningococcal vaccine data	
VEGF inhibitors		
VEGFR inhibitors	Very small numbers, influenza vaccine only	
ErbB2/HER2 inhibitors	Small numbers, influenza vaccine only	
ErbB receptor tyrosine kinase	Influenza vaccine only	
BCR-ABL tyrosine kinase	Influenza vaccine only	Report from 4 patients
Burton tyrosine kinase	Influenza vaccine only	
PI3K inhibitors	PCV-13 vaccine only	
Janus kinase inhibitors		
Anti-CD20		
Alemtuzumab		
Anti-CD-38	Very limited data	
CTLA-4 inhibitors		
PD-1 and PD-1 ligand inhibitors	¼ studies showing increased adverse events	
LFA-3 inhibitor	One study only	
Alpha 4-integrin and LFA-1 inhibitors		One report of measles post vaccine; no yellow fever vaccine-related illness
Sphingosine 1-phosphate receptor inhibitors		
Proteosome inhibitors	Pneumococcal conjugate vaccine only	MMR vaccine

Legend:

- Preserved response, safe
- Preserved response for some vaccines and decreased in others, but safe
- Decreased response, but safe
- Preserved response, but reports of increased adverse events
- Reports of vaccine strain infection/ serious adverse events
- No data
- Safe but no/ limited data on response

A. Sonpar (✉)
Division of Infectious Diseases, University of Alberta, Edmonton, AB, Canada
e-mail: sonpar@ualberta.ca

C. Cervera, J. M. Aguado (eds.), *Infectious Complications in Biologic and Targeted Therapies*, https://doi.org/10.1007/978-3-031-11363-5_3

Evidence Summary by Medication Class

TNF-Alpha Inhibitors and Abatacept

Hepatitis B (HBV) Vaccine

Patients on TNF inhibitors may have a lower response rate to HBV vaccine that is not significantly improved by using high dose vaccine. The general trend of declining response with age is seen in these patients as well.

HBV vaccine is more than 90% effective in healthy young adults and 95% effective in infants, children, and adolescents after three doses. However, after age 40 only 90% respond with protective titers with a further decline to 75% by age 60. It is recommended that patients on renal replacement therapy receive high dose HBV vaccine. This recommendation may be applicable to other immunocompromised patients, but specific groups are not mentioned [1].

In a study looking at high dose (HD) vs. standard dose (SD) HBV vaccine with patients on TNF inhibition, no significant difference was found (61.1% in HD, 49.3% in SD) [2].

In a retrospective chart review using healthy hospital employees as controls, 60.8% of chronic inflammatory disease patients responded to HBV vaccine vs. 94.3% of healthy controls. 33–80% of patients on anti-TNF therapy had protective titers, depending on which TNF inhibitor was prescribed (infliximab and certolizumab had the lowest seroconversion rate). Increasing age and longer time on biologics tended to cause decreased response rates [3]. In a subset of patients ($N = 4$) receiving anti-TNF therapy, all 4 responded to HBV vaccine with only mild side effects. One patient had a disease flare unrelated to the vaccine [4]. In another cohort study, response rates to HBV vaccine varied by biologic prescribed but ranged from 67% to 100% (lowest were abatacept and adalimumab). Older patients were more likely to be nonresponders [5].

Among children receiving HBV vaccine on TNF inhibition—lower titers were observed; however, overall seroprotective titer rate was similar. There may be a faster decline in titers, but 74% of children responded to boosters. No safety concerns were noted [6].

Pneumococcal Vaccine

There is some conflicting evidence, but patients on abatacept may have decreased response to pneumococcal vaccination with preserved response in patients on TNF-inhibitors. Patients on TNF inhibition, but not abatacept, responded to boosting PCV-13 with PPSV-23.

In a study of patients with inflammatory rheumatic diseases, fewer patients on abatacept responded to PCV13 and PPSV23 than controls or patients on cDMARDs. Antibody increase was seen post PCV-13, but not PPSV-23 in the abatacept group. Antibody functionality (as measured by opsonophagocytosis) was also reduced [7]. In contrast, in a systematic review and meta-analysis more patients on TNF inhibitors seroconverted post PPSV-23 suggesting some benefit of boosting PCV-13 response with PPSV-23. In the same meta-analysis, older patients, longer disease history, and higher disease activity score correlated with nonresponse [8].

In a study of 88 rheumatoid arthritis (RA) patients, 17 receiving abatacept, response to PCV-13 was lower in the abatacept group compared to controls. For one strain, response was better than the methotrexate only group [9]. In another study of 149 RA patients—50 on combination therapy with methrotrexate and TNF-i and 62 on TNF-i alone—compared to healthy controls, all groups had similar response rates to PPSV-23. Interestingly, the methotrexate group had the lowest response rate, although this was not statistically significant [10]. An additional study of 22 RA patients receiving etanercept (with or without methotrexate) compared with 24 osteoarthritis controls showed greater than twofold increases in IgG titers in both groups after PCV-13 vaccination. The control group had higher titers than the etanercept group [11]. In 96 IBD patients, response and antibody titer to PPSV-23 was lower in infliximab and combination therapy groups (infliximab + cDMARD). Disease activity was not found to correlate in multivariate analysis. Vaccine was well tolerated with only two mild reactions noted and no disease flare post vaccine [12].

Influenza Vaccine

Influenza vaccine is safe and well tolerated with some conflicting evidence on efficacy (most studies showing no difference in seroresponders). Antibody titers may be improved by high dose vaccine; they may not last as long as in immunocompetent patients. Vaccination reduces the number of influenza-related adverse events.

In a study of patients with chronic inflammatory diseases, there were no differences between TNF-I, abatacept, tocilizumab, and anakinra groups with lower response rates in the rituximab group. No healthy control or disease control groups were analyzed [13]. In another study looking at TNF-i, TNF-i plus other immunosuppression, or healthy controls there was no difference in number of patients with seroprotective titers post influenza vaccination. However, seroconversion rate (measured as >fourfold rise in titer) was lower in the TNF and combination therapy groups. Vaccine was safe and well tolerated with four mild adverse reactions and no disease flares [14]. Similar results were found in a systematic review of RA patients on TNF inhibition compared to healthy controls [15] and other studies [16, 17], although response on abatacept was lower in one ($N = 20$) [16]. Conversely, two studies found decreased seroprotection rates in patients on TNF-i compared to healthy controls, especially with influenza B [18, 19] and an additional study with decreased rates against H1 Influenza compared to healthy controls but not methotrexate [20]. No serious adverse events or disease flares were reported.

In a study of 40 patients on TNF inhibition comparing high dose versus standard dose vaccine, high dose vaccine was associated with higher seroprotection and seroconversion rates [21].

Lokota et al. studied the effects of using a pandemic influenza vaccine post trivalent vaccine with another booster a few weeks later. Again, seroprotective rates were similar in TNF-i, tocilizumab, and healthy controls but titers waned more quickly in the immunosuppressant group. The booster dose did not significantly change the number of patients with seroprotective titers or increase longevity of antibody response [22].

In a study looking at the long-term effects of adalimumab, a sub-group of vaccinated vs. unvaccinated patients was analyzed for influenza-related adverse events. These occurred in 14% of unvaccinated patients compared to 5% of vaccinated patients [23].

Live Vaccines

Live vaccines are likely safe up to 14 days prior to biologic start. Although there are limited data, MMR and varicella vaccine may be safely administered on therapy. There are case reports of vaccine strain-related yellow fever infections, although revaccination may be tolerated. BCG vaccination can lead to vaccine strain disease.

In a review of children on biologic medications, overall data suggests VZV vaccine has maintained efficacy with mild reactions (no reaction to mild self-limiting vesicular rash noted). No flares were noted. Similarly, there were no safety concerns with the MMR vaccine. Seroprotective rates were similar to non-immunocompromised vaccine recipients, with a trend to lower antibody titers [6, 24].

There are two studies published on the use of live vaccines (Measles, mumps, rubella, varicella, and rotavirus vaccines) prior to infliximab (14–90 days prior) for Kawasaki's disease. No serious vaccine-related adverse events were reported; however, patients received vaccine prior to biologic start and most received only one dose of infliximab [25, 26].

A few case reports of yellow fever following yellow fever vaccination in patients on TNF inhibition or adalimumab. One patient recovered without need for hospitalization and only noted prolonged fatigue. Seroprotective antibodies persisted for at least 10 months (no further measurements reported) [27]. Another developed fever and increased liver enzymes with no other complications and development of protective antibodies [28], and a third had no illness reported with protective antibodies measured 2 years post vaccine [29].

The preceding three cases were reported from areas not endemic for yellow fever. There are two reports from Brazil—one with 31 patients with rheumatic illness including three on infliximab. There were only mild adverse events noted, with titers lower than in healthy controls [30]. The other report included 17 patients on infliximab and methotrexate revaccinated during the outbreak (preceding vaccine was 10–22 years prior) with only two patients having no detectable titers prior to vaccine. All but one patient responded to vaccine with a trend to lower titers in the immunosuppressed group. No safety concerns were noted [31].

A Crohn's patient on infliximab inadvertently injected with BCG vaccine developed an abscess at the injection site requiring drainage and systemic therapy for 6 months [32]. Another patient on infliximab given BCG vaccine had no symptoms up to 9 months later [33].

IL-1 Inhibitors

Data found only for canakinumab. No difference in vaccine response or increase in adverse events even in cases of live vaccines (N = 3), except unusual severe inflammatory reaction noted with pneumococcal vaccines in patients with CAPS.

In a study of 51 healthy volunteers (25 given canakinumab and 26 controls), there was no difference in response to influenza or meningococcal vaccine. No serious adverse events were noted [34].

Analysis of vaccine response in 68 cryopyrin associated periodic syndrome (CAPS) patients from a registry being treated with canakinumab. Fifty-five patients received influenza vaccine (107 vaccines administered) with 7 mild reactions. Twelve patients received tetanus and diphtheria vaccine with mild reactions noted. Eleven patients received 21 other vaccines (6 HBV, 5 HAV, 3 typhoid, 2 tick borne encephalitis, 1 polio, 1 MMR, 1 HPV, 1 Lyme disease, and 1 cholera) with 21 non-severe reactions noted. Eighteen patients received 19 pneumococcal vaccines (2 PCV-13, 15 PPSV-23, 2 unknown) with 5 serious adverse reactions to PPSV-23, 3 of these requiring hospitalization (1 non-resolving fever, 2 headache and nausea (1 possible meningitis)) [35].

Two more reports of CAPS patients (one in age 5 and younger and the other in pediatric and adult patients) reported good vaccine seroconversions rates with no adverse events, including in the patients receiving pneumococcal vaccines. One live vaccine (MMR) was administered [36, 37]. There is an additional case report of live vaccines administered while on canakinumab—measles, mumps, rubella, and varicella with no adverse effects and documented seroconversion [38].

In a report of 7 patients with CAPS (6 receiving canakinumab), 2 had systemic reactions, including one meningitis, post pneumococcal vaccination (1 PPSV and 1 PCV13), and 5 had severe local reactions. The authors hypothesize that this could be due to stimulation of TLR-2 and TLR-4, as this reaction was not seen with other vaccines in the same patients [39].

IL-6

Small numbers for each individual vaccine, but most studies show little impact on post vaccine titers. Data is from tocilizumab patients only.

HBV Vaccine

Within a larger cohort of patients on various immunosuppressive agents given HBV vaccine—7/9 (78%) of patients on tocilizumab responded with protective titers [5].

Pneumococcal Vaccine

Sixteen patients treated with tocilizumab within 88 RA patient cohort receiving PCV-13 showed the same number of seroresponders as control. Absolute titers were lower in the tocilizumab group [9]. Ninety one patients receiving tocilizumab plus methotrexate showed numerically lower response rates than methotrexate alone for PPSV-23 (60% vs. 70.8%), but this did not reach significance [40]. In other studies, all 21 patients receiving tocilizumab responded to PPSV-23 [41], and there was no difference in response rates between tocilizumab and RA control patients [42].

Influenza

Six studies for influenza vaccine included patients on tocilizumab. Two studies showed equal seroprotective rates compared to control for influenza A [22, 43]; however, titers waned more quickly compared to control [22]. Seroresponse rate was slightly decreased for Influenza B in one study [43]. One study ($N = 5$ patients on tocilizumab) showed decreased response compared to other immunosuppressants (methotrexate and TNF-inhibitors) [16]. Three other studies (one in JIA patients, two in RA patients) showed no difference in response on tocilizumab compared to age matched controls (JIA) or other DMARDs (RA patients) [41, 44, 45].

There were no serious adverse events or disease flares noted in the above studies, but there is one case report in a JIA patient with disease flares post both doses of influenza vaccine [46].

Tetanus

Tetanus vaccine seroconversion was similar between both groups (42% for combination and 39.1% in methotrexate alone) [40].

Live Vaccines

In two studies on juvenile idiopathic arthritis patients (only three patients total on tocilizumab), no safety issues or vaccine strain disease was noted. Varicella antibodies titers were low 11 and 27 months post vaccine [47, 48].

IL-12/23

Few studies involved patients on Ustekinumab but the response rates were similar to controls except for hepatitis B vaccine.

Twenty-five patients on Ustekinumab among 109 patients with inflammatory disease were vaccinated against hepatitis B. There was a 72% response rate in the Ustekinumab group. Overall, there was no improvement in response rate with a higher dose [2].

Sixty psoriasis patients on Ustekinumab were compared to 50 patients not on systemic therapy after PPSV-23 and tetanus vaccines. There was no difference in vaccine response [49].

Twenty-seven patients with Crohn's disease (15 Ustekinumab, 12 adalimumab) and 20 healthy controls were vaccinated with the seasonal influenza vaccine. No difference in titers between ustekinumab patients and healthy controls, and post vaccine T-cell responses were also similar [50].

IL-17

Only a few studies are available, but the evidence suggests no impact on vaccine response rates. No data available for live vaccines.

Three studies compared influenza vaccine in patients receiving secukinumab (two in psoriasis patients and one in healthy volunteers). No differences in post vaccine titer or response and no serious adverse events or disease flares were recorded [51–53].

The study with healthy volunteers also looked at the group C meningococcal vaccine response. Again, responses between the secukinumab and control groups were similar [51].

One study with ixekizumab looked at responses to PPSV-23 and tetanus vaccine in healthy volunteers. No differences in response rates were noted. All adverse events were mild—mostly headache, injection site erythema, and fatigue [54].

Eculizumab

Patients on eculizumab are at extremely high risk of invasive meningococcal disease. These patients should receive both the quadrivalent and MenB vaccines prior to therapy initiation. Given the breakthrough infections, sub-optimal vaccine response, and non-vaccine strains causing critical (and occasionally fatal) disease, consideration should be given to antimicrobial prophylaxis.

Current recommendations include immunization against meningococcal disease using both quadrivalent (MenACYW) and MenB vaccine [55–57]. Booster vaccines are recommended while patients continue on eculizumab, as rates of disease as well as mortality are higher compared to the general population. Preferably, vaccination series should be completed at least 2 weeks prior to the first dose of eculizumab, but if treatment is urgent, antimicrobial prophylaxis should be provided for at least 2 weeks [58].

Studies looking at titers post vaccination show a general trend of lower titers and response rates. Nine patients with cold agglutinin disease were vaccinated for MenACYW and response rates were 25%, 37.5%, 75%, and 62.5% to group A, C, Y, and W respectively. Patients with prior B cell therapy (like rituximab) were less likely to respond. No cases of meningococcal disease were reported [59]. In another study of 23 patients with PNH, overall response rates were 78%, 87%, 48%, and 70% for groups A, C, Y, and W respectively [60]. In a subset of pediatric patients with splenic or complement deficiencies, the eight patients on eculizumab had lower response rates compared to the other children [61]. In 25 patients receiving eculizumab for aHUS, only 20% showed a full response after the first dose of quadrivalent meningococcal vaccine, a further 36% responded after the second dose. Incomplete response was seen in 52% after the first dose and 29% of the revaccinated patients [62].

Response to the menB vaccine is likely also reduced. In a study of 15 patients with aHUS (5 on eculizimab at time of vaccination), response rates were only 50%.

Titers were measured when patients were off eculizumab as human complement is needed to judge response (which is blocked by eculizumab) [63]. In 43 patients with PNH, IgG, and IgG binding post MenB vaccine was similar to healthy controls. However, no whole blood killing was noted. Therefore despite adequate titers, there may be an impaired response when exposed [64].

Meningococcemia has been noted even in immunized patients [65–67] and occasionally despite prophylactic antimicrobials [68, 69]. Fatal sepsis from non-vaccine strains has also been reported [70].

VEGF Inhibitors (Bevacizumab, Aflibercept)

Very little data, therefore no comment can be made for efficacy compared to other oncology patients. No serious adverse events reported for the 3 bevacizumab patients.

Ninety-five oncology patients treated with various chemotherapy agents, including 3 on bevacizumab, were given seasonal influenza, pandemic influenza, and PPSV 23 vaccine. Response rates were divided into rituximab and non-rituximab patients with no further breakdown. In the 83 patients not on rituximab, 62% and 87% responded after dose 1 and 2 of the pandemic influenza vaccine. Response rate for the seasonal influenza was 70% for H1N1, 58% for H3N2, and 43% for the PPSV-23 vaccine. No serious adverse events were reported [71].

VEGF-R Inhibitors (Sorafenib, Sunitinib, Axitinib, Pazopanib, Regorafenib, Vandetanib, Cabozantinib, Ramucirumab)

Influenza vaccine appears to have the same response in patients on sorafenib and sunitinib as healthy control in a very small number of patients. No serious adverse events were mentioned in the study.

In the previously mentioned study, one patient was on sunitinib. Since no breakdown of the non-rituximab patients was reported, no comment on efficacy can be made. No serious adverse events were reported [71].

Sixteen sunitinib and six sorafenib patients were compared to 11 healthy control and seven patients with metastatic RCC without systemic therapy. There was no difference in titers measured post vaccination between groups, but the patients on sorafenib had lower interferon gamma production and lymphocyte proliferation. Adverse event rates were not mentioned [72].

ErbB2/HER2 Inhibitors (Trastuzumab, Pertuzumab)

In a small number of patients on trastuzumab only, influenza vaccine had the same response rate as healthy controls and was well tolerated.

Influenza vaccine was given to 37 patients on trastuzumab vs. 20 healthy controls and titers were checked post immunization. Patients on any other immunosuppressive therapy, metastatic cancer, and dual HER2 blockade patients were excluded. Similar seroconversion and seroprotective rates between groups for the H1N1 and influenza B strains after adjusting for baseline titer differences, five patients had mild adverse events that resolved within 48 h (local pain, arthalgias, myalgias, chills), and one skin and skin structure infection unrelated to vaccine site. No influenza like illness was reported in either group during the follow-up period [73].

ErbB Receptor Tyrosine Kinases (Erlotinib, Gefitinib, Afatinib, Osimertinib, Lapatinib, Neratinib)

Very little data, but only a few mild reactions in a small number of erlotinib patients receiving influenza vaccine.

Fourteen patients with NSCLC on erlotinib received seasonal influenza vaccine (11 vaccines) and pandemic H1N1 vaccine (seven vaccines). No data on immunogenicity, but only two mild reactions were observed (pain at injection site and rash). No patients developed influenza [74].

BCR-ABL Tyrosine Kinase Inhibitors (Imatinib, Dasatinib, Nilotinib, Bosutinib, Ponatinib)

With the limited data available, influenza vaccine appears to be safe. Seroprotective rates are similar to other patients on chemotherapy, but rates are lower than reports from other biologics or immunocompetent patients. A few live virus vaccines were administered to CML patients with some efficacy and no adverse events.

Four patients with CML (age 12–15) on imatinib were vaccinated against measles and varicella. Fifty percent had stable seroconversion, one did not seroconvert for varicella, and one lost immunity and so was re-immunized. No adverse vaccine events were reported, and imatinib was held for only one patient for 1 week pre- and 2 weeks post-vaccine. All patients had stable disease (ratio BCR-ABL1/ABL1 = 1% or lower with lymphocyte counts >1500 cells/μL) at the time of vaccination [75].

In a study on response to Influenza vaccine, 33% of patients on tyrosine kinase inhibitors responded with protective titers against all three strains compared to 27% of patients on other chemotherapies. No serious adverse events were reported, two patients had injection site pain and fever. Two influenza infections occurred in this patient population, but not in patients with protective titers [76].

Burton Tyrosine Kinase Inhibitors (Ibrutinib, Acalabrutinib)

Data only for ibrutinib. Small numbers, but data suggests decreased vaccine response for influenza, PCV-13, and hepatitis B vaccine.

Two studies looked at the response to influenza vaccine in patients on ibrutinib (almost all CLL, 1 Waldenstrom's macroglobulinemia). Influenza response was lower in the ibrutinib group ($N = 14$) compared to healthy controls. Five infections were reported in the ibrutinib group, only one was confirmed as influenza B [77]. Another study with 19 patients showed that 74% of patients had seroprotective titers post immunization, although only five patients had increasing antibody levels enough to seroconvert. Seven patients developed ILI—one confirmed influenza B, the others were mild and not lab-confirmed [78]. No mention of vaccine-related side effects in either study.

In a subgroup analysis of CLL patients treated with ibrutinib ($N = 34$), only one patient had an immune response to PCV13 based on IgG measurements. Side effects were seen in four patients and were mild. Another study compared patients with CLL on ibrutinib to controls—none of the patients in the ibrutinib group responded to PCV-13, whereas all four of the control patients did. All the ibrutinib patients were also on rituximab, so that may have confounded the findings [79].

A total of 315 lymphoma patients were vaccinated with hepatitis B vaccine—118 in the low dose group, 118 in the high dose group, and 79 in the high dose, high frequency group. Response rates were 68.8%, 81.4%, and 82.3% respectively. Only 47.4% of the ibrutinib patients responded to vaccine [80].

PI3K Inhibitors Idelalisib, Buparlisib, Rigosertib, Duvelisib

One study with PCV-13 in ten patients suggests decreased ability to respond to vaccines.

In a subgroup analysis of CLL patients treated with idelalisib ($N = 10$), none had a response to PCV13 as measured by IgG response. Vaccine-related adverse events were mild [81].

Janus Kinase Inhibitors (Ruxolitinib, Tofacitinib, Baricitinib)

Vaccine response may be blunted for patients on Janus kinase inhibitors, especially when used with methotrexate. Live vaccines administered prior to biologic start are safe.

Pneumococcal Vaccine

Response to PCV13 was tested in 60 patients on tofacitinib for psoriasis. More than 80% of patients responded adequately, with no difference found in the subgroup of lymphopenic patients. 37.7% of patients reported adverse events, but all were mild reactions [82]. In another study comparing patients on tofacitinib to placebo, fewer patients in the tofacitinib group responded to PPSV-23 (45.1% vs. 68.4%). In the subset of patients only on tofacitinib (without methotrexate) compared to no DMARD, the response was still slightly lower (62.2% vs. 76.7%) [83].

In the same study, the investigators compared vaccine response when tofacitinib was interrupted vs. continued. The response was 75% in the continuous vs. 84.6% in the interrupted group. Again, response rates were higher if the patients were not on concomitant methotrexate (89.2% vs. 91.7%) [83].

One hundred and six rheumatoid arthritis patients on baracitinib (89% also on methotrexate) were vaccinated with PCV-13. Sixty-eight percent of patients had a response that was maintained for at least 3 months. Older age was inversely correlated with response. Adverse effects were all mild [84].

Influenza

Winthrop et al. also compared the reaction to influenza vaccine alongside PPSV-23. The response was 56.9% vs. 62.2% in the tofacitinib and placebo groups, with a higher response seen in the subset of patients not on methotrexate (64.4% vs. 67.4%). The proportion of patients with seroprotective titers was higher in the placebo group (91.8% vs. 76.5%).

Response to influenza in the interrupted arm was 63.7% compared to 66.3%, with seroprotective titers of 75% in the interrupted arm compared to 82.4% [83].

Tetanus

Two studies compared the response to tetanus vaccine—one with tofacitinib and one with baricitinib. Eighty-eight percent of tofacitinib patients had an adequate response and 74% of baricitinib patients. No control group was included. Adverse events were all mild [82, 84].

Live Zoster Vaccine

Two studies compared safety and efficacy of live zoster vaccine (LZV) either 2 or 4 weeks prior to tofacitinib start. In the first, a post hoc analysis of a randomized control trial, 3 (1.4%) patients in the vaccinated arm had herpes zoster compared to 15 (1.6%) in the unvaccinated arm. This was not statistically significant. Only one infection was multidermatomal but none were serious. The vaccine was well tolerated with no vesicular lesions within 42 days of vaccine [85].

The other study looked at 112 patients—55 on tofacitinib and 57 on placebo. Both groups were given LZV 2 weeks prior to tofacitinib start. Judging response by mean fold rise in IgG titers, both groups were similar at week 2, 6, and 14. Seven nonserious adverse events were reported in the tofacitinib group and five in placebo group. An additional three serious events occurred in the tofacitinib group—bronchitis, cholangitis, and primary varicella (in a patient later found to have no primary immunity) [86].

mTOR Inhibitors (Everolimus, Temsirolimus)

In a study of pandemic strain influenza vaccine (2009), seroprotection and seroconversion rates were similar to other solid organ transplant recipients but titers were lower. Four patients were infected with influenza, but none had protective antibodies even post infection. No safety concerns were noted (rejection or vaccine adverse events) [87].

Anti-CD20 (Rituximab, 90Y-Ibritumomab Tiuxetan, Ofatumumab, Ocrelizumab, Veltuzumab, 131I-Tositumomab, Obinutuzumab, Ocaratuzumab, Ublituximab)

Overall results show dramatic decrease in vaccine response lasting months beyond last dose. No increase in adverse events for inactivated vaccines.

Pneumococcal Vaccine

Sixty-eight ocrelizumab patients in the VELOCE study (relapsing multiple sclerosis) were vaccinated with PPSV-23 and PCV-13 (as a booster to PPSV-23). Positive response to PPSV-23 was 71.6% compared to 100% in the control group. PCV-13 did not boost response to PPSV-23 for ocrelizumab patients [88]. Reduction in response to PPSV-23 was also seen in a study of rheumatoid arthritis patients on Rituximab (57% vs. 82%) [89]. Other studies in different diseases also show reduction or no response in response to both PPSV-23 and PCV-13 while on rituximab [7–9, 81, 90].

Similar results are found in pediatric lupus patients given PCV-13—among the nine patients on rituximab, only one responded and reached protective titers. Another patient remotely exposed to rituximab (>2 years ago) with hypogammaglobulinemia had a fourfold increase in titers but did not reach protective levels. All control pediatric patients responded to the vaccine [91].

Influenza

Decreased influenza response was noted across many studies and patient populations, with a trend to increasing response with more time between vaccine and rituximab dose. No serious adverse events noted in studies and no disease flares [13, 15, 16, 22, 71, 92–95].

Hepatitis B Vaccine

Significantly fewer patients on rituximab responded to Hepatitis B vaccine. Response rates varied from 25% to 69.5%. Vaccine was well tolerated with only mild adverse effects noted and no disease flares [4, 5, 80, 96].

Tetanus

Decreased tetanus response was compared to control with ocrelizumab (23.9% vs. 54.5%) [88]. Response to vaccine on rituximab was similar to patients on methotrexate (39.1% vs. 42.3%) [89].

Varicella

Case report of a patient on ocrelizumab vaccinated with varicella vaccine with seroconversion to positive IgG (VZV IgG). After receiving ocrelizumab, titers of VZV

IgG declined to nonprotective levels. Repeat vaccination was attempted, but with no response (given 7 months post ocrelizumab dose).

Hematological malignancy patients on anti-CD20 were given a four-dose regimen of the inactivated herpes zoster vaccine. There was a fourfold rise in titer from baseline suggestive of immunogenicity. Most reactions were mild and, while 18 serious adverse events were noted, only one was thought to be vaccine-related (seizures). Five patients reported a vesicular rash [97].

Alemtuzumab

Small amount of data, but vaccine response likely to be reduced especially if within 6 months of alemtuzumab infusion.

Twenty-four multiple sclerosis patients on alemtuzumab (median time since last infusion 18 months) were given multiple vaccines to measure antibody response. Twenty-two patients received diphtheria and tetanus vaccine, 21 received inactivated polio vaccine, 23-valent polysaccharide pneumococcal vaccine (PPSV-23), Haemophilus vaccine, and meningococcal C vaccine. All vaccinated patients had positive IgG to diphtheria and tetanus prior to vaccine, therefore no comment on vaccine effect can be made. Polio seroprotective rate improved from 95% to 100% for type 1 poliovirus, and from 77% to 95% for type 3 poliovirus. Response in patients receiving PPSV-23 exceeded literature controls. Seropositivity for Haemophilus increased from 13% to 74% and from 91% to 100% for meningococcal C vaccine. Overall trend towards decreased vaccine response if within 6 months of alemtuzumab infusion [89, 98].

In 61 islet cell transplant patients, lower seroconversion and seroprotection rates were seen for 2010–2011 influenza vaccine compared to published rates for healthy controls. There was a trend towards lower response if patients received alemtuzumab for induction therapy, regardless of time from transplant. There was a significantly lower response rate in patients who were less than 1 year from their transplant [99].

Anti CD-38 (Daratumumab, Isatuxumab)

Very limited data on a small number of patients with confounding immune system abnormalities. No further decrease in response to pneumococcal vaccine compared to other patients with the same chronic illness. One case report suggesting recombinant zoster vaccine is ineffective.

In a series of multiple myeloma patients (17 on daratumumab, 10 on other immunomodulators) vaccinated against pneumococcal disease, response rates to PCV-13 and PPSV-23 were comparable between the two groups [100].

One case report of a 65-year-old with prior stem cell transplant on daratumumab with a vesicular rash, hypoxic respiratory failure, and subsequent retinitis secondary to VZV. She was vaccinated with recombinant zoster vaccine 6 months prior to presentation and 2 months prior to daratumumab. Virus was sequenced and found to be wild-type, suggesting the vaccine is not effective in all patients [101].

CTLA-4 Inhibitors (Ipilimumab, Tremelimumab)

No increased adverse events noted post influenza vaccine with a lower rate of influenza compared to institutional average.

A retrospective review was done over three influenza seasons (2014–2017) in patients receiving Influenza vaccine within 65 days of immune checkpoint inhibitor. Most patients received PD-1 inhibitors only, but 81 patients received combination therapy with ipilimumab. Only four patients received monotherapy with ipilimumab. 20% of patients experienced immune-related adverse events (IRAEs); the majority were Grade 2–3 in severity. Patients receiving combination therapy had a higher likelihood of having an IRAE and it being more severe. There were no large local reactions or severe post vaccine events. These rates are not higher than published literature for the medications alone, leading the authors to conclude that vaccination did not lead to increased IRAEs. The rate of influenza in these vaccinated patients over 3 years was 3.5% compared to the institutional incidence of 10.7% [102].

PD-1 and PD-1 Ligand Inhibitors (Nivolumab, Pembrolizumab, Atezolizumab)

Data mostly on Influenza vaccine—high baseline immune-related adverse events, but these were not worse with vaccine administration in all but one study.

Influenza Vaccine

The retrospective review mentioned above included patients mostly on PD-1 inhibitors. As noted earlier, no increased IRAEs were noted in the influenza-vaccinated patients compared to the published literature. The rate of influenza in these vaccinated patients over 3 years was 3.5% compared to the institutional incidence of 10.7% [102]. In two cohort studies, the incidence of IRAEs was not higher in the vaccinated group. There was also no increased risk if the vaccine was given in between doses [103, 104].

One study with 23 patients compared to 11 healthy controls found a slightly lower seropositivity rate in treated patients (not significant). IRAEs occurred in 52.2% of patients with 26.1% of patients having grade 3–4 reactions, including 3 neurological reactions (2 encephalitis and 1 peripheral neuropathy). This rate was higher than the published literature for PD-1 inhibitors [105]. Additionally, there was one report on a patient with Guillain-Barre syndrome (GBS) with symptoms starting 3 weeks post influenza vaccine. Unfortunately, the patient worsened and passed away. The differential for his symptoms included vaccine-related GBS, but also worsening melanoma with brain metastases and nivolumab-associated neurological IRAE [106].

Recombinant Zoster Vaccine

A patient receiving pembrolizumab developed oral and skin lesions suggestive of Stevens-Johnson syndrome 7 days post vaccination with recombinant zoster vaccine. The patient improved on steroids but was not given the second dose of vaccine [107].

LFA-3 Inhibitor (Alefacept)

Data from one study in patients with psoriasis shows polysaccharide pneumococcal vaccine is safe with no loss in efficacy (when compared to patients on other immunomodulators).

Forty-two patients with psoriasis were given PPSV-23 in the middle of 12 weekly doses of Alefacept. Serial antibody titers showed 86% and 78% of patients had a twofold rise at 3 and 6 months, and 57% and 47% of patients had a fourfold rise. This is compared to a baseline rate of 34.5% response for patients on methotrexate and anti-TNF agents. Adverse events were generally mild [108].

Alpha 4-Integrin and LFA-1 Inhibitors (Natalizumab, Vedolizumab, Efalizumab)

Influenza Vaccine

Likely lower response in patients on natalizumab; no difference in one study done for patients on vedolizumab.

Seventeen patients on Natalizumab had no significant difference in Influenza A and B antibody titers post vaccine compared to ten healthy controls. There was a trend towards lower titers in the natalizumab group, but overall small numbers and the groups were not well matched [109]. In another study with 113 patients on immunomodulators (17 on natalizumab and 36 on interferon) compared to 216 healthy controls, response to 2009 H1N1 influenza vaccine was lower in the natalizumab group compared to the interferon or health control groups [89]. A similar trend was found in two other studies comparing 14 patients on natalizumab to patients on interferon [110] and 12 patients on natalizumab compared to 53 controls [111]. In contrast, a study of patient 19 patients on vedolizumab receiving standard dose influenza vaccine showed no difference in seroprotection or seroconversion rates compared to healthy controls [21].

Other Vaccines

Small numbers, but trend suggestive of preserved response to tetanus vaccine and hepatitis B vaccine.

Sixty patients (30 natalizumab, 30 control) were evaluated for their response to tetanus vaccine and keyhole limpet hemocyanin (KLH, a neoantigen). No significant differences were observed between natalizumab and control groups, although the number of patients that responded was slightly lower in the natalizumab group [112]. Similar results were seen in a study with 41 patients on efalizumab compared to 22 controls receiving tetanus vaccine. Antibody titers were slightly lower in the efalizumab group, but seroprotection rates were equivalent [113].

Hepatitis B and oral cholera vaccine responses were assessed in 127 healthy volunteers (64 vedolizumab and 63 placebo). Response to hepatitis B vaccine was preserved, but response to oral cholera vaccine was lower in the vedolizumab group. Adverse events were similar in both groups [114].

Live Vaccines

No disease flare or vaccine illness noted post yellow fever vaccine, but one case report of likely vaccine strain measles.

Twenty-three multiple sclerosis patients on natalizumab received yellow fever vaccine with no adverse events and no flares post vaccine. All patients were from Switzerland and received vaccine for travel reasons. Therefore, they would be unlikely to have prior immunity or exposure [115].

One case report of a patient on natalizumab developing non-severe measles 7 days post vaccine. No typing was done, but the diagnosis was confirmed by PCR. However, the report is from Switzerland with no known community measles contact, making it more likely that this is vaccine strain disease [116].

Sphingosine 1-Phosphate Receptor Inhibitor (Fingolimod, Siponimod)

Data suggests lowered vaccine response, and possible loss of protective antibodies from prior vaccines.

A review of multiple sclerosis patients on immunomodulators had conflicting evidence regarding patients on fingolimod receiving Influenza vaccine—two studies showing no difference in efficacy (with lower absolute antibody titers) and two studies showing lowered seroprotection (smaller numbers) [89]. A study of Siponimod in healthy persons receiving influenza vaccine and polysaccharide pneumococcal vaccine showed decreased response to Influenza B in the continued therapy and interrupted therapy groups. All groups responded well to the pneumococcal vaccine [117].

Two patients on fingolimod vaccinated against tick-borne encephalitis had the lowest antibody increase compared to 18 other multiple sclerosis patients. It is unknown if they developed protective (but low) titers [118]. Out 23 patients vaccinated for varicella zoster virus (VZV) prior to therapy, 7 lost detectable antibody. Out of three patients that stopped fingolimod due to side effects, two recovered varicella antibody and one developed chickenpox 1 year post fingolimod [119]. There is also one case report of a patient on fingolimod developing VZV encephalitis despite history of chickenpox and prior vaccination. This patient was also previously treated with natalizumab [120].

Proteosome Inhibitors (Bortezomib, Carfilzomib, Ixazomib)

No data on efficacy, but MMR vaccine may be tolerated while on proteosome inhibitors. One study showing clinical benefit with pneumococcal vaccine.

Thirteen multiple myeloma patients post stem cell transplant on bortezomib were vaccinated for the measles, mumps, and rubella (MMR) vaccine 25 months post transplant. Three patients had mild adverse events, but there was no vaccine strain disease, no fevers, no hospitalizations, and no deaths. No titers were done to look at efficacy [121]. In a study looking at conjugate pneumococcal vaccine efficacy, 18 vaccinated multiple myeloma patients (11 on bortezomib and 2 on ixazomib) were compared to 18 unvaccinated multiple myeloma patients (9 on bortezomib and 5 on ixazomib). The rate of pneumonia over 1 year was 16.7% in the vaccinated group and 50% in the unvaccinated group, suggesting that pneumococcal vaccine is effective at preventing clinical disease. No adverse vaccine events were documented in the study. The dosing of vaccine was unusual (three doses given 1 month apart) [122].

References

1. Hamborsky J, Kroger A, Wolfe S, editors. Centers for Disease Control and Prevention. Epidemiology and prevention of vaccine-preventable diseases. 13th ed. Washington, DC: Public Health Foundation; 2015.
2. Haykir Solay A, Eser F. High dose hepatitis B vaccine is not effective in patients using immunomodulatory drugs: a pilot study. Hum Vaccin Immunother. 2019;15(5):1177–82.
3. Okay G, Biberci Keskin E, Akkoyunlu Y, Bolukcu S, Betul Uslu A, Meric Koc M. Evaluation of hepatitis B vaccine efficacy and factors affecting vaccine nonresponse in patients receiving anti-tumor necrosis factor agents. Eur J Gastroenterol Hepatol. 2020;33(8):1091–6.
4. Intongkam S, Samakarnthai P, Pakchotanon R, Narongroeknawin P, Assavatanabodee P, Chaiamnuay S. Efficacy and safety of hepatitis B vaccination in rheumatoid arthritis patients receiving disease-modifying antirheumatic drugs and/or biologics therapy. J Clin Rheumatol. 2018;25(8):329–34.
5. Richi P, Alonso O, Martin MD, Gonzalez-Hombrado L, Navio T, Salido M, et al. Evaluation of the immune response to hepatitis B vaccine in patients on biological therapy: results of the RIER cohort study. Clin Rheumatol. 2020;39(9):2751–6.
6. Tse HN, Borrow R, Arkwright PD. Immune response and safety of viral vaccines in children with autoimmune diseases on immune modulatory drug therapy. Expert Rev Vaccines. 2021;19(12):1115–27.
7. Nived P, Jonsson G, Settergren B, Einarsson J, Olofsson T, Jorgensen CS, et al. Prime-boost vaccination strategy enhances immunogenicity compared to single pneumococcal conjugate vaccination in patients receiving conventional DMARDs, to some extent in abatacept but not in rituximab-treated patients. Arthritis Res Ther. 2020;22(1):36.
8. van Aalst M, Langedijk AC, Spijker R, de Bree GJ, Grobusch MP, Goorhuis A. The effect of immunosuppressive agents on immunogenicity of pneumococcal vaccination: a systematic review and meta-analysis. Vaccine. 2018;36(39):5832–45.

9. Crnkic Kapetanovic M, Saxne T, Jonsson G, Truedsson L, Geborek P. Rituximab and abatacept but not tocilizumab impair antibody response to pneumococcal conjugate vaccine in patients with rheumatoid arthritis. Arthritis Res Ther. 2013;15(5):R171.
10. Kapetanovic MC, Saxne T, Sjoholm A, Truedsson L, Jonsson G, Geborek P. Influence of methotrexate, TNF blockers and prednisolone on antibody responses to pneumococcal polysaccharide vaccine in patients with rheumatoid arthritis. Rheumatology (Oxford). 2006;45(1):106–11.
11. Rakoczi E, Perge B, Vegh E, Csomor P, Pusztai A, Szamosi S, et al. Evaluation of the immunogenicity of the 13-valent conjugated pneumococcal vaccine in rheumatoid arthritis patients treated with etanercept. Jt Bone Spine. 2016;83(6):675–9.
12. Fiorino G, Peyrin-Biroulet L, Naccarato P, Szabo H, Sociale OR, Vetrano S, et al. Effects of immunosuppression on immune response to pneumococcal vaccine in inflammatory bowel disease: a prospective study. Inflamm Bowel Dis. 2012;18(6):1042–7.
13. Richi P, Martin MD, Navio MT, Gonzalez-Hombrado L, Salido M, Llorente J, et al. Antibody responses to influenza vaccine in patients on biological therapy: results of RIER cohort study. Med Clin (Barc). 2019;153(10):380–6.
14. Andrisani G, Frasca D, Romero M, Armuzzi A, Felice C, Marzo M, et al. Immune response to influenza A/H1N1 vaccine in inflammatory bowel disease patients treated with anti TNF-alpha agents: effects of combined therapy with immunosuppressants. J Crohns Colitis. 2013;7(4):301–7.
15. Huang Y, Wang H, Tam WWS. Is rheumatoid arthritis associated with reduced immunogenicity of the influenza vaccination? A systematic review and meta-analysis. Curr Med Res Opin. 2017;33(10):1901–8.
16. Adler S, Krivine A, Weix J, Rozenberg F, Launay O, Huesler J, et al. Protective effect of A/H1N1 vaccination in immune-mediated disease—a prospectively controlled vaccination study. Rheumatology (Oxford). 2012;51(4):695–700.
17. Elkayam O, Bashkin A, Mandelboim M, Litinsky I, Comaheshter D, Levartovsky D, et al. The effect of infliximab and timing of vaccination on the humoral response to influenza vaccination in patients with rheumatoid arthritis and ankylosing spondylitis. Semin Arthritis Rheum. 2010;39(6):442–7.
18. Salemi S, Picchianti-Diamanti A, Germano V, Donatelli I, Di Martino A, Facchini M, et al. Influenza vaccine administration in rheumatoid arthritis patients under treatment with TNFalpha blockers: safety and immunogenicity. Clin Immunol. 2010;134(2):113–20.
19. Mamula P, Markowitz JE, Piccoli DA, Klimov A, Cohen L, Baldassano RN. Immune response to influenza vaccine in pediatric patients with inflammatory bowel disease. Clin Gastroenterol Hepatol. 2007;5(7):851–6.
20. Fomin I, Caspi D, Levy V, Varsano N, Shalev Y, Paran D, et al. Vaccination against influenza in rheumatoid arthritis: the effect of disease modifying drugs, including TNF alpha blockers. Ann Rheum Dis. 2006;65(2):191–4.
21. Caldera F, Hillman L, Saha S, Wald A, Grimes I, Zhang Y, et al. Immunogenicity of high dose influenza vaccine for patients with inflammatory bowel disease on anti-TNF monotherapy: a randomized clinical trial. Inflamm Bowel Dis. 2020;26(4):593–602.
22. Lakota K, Perdan-Pirkmajer K, Sodin-Semrl S, Cucnik S, Subelj V, Prosenc K, et al. The immunogenicity of seasonal and pandemic influenza vaccination in autoimmune inflammatory rheumatic patients-a 6-month follow-up prospective study. Clin Rheumatol. 2019;38(5):1277–92.
23. Burmester GR, Landewe R, Genovese MC, Friedman AW, Pfeifer ND, Varothai NA, et al. Adalimumab long-term safety: infections, vaccination response and pregnancy outcomes in patients with rheumatoid arthritis. Ann Rheum Dis. 2017;76(2):414–7.
24. Borte S, Liebert UG, Borte M, Sack U. Efficacy of measles, mumps and rubella revaccination in children with juvenile idiopathic arthritis treated with methotrexate and etanercept. Rheumatology (Oxford). 2009;48(2):144–8.

25. Miura M, Kobayashi T, Igarashi T, Hamada H, Iwata N, Sasaki Y, et al. Real-world safety and effectiveness of infliximab in pediatric patients with acute Kawasaki disease: a postmarketing surveillance in Japan (SAKURA study). Pediatr Infect Dis J. 2020;39(1):41–7.
26. Lee AM, Burns JC, Tremoulet AH. Safety of infliximab following live virus vaccination in Kawasaki disease patients. Pediatr Infect Dis J. 2017;36(4):435–7.
27. Ekenberg C, Friis-Moller N, Ulstrup T, Aalykke C. Inadvertent yellow fever vaccination of a patient with Crohn's disease treated with infliximab and methotrexate. BMJ Case Rep. 2016;2016.
28. Ruddel J, Schleenvoigt BT, Schuler E, Schmidt C, Pletz MW, Stallmach A. Yellow fever vaccination during treatment with infliximab in a patient with ulcerative colitis: a case report. Z Gastroenterol. 2016;54(9):1081–4.
29. Nash ER, Brand M, Chalkias S. Yellow fever vaccination of a primary vaccinee during adalimumab therapy. J Travel Med. 2015;22(4):279–81.
30. Oliveira ACV, Mota LMH, Santos-Neto LL, Simoes M, Martins-Filho OA, Tauil PL. Seroconversion in patients with rheumatic diseases treated with immunomodulators or immunosuppressants, who were inadvertently revaccinated against yellow fever. Arthritis Rheumatol. 2015;67(2):582–3.
31. Scheinberg M, Guedes-Barbosa LS, Mangueira C, Rosseto EA, Mota L, Oliveira AC, et al. Yellow fever revaccination during infliximab therapy. Arthritis Care Res (Hoboken). 2010;62(6):896–8.
32. Aegerter JP, Christin L, Guyot J, Zellweger J. Bacille Calmette-Guerin injection instead of purified protein derivative injection in an infliximab treated patient. Int J Tuberc Lung Dis. 2016;20(7):990–1.
33. Toussirot E, Wendling D. Bacillus Calmette-Guerin vaccination in a patient treated with infliximab. J Rheumatol. 2005;32(12):2500–1.
34. Chioato A, Noseda E, Felix SD, Stevens M, Del Giudice G, Fitoussi S, et al. Influenza and meningococcal vaccinations are effective in healthy subjects treated with the interleukin-1 beta-blocking antibody canakinumab: results of an open-label, parallel group, randomized, single-center study. Clin Vaccine Immunol. 2010;17(12):1952–7.
35. Jaeger VK, Hoffman HM, van der Poll T, Tilson H, Seibert J, Speziale A, et al. Safety of vaccinations in patients with cryopyrin-associated periodic syndromes: a prospective registry based study. Rheumatology (Oxford). 2017;56(9):1484–91.
36. Brogan PA, Hofer M, Kuemmerle-Deschner JB, Kone-Paut I, Roesler J, Kallinich T, et al. Rapid and sustained long-term efficacy and safety of canakinumab in patients with cryopyrin-associated periodic syndrome ages five years and younger. Arthritis Rheumatol. 2019;71(11):1955–63.
37. Kuemmerle-Deschner JB, Hachulla E, Cartwright R, Hawkins PN, Tran TA, Bader-Meunier B, et al. Two-year results from an open-label, multicentre, phase III study evaluating the safety and efficacy of canakinumab in patients with cryopyrin-associated periodic syndrome across different severity phenotypes. Ann Rheum Dis. 2011;70(12):2095–102.
38. Watanabe M, Nishikomori R, Fujimaki Y, Heike T, Ohara A, Saji T. Live-attenuated vaccines in a cryopyrin-associated periodic syndrome patient receiving canakinumab treatment during infancy. Report No.: 5.
39. Walker UA, Hoffman HM, Williams R, Kuemmerle-Deschner J, Hawkins PN. Brief report: severe inflammation following vaccination against Streptococcus pneumoniae in patients with cryopyrin-associated periodic syndromes. Arthritis Rheumatol. 2016;68(2):516–20.
40. Bingham CO, Rizzo W, Kivitz A, Hassanali A, Upmanyu R, Klearman M. Humoral immune response to vaccines in patients with rheumatoid arthritis treated with tocilizumab: results of a randomised controlled trial (VISARA). Ann Rheum Dis. 2015;74(5):818–22.
41. Tsuru T, Terao K, Murakami M, Matsutani T, Suzaki M, Amamoto T, et al. Immune response to influenza vaccine and pneumococcal polysaccharide vaccine under IL-6 signal inhibition therapy with tocilizumab. Mod Rheumatol. 2014;24(3):511–6.

42. Mori S, Ueki Y, Akeda Y, Hirakata N, Oribe M, Shiohira Y, et al. Pneumococcal polysaccharide vaccination in rheumatoid arthritis patients receiving tocilizumab therapy. Ann Rheum Dis. 2013;72(8):1362–6.
43. Mori S, Ueki Y, Hirakata N, Oribe M, Hidaka T, Oishi K. Impact of tocilizumab therapy on antibody response to influenza vaccine in patients with rheumatoid arthritis. Ann Rheum Dis. 2012;71(12):2006–10.
44. Shinoki T, Hara R, Kaneko U, Miyamae T, Imagawa T, Mori M, et al. Safety and response to influenza vaccine in patients with systemic-onset juvenile idiopathic arthritis receiving tocilizumab. Mod Rheumatol. 2012;22(6):871–6.
45. Kapetanovic MC, Kristensen L, Saxne T, Aktas T, Morner A, Geborek P. Impact of anti-rheumatic treatment on immunogenicity of pandemic H1N1 influenza vaccine in patients with arthritis. Arthritis Res Ther. 2014;16(1):R2.
46. Shimizu M, Ueno K, Yachie A. Relapse of systemic juvenile idiopathic arthritis after influenza vaccination in a patient receiving tocilizumab. Clin Vaccine Immunol. 2012;19(10):1700–2.
47. Uziel Y, Moshe V, Onozo B, Kulcsar A, Trobert-Sipos D, Akikusa JD, et al. Live attenuated MMR/V booster vaccines in children with rheumatic diseases on immunosuppressive therapy are safe: Multicenter, retrospective data collection. Vaccine. 2020;38(9):2198–201.
48. Toplak N, Avcin T. Long-term safety and efficacy of varicella vaccination in children with juvenile idiopathic arthritis treated with biologic therapy. Vaccine. 2015;33(33):4056–9.
49. Brodmerkel C, Wadman E, Langley RG, Papp KA, Bourcier M, Poulin Y, et al. Immune response to pneumococcus and tetanus toxoid in patients with moderate-to-severe psoriasis following long-term ustekinumab use. J Drugs Dermatol. 2013;12(10):1122–9.
50. Doornekamp L, Goetgebuer RL, Schmitz KS, Goeijenbier M, van der Woude CJ, Fouchier R, et al. High immunogenicity to influenza vaccination in Crohn's disease patients treated with ustekinumab. Vaccines (Basel). 2020;8(3):455.
51. Chioato A, Noseda E, Stevens M, Gaitatzis N, Kleinschmidt A, Picaud H. Treatment with the interleukin-17A-blocking antibody secukinumab does not interfere with the efficacy of influenza and meningococcal vaccinations in healthy subjects: results of an open-label, parallel-group, randomized single-center study. Clin Vaccine Immunol. 2012;19(10):1597–602.
52. Richi P, Martin MD, de Ory F, Gutierrez-Larraya R, Casas I, Jimenez-Diaz AM, et al. Secukinumab does not impair the immunogenic response to the influenza vaccine in patients. RMD Open. 2019;5(2):e001018.
53. Furer V, Zisman D, Kaufman I, Arad U, Berman M, Sarbagil-Maman H, et al. Immunogenicity and safety of vaccination against seasonal influenza vaccine in patients with psoriatic arthritis treated with secukinumab. Vaccine. 2020;38(4):847–51.
54. Gomez EV, Bishop JL, Jackson K, Muram TM, Phillips D. Response to tetanus and pneumococcal vaccination following administration of ixekizumab in healthy participants. BioDrugs. 2017;31(6):545–54.
55. Immunisation of individuals with underlying medical conditions: the green book, chapter 7 - GOV.UK (2020) https://www.gov.uk/government/publications/immunisation-of-individuals-with-underlying-medical-conditions-thegreen-book-chapter-7 (accessed August 29, 2022).
56. Manage Meningococcal Disease Risk in Patients Taking Eculizumab | CDC n.d. https://www.cdc.gov/meningococcal/clinical/eculizumab.html (accessed August 29, 2022).
57. Meningococcal vaccine: Canadian Immunization Guide - Canada.ca n.d. https://www.canada.ca/en/publichealth/services/publications/healthy-living/canadian-immunization-guide-part-4-active-vaccines/page-13-meningococcal-vaccine.html#p4c12a5c1 (accessed August 29, 2022).
58. Pittock SJ, Weitz I, Howard JF, Sabatella G, Mehta S, Franklin J. Response to: eculizumab package insert recommendations for meningococcal vaccinations: call for clarity and a targeted approach for use of the drug in neuromyelitis optica spectrum disorder. CNS Spectr. 2020;26(3):195–6.
59. Alashkar F, Vance C, Herich-Terhurne D, Turki AT, Schmitz C, Bommer M, et al. Serologic response to meningococcal vaccination in patients with cold agglutinin disease (CAD) in the novel era of complement inhibition. Vaccine. 2019;37(44):6682–7.

60. Alashkar F, Vance C, Herich-Terhurne D, Preising N, Duhrsen U, Roth A. Serologic response to meningococcal vaccination in patients with paroxysmal nocturnal hemoglobinuria (PNH) chronically treated with the terminal complement inhibitor eculizumab. Ann Hematol. 2017;96(4):589–96.
61. Martinon-Torres F, Bernatowska E, Shcherbina A, Esposito S, Szenborn L, Marti MC, et al. Meningococcal B vaccine immunogenicity in children with defects in complement and splenic function. Pediatrics. 2018;142(3):09.
62. Gackler A, Kaulfus M, Rohn H, Vogel U, Claus H, Feldkamp T, et al. Failure of first meningococcal vaccination in patients with atypical haemolytic uraemic syndrome treated with eculizumab. Nephrol Dial Transplant. 2020;35(2):298–303.
63. Mulling N, Rohn H, Vogel U, Claus H, Wilde B, Eisenberger U, et al. Low efficacy of vaccination against serogroup B meningococci in patients with atypical hemolytic uremic syndrome. Biosci Rep. 2020;40(3):BSR20200177.
64. Langereis JD, van den Broek B, Franssen S, Joosten I, Blijlevens NMA, de Jonge MI, et al. Eculizumab impairs Neisseria meningitidis serogroup B killing in whole blood despite 4CMenB vaccination of PNH patients. Blood Adv. 2020;4(15):3615–20.
65. Reher D, Fuhrmann V, Kluge S, Nierhaus A. A rare case of septic shock due to Neisseria meningitidis serogroup B infection despite prior vaccination in a young adult with paroxysmal nocturnal haemoglobinuria receiving eculizumab. Vaccine. 2018;36(19):2507–9.
66. Lebel E, Trahtemberg U, Block C, Zelig O, Elinav H. Post-eculizumab meningococcaemia in vaccinated patients. Clin Microbiol Infect. 2018;24(1):89–90.
67. Struijk GH, Bouts AHM, Rijkers GT, Kuin EAC, ten Berge IJM, Bemelman FJ. Meningococcal sepsis complicating eculizumab treatment despite prior vaccination. Am J Transplant. 2013;13(3):819–20.
68. Polat M, Yuksel S, Sahin NU. Fatal meningococcemia due to Neisseria meningitidis serogroup Y in a vaccinated child receiving eculizumab. Hum Vaccin Immunother. 2018;14(11):2802.
69. Parikh SR, Lucidarme J, Bingham C, Warwicker P, Goodship T, Borrow R, et al. Meningococcal B vaccine failure with a penicillin-resistant strain in a young adult on long-term eculizumab. Pediatrics. 2017;140(3):e20162452.
70. Nolfi-Donegan D, Konar M, Vianzon V, MacNeil J, Cooper J, Lurie P, et al. Fatal nongroupable Neisseria meningitidis disease in vaccinated patient receiving eculizumab. Emerg Infect Dis. 2018;24(8):08.
71. Berglund A, Willen L, Grodeberg L, Skattum L, Hagberg H, Pauksens K. The response to vaccination against influenza A(H1N1) 2009, seasonal influenza and Streptococcus pneumoniae in adult outpatients with ongoing treatment for cancer with and without rituximab. Acta Oncol. 2014;53(9):1212–20.
72. Mulder SF, Jacobs JFM, Olde Nordkamp MAM, Galama JMD, Desar IME, Torensma R, et al. Cancer patients treated with sunitinib or sorafenib have sufficient antibody and cellular immune responses to warrant influenza vaccination. Clin Cancer Res. 2011;17(13):4541–9.
73. Joona TB, Digkas E, Wennstig A, Nystrom K, Nearchou A, Nilsson C, et al. Influenza vaccination in breast cancer patients during subcutaneous trastuzumab in adjuvant setting. Breast Cancer Res Treat. 2020;184(1):45–52.
74. Spitaleri G, Delmonte A, Toffalorio F, De Pas TM, Gregorc V. Safety of concomitant administration of seasonal and/or H1N1 flu vaccination in patients receiving erlotinib for advanced non-small cell lung cancer. J Thorac Oncol. 2010;5(5):752–4.
75. Bettoni da Cunha-Riehm C, Hildebrand V, Nathrath M, Metzler M, Suttorp M. Vaccination with live attenuated vaccines in four children with chronic myeloid leukemia while on imatinib treatment. Front Immunol. 2020;11:628.
76. Sanada Y, Yakushijin K, Nomura T, Chayahara N, Toyoda M, Minami Y, et al. A prospective study on the efficacy of two-dose influenza vaccinations in cancer patients receiving chemotherapy. Jpn J Clin Oncol. 2016;46(5):448–52.
77. Douglas AP, Trubiano JA, Barr I, Leung V, Slavin MA, Tam CS. Ibrutinib may impair serological responses to influenza vaccination. Haematologica. 2017;102(10):e397–9.

78. Sun C, Gao J, Couzens L, Tian X, Farooqui MZ, Eichelberger MC, et al. Seasonal influenza vaccination in patients with chronic lymphocytic leukemia treated with ibrutinib. JAMA Oncol. 2016;2(12):1656–7.
79. Andrick B, Alwhaibi A, DeRemer DL, Quershi S, Khan R, Bryan LJ, et al. Lack of adequate pneumococcal vaccination response in chronic lymphocytic leukaemia patients receiving ibrutinib. Br J Haematol. 2018;182(5):712–4.
80. Zhuang W, Wang Y. Analysis of the immunity effects after enhanced hepatitis B vaccination on patients with lymphoma. Leuk Lymphoma. 2020;61(2):357–63.
81. Mauro FR, Giannarelli D, Galluzzo CM, Vitale C, Visentin A, Riemma C, et al. Response to the conjugate pneumococcal vaccine (PCV13) in patients with chronic lymphocytic leukemia (CLL). Leukemia. 2020;35:737–46.
82. Winthrop KL, Korman N, Abramovits W, Rottinghaus ST, Tan H, Gardner A, et al. T-cell-mediated immune response to pneumococcal conjugate vaccine (PCV-13) and tetanus toxoid vaccine in patients with moderate-to-severe psoriasis during tofacitinib treatment. J Am Acad Dermatol. 2018;78(6):1149–55.e1.
83. Winthrop KL, Silverfield J, Racewicz A, Neal J, Lee EB, Hrycaj P, et al. The effect of tofacitinib on pneumococcal and influenza vaccine responses in rheumatoid arthritis. Ann Rheum Dis. 2016;75(4):687–95.
84. Winthrop KL, Bingham CO, Komocsar WJ, Bradley J, Issa M, Klar R, et al. Evaluation of pneumococcal and tetanus vaccine responses in patients with rheumatoid arthritis receiving baricitinib: results from a long-term extension trial substudy. Arthritis Res Ther. 2019;21(1):102.
85. Calabrese LH, Abud-Mendoza C, Lindsey SM, Lee S, Tatulych S, Takiya L, et al. Live zoster vaccine in patients with rheumatoid arthritis treated with tofacitinib with or without methotrexate, or adalimumab with methotrexate: a post hoc analysis of data from a phase IIIb/IV randomized study. Arthritis Care Res (Hoboken). 2020;72(3):353–9.
86. Winthrop KL, Wouters AG, Choy EH, Soma K, Hodge JA, Nduaka CI, et al. The safety and immunogenicity of live zoster vaccination in patients with rheumatoid arthritis before starting tofacitinib: a randomized phase II trial. Arthritis Rheumatol. 2017;69(10):1969–77.
87. Cordero E, Perez-Ordonez A, Aydillo TA, Torre-Cisneros J, Gavalda J, Lara R, et al. Therapy with m-TOR inhibitors decreases the response to the pandemic influenza A H1N1 vaccine in solid organ transplant recipients. Am J Transplant. 2011;11(10):2205–13.
88. Bar-Or A, Calkwood JC, Chognot C, Evershed J, Fox EJ, Herman A, et al. Effect of ocrelizumab on vaccine responses in patients with multiple sclerosis: the VELOCE study. Neurology. 2020;95(14):e1999–2008.
89. Ciotti JR, Valtcheva MV, Cross AH. Effects of MS disease-modifying therapies on responses to vaccinations: a review. Mult Scler Relat Disord. 2020;45:102439.
90. Nived P, Nagel J, Saxne T, Geborek P, Jonsson G, Skattum L, et al. Immune response to pneumococcal conjugate vaccine in patients with systemic vasculitis receiving standard of care therapy. Vaccine. 2017;35(29):3639–46.
91. Gorelik M, Elizalde A, Wong Williams K, Gonzalez E, Cole JL. Immunogenicity of sequential 13-valent conjugated and 23-valent unconjugated pneumococcal vaccines in a population of children with lupus. Lupus. 2018;27(14):2228–35.
92. Oren S, Mandelboim M, Braun-Moscovici Y, Paran D, Ablin J, Litinsky I, et al. Vaccination against influenza in patients with rheumatoid arthritis: the effect of rituximab on the humoral response. Ann Rheum Dis. 2008;67(7):937–41.
93. van Assen S, Holvast A, Benne CA, Posthumus MD, van Leeuwen MA, Voskuyl AE, et al. Humoral responses after influenza vaccination are severely reduced in patients with rheumatoid arthritis treated with rituximab. Arthritis Rheum. 2010;62(1):75–81.
94. Bedognetti D, Zoppoli G, Massucco C, Zanardi E, Zupo S, Bruzzone A, et al. Impaired response to influenza vaccine associated with persistent memory B cell depletion in non-Hodgkin's lymphoma patients treated with rituximab-containing regimens. J Immunol. 2011;186(10):6044–55.

95. Ide Y, Imamura Y, Ohfuji S, Fukushima W, Ide S, Tsutsumi C, et al. Immunogenicity of a monovalent influenza A(H1N1)pdm09 vaccine in patients with hematological malignancies. Hum Vaccin Immunother. 2014;10(8):2387–94.
96. Intongkam S, Samakarnthai P, Pakchotanon R, Narongroeknawin P, Assavatanabodee P, Chaiamnuay S. Efficacy and safety of hepatitis B vaccination in rheumatoid arthritis patients receiving disease-modifying antirheumatic drugs and/or biologics therapy. J Clin Rheumatol. 2019;25(8):329–34.
97. Parrino J, McNeil SA, Lawrence SJ, Kimby E, Pagnoni MF, Stek JE, et al. Safety and immunogenicity of inactivated varicella-zoster virus vaccine in adults with hematologic malignancies receiving treatment with anti-CD20 monoclonal antibodies. Vaccine. 2017;35(14):1764–9.
98. McCarthy CL, Tuohy O, Compston DAS, Kumararatne DS, Coles AJ, Jones JL. Immune competence after alemtuzumab treatment of multiple sclerosis. Neurology. 2013;81(10):872–6.
99. Silva M, Humar A, Shapiro AMJ, Senior P, Hoschler K, Baluch A, et al. Humoral immune response following seasonal influenza vaccine in islet transplant recipients. Cell Transplant. 2013;22(3):469–76.
100. Frerichs KA, Bosman PWC, van Velzen JF, Fraaij PLA, Koopmans MPG, Rimmelzwaan GF, et al. Effect of daratumumab on normal plasma cells, polyclonal immunoglobulin levels, and vaccination responses in extensively pre-treated multiple myeloma patients. Haematologica. 2020;105(6):e302–6.
101. Chen RI, Deaner JD, Srivastava SK, Lowder CY. Acute retinal necrosis following recombinant subunit varicella-zoster virus vaccine. United States: 2020. Report No.: 20.
102. Chong CR, Park VJ, Cohen B, Postow MA, Wolchok JD, Kamboj M. Safety of inactivated influenza vaccine in cancer patients receiving immune checkpoint inhibitors. Clin Infect Dis. 2020;70(2):193–9.
103. Failing JJ, Ho TP, Yadav S, Majithia N, Riaz IB, Shin JY, et al. Safety of influenza vaccine in patients with cancer receiving pembrolizumab. JCO Oncol Pract. 2020;16(7):e573–80.
104. Wijn DH, Groeneveld GH, Vollaard AM, Muller M, Wallinga J, Gelderblom H, et al. Influenza vaccination in patients with lung cancer receiving anti-programmed death receptor 1 immunotherapy does not induce immune-related adverse events. Eur J Cancer. 2018;104:182–7.
105. Läubli H, Balmelli C, Kaufmann L, Stanczak M, Syedbasha M, Vogt D, et al. Influenza vaccination of cancer patients during PD-1 blockade induces serological protection but may raise the risk for immune-related adverse events. J Immunother Cancer. 2018;6(1):40.
106. Yuen C, Kamson D, Soliven B, Kramer C, Goldenberg F, Rezania K. Severe relapse of vaccine-induced Guillain-Barre syndrome after treatment with nivolumab. J Clin Neuromuscul Dis. 2019;20(4):194–9.
107. Riano I, Cristancho C, Treadwell T. Stevens-Johnson syndrome-like reaction after exposure to pembrolizumab and recombinant zoster vaccine in a patient with metastatic lung cancer. J Investig Med High Impact Case Rep. 2020;(8):2324709620914796.
108. Lynde C, Krell J, Korman N, Mathes B. Vaccine Study Investigators. Immune response to pneumococcal polysaccharide vaccine in adults with chronic plaque psoriasis treated with alefacept. J Am Acad Dermatol. 2011;65(4):799–806.
109. Vagberg M, Kumlin U, Svenningsson A. Humoral immune response to influenza vaccine in natalizumab-treated MS patients. Neurol Res. 2012;34(7):730–3.
110. Metze C, Winkelmann A, Loebermann M, Hecker M, Schweiger B, Reisinger EC, et al. Immunogenicity and predictors of response to a single dose trivalent seasonal influenza vaccine in multiple sclerosis patients receiving disease-modifying therapies. CNS Neurosci Ther. 2019;25(2):245–54.
111. Olberg HK, Eide GE, Cox RJ, Jul-Larsen A, Lartey SL, Vedeler CA, et al. Antibody response to seasonal influenza vaccination in patients with multiple sclerosis receiving immunomodulatory therapy. Eur J Neurol. 2018;25(3):527–34.
112. Kaufman M, Pardo G, Rossman H, Sweetser MT, Forrestal F, Duda P. Natalizumab treatment shows no clinically meaningful effects on immunization responses in patients with relapsing-remitting multiple sclerosis. J Neurol Sci. 2014;341(1):22–7.

113. Krueger JG, Ochs HD, Patel P, Gilkerson E, Guttman-Yassky E, Dummer W. Effect of therapeutic integrin (CD11a) blockade with efalizumab on immune responses to model antigens in humans: results of a randomized, single blind study. J Invest Dermatol. 2008;128(11):2615–24.
114. Wyant T, Leach T, Sankoh S, Wang Y, Paolino J, Pasetti MF, et al. Vedolizumab affects antibody responses to immunisation selectively in the gastrointestinal tract: randomised controlled trial results. Gut. 2015;64(1):77–83.
115. Huttner A, Eperon G, Lascano AM, Roth S, Schwob J, Siegrist C, et al. Risk of MS relapse after yellow fever vaccination: a self-controlled case series. Neurol Neuroimmunol Neuroinflamm. 2020;7(4):07.
116. Miauton A, Tan R, Pantazou V, Du Pasquier R, Genton B. Vaccine-associated measles in a patient treated with natalizumab: a case report. BMC Infect Dis. 2020;20(1):753.
117. Ufer M, Shakeri-Nejad K, Gardin A, Su Z, Paule I, Marbury TC, et al. Impact of siponimod on vaccination response in a randomized, placebo-controlled study. Neurol Neuroimmunol Neuroinflamm. 2017;4(6):e398.
118. Winkelmann A, Metze C, Frimmel S, Reisinger EC, Zettl UK, Loebermann M. Tick-borne encephalitis vaccination in multiple sclerosis: a prospective, multicenter study. Neurol Neuroimmunol Neuroinflamm. 2020;7(2):01.
119. Signoriello E, Bonavita S, Sinisi L, Russo CV, Maniscalco GT, Casertano S, et al. Is antibody titer useful to verify the immunization after VZV vaccine in MS patients treated with fingolimod? A case series. Netherlands: 2020. Report No.: 40.
120. Issa NP, Hentati A. VZV encephalitis that developed in an immunized patient during fingolimod therapy. Neurology. 2015;84(1):99–100.
121. Pandit A, Leblebjian H, Hammond SP, Laubach JP, Richardson PG, Baden LR, et al. Safety of live-attenuated measles-mumps-rubella and herpes zoster vaccination in multiple myeloma patients on maintenance lenalidomide or bortezomib after autologous hematopoietic cell transplantation. Bone Marrow Transplant. 2018;53(7):942–5.
122. Stoma I, Karpov I, Iskrov I, Lendina I, Uss A. Clinical efficacy of pneumococcal vaccination in multiple myeloma patients on novel agents: results of a prospective clinical study. Vaccine. 2020;38(30):4713–6.

Travel and Risk of Infections

4

Diego Viasus, Emiro Buendia, and Jordi Carratalà

Introduction

The increasing interdependence of countries, the easy availability of tourist routes around the world, the provision of health services to foreign patients, and the government sponsorship for travel are unprecedented in human history [1]. National and international travel is therefore undertaken with increasing frequency by large numbers of individuals for professional, social, entertaining, and cooperative purposes. Recreation and holidays account for nearly 50% of all international travel, with 15% of travel for business and professional purposes and 27% for other reasons, such as visiting relatives and friends, religion, or health tourism. Europe is the most common destination for international travelers, but travelers are increasingly visiting regions with emerging economies. Indeed, travel to Latin America, Asia, Africa, and the Middle East is expected to increase over the coming years [2], exposing travelers to unfamiliar environments and a new set of health risks. All individuals planning travel should seek guidance on the potential risks in the destination country and recognize how best to protect their health and minimize the risk of acquiring disease [3]. Certain particularities must also be considered in this planning, such as their previous health status, immunocompetence, comorbidities, and

D. Viasus · E. Buendia
Division of Health Sciences, Department of Medicine, Universidad del Norte and Hospital Universidad del Norte, Barranquilla, Colombia
e-mail: dviasus@uninorte.edu.co; erbuendia@uninorte.edu.co

J. Carratalà (✉)
Department of Infectious Diseases, Hospital Universitari de Bellvitge—IDIBELL, Centro de Investigación Biomédica en Red de Enfermedades Infecciosas (CIBERINFEC), Barcelona, Spain

Department of Clinical Sciences, Faculty of Medicine, University of Barcelona, Barcelona, Spain
e-mail: jcarratala@bellvitgehospital.cat

C. Cervera, J. M. Aguado (eds.), *Infectious Complications in Biologic and Targeted Therapies*, https://doi.org/10.1007/978-3-031-11363-5_4

Table 4.1 Key websites for travelers

Website	URL
Centers for Disease Control and Prevention (CDC): Travelers' Health	https://wwwnc.cdc.gov/travel/
World Health Organization. International travel and health	https://www.who.int/ith/en/
European Centre for Disease Prevention and Control	https://www.ecdc.europa.eu/en/travelers-health
The International Society of Travel Medicine	https://www.istm.org
National Travel Health Network and Centre (NaTHNaC)	https://travelhealthpro.org.uk/

the planned type of tourism [3]. Important websites that contain key information for travelers are shown in Table 4.1.

The spectrum of disease is variable among travelers, but infective etiologies are the most common [3, 4], typically presenting as systemic febrile illness, acute diarrhea, respiratory infections, or dermatologic disorders [3]. However, there is no precise information on the proportion of international travelers who acquire disease while abroad. Estimating this proportion is complicated by the fact that many ill travelers will not seek medical care if they have minor symptoms or do not know where or how to access care in the country they are visiting. Travelers may also fail to attribute their illness to travel, especially if it has a long incubation period or if symptoms develop weeks or months after returning home [2].

Novel biologic therapies constitute a field of medicine that has increased exponentially over recent years. Although these therapies have improved the quality of life of patients and could facilitate travel to exotic destinations, this latter aspect places them at risk of a various infections that had not previously been a major concern. There have been few studies regarding travel and risk of infection among recipients of biological and targeted therapies, with much of the current data being extrapolated from studies in all travelers. Although infection rates are not necessarily higher in immunosuppressed travelers, the severity of disease can be increased [5].

Health risks can be diminished by appropriate intervention before, during, and after travel. As part of this, it is increasingly important for travel medicine to counsel people to avoid travel-associated disease [6, 7]. In this chapter, we review the most relevant infectious etiologies in travelers, together with the related factors that modify the risk of infection.

Infectious Diseases and Risks Factors for Travelers

The risk of infection for travelers varies with their medical history, the travel destination, the geographical features of that destination, the time spent traveling, the type of tourist activities to be engaged in, and the accommodation used [8]. General precautions can significantly decrease the risk of exposure to infectious pathogens regardless of whether vaccinations or medication are given. These general recommendations should always be given for visits to any destination where there is a substantial risk of exposure.

Modes of Transmission of Infections

The modes of transmission for different infectious diseases are shown in Table 4.2. In general, most infections in travelers are acquired by consuming contaminated food and drink (foodborne and waterborne diseases) or by airborne transmission (droplets are disseminated by air and inhaled or contracted by contact between contaminated surfaces and mucous membranes of the nose, mouth, or conjunctivae). A few serious infections are also transmitted by insects, such as mosquitos or ticks. Similarly, as described in Table 4.2, different general precautions can be taken to reduce the risk of acquiring some of these infectious diseases according to their mode of transmission.

Table 4.2 The modes of transmission for different infectious diseases in travelers

Mode of transmission	Precautions	Examples
Foodborne and waterborne diseases (contaminated food and drink)	Precautions with all food and drinking water and avoid contact with polluted recreational waters	Traveler's diarrhea, hepatitis A, typhoid fever, and cholera
Vector-borne diseases (insects, such as mosquitos and ticks)	Avoid insect bites and contact with other vectors: Use insect repellent and cover exposed skin	Malaria, yellow fever, dengue, Japanese encephalitis, chikungunya, Zika, and tick-borne encephalitis
Zoonoses (animal bites or contact with animals or by consumption of foods of animal origin, particularly meat and milk products)	Avoid close contact with any animals (including wild, captive, and domestic animals) and take precautions with all food and drink	Rabies, tularemia, brucellosis, and leptospirosis
Sexually transmitted infections	Avoid unprotected sexual intercourse	Hepatitis B, syphilis, and HIV/AIDS
Blood-borne diseases (contact with infected blood or other body fluids)	Avoid direct contact with blood and body fluids (needles and syringes for injection or any other medical or cosmetic procedure that penetrates the skin) and by avoiding transfusion of unsafe blood	Hepatitis B and C, HIV/AIDS, and malaria.
Soil-transmitted diseases	Protecting the skin from direct contact with soil	Anthrax, tetanus, and some intestinal parasitic infections (e.g., ascariasis and trichuriasis)
Airborne diseases	Avoiding infected individuals when coughing, sneezing, or talking, and avoiding artificial water reservoirs (e.g., cooling towers, whirlpool spas, warm-water baths, or decorative fountains)	Pulmonary tuberculosis, measles, varicella (chickenpox), legionellosis, diphtheria, influenza, mumps, meningitis, pertussis, and SARS

Risks Factors for Travelers

Some factors are critical for evaluating infections in travelers. The travel itinerary is important because probable exposure varies by the region of travel. A study from the GeoSentinel Surveillance Network, for example, confirmed that the occurrence of certain illnesses varied with the region of the world visited. Here, travelers presenting with fevers after travel to from Africa were diagnosed more frequently with malaria than travelers from Asia, in whom dengue fever was diagnosed more often [3, 6]. The length of travel is also important, with studies having found that the risk of acquiring some illnesses increases with the duration of a trip. Accommodation types can also affect the risk of infection while abroad, evidence showing that travelers visiting rural areas tend to be at higher risk of certain infections than those staying in hotels. Moreover, travelers who visit relatives are at higher risk because they stay longer, go to more remote destinations, have more contact with local water sources, and seek pre-travel advice less frequently.

The underlying diseases of travelers can also modify their vulnerability to infection and the subsequent clinical features and severity of disease. A growing number of immunosuppressed individuals are currently able to travel internationally despite organ transplantation, biological therapy, HIV infection, or other primary or acquired immunodeficiencies. These patients are just as at risk from exposures and behaviors during travel, such as insect or animal bites, contaminated food or water ingestion, or freshwater swimming.

The history of pre-travel advice, vaccinations, and antimalarial prophylaxis should be reviewed when evaluating the risk of infection in travelers. However, it has been documented that fewer than half of US travelers to developing countries seek pre-travel medical advice and may not have received vaccines or taken antimalarial drugs. In one study, the most common vaccine-preventable diseases among returned travelers seeking care at a GeoSentinel clinic between 1997 and 2010 were typhoid fever, hepatitis A, hepatitis B, and influenza. Significantly, more than half of these patients required hospitalization [9].

Common Infectious Diseases in Travelers

Gastrointestinal Infections

Gastrointestinal infections are common in travelers, diarrhea developing in nearly 60% visiting tropical and subtropical regions. The principal source of traveler's diarrhea is the fecal-oral route after consuming contaminated water or food. The morbidity associated with gastrointestinal infection is broad, and only some will develop a more serious or more prolonged disease course. Enteric bacteria, including *Escherichia coli*, *Campylobacter*, *Salmonella*, and *Shigella*, as well as parasites, such as giardiasis and amebiasis, are the most prevalent infectious etiologies. However, no pathogen is identified in up to 50%. Traveler's diarrhea usually occurs a few weeks after arrival at a destination, and risk is lower with shorter stays [10]. The condition is generally self-limiting and does not need special health care interventions. In severe cases, traveler's diarrhea can be treated effectively with antibiotics such as rifaximin, ciprofloxacin, or azithromycin [11, 12], while parasitic infection responds to metronidazole and albendazole [13].

Other parasitic infections are important causes of disease in travelers worldwide. Soil-transmitted helminth infections are prevalent in underdeveloped countries with poor sanitation, no clean or secure water supply, and inadequate sewage disposal [14]. The main etiological organisms are *Ascaris lumbricoides*, *Trichuris trichiura*, *Ancylostoma duodenale*, *Necator americanus*, and *Strongyloides stercoralis*, which complete a stage of their life cycle in the soil and are transmitted to humans by the fecal-oral route by consuming contaminated water or food and/or by penetrating the skin [15]. Infection prevention relies on hand washing, drinking sanitized water, drug prophylaxis, and wearing appropriate footwear [16–18].

Given the lack of licensed vaccines for most etiologies of traveler's diarrhea, prevention is mainly by improving hygiene when staying at the destination. For high-risk travelers, oral cholera and salmonella vaccines could be an option before travel [19].

Respiratory Infections

Respiratory tract infections are the second most frequent cause of illness in travelers and of fever in returned travelers [20]. Acute respiratory tract infections occur in 10–20% of all travelers, and outbreaks of respiratory infection have been described on cruise ships. The possible public health significance of imported infections includes the introduction and transmission of new strains of respiratory pathogens into susceptible populations upon return [21]. Data accumulated from several geographically distinct sites by the GeoSentinel Surveillance Network provide a global perspective on the spectrum and relative frequency of respiratory infections encountered during travel [20].

Respiratory infections caused by *Streptococcus pneumoniae*, *Mycoplasma pneumoniae*, *Haemophilus influenzae*, and *Chlamydophila pneumoniae* seem to be the most common bacterial etiologies of pneumonia worldwide [22, 23]. However, depending on the country visited, *Coxiella burnetii* (Q fever), *Legionella pneumophila* (legionellosis), *Bordetella pertussis* (pertussis), *Corynebacterium diphtheriae* (diphtheria), and *Leptospira spp.* should also be considered [21, 24]. In travelers who return with fever and respiratory symptoms, infectious pneumonia should be considered and evaluated systematically [25]. Fungal etiologies also need to be considered depending on the local epidemiology of the destination country and the time to symptom presentation [24].

Given the recent coronavirus pandemic, the role of these viruses as important causes of severe pneumonia in humans has come to the fore. Middle East respiratory syndrome coronavirus (MERS-CoV), and more recently, severe acute respiratory syndrome coronavirus 2 (SARS-CoV-2) are the most important etiologic agents to date [26]. MERS-CoV is a zoonotic virus that has infected humans via direct or indirect contact with infected dromedary camels, mainly in the Arabian Peninsula. Although human-to-human transmission has been rare, it can occur in health care settings when infection prevention and control measures are unsatisfactory. There have been imported cases reported outside the Middle East region, including in the United States, China, the Republic of Korea, Thailand, Austria, France, Germany, Greece, Italy, the Netherlands, Turkey, and the United Kingdom. The MERS-CoV is more lethal than SARS-CoV-2 [27, 28]. Moreover, SARS-CoV-2 caused an outbreak of respiratory disease in China in December 2019 that has rapidly spread throughout the world [29, 30]. The number of hospitalizations and deaths increased continuously through 2020, with a substantial number of patients with severe illness requiring intensive care unit admission and ventilator support. Mortality has been related to male sex, older age, and the presence of comorbidities, such as obesity, diabetes mellitus, cancer, and chronic cardiovascular and pulmonary diseases [30, 31]. During the coronavirus disease 2019 (COVID-19) pandemic, biosecurity measures and travel restrictions have been put in place to help prevent the spread of SARS-CoV-2.

Increasing age and male sex are associated with a greater risk of lower respiratory tract infection, particularly pneumonia and bronchitis. Moreover, timing and reason for travel affect the infection type, with influenza common among travelers to the Northern Hemisphere from December through February and travelers to the Southern Hemisphere from June through August (the respective influenza seasons). In addition, people visiting friends or relatives, and those with long trips are more likely to develop influenza than other types of travelers. This is most likely to result from the closer contact between these travelers and the local populations. Several outbreaks of influenza have previously been reported to be associated with travel [32, 33]. Travelers with some of these risk factors should be considered specifically for pre-travel influenza vaccination.

Vector-Borne Infections

Vector-borne infections are human illnesses caused by parasites, viruses, or bacteria transmitted to humans and other animals by blood-feeding arthropods, such as mosquitos, ticks, and fleas. Travelers should adhere to mosquito-avoidance measures, such as wearing clothes that do not expose skin, using an insect repellent, and sleeping under a bed net. Moreover, the prevention of some vector-borne viral infections is possible through vaccination.

Dengue, Zika, chikungunya, yellow fever, Usutu, Japanese encephalitis, and Venezuelan equine encephalitis are important infectious etiologies of fever in Asia, Africa, America, and the Caribbean [34, 35]. All are transmitted by the mosquitos *Aedes aegypti* and/or *Culex* spp., which are especially suited to surviving in warm and humid tropical regions and transmit the virus through bites. Other mechanisms of transmission, as is the case for Zika virus, include sexual and vertical transmission [36]. A study of the features of travelers returning to Canada with Zika infection acquired in the Americas revealed that Zika infection was as common as dengue (nearly 4% in both cases) [37]. Zika virus was acquired mainly by people visiting friends and relatives in South America and by tourists in the Caribbean, and typically by probable mosquito exposure (one case had confirmed sexual acquisition). The clinical spectrum of acute infection comprised adverse fetal and neurologic outcomes.

Rickettsiosis, caused by the genera *Rickettsia* spp., is an emerging and relevant infection in travelers worldwide [38, 39]. This vector-borne infection is transmitted via ticks, lice, fleas, and mites, and it presents clinically with fever and vasculitis-looking skin manifestations [40]. In other aspects, its presentation is similar to other tropical hemorrhagic fevers, and it is often mistakenly diagnosed as malaria [41]. Doxycycline is the first-line treatment for rickettsiosis, but fluoroquinolones and chloramphenicol are other viable options [38].

Malaria is a parasitic infection that is endemic to various regions of South America, Africa, and Asia [42]. Five species may infect humans, all being transmitted by the bite of *Anopheles spp.* mosquitos. *Plasmodium falciparum* and *Plasmodium knowlesi* cause the most severe forms of disease, whereas *Plasmodium malariae, Plasmodium ovale*, and *Plasmodium vivax* cause milder forms. However, without adequate treatment, all may cause death, especially in children [43]. In the absence of an effective malaria vaccine [44], efforts focus on preventing infection in travelers through chemoprophylaxis [8]. The risk of travelers getting infected with the malaria parasite when not receiving chemoprophylaxis is 3.4% per month for West Africa, 0.34% for the Indian subcontinent, and 0.034% for South America [8]. Drug prophylaxis schemes for those traveling to areas with high transmission include daily atovaquone–proguanil, doxycycline, mefloquine, or primaquine, though fewer adverse effects have been observed with atovaquone–proguanil [43, 45, 46]. In those traveling to low-risk areas, self-treatment is possible with atovaquone–proguanil or artemether–lumefantrine in the event of symptomatic infection when it is not possible to access a hospital with the capacity to diagnose and treat malaria [47].

Leishmaniasis is another vector-borne infectious disease endemic to underdeveloped countries in Southern Europe, the Middle East, central Asia, South America, and Central America. This zoonosis is also an emerging problem in travelers, and, as such, warrants consideration as a diagnosis in those returning with fever and splenomegaly or skin ulcers [25, 48, 49]. The vectors are *Phlebotomus* sp. and *Lutzomyia* sp. sandflies, with transmission occurring when they bite the host, typically outdoors. Visceral, cutaneous and post-kala-azar dermal leishmaniasis are the main clinical presentations in humans [50]. There is no licensed vaccine for its prevention in humans, but ChAd63-KH developed by York University, has shown promise as a candidate vaccine [51]. Travel-related data on returned international travelers diagnosed with cutaneous leishmaniasis were reported in a GeoSentinel Surveillance Network analysis for 1997 and 2017 [52]. Common source countries were Bolivia, Costa Rica, Syria, and Afghanistan, with 10% of cases of mucocutaneous leishmaniasis acquired in Africa, Asia, and Europe.

The filaria *Onchocerca volvulus* [53] is other important vector-borne infections in travelers [54]. Filariasis is prevalent in some American and African countries [55, 56].

Skin Infections

Skin disease ranks third among all medical visits for travelers. The most common skin-related diagnoses in this group are cutaneous larva migrans, insect bites (including superinfected bites), skin abscesses, and allergic reactions. Pediatric travelers more frequently suffer dog bites and cutaneous larva migrans, but less frequently suffer insect bites, compared with adult travelers [57]. Cutaneous larva migrans is one of the most common skin infections among returning travelers, accounting for about 10% of all skin diseases. It is most often acquired in Asia, Africa, South and Central America, and the Caribbean. The main clinical feature is the presence of extremely pruritic linear or serpiginous erythematous tracts through the epidermis, typically on the feet, thighs, or legs. Possible complications include superinfection/impetigo, bullae, and papular urticaria [58]. Scabies, caused by the mite *Sarcoptes scabiei* [59], is also common in travelers. Clinical manifestation comprises itching and localized maculopapular lesions that occur 3–6 weeks after infestation due to an allergic response to the ectoparasite, though this can occur earlier in cases of reinfestation [58, 60]. The main route of infestation is skin to skin contact or through contact with infested clothes or bed sheets [61].

Moreover, wound myiasis occurs when a fly infests open wounds and mucous membranes. The female fly lays eggs around wounds or on mucous membranes, particularly the nose. Eggs hatch in 1–2 days and the larvae feed on tissue, which can increase the size of the wound. Myiasis represents 1–5% of illness in travelers returning from sub-Saharan Africa, Latin America, and the Caribbean, but fewer from northeast Asia. However, myiasis has also been reported across North America and Southern Europe [58]. Tungiasis is another relevant infestation caused by the sand flea *Tunga penetrans*. In this infestation, the female extrudes more than 100 eggs in the skin, which then fall to the ground. The flea grows approximately 2000-fold in size in the skin and remains in the host for approximately 4–6 weeks. The parasite can also be carried by animal hosts, including dogs, pigs, cows, and rats, which can lead to the organism persisting in rural communities. Tungiasis is found worldwide in both the eastern and the western hemispheres, including sub-Saharan Africa, India, Pakistan, and especially in the Caribbean [58].

Sexually Transmitted Infections

Travel is assumed to be a risk factor for sexually transmitted infections because individuals modify their usual sexual practices. In a study of 112,180 travelers who developed an illness between 1996 and 2010, nearly 1% had a sexually transmitted infection [62]. Non-gonococcal or unspecified urethritis, acute HIV infection, and syphilis were the most common diagnoses. Male sex, traveling to visit friends or relatives, not having a pre-travel consultation, and travel for fewer than 30 days were independently associated with sexually transmitted infection in a multivariate analysis. Post-travel screening is recommended for travelers engaging in unprotected casual sex during travel (including commercial sex workers), including screening for sexually transmitted infections more frequent in tropical areas (e.g. chancroid).

Other Infections

Hepatitis caused by hepatitis A, B, and C viruses are prevalent worldwide and are of special concern in travelers because they have such varied routes of infection

[63]. Hepatitis A virus is transmitted by the fecal-oral route, whereas hepatitis B and C viruses are transmitted sexually and bloodborne (the latter by sharing syringes or by contaminated blood products) [64]. Acute and chronic viral hepatitis and their long-term complications affect people of all ages [65, 66] and geographies, making their elimination a worldwide public health priority [67, 68]. Since there are vaccines available to induce protective immunity against some of these viral etiologies, pre-travel vaccination is the main preventive strategy for travelers [69]. Other viruses that should be considered among travelers include enteroviruses, cytomegalovirus, varicella zoster virus, human herpes viruses, and various arboviruses, which are important causes of meningitis and encephalitis [70, 71]. Rabies is also an important and deadly zoonosis that causes encephalitis [72] and should be considered in travelers presenting with psychosis and focal neurologic symptoms after exploring forests and wildlife [73]. Pre- and post-exposure vaccination is recommended as the best available primary prevention against rabies in travelers [74, 75].

Fever in Travelers

Fever is a marker of potentially serious illness in a returned traveler. However, assessment is complicated not only because diseases vary by the geographic region visited and because travelers frequently visit numerous areas but also because incubation periods for travel-related infections can range from a few days to more than a year. Although a returned traveler may have disease due to typical, globally distributed pathogens of the respiratory and urinary tract, they may acquire infections that are unfamiliar to most clinicians. Therefore, knowledge of disease risk by country or geographic region can help to guide decisions about diagnostic testing and treatment. However, many returned travelers with fever often have a febrile illness of indeterminate origin [25].

It has been reported that the predominant pathogen in febrile illness varies markedly by geographic region [25]. In ill travelers from Oceania (predominantly Papua New Guinea) and sub-Saharan Africa, malaria was the primary diagnosis in travelers who returned with fever. By contrast, dengue was the most frequent cause of febrile illness in those who had stayed in Southeast Asia, while enteric fever was most frequent among those returning from south-central Asia. Of note, mononucleosis syndromes (e.g., Epstein-Barr virus infection, cytomegalovirus infection, acute HIV infection, or toxoplasmosis) occurred less frequently in patients with systemic febrile illnesses. Uncommon causes of systemic illness include leptospirosis, brucellosis, amebic liver abscess, and viral meningitis. Among those who experience respiratory illness and fever, influenza or influenza-like illness was the most frequent etiology. Upper respiratory infections occurred in more than half of patients who had respiratory illness and fever, with bacterial pneumonia being less frequent [20].

Health Tourism and Infectious Diseases

Health tourism refers to the practice of people traveling to other countries for non-emergency medical care. Comprehensive data on health tourism, services, destinations, and procedures are currently unavailable [76, 77]. Similarly, evidence about the risks facing medical tourists is limited. However, we do know that the main health tourism destinations are Asia (India, Thailand, China, and Singapore), America (Mexico, Brazil, and the Caribbean), and Europe [77]. Principal procedures include dental work, bariatric, cosmetic, and cardiac surgery, as well as arthroplasty, reproductive care, and organ transplantation [77].

Most data suggest that procedures performed abroad are associated with higher rates of infections and complications. Health tourists are at risk of infectious diseases, either those specific to their surgical procedure or specific to the region of travel. In addition, many countries with robust medical tourism programs are in tropical and subtropical regions where malaria, dengue fever, enteric fever, and other infections are endemic. Many also have high background rates of tuberculosis, hepatitis B and C, and HIV. Moreover, medical tourism is accompanied by the risk of transmission of multi-resistant organisms from the country where the procedure is performed [78].

Transplant tourism, defined as travel with the intent of receiving or donating an organ, has grown over recent decades [79], but it is important to consider that transplanted organs can be sources of infection and complications. Some documented transplant-associated infections are geographically restricted, including human T-lymphotropic virus types 1 and 2, West Nile virus, rabies, malaria, *Leishmania*, *Trypanosoma cruzi*, and several fungi [80]. "Cosmetic tourism," the process of traveling overseas for cosmetic procedures, is another expanding global phenomenon. Although the main infective pathogens are Streptococci and Staphylococci, cases of infection by fungi and multi-resistant organisms also have been reported, including clusters of wound infection caused by *Mycobacterium abscessus* (e.g., following abdominoplasty, breast surgery, and liposuction) [81, 82].

Vaccine-Preventable Diseases and Vaccines

Vaccination is an effective method of preventing certain infectious diseases, helping travelers to avoid several hazardous illnesses. Vaccination in patients receiving biologic and immune-targeted therapies is discussed in Chap. 3, but some specific considerations apply to travelers. Although vaccines are usually safe and rarely produce serious adverse events, they are yet to be developed against some of the most serious infections, including malaria and HIV. When used, the vaccinated traveler should be counseled that, despite their success in preventing disease, there remains some risk of catching the disease against which he/she has been vaccinated (i.e., vaccines are not 100% effective).

A published study by the GeoSentinel Surveillance Network showed that 3% of ill travelers presenting with fever had a vaccine-preventable disease on returning home [9]. However, the overall burden of vaccine-preventable disease among all ill travelers on return home is unknown. The most common diagnoses are enteric fever, acute viral hepatitis, and influenza. Travel to south-central Asia has been associated with *S. typhi*, business travel with influenza, and longer travel with hepatitis A. Nearly 55% of those with vaccine-preventable diseases require hospital admission compared with 9.5% of those with non-vaccine-preventable diseases.

Before departure, travelers should be counseled about the risk of disease in the destination country or countries and be given targeted advice to prevent illness. Pre-travel services, including vaccination, should be readily available to all travelers (Table 4.3) and tailored based on their immunization history, the countries to be visited, the type and duration of travel, and the amount of time available before departure. Incompletely vaccinated travelers should be offered all routine vaccinations in addition to those required for travel. Travelers are recommended to consult 2–3 months before departure to allow sufficient time for optimal immunization schedules. However, even when travel is imminent, there is still time to provide advice and some vaccinations.

Vaccination is the best preventive strategy for immunosuppressed patients, including those receiving and/or planning to start biologic or targeted therapies [83, 84]. Most recombinant vaccines are safe in those individuals, with some schedules

Table 4.3 Vaccines for travelers [91]

Category	Vaccines
Routine vaccines (recommended for everyone in most countries and based on age, health status, and other risk factors)	• Diphtheria, tetanus, and pertussis • Hepatitis B • Haemophilus influenzae type b • Human papillomavirus • Influenza (seasonal) • Measles, mumps, and rubella • Pneumococcal • Polio • Rotavirus • Tuberculosis • Varicella
Required vaccine (those needed to enter a given country based on government regulations in that country)	• Polio vaccine • Yellow fever • Meningococcal vaccine (pilgrims to Saudi Arabia)
Recommended vaccines for certain destinations (advised by various institutions to protect the health of travelers, but not required to enter the destination country)	• Cholera • Hepatitis A and/or E • Typhoid fever • Yellow fever • Japanese encephalitis • Meningococcal • Polio (adult booster dose) • Rabies • Tick-borne encephalitis

recommended before and after starting treatment [85, 86], but live attenuated vaccines are not recommended [85]. The vaccination schedules in immunosuppressed patients who travel are otherwise similar to those for the general population [87]. Some schedules are recommended independently of the destination, but other vaccines are recommended depending on destinations [88, 89]. It is important to note that vaccine immunogenicity can be attenuated by biological therapies, resulting in reduced vaccine efficacy and protection [90].

Advice for Healthcare Workers to Give Travelers

The following recommendations are proposed to tackle infection among patients receiving biological and targeted therapies who travel abroad:

- *Visit a travel health clinic ideally 2–3 months prior to the planned trip.* Patients should receive advice regarding travel-related infections and their prevention, including the endemic and tropical infections that can occur in the target countries. All routine and travel-related vaccines should be updated as needed before travel. When possible, get vaccinations at least 2–3 months in advance of the planned trip.
- *Obtain targeted information.* This should include the need and type of prophylactic medication specific to the patient and travel destination.
- *Take precautions with all food and drinking-water during travel.* Drinking bottled or boiled water is advised, as is avoiding food that is uncooked or partially cooked, from street vendors, or from markets. Unpasteurized milk products may carry bacteria such as *Listeria* and *Brucella*. Foods with raw eggs put travelers at risk for salmonella infection. Fresh fruits that can be peeled are considered safe.
- *Avoid insect bites and contact with other vectors: use insect repellent and cover exposed skin.*
- *Avoid close contact with any animals (including wild, captive, and domestic animals).*
- *Avoid unprotected sexual intercourse.*
- *Avoid direct contact with blood and body fluids.* This includes avoiding the transfusion of unsafe blood and the use of needles, syringes, or any other medical or cosmetic device/procedure that penetrates the skin.
- *Practice biosecurity measure during pandemics.* Use respirators or surgical masks, perform hand hygiene, and maintain physical distancing (6 ft between people). Avoid contact with infected individuals who are coughing, sneezing, or talking.
- *Have a plan.* Develop a plan in case of sickness when at the destination (e.g., know the clinic or hospital that is able to care for an immunocompromised host) and get suitable travel insurance.
- *Medication precautions.* Keep all prescribed medicines in their original bottles and bring extra in case of travel delays. Avoid taking medicines obtained at the

destination to avoid issues with potential drug interactions or falsified medical products.

– *All medical centers should have a predefined approach to the management of travelers who seek medical attention:* Guidelines for the diagnosis and treatment of clinical syndromes among ill travelers (systemic febrile illness, acute diarrhea, respiratory infections, and dermatological disorders); in some cases, screening for blood-borne pathogens, including HIV, HBV, HCV, and other pathogens should be considered depending on the place visited (e.g., malaria, tuberculosis, or Chagas disease); and patients should be evaluated by an infectious disease specialist as soon as possible after returning home.

References

1. OECD. Tourism 2020: policies to promote competitive and sustainable tourism. OECD Tour. Trends Policies; 2010.
2. Angelo KM, Kozarsky PE, Ryan ET, Chen LH, Sotir MJ. What proportion of international travellers acquire a travel-related illness? A review of the literature. J Travel Med. 2017;24(5). https://doi.org/10.1093/jtm/tax046.
3. Freedman DO, Weld LH, Kozarsky PE, Fisk T, Robins R, Von Sonnenburg F, Keystone JS, Pandey P, Cetron MS. Spectrum of disease and relation to place of exposure among ill returned travelers. N Engl J Med. 2006;354(2):119–30. https://doi.org/10.1056/NEJMoa051331.
4. Gautret P, Gaudart J, Leder K, et al. Travel-associated illness in older adults (>60 y). J Travel Med. 2012;19(3):169–77. https://doi.org/10.1111/j.1708-8305.2012.00613.x.
5. Beeching NJ, Carratalà J, Razonable RR, Oriol I, Vilela EG. Traveler's diarrhea recommendations for solid organ transplant recipients and donors. Transplantation. 2018;102(2S Suppl 2):S35–41. https://doi.org/10.1097/TP.0000000000002015.
6. Leder K, Torresi J, Libman MD, et al. GeoSentinel surveillance of illness in returned travelers, 2007-2011. Ann Intern Med. 2013;158(6):456–68. https://doi.org/10.7326/0003-4819-158-6-201303190-00005.
7. Paudel P, Raina C, Zwar N, Seale H, Worth H, Sheikh M, Heywood AE. Risk activities and pre-travel health seeking practices of notified cases of imported infectious diseases in Australia. J Travel Med. 2017;24(5). https://doi.org/10.1093/jtm/tax044.
8. Galán-Puchades MT, Osuna A. Medical considerations before international travel. N Engl J Med. 2016;375(3):247–60. https://doi.org/10.1056/NEJMc1610671.
9. Boggild AK, Castelli F, Gautret P, et al. Vaccine preventable diseases in returned international travelers: results from the GeoSentinel Surveillance Network. Vaccine. 2010;28(46):7389–95. https://doi.org/10.1016/j.vaccine.2010.09.009.
10. Shah N, Ldupont H, Ramsey DJ. Global etiology of travelers' diarrhea: systematic review from 1973 to the present. Am J Trop Med Hyg. 2009;80(4):609–14. https://doi.org/10.4269/ajtmh.2009.80.609.
11. Cavalcanti A, Clemens SAC, Von Sonnenburg F, Collard F, De Clercq N, Steffen R, Clemens R. Traveler's diarrhea: epidemiology and impact on visitors to Fortaleza, Brazil. Rev Panam Salud Publica/Pan Am J Public Heal. 2002;11(4):245–52. https://doi.org/10.1590/S1020-49892002000400006.
12. Kollaritsch H, Paulke-Korinek M, Wiedermann U. Traveler's diarrhea. Infect Dis Clin North Am. 2012;26(3):691–706. https://doi.org/10.1016/j.idc.2012.06.002.
13. Okhuysen PC. Traveler's diarrhea due to intestinal protozoa. Clin Infect Dis. 2001;33(1):110–4. https://doi.org/10.1086/320894.

14. Ediriweera DS, Gunawardena S, Gunawardena NK, Iddawela D, Kannathasan S, Murugananthan A, Yahathugoda C, Pathmeswaran A, Diggle PJ, de Silva N. Reassessment of the prevalence of soil-transmitted helminth infections in Sri Lanka to enable a more focused control programme: a cross-sectional national school survey with spatial modelling. Lancet Glob Heal. 2019;7:e1237–46. https://doi.org/10.1016/S2214-109X(19)30253-0.
15. Chammartin F, Scholte RGC, Guimarães LH, Tanner M, Utzinger J, Vounatsou P. Soil-transmitted helminth infection in South America: a systematic review and geostatistical meta-analysis. Lancet Infect Dis. 2013;13(6):507–18. https://doi.org/10.1016/S1473-3099(13)70071-9.
16. Bieri FA, Gray DJ, Williams GM, et al. Health-education package to prevent worm infections in Chinese schoolchildren. N Engl J Med. 2013;368(17):1603–12. https://doi.org/10.1056/NEJMoa1204885.
17. Knopp S, Steinmann P, Keiser J, Utzinger J. Nematode infections. Soil-transmitted helminths and trichinella. Infect Dis Clin North Am. 2012;26(2):341–58. https://doi.org/10.1016/j.idc.2012.02.006.
18. Clarke NE, Clements ACA, Doi SA, Wang D, Campbell SJ, Gray D, Nery SV. Differential effect of mass deworming and targeted deworming for soil-transmitted helminth control in children: a systematic review and meta-analysis. Lancet. 2017;389(10066):287–97. https://doi.org/10.1016/S0140-6736(16)32123-7.
19. Hill DR, Ford L, Lalloo DG. Oral cholera vaccines: use in clinical practice. Lancet Infect Dis. 2006;6(6):361–73. https://doi.org/10.1016/S1473-3099(06)70494-7.
20. Leder K, Sundararajan V, Weld L, Pandey P, Brown G, Torresi J. Respiratory tract infections in travelers: a review of the GeoSentinel surveillance network. Clin Infect Dis. 2003;36(4):399–406. https://doi.org/10.1086/346155.
21. Ansart S, Pajot O, Grivois JP, Zeller V, Klement E, Perez L, Bossi P, Bricaire F, Caumes E. Pneumonia among travelers returning from abroad. J Travel Med. 2004;11(2):87–91. https://doi.org/10.2310/7060.2004.17055.
22. Olson G, Davis AM. Diagnosis and treatment of adults with community-acquired pneumonia. JAMA. 2020;200(7):e45–67. https://doi.org/10.1001/jama.2019.21118.
23. Prina E, Ranzani OT, Torres A. Community-acquired pneumonia. Lancet. 2015;386(9998):1097–108. https://doi.org/10.1016/S0140-6736(15)60733-4.
24. Trimble A, Moffat V, Collins AM. Pulmonary infections in the returned traveller. Pneumonia. 2017;9:1. https://doi.org/10.1186/s41479-017-0026-1.
25. Thwaites GE, Day NPJ. Approach to fever in the returning traveler. N Engl J Med. 2017;376(18):1797. https://doi.org/10.1056/NEJMra1508435.
26. Berlin DA, Gulick RM, Martinez FJ. Severe Covid-19. N Engl J Med. 2020;383:2451–60. https://doi.org/10.1056/nejmcp2009575.
27. Petersen E, Koopmans M, Go U, Hamer DH, Petrosillo N, Castelli F, Storgaard M, Al Khalili S, Simonsen L. Comparing SARS-CoV-2 with SARS-CoV and influenza pandemics. Lancet Infect Dis. 2020;21(4):e77. https://doi.org/10.1016/S1473-3099(20)30484-9.
28. World Health Organization. Coronavirus disease (COVID-19) situation report – 198; 2020.
29. Wiersinga WJ, Rhodes A, Cheng AC, Peacock SJ, Prescott HC. Pathophysiology, transmission, diagnosis, and treatment of coronavirus disease 2019 (COVID-19): a review. JAMA. 2020;324(8):782–93. https://doi.org/10.1001/jama.2020.12839.
30. Qiu P, Zhou Y, Wang F, Wang H, Zhang M, Pan X, Zhao Q, Liu J. Clinical characteristics, laboratory outcome characteristics, comorbidities, and complications of related COVID-19 deceased: a systematic review and meta-analysis. Aging Clin Exp Res. 2020;32(9):1869–78. https://doi.org/10.1007/s40520-020-01664-3.
31. Liang W, Liang H, Ou L, et al. Development and validation of a clinical risk score to predict the occurrence of critical illness in hospitalized patients with COVID-19. JAMA Intern Med. 2020;180(8):1081–9. https://doi.org/10.1001/jamainternmed.2020.2033.
32. Payne M, Skowronski D, Sabaiduc S, Merrick L, Lowe C. Increase in hospital admissions for severe influenza A/B among travelers on cruise ships to Alaska, 2015. Emerg Infect Dis. 2018;24(3):566–8. https://doi.org/10.3201/eid2403.171378.

33. Goeijenbier M, van Genderen P, Ward BJ, Wilder-Smith A, Steffen R, Osterhaus ADME. Travellers and influenza: risks and prevention. J Travel Med. 2017;24(1):taw078. https://doi.org/10.1093/jtm/taw078.
34. Pierson TC, Diamond MS. The continued threat of emerging flaviviruses. Nat Microbiol. 2020;5(6):796–812. https://doi.org/10.1038/s41564-020-0714-0.
35. Aguilar PV, Estrada-Franco JG, Navarro-Lopez R, Ferro C, Haddow AD, Weaver SC. Endemic Venezuelan equine encephalitis in the Americas: hidden under the dengue umbrella. Future Virol. 2011;6(6):721–40. https://doi.org/10.2217/fvl.11.50.
36. Musso D, Ko AI, Baud D. Zika virus infection—after the pandemic. N Engl J Med. 2019;381(15):1444–57. https://doi.org/10.1056/NEJMra1808246.
37. Boggild AK, Geduld J, Libman M, et al. Surveillance report of Zika virus among Canadian travellers returning from the Americas. CMAJ. 2017;189(9):E334–40. https://doi.org/10.1503/cmaj.161241.
38. Blanton LS. Rickettsial infections in the tropics and in the traveler. Curr Opin Infect Dis. 2013;26(5):435–40. https://doi.org/10.1097/QCO.0b013e328363811b.
39. Cazorla C, Socolovschi C, Jensenius M, Parola P. Tick-borne diseases: tick-borne spotted fever rickettsioses in Africa. Infect Dis Clin North Am. 2008;22(3):531–44. https://doi.org/10.1016/j.idc.2008.03.009.
40. Walker DH, Ismail N. Emerging and re-emerging rickettsioses: endothelial cell infection and early disease events. Nat Rev Microbiol. 2008;6(5):375–86. https://doi.org/10.1038/nrmicro1866.
41. Acestor N, Cooksey R, Newton PN, Ménard D, Guerin PJ, Nakagawa J, Christophel E, González IJ, Bell D. Mapping the aetiology of non-malarial febrile illness in Southeast Asia through a systematic review—terra incognita impairing treatment policies. PLoS One. 2012;7(9):e44269. https://doi.org/10.1371/journal.pone.0044269.
42. Phillips MA, Burrows JN, Manyando C, Van Huijsduijnen RH, Van Voorhis WC, Wells TNC. Malaria. Nat Rev Dis Prim. 2017;3:17050. https://doi.org/10.1038/nrdp.2017.50.
43. White NJ, Pukrittayakamee S, Hien TT, Faiz MA, Mokuolu OA, Dondorp AM. Malaria. Lancet. 2014;383(9918):723–35. https://doi.org/10.1016/S0140-6736(13)60024-0.
44. Efficacy and safety of RTS,S/AS01 malaria vaccine with or without a booster dose in infants and children in Africa: final results of a phase 3, individually randomised, controlled trial. Lancet. 2015;386(9988):31–45. https://doi.org/10.1016/S0140-6736(15)60721-8.
45. Schlagenhauf P, Hatz C, Behrens R, et al. Mefloquine at the crossroads? Implications for malaria chemoprophylaxis in Europe. Travel Med Infect Dis. 2015;13(2):192–6. https://doi.org/10.1016/j.tmaid.2015.03.010.
46. Price RN, von Seidlein L, Valecha N, Nosten F, Baird JK, White NJ. Global extent of chloroquine-resistant Plasmodium vivax: a systematic review and meta-analysis. Lancet Infect Dis. 2014;14(10):982–91. https://doi.org/10.1016/S1473-3099(14)70855-2.
47. Schlagenhauf P, Petersen E. Standby emergency treatment of malaria in travelers: experience to date and new developments. Expert Rev Anti-Infect Ther. 2012;10(5):537–46. https://doi.org/10.1586/eri.12.42.
48. Pavli A, Maltezou HC. Leishmaniasis, an emerging infection in travelers. Int J Infect Dis. 2010;14(12):e1032–9. https://doi.org/10.1016/j.ijid.2010.06.019.
49. Mansueto P, Seidita A, Vitale G, Cascio A. Leishmaniasis in travelers: a literature review. Travel Med Infect Dis. 2014;12(6 Pt A):563–81. https://doi.org/10.1016/j.tmaid.2014.09.007.
50. Burza S, Croft SL, Boelaert M. Leishmaniasis. Lancet. 2018;392(10151):951–70. https://doi.org/10.1016/S0140-6736(18)31204-2.
51. Osman M, Mistry A, Keding A, et al. A third generation vaccine for human visceral leishmaniasis and post kala azar dermal leishmaniasis: first-in-human trial of ChAd63-KH. PLoS Negl Trop Dis. 2017;11(5):e0005527. https://doi.org/10.1371/journal.pntd.0005527.
52. Boggild AK, Caumes E, Grobusch MP, et al. Cutaneous and mucocutaneous leishmaniasis in travellers and migrants: a 20-year GeoSentinel Surveillance Network analysis. J Travel Med. 2019;26(8):taz055. https://doi.org/10.1093/jtm/taz055.

53. Taylor MJ, Bockarie M, Taylor MJ, Hoerauf A, Bockarie M. Lymphatic filariasis and onchocerciasis. Parasite biology and epidemiology. Lancet. 2010;376(9747):1175–85. https://doi.org/10.1016/S0140-6736(10)60586-7.
54. Lipner EM, Law MA, Barnett E, et al. Filariasis in travelers presenting to the GeoSentinel Surveillance Network. PLoS Negl Trop Dis. 2007;1(3):e88. https://doi.org/10.1371/journal.pntd.0000088.
55. Deshpande A, Miller-Petrie MK, Lindstedt PA, et al. The global distribution of lymphatic filariasis, 2000–18: a geospatial analysis. Lancet Glob Heal. 2020;8(9):e1186–94. https://doi.org/10.1016/S2214-109X(20)30286-2.
56. Ndeffo-Mbah ML, Galvani AP. Global elimination of lymphatic filariasis. Lancet Infect Dis. 2017;17(4):358–9. https://doi.org/10.1016/S1473-3099(16)30544-8.
57. Vasievich MP, Villarreal JDM, Tomecki KJ. Got the travel bug? A review of common infections, infestations, bites, and stings among returning travelers. Am J Clin Dermatol. 2016;17(5):451–62. https://doi.org/10.1007/s40257-016-0203-7.
58. Chosidow O. Scabies. N Engl J Med. 2006;354(16):1718–27. https://doi.org/10.1056/NEJMcp052784.
59. Hochedez P, Vinsentini P, Ansart S, Caumes E. Changes in the pattern of health disorders diagnosed among two cohorts of French travelers to Nepal, 17 years apart. J Travel Med. 2004;11(6):341–6. https://doi.org/10.2310/7060.2004.19201.
60. Bhat SA, Mounsey KE, Liu X, Walton SF. Host immune responses to the itch mite, Sarcoptes scabiei, in humans. Parasit Vectors. 2017;10:385. https://doi.org/10.1186/s13071-017-2320-4.
61. Hochedez P, Caumes E. Common skin infections in travelers. J Travel Med. 2008;15(4):252–62. https://doi.org/10.1111/j.1708-8305.2008.00206.x.
62. Matteelli A, Schlagenhauf P, Carvalho ACC, et al. Travel-associated sexually transmitted infections: an observational cross-sectional study of the GeoSentinel surveillance database. Lancet Infect Dis. 2013;3(3):205–13. https://doi.org/10.1016/S1473-3099(12)70291-8.
63. Khuroo MS. Viral hepatitis in international travellers: risks and prevention. Int J Antimicrob Agents. 2003;21(2):143–52. https://doi.org/10.1016/S0924-8579(02)00290-X.
64. Smith S, Harmanci H, Hutin Y, et al. Global progress on the elimination of viral hepatitis as a major public health threat: an analysis of WHO Member State responses 2017. JHEP Rep. 2019;1(2):81–9. https://doi.org/10.1016/j.jhepr.2019.04.002.
65. Indolfi G, Easterbrook P, Dusheiko G, et al. Hepatitis B virus infection in children and adolescents. Lancet Gastroenterol Hepatol. 2019;4(6):466–76. https://doi.org/10.1016/S2468-1253(19)30042-1.
66. Indolfi G, Easterbrook P, Dusheiko G, et al. Hepatitis C virus infection in children and adolescents. Lancet Gastroenterol Hepatol. 2019;4(6):477–87. https://doi.org/10.1016/S2468-1253(19)30046-9.
67. Thomas DL. Global elimination of chronic hepatitis. N Engl J Med. 2019;380:2041–50. https://doi.org/10.1056/NEJMra1810477.
68. Brierley R. Elimination of viral hepatitis by 2030: ambitious, but achievable. Lancet Gastroenterol Hepatol. 2019;4(2):88–9. https://doi.org/10.1016/S2468-1253(18)30420-5.
69. Steffen R, Kane MA, Shapiro CN, Billo N, Schoellhorn KJ, Van Damme P. Epidemiology and prevention of hepatitis A in travelers. JAMA. 1994;20(6):394–9. https://doi.org/10.1001/jama.1994.03520110065031.
70. McGill F, Griffiths MJ, Solomon T. Viral meningitis: current issues in diagnosis and treatment. Curr Opin Infect Dis. 2017;30(2):248–56. https://doi.org/10.1097/QCO.0000000000000355.
71. Tyler KL. Acute viral encephalitis. N Engl J Med. 2018;379(6):557–66. https://doi.org/10.1056/NEJMra1708714.
72. Fooks AR, Cliquet F, Finke S, et al. Rabies. Nat Rev Dis Primers. 2017;3:17091. https://doi.org/10.1038/nrdp.2017.91.
73. Hemachudha T, Ugolini G, Wacharapluesadee S, Sungkarat W, Shuangshoti S, Laothamatas J. Human rabies: neuropathogenesis, diagnosis, and management. Lancet Neurol. 2013;12(5):498–513. https://doi.org/10.1016/S1474-4422(13)70038-3.

74. Fooks AR, Johnson N, Brookes SM, Parsons G, McElhinney LM. Risk factors associated with travel to rabies endemic countries. J Appl Microbiol. 2003;94 Suppl:31S–6S. https://doi.org/10.1046/j.1365-2672.94.s1.4.x.
75. Li J, Ertel A, Portocarrero C, Barkhouse DA, Dietzschold B, Hooper DC, Faber M. Postexposure treatment with the live-attenuated rabies virus (RV) vaccine TriGAS triggers the clearance of wild-type RV from the central nervous system (CNS) through the rapid induction of genes relevant to adaptive immunity in CNS tissues. J Virol. 2012;86(6):3200–10. https://doi.org/10.1128/jvi.06699-11.
76. MacReady N. Developing countries court medical tourists. Lancet. 2007;369(9576):1849–50. https://doi.org/10.1016/S0140-6736(07)60833-2.
77. Chen LH, Wilson ME. The globalization of healthcare: implications of medical tourism for the infectious disease clinician. Clin Infect Dis. 2013;57(12):1752–9. https://doi.org/10.1093/cid/cit540.
78. Chan HLE, Poon LM, Chan SG, Teo JWP. The perils of medical tourism: NDM-1-positive Escherichia coli causing febrile neutropenia in a medical tourist. Singapore Med J. 2011;52(4):299–302.
79. Kotton CN, Hibberd PL. Travel medicine and transplant tourism in solid organ transplantation. Am J Transplant. 2013;13(Suppl 4):337–4. https://doi.org/10.1111/ajt.12125.
80. Martín-Dávila P, Fortún J, López-Vélez R, et al. Transmission of tropical and geographically restricted infections during solid-organ transplantation. Clin Microbiol Rev. 2008;21(1):60–96. https://doi.org/10.1128/CMR.00021-07.
81. Centers for Disease Control and Prevention (CDC). Nontuberculous mycobacterial infections after cosmetic surgery—Santo Domingo, Dominican Republic, 2003–2004. MMWR Morb Mortal Wkly Rep. 2004;53(23):509.
82. Cai SS, Chopra K, Lifchez SD. Management of Mycobacterium abscessus infection after medical tourism in cosmetic surgery and a review of literature. Ann Plast Surg. 2016;77(6):678–82. https://doi.org/10.1097/SAP.0000000000000745.
83. Askling HH, Dalm VASH. The medically immunocompromised adult traveler and pre-travel counseling: status quo 2014. Travel Med Infect Dis. 2014;12(3):219–28. https://doi.org/10.1016/j.tmaid.2014.04.009.
84. Buchan CA, Kotton CN. Travel medicine, transplant tourism, and the solid organ transplant recipient—guidelines from the American Society of Transplantation Infectious Diseases Community of Practice. Clin Transpl. 2019;33(9):e13529. https://doi.org/10.1111/ctr.13529.
85. Papp KA, Haraoui B, Kumar D, et al. Vaccination guidelines for patients with immune-mediated disorders on immunosuppressive therapies. J Cutan Med Surg. 2019;23(1):50–74. https://doi.org/10.1177/1203475418811335.
86. Mikulska M, Cesaro S, de Lavallade H, et al. Vaccination of patients with haematological malignancies who did not have transplantations: guidelines from the 2017 European Conference on Infections in Leukaemia (ECIL 7). Lancet Infect Dis. 2019;19(6):e188–99. https://doi.org/10.1016/S1473-3099(18)30601-7.
87. Freedman M, Kroger A, Hunter P, et al. Recommended adult immunization schedule, United States, 2020. Ann Intern Med. 2020;172(5):337–47. https://doi.org/10.7326/M20-0046.
88. Yates JA, Rao SR, Walker AT, Esposito DH, Sotir M, Larocque RC, Ryan ET. Characteristics and preparation of the last-minute traveler: analysis of vaccine usage in the Global TravEpiNet Consortium. J Travel Med. 2019;26(6):taz031. https://doi.org/10.1093/jtm/taz031.
89. Mackell SM. Vaccinations for the pediatric traveler. Clin Infect Dis. 2003;37(11):1508–16. https://doi.org/10.1086/379515.
90. Hall V, Johnson D, Torresi J. Travel and biologic therapy: travel-related infection risk, vaccine response and recommendations. J Travel Med. 2018;25(1). https://doi.org/10.1093/jtm/tay018.
91. World Health Organization. Vaccine preventable diseases and vaccines. In: International travel and health. WHO; 2012.

Part II

Specific Agents and Risk of Infections

Anti-tumor Necrosis Factor-Alpha Agents

5

Joel V. Chua and John W. Baddley

Introduction

Tumor necrosis factor-α (TNF-α) plays a central role in the immunopathogenesis of a wide variety of inflammatory conditions from diseases such as rheumatoid arthritis (RA) to inflammatory bowel diseases (IBD). Development of TNF-α inhibitors (TNFI) has revolutionized the ability treat these conditions resulting in substantial improvement in outcomes [1–3]. Since the introduction of infliximab and etanercept in 1998, indications for the use of TNFI have expanded, and these medications are predominately prescribed by rheumatologists, dermatologists, and gastroenterologists for moderate to severe inflammatory and autoimmune diseases. Although these drugs have had a substantial impact in the treatment of many diseases, there are important safety concerns, the foremost of which is increased risk of infection caused by bacterial, mycobacterial, fungal, and viral pathogens [4]. Herein, we will review available data on the epidemiology of infectious complications in patients receiving TNFI for the treatment of inflammatory conditions.

J. V. Chua · J. W. Baddley (✉)
Division of Infectious Diseases, Institute of Human Virology, University of Maryland School of Medicine, Baltimore, MD, USA
e-mail: jchua@ihv.umaryland.edu; jbaddley@ihv.umaryland.edu

C. Cervera, J. M. Aguado (eds.), *Infectious Complications in Biologic and Targeted Therapies*, https://doi.org/10.1007/978-3-031-11363-5_5

Tumor Necrosis Factor-Alpha and the Innate Immune System

Tumor necrosis factor-α, primarily produced by macrophages and T-lymphocytes, is the principal endogenous regulator of inflammation and immune responses. First described in 1975 and named after its ability to cause tumor apoptosis in vitro, TNF-α is found constitutively in macrophages as a 233-amino acid transmembrane protein. Monomeric membrane-bound TNF-α aggregates into metabolically active homotrimers. When cleaved by the membrane-bound metalloprotease TNF-α converting enzyme (TACE), a soluble 157-amino acid TNF-α residue is released into circulation [5]. Only in the homotrimeric form is soluble TNF-α able to bind to its target receptors (Fig. 5.1). The activity of TNF-α is mediated by two types of receptors: tumor necrosis factor receptor 1 (TNFR1, also known as p55) and 2 (TNFR2, also known as p75). Although both receptors are structurally related, they are functionally distinct receptors mediating the activity of TNF-α in cells [6]. TNFR1 is found in a broad array of cells including macrophages, while TNFR2 is expressed predominantly in endothelial cells and lymphocytes [6]. Activation of TNFR1, which contains an intracellular death domain, results in induction of a signaling cascade with pleotropic effect that includes cell proliferation, apoptosis, and cytokine secretion [7]. TNFR2 does not contain a death domain and its stimulation can result in proliferation, migration, and production of cytokines such as interleukins -1 (IL-1) or -6 (IL-6), both important mediators of inflammation [7].

The activation of the innate immune response by an infectious pathogen includes release of TNF-α by activated macrophages into the affected tissue. The subsequent activation of TNFR1 and TNFR2 by binding with the homotrimer TNF-α results in a torrent of inflammatory events that includes release of inflammatory cytokines IL-1β, IL-6, IL-8, and granulocyte-macrophage colony stimulating factor (GM-CSF); upregulation of adhesion molecules, including intracellular adhesion molecule-1 (ICAM-1), vascular cell adhesion molecule-1 (VCAM-1), and E selectin (also known as endothelial leukocyte adhesion molecule-1, or ELAM-1); and increased expression of chemokines (e.g. RANTES, MCP-1, MIP-2) [8–13]. The combined effect results in vasodilatation at the infection site, coordinated recruitment, and migration of leukocytes to the target site, and activation of efficient phagocytosis of the pathogens resulting in successful host defense [13, 14].

TNF-α is essential for mounting effective host defense against pathogens that require granuloma formation for control [13]. These pathogens, which include Mycobacterium species including *M. tuberculosis* (TB), *M. avium*, and fungal pathogens such as *Histoplasma capsulatum*, *Aspergillus fumigatus*, and *Cryptococcus neoformans*, are not easily eradicated by host defense mechanisms and require sequestration into granulomas [13, 15–19]. TNF-α coordinates the organized formation of granulomas initially with chemokine production, phagosome activation, and leukocyte recruitment and differentiation, and subsequent leukocyte aggregation into function granulomas that can control infectious pathogens [13, 14].

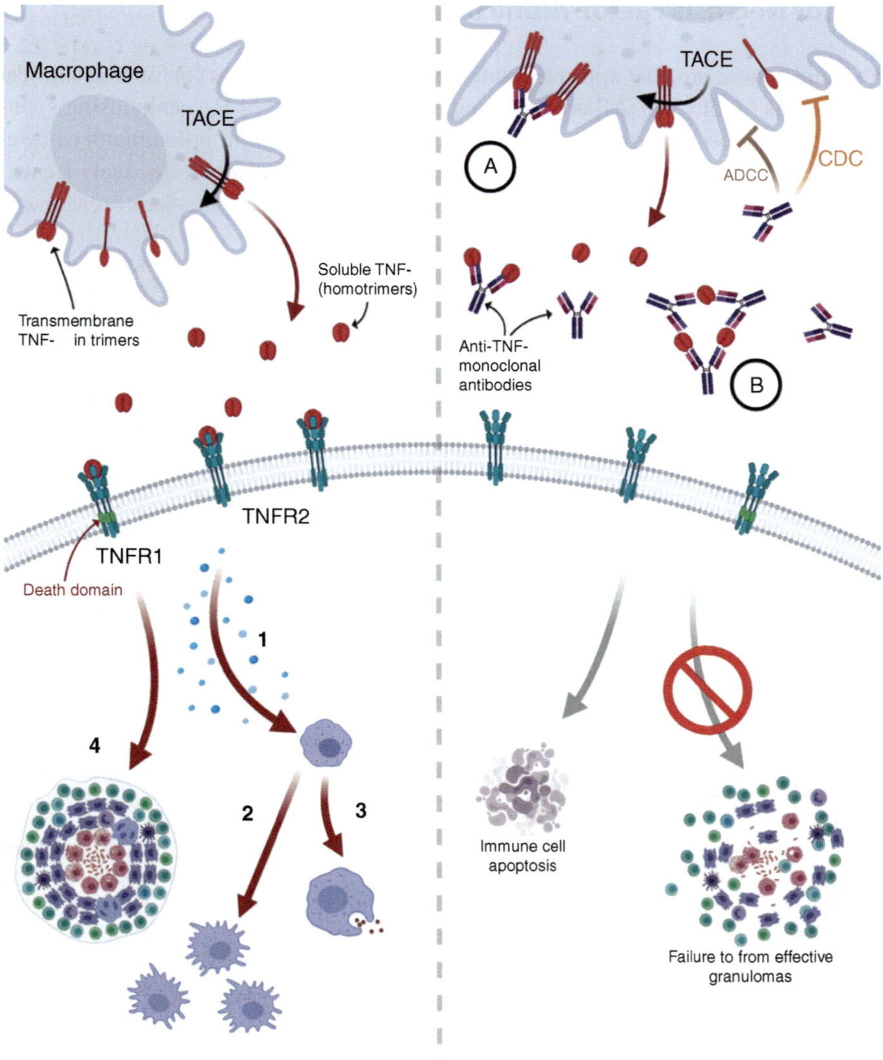

Fig. 5.1 Overview of the TNF-α cascade in the presence of TNF-α inhibitors. *Left half*: Transmembrane TNF-α found on cell membranes of macrophages and other immune cells forms trimers and are released as biologically active homotrimeric soluble form via cleavage by TNF-α converting enzyme (TACE). Both soluble and transmembrane TNF-α homotrimers can bind to their ligand receptors (TNFR1 and TNFR2) found in a wide variety of cells throughout the body. The effect of which is a cascade of cell signaling that includes (1) cytokine and chemokine release; (2) maturation, proliferation, and migration of macrophages and other immune cells; (3) increased phagocytic activity of macrophages; and (4) formation and maintenance of granuloma. *Right half*: TNF-α inhibitors (TNFI) act by either binding transmembrane (A) and/or soluble (B) TNF-α. TNFI with IgG1 Fc region contains a CH1 domain that in the presence of complements can induce complement-dependent cytotoxicity (CDC) and antibody-dependent cell-mediated cytotoxicity (ADCC) leading to apoptosis of cells expressing transmembrane TNF-α (e.g. macrophages). (Illustration created by authors with BioRender.com)

Tumor Necrosis Factor-Alpha Inhibitors (TNFI)

Currently there are five approved anti-TNF-α agents available for various clinical indications (Table 5.1). All are indicated for the treatment of RA, ankylosing spondylitis, and psoriatic arthritis [2, 3, 20]. Except for etanercept, inflammatory bowel diseases (namely, Crohn's disease and ulcerative colitis) can be effectively treated

Table 5.1 Summary of approved tumor necrosis factor-α inhibitors

Agent	Route	FDA approval	EMA approval	Structure	Approved indications
Infliximab	IV	1998	1999	Chimeric (mouse/human) anti-TNF-α monoclonal antibody. Human IgG1 Fc region coupled with mouse anti-TNF-α Fab region	Rheumatoid arthritis Ankylosing spondylitis Psoriatic arthritis Crohn's disease Ulcerative colitis Plaque psoriasis
Etanercept	SC	1998	2000	Soluble fusion protein with 2 human TNF-α receptor (TNFR2) bound to the Fc region of a human IgG1	Rheumatoid arthritis Ankylosing spondylitis Psoriatic arthritis Juvenile idiopathic arthritis Plaque psoriasis
Adalimumab	SC	2002	2003	Fully human monoclonal anti-TNF-α antibody (both Fc and Fab regions are human)	Rheumatoid arthritis Psoriatic arthritis Ankylosing spondylitis Juvenile idiopathic arthritis Crohn's disease Ulcerative colitis Plaque psoriasis Hidradenitis suppurativa Noninfectious uveitis

Table 5.1 (continued)

Agent	Route	FDA approval	EMA approval	Structure	Approved indications
Certolizumab pegol	SC	2008	2009	Pegylated Fab fragment of a humanized monoclonal antibody (No Fc portion = does not induce complement activation, antibody-dependent cellular toxicity, or apoptosis)	Rheumatoid arthritis Ankylosing spondylitis Psoriatic arthritis Crohn's disease
Golimumab	SC	2013	2013	Human IgG1 kappa monoclonal anti-TNF-α antibody (binds to both soluble and transmembrane bioactive forms of human TNF-α)	Rheumatoid arthritis Ankylosing spondylitis Psoriatic arthritis Ulcerative colitis

EMA European Medicines Agency, *FDA* U.S. Food and Drug Administration, *IV* intravenous, *SC* subcutaneous

with TNFI [21, 22]. Other TNFI indications include treatment of inflammation of the skin (plaque psoriasis and hidradenitis suppurativa) and the eye (uveitis) [23–25].

Etanercept and Infliximab were the earliest developed TNFI for clinical use and both were approved in 1998. Etanercept is a soluble fusion protein consisting of two human TNF-α receptor-2 (TNFR2) bound to the constant (Fc) region of a human IgG1 that acts as a decoy and binds both soluble forms of TNF-α and TNF-β, the latter is a related cytokine that utilizes the same receptors as TNF-α [26]. In contrast, infliximab is a chimeric monoclonal antibody consisting of a mouse anti-TNF-α variable (Fab′) region coupled with a human IgG Fc region. Adalimumab and Golimumab are both fully human IgG monoclonal anti-TNF-α antibodies with both humanized Fab′ and Fc regions [26]. As IgG1 monoclonal antibodies, infliximab, adalimumab, and golimumab can inhibit both soluble and membrane-bound forms of TNF-α but do not neutralize TNF-β [27]. As the Fc region of IgG1 contains a CH2 domain that is responsible for the activation of C1 (first component of the classical pathway of complement activation), both the full chain IgG monoclonal antibodies (infliximab, adalimumab, and golimumab) and etanercept in the presence of complements can induce both complement-dependent cytotoxicity (CDC) and antibody-dependent cell-mediated cytotoxicity (ADCC) with subsequent lysis of membrane-bound TNF-α expressing cells [26–28]. Lacking a CH1 domain that serves as the platform for C3 activation (the most vital step in the complement cascade), etanercept induces significantly less CDC on membrane-bound TNF-α-expressing cells [27, 28].

Certolizumab is a PEGylated Fab′ fragment of a humanized monoclonal anti-TNF-α antibody. The attachment of the Fab′ fragment to a 40-kDa polyethylene glycol moiety markedly increases the half-life of certolizumab compared to other TNFIs [29]. Like the full-chain anti-TNF-α monoclonal antibodies, certolizumab inhibits both soluble and membrane-bound TNF-α and lacks activity against TNF-β [29]. But in contrast to other inhibitors, certolizumab does not contain the crystallizable IgG Fc fragment and does not cause complement fixation, thus it does not induce CDC and ADCC in vitro [27–29].

Risk of Infection

Data evaluating infection risk are derived from a variety of sources, including clinical trials, meta-analyses, observational studies, and registries [30–34] (Table 5.2). In general, there is increased risk of infection with TNFI use, especially for tuberculosis, bacterial infections, and fungal infections. Several studies report a higher

Table 5.2 Selected studies of infections associated with TNFI

Reference, year	Study Information	Infection type
Singh et al., 2011 [30]	Meta-analysis of 163 RCTs and 46 OLEs (*N* = 61,964); biological vs. nonbiological DMARDs until 2010	Serious infection Tuberculosis
Singh et al., 2015 [31]	Meta-analysis of 106 RCTs; only RA (*N* = 42,330); biological vs. nonbiological DMARDs until 2014	Serious infection
Grijalva et al., 2011 [32]	Multicenter retrospective cohort (*N* = 10,484 RA pts, 3215 pts with other conditions); anti-TNFs vs. nonbiologicals from 1998 to 2007	Serious infection
Galloway et al., 2011 [48]	Multicenter registry (*N* = 1809) in RA patients treated with TNFI or nonbiologic DMARDs	Serious infection
Fouque-Aubert et al., 2012 [50]	Systematic review of 14 RCTs in patients with ankylosing spondylitis with and without use of TNFI	Serious infection
Minozzi et al., 2016 [33]	Meta-analysis of 71 RCTs plus 7 OLEs; RA, PsA and AS (*N* = 22,760 plus 2236); infliximab, adalimumab, etanercept, golimumab, certolizumab vs. no anti-TNFs until 2014	Serious infection Tuberculosis Opportunistic infection
Bonovas et al., 2016 [51]	Meta-analysis of 49 RCTs; IBD (*N* = 8897) different TNFI until 2016	Serious infections Tuberculosis Opportunistic infection
Kourbeti et al., 2014 [34]	Meta-analysis of 70 trials in patients receiving biologic agents. RA patients only	Opportunistic infections Tuberculosis Fungal infections Viral infections Herpes Zoster Pneumocystis pneumonia
Ai et al., 2015 [39]	Meta-analysis of 50 RCTs and 13 registries and cohort studies; only RA (*N* = 82,590); infliximab, etanercept, adalimumab, golimumab and certolizumab vs. no TNFI or general population	Tuberculosis
Zheng et al., 2017 [41]	Meta-analysis of 29 RCTs (*N* = 11,879) on use of TNFI vs. placebo or SOC	Tuberculosis

Table 5.2 (continued)

Reference, year	Study Information	Infection type
Cao et al., 2018 [38]	Meta-analysis of 23 placebo controlled RCTs on use of TNFI on Crohn's disease (*N* = TNFI 1113 vs. placebo 822)	Tuberculosis
Tubach et al., [40]	French RATIO registry collected TB cases in pts on TNFI over 3 years (TB *N* = 69)	Tuberculosis
Winthrop et al., 2013 [43]	Multicenter registry (*N* = 8418); infliximab, etanercept or adalimumab vs. no anti-TNFI	Tuberculosis Nontuberculous mycobacteria
Lan et al., 2011 [62]	Retrospective cohort (Taiwan, 2006–2009) *N* = 88 anti-HBc+ RA on TNFI	Hepatitis B
Tamori et al., 2011 [65]	Prospective cohort (Japan) *N* = 50 anti-HBc+ RA on >1 year of TNFI	Hepatitis B
Pauly et al., 2018 [63]	Retrospective cohort (Kaiser, 2001–2012) *N* = 4267 rheumatologic disease on TNFI	Hepatitis B
Barone M et al., 2015 [66]	Prospective cohort (Italy, 2001–2012) of anti-HBc+ with rheumatologic disease on TNFI (*N* = 146).	Hepatitis B
Ferri et al., 2008 [98]	Prospective cohort (Italy, April–June 2007) *N* = 31 RA with HCV on TNFI	Hepatitis C
Strangfeld et al. 2009 [72]	Prospective cohort (Germany, 2001–2006) on TNFI vs. DMARDs (*N* = 5040)	Herpes zoster
García-Doval et al. 2010 [74]	BIOBADASER national registry (Spain, 2000–2010) on TNFI, *N* = 5040	Herpes zoster
Winthrop et al., 2013 [71]	Large retrospective cohort (U.S., 1998–2007) pts with RA, PsA, AS, psoriasis, and IBD on TNFI (*N* = 33,324)	Herpes zoster
Baddley 2014 [89]	Multicenter retrospective cohort (10,484 RA pts, 3215 pts with other conditions); anti-TNFs vs. nonbiologicals from 1998 to 2007	Opportunistic infection Fungal infection
Olson 2011 [94]	Single center review of RA patients on TNFI	Histoplasmosis
Takeuchi 2008 [95]	Post-marketing surveillance study in Japan *N* = 5000 with RA who received infliximab	Pneumocytsosis Tuberculosis Bacterial pneumonia

Anti-HBc+ hepatitis B core antibody positive, *AS* ankylosing spondylitis, *DMARDs* disease-modifying antirheumatologic drugs, *HCV* hepatitis C virus, *IBD* inflammatory bowel disease, *OLEs* open-label extension studies, *PsA* psoriatic arthritis, *RA* rheumatoid arthritis, *RCT* randomized controlled trial, *SOC* standard of care, *TB* tuberculosis, *TNFI* tumor necrosis factor-α inhibitor

infection risk with infliximab when compared to adalimumab or etanercept [32, 35, 36]. However, there are several important limitations. Clinical trials may be limited by small sample sizes, inclusion of healthier patients, and insufficient statistical power to detect uncommon infection events. In observational studies, due to lack of randomization, confounding factors can impact results. Patients with autoimmune diseases enrolled in trials may be receiving corticosteroids or other medications that increase risk of infection, making attribution of infection risk to a particular TNFI challenging. Another important limitation in identifying TNFI infection risk in populations is related to underlying diseases that may impact infection risk. For example, patients with RA have an increased risk of infection compared with non-RA controls [37].

Mycobacterial Infections

Effective host immune response against *Mycobacterium tuberculosis* involves TNF-α-mediated formation of organized granulomas for control and prevention of dissemination. Studies including meta-analyses of randomized controlled trials, retrospective and prospective cohorts, and post-marketing registries have consistently shown increased risk for active tuberculosis (TB) in people on TNFI [30, 33, 38–41]. Patients with latent tuberculosis infection (LTBI) receiving TNFI therapy for RA, ankylosing spondylitis, or psoriatic arthritis have an estimated fourfold increased risk of TB reactivation as compared to controls [4, 30, 39, 41]. In a recent publication, Cao and colleagues reviewed 23 placebo-controlled clinical trials and similar increased odds of active tuberculosis were seen in patients with Crohn's disease receiving TNFI [38]. All TB reactivation cases occurred in the TNFI arm and none in the placebo controls, with an odds ratio (OR) of 4.85 with a 95% confidence interval (CI) between 1.02 and 22.99 [38].

The risk of active TB may be different among TNFI [39, 40]. A systematic review in patients with RA treated with TNFI showed higher risk of tuberculosis with the use of adalimumab and infliximab compared to etanercept, with OR of 3.88 and 2.78, respectively [39]. The French RATIO registry reported a significantly higher odds ratio with adalimumab (OR 17.08) and infliximab (OR 13.29) when compared to etanercept [40]. Tuberculosis reactivation occurred five times higher during the first year of initiating TNFI therapy [40]. Latent TB infection screening and treatment for patients who will be receiving TNFI therapy can reduce risk of reactivation by 65% [39].

Nontuberculous mycobacteria (NTM) can cause a variety of human diseases particularly of the lungs in people with underlying lung conditions. Few data exist on the risk of NTM in patients on TNFI. The U.S. Food and Drug Administration (FDA) MedWatch database report in 2009 found 105 cases of NTM related to TNFI use. The majority were women (65%), had rheumatoid arthritis (70%), and most were receiving infliximab (70%) [42]. Half of the NTM infections were due to *Mycobacterium avium*, and though 56% were lung infections, extrapulmonary infections were not uncommon [42].

Mycobacterial infection rates in patients who used TNFI were evaluated using the Kaiser Permanente database [43]. TNFI-associated rates of NTM were 49 per 100,000 person years, greater than in unexposed RA patients (19.2 per 100,000 person years) or the general population (4.1 per 100,000 person years). NTM rates were lower for users of etanercept, when compared with infliximab or adalimumab [43].

Bacterial and Other Serious Infections

Many studies have reported data on TNFI use and serious (hospitalized) infections, which include a variety of organisms, but most frequently refer to bacterial infections [4, 30–32]. However, fewer details have been captured on specific bacteria causing an infection or infectious syndrome. Typically, pneumonia, skin, and soft tissue and urinary tract infections are the most common serious infections observed in adults, similar to the pre-biologic era [37]. In children, skin/soft tissue and respiratory infections are common [44].

In general, when comparing patients on TNFI to those receiving conventional disease modifying anti-rheumatic drugs (DMARDs), there is an increased risk of serious infection, with adjusted rate ratios ranging from 1.5 to 5.0, and infections per 100 person-years ranging from 2 to 15 [32, 33, 45–47]. It is important to note that timing of risk assessment is important, as studies focused on the first year of TNFI therapy show adjusted increased rate ratios, where a decline in absolute and relative risk of infection is typically seen after 1 year [32, 46–48].

A 2011 network meta-analysis of RCTs and extension studies found that TNFIs increased serious infection risk [30]. Certolizumab pegol was the only individual TNFI agent that significantly increased the risk of serious infection compared to control (OR 3.51; 95% CI 1.59–7.79). Another recent meta-analysis of 106 RCTs of targeted therapies (mostly TNFI) in RA patients demonstrated an increased risk of serious infections (OR 1.31, 95% CI 1.09–1.58) in patients who received standard dose TNFIs compared with traditional DMARDS. The risk was more pronounced (OR 1.9, 95% CI 1.50–2.39) in patients receiving high doses [31].

Studies in other populations have shown a variability in risk estimates. A meta-analysis evaluating patients with psoriatic arthritis reported a crude OR for infection of 1.18 (95% CI: 1.05–1.33) in patients exposed to TNFI (versus controls) [49]. In a meta-analysis among patients with ankylosing spondylitis, the risk of serious infection related to TNFI was low and was not significantly increased compared to untreated controls [50]. Two meta-analyses in patients with inflammatory bowel disease concluded that the risk of serious infection with TNFI was not increased [51, 52].

Many randomized controlled trials and observational studies fail to detail the precise nature of infectious syndromes or the causative agents. However, some series have reported either site-specific infections or data on specific pathogens. Risk for septic arthritis in RA with use of TNFI was evaluated in the British Society for Rheumatology Biologics Register. The adjusted hazard ratio for septic arthritis was 2.3 (95% CI: 1.2–4.4) for TNFI compared with traditional DMARDs. *Staphylococcus aureus* was the most common cause of septic arthritis [53].

Several studies have evaluated TNFI use and risk of listeriosis, one of which described a fourfold increased risk of severe listeriosis with TNFI in comparison with the general population [54–56]. There is a risk for legionellosis and TNFI, with one study finding the incidence rate of legionellosis in patients in TNFI to be 46.7 per 100,000 person-years and greater than the general population [57].

Viral Infections

Hepatitis B

TNF-α stimulates hepatitis B (HBV)-specific T-cell responses, inhibits HBV replication, and mediates HBV clearance in infected hepatocytes [58, 59]. Hepatitis

B reactivation is the result of the loss of HBV immune control and is defined as an increase in HBV DNA level of either: (1) ≥2 log (100-fold) compared to baseline, (2) ≥2 log (1000) IU/mL in a previously undetectable level, or (3) ≥4 log (10,000) IU/mL if baseline not available [60]. HBV reactivation is a well-known complication in patients receiving TNFI [61–65]. In a retrospective Taiwanese study, HBV reactivation occurred in 5 (28%) of 18 hepatitis B surface antigen (HBsAg)-positive patients and 1 (25%) in 4 patients with occult HBV infection during the first year of TNFI therapy [62]. In addition, HBV reactivation occurs in previously inactive HBsAg carriers occurs following TNFI therapy [61]. A prospective Japanese cohort of 50 anti-HBc-positive RA patients on TNFI therapy followed up to 32 months, HBV reactivation was seen in 2 of 5 (40%) of HBsAg-positive patients and only 1 of 45 (2%) HBsAg [65]. In patients with previously resolved HBV infection, TNFI therapy was found to be safe, with no HBV seroconversion or reactivation observed [66]. Prophylactic antiviral therapy is effective in preventing reactivation [62, 67].

Guidelines consider use of TNFI as a moderate risk category with regards to HBV reactivation. Patients who are to start TNFI should at least have a baseline HBV serology that includes HBV surface antigen (HBsAg) and total HBV core antibody (anti-HBc) [67]. In HBV-endemic areas, HBV DNA should also be checked at baseline to detect occult HBV infections. In patients with either positive HBsAg or HBV DNA, preemptive anti-HBV antivirals with high barrier to resistance, such as tenofovir or entecavir, should be considered until 6–12 months after the last TNFI dose. Serial monitoring of HBV while on TNFI therapy every 6–12 months even for those with resolved HBV infections (anti-HBc positive but negative for HBsAg and HBV DNA) is recommended.

Hepatitis C

Evidence supports a TNF-α role in mediating inflammatory responses to hepatitis C (HCV) such as enabling apoptosis of infected cells, but it does not appear to play a pivotal role in the control of HCV replication [68]. In addition, TNF-α polymorphism has no significant effect to HCV susceptibility or viral clearance [68]. Data on the safety of TNFI use in patients with chronic HCV is limited and mostly derived from small cohorts and aggregates of case reports and case series. In a small cohort of 29 patients with both active RA and mild chronic HCV, use of etanercept was observed to be safe, with no increased risk of hepatic flare related to HCV replication [69]. A literature review found 216 patients with HCV who received TNFI (either etanercept, infliximab, or adalimumab) with mean observation time of 1.2 years and found only three patients needing TNFI withdrawal due to suspected HCV reactivation [70]. The limited data available supports that TNFI use in HCV patients is at least safe in the short-term [69, 70]. With the availability of safe and effective direct acting antivirals (DAAs) for HCV, treatment should be considered for patients planning to receive or receiving TNFI.

Herpes Zoster

Numerous studies have evaluated risk of herpes zoster with TNFI use, but evidence of risk of herpes zoster and TNFI therapy have been conflicting. A large U.S. multicenter cohort study [71] involving more than 33,000 patients with RA and other inflammatory diseases showed no increased risk of HZ when treated with TNFI. However, European registries [35, 72–74] and an Asian case-control study [75] showed an approximate twofold increase risk. Moreover, patients on TNFI had almost a ten times higher rate of hospitalization related to zoster when compared to the general population (32 vs. 3.4 cases per 100,000 patient-years) in a Spanish registry [74]. An international prospective registry study of patients with psoriasis showed that TNFI was not significantly associated with an increased risk of HZ, although the adjusted hazard ratio was 2.73 (95% CI 0.98–7.58) [76]. A British registry study found that zoster was highest among patients on infliximab (hazard risk [HR] of 2.2; 95% confidence interval [CI] 1.4–3.4) and lowest with adalimumab use (HR 1.5; 95% CI 1.1–2.0) [35].

Herpes zoster is a vaccine preventable disease. Shingrix, an adjuvanted recombinant zoster vaccine, significantly reduced risk of shingles by 94–97% compared to placebo in immunocompetent adults 50 years or older [77]. In a pooled post hoc analysis of participants with autoimmune diseases from two phase 3 trials showed overall vaccine efficacy of Shingrix at 90.5% (95% CI: 73.5–97.5%) [78]. This vaccine given in two doses 2–6 months apart is currently recommended for adults age 50 including those who are on low dose immunosuppression or anticipating being on immunosuppressive therapy [79, 80]. Although no head-to-head studies present, Shingrix is preferred over the live attenuated HZ vaccine, Zostavax, due to the latter lower efficacy rates especially in the older at-risk groups [77, 81, 82]. Zostavax is no longer available in the United States.

Fungal Infections

Tumor necrosis factor-α plays an important role in the control of infection due to fungi; however, fungal infections complicating TNFI use are relatively uncommon. Most reports detail impact on histoplasmosis, coccidioidomycosis, aspergillosis, and *Pneumocystis jirovecii* pneumonia (PCP) [34, 83–88]. The precise risk of TNFI use and fungal infection is difficult to acertain, as the concomitant use of other immunosuppressive therapies, especially corticosteroids, renders risk interpretation problematic. A recent meta-analysis reported the risks of opportunistic infections in RA patients from clinical trial data of biologic use, mostly TNFI [34]. Biologic use did not significantly increase the risk for all fungal (superficial or invasive) infections (odds ratio 1.31, 95% CI 0.46–3.72), invasive fungal infections (odds ratio 2.58; 95% confidence interval 0.68–11.91), or PCP (odds ratio 1.77, 95% confidence interval 0.42–7.47). A large US cohort study evaluated new users of TNFI and investigated the incidence of nonviral opportunistic infections among patients with RA, ankylosing spondylitis, psoriatic arthritis, psoriasis, and IBD [89]. Among

33,324 new users of TNFI, 80 nonviral OIs were identified. Of these, 32 (40%) were caused by fungi, with a crude incidence rate of 112 cases per 100,000 person-years. The most common fungal infections were pneumocystosis (16 cases) and histoplasmosis (9 cases).

The estimated incidence of aspergillosis is approximately seven cases per 100,000 persons treated with TNFI [85, 88]. A case series was published by Tsiodras and colleagues, who reviewed publications up to June 1, 2007 to determine the association of fungal infections with TNF-α blockade [90]. Sixty-four cases of aspergillosis, mostly invasive pulmonary disease, were identified. The most common TNFI used was infliximab in 48 cases (75%), followed by etanercept in 14 (22%), and adalimumab in three cases (3%) [90].

The incidence of coccidioidomycosis in patients receiving TNFI is estimated to range up to 5.58 per 100,000 persons treated with infliximab and 0.88 per 100,000 persons treated with etanercept [91]. Bergstrom and colleagues described 13 cases among patients receiving TNFI from in areas endemic for coccidioidomycosis [92]. The interval between TNFI and infection ranged from 1 to 96 weeks (mean, 27 weeks), and two cases were likely due to reactivation. All patients had pneumonia on presentation, with 4 (30.7%) having disseminated disease. The risk of infliximab in development of symptomatic coccidioidomycosis when compared to other agents was greater (RR 5.23, 95% CI 1.54–17.71; $p < 0.01$).

Taroumian and colleagues described 44 patients with rheumatologic disease treated with nonbiologic DMARDS and/or biologic therapies in Tucson, Arizona [93]. Twenty-nine patients had pulmonary coccidioidomycosis, nine patients had disseminated disease, and six had asymptomatic coccidioidomycosis based on positive serology. With continuation or resuming biologic therapy after treatment, no patients had subsequent dissemination or complications of coccidioidomycosis.

Histoplasmosis is one of the most common fungal infections in patients receiving TNFI [84, 85]. Wallis and colleagues collected data from cases reported to FDA Adverse Event Reporting System (AERS) from January 1998 through September 2002 and identified 40 cases of histoplasmosis. The estimated rate of histoplasmosis per 100,000 patients treated was 18.78 in patients treated with infliximab and 2.65 in patients treated with etanercept [85]. Vergidis and colleagues described 98 patients diagnosed with histoplasmosis while receiving TNF-α inhibitors from January 2000 to June 2011. Seventy-four (76%) patients presented with disseminated histoplasmosis; pulmonary involvement was present in 78 (80%) patients. The median time to diagnosis after TNFI initiation was 15.5 months (range of 1–88 months) [84]. Rheumatoid arthritis was the most common underlying disease, and infliximab (67.3%) was most used. TNFI therapy was initially discontinued in 96.9% of patients but resumed in 33% of patients at a median of 12 months. The recurrence rate at follow-up was 3.2%.

Olson and colleagues found that 15 of 26 patients with RA who developed disseminated histoplasmosis from 1998 to 2009 were on TNFI and had a median time on TNFI to histoplasmosis diagnosis of 15 months (range, 2–132 months) [94]. Most patients were treated with at least 6 months of antifungal therapy. In this study,

TNFI were discontinued at the time of infection in 14 patients and was restarted successfully in 4/15 with recurrence of disease in only one patient [94].

Pneumocystis Pneumonia

Pneumocystis jirovecii pneumonia (PCP) complicating patients receiving TNFI is uncommon, with variability in incidence rates depending on the population studied and diagnostic method used. Observational studies have reported incidence rates of up to 8.8 cases per 1000 patient-years [95–97]. Takeuchi and colleagues examined the incidence of adverse events in Japanese patients with RA for their first 6 months on infliximab as post-marketing surveillance [95]. The diagnosis of suspected PCP was made in 22 (0.4%) patients, with many cases diagnosed by PCR for *P jirovecii* DNA from bronchoalveolar lavage fluid.

The National Institutes of Health conducted a population-based study to determine if the incidence of PCP in patients with RA had changed significantly from 1996 to 2007 using data from the Nationwide Inpatient Sample and the California Office of Statewide Health Planning and Development [97]. They found no significant change in the number of patients with RA and PCP diagnoses over this period.

Conclusion

Tumor necrosis factor-α inhibitors have become an important class of drugs and will continue to be used widely in the treatment of autoimmune and inflammatory diseases. Although uncommon, increased risk of infection caused by bacterial, mycobacterial, fungal, and viral pathogens have the potential for increased morbidity and mortality. Risk of infection is often difficult to characterize, as it may differ with underlying patient comorbidities, concomitant medications, and the specific TNFI agent. Use of TNFI will warrant clinician vigilance and continued infection surveillance.

Potential Conflicts of Interest

JVC: *Research grants from Gilead Sciences, Inc.*

JWB*:* *Consultation for Eli Lilly and Viela Bio.*

References

1. Hanauer SB, Feagan BG, Lichtenstein GR, Mayer LF, Schreiber S, Colombel JF, et al. Maintenance infliximab for Crohn's disease: the ACCENT I randomised trial. Lancet. 2002;359(9317):1541–9.
2. Aaltonen KJ, Virkki LM, Malmivaara A, Konttinen YT, Nordström DC, Blom M. Systematic review and meta-analysis of the efficacy and safety of existing TNF blocking agents in treatment of rheumatoid arthritis. PLoS One. 2012;7(1):e30275.

3. Corbett M, Soares M, Jhuti G, Rice S, Spackman E, Sideris E, et al. Tumour necrosis factor-α inhibitors for ankylosing spondylitis and non-radiographic axial spondyloarthritis: a systematic review and economic evaluation. Health Technol Assess (Rockv). 2016;20(9):333.
4. Baddley JW, Cantini F, Goletti D, Gómez-Reino JJ, Mylonakis E, San-Juan R, et al. ESCMID Study Group for Infections in Compromised Hosts (ESGICH) consensus document on the safety of targeted and biological therapies: an infectious diseases perspective (soluble immune effector molecules [I]: anti-tumor necrosis factor-α agents). Clin Microbiol Infect. 2018;24:S10–20.
5. Black RA, Rauch CT, Kozlosky CJ, Peschon JJ, Slack JL, Wolfson MF, et al. A metalloproteinase disintegrin that releases tumour-necrosis factor-∅ from cells. Nature. 1997;385(6618):729–33.
6. Walczak H. TNF and ubiquitin at the crossroads of gene activation, cell death, inflammation, and cancer. Immunol Rev. 2011;244(1):9–28.
7. Billmeier U, Dieterich W, Neurath MF, Atreya R. Molecular mechanism of action of anti-tumor necrosis factor antibodies in inflammatory bowel diseases. World J Gastroenterol. 2016;22(42):9300–13.
8. Kaushansky K, Broudy VC, Harlan JM, Adamson JW. Tumor necrosis factor-γ and tumor necrosis factor-β (lymphotoxin) stimulate the production of granulocyte-macrophage colony-stimulating factor, macrophage colony-stimulating factor, and IL-1 in vivo. J Immunol. 1988;141(10):3410–5.
9. Shalaby MR, Aggarwal BB, Rinderknecht E, Svedersky LP, Finkle BS, Palladino MA. Activation of human polymorphonuclear neutrophil functions by interferon-gamma and tumor necrosis factors. J Immunol. 1985;135(3):2069–73. http://www.ncbi.nlm.nih.gov/pubmed/3926894.
10. Sumagin R, Sarelius IH. TNF-α activation of arterioles and venules alters distribution and levels of ICAM-1 and affects leukocyte-endothelial cell interactions. Am J Physiol Heart Circ Physiol. 2006;291(5):H2116.
11. Murao K, Ohyama T, Imachi H, Ishida T, Cao WM, Namihira H, et al. TNF-α stimulation of MCP-1 expression is mediated by the Akt/PKB signal transduction pathway in vascular endothelial cells. Biochem Biophys Res Commun. 2000;276(2):791–6.
12. Victor FC, Gottlieb AB. TNF-alpha and apoptosis: implications for the pathogenesis and treatment of psoriasis. J Drugs Dermatol. 2002;1:264–75.
13. Roach DR, Bean AGD, Demangel C, France MP, Briscoe H, Britton WJ. TNF regulates chemokine induction essential for cell recruitment, granuloma formation, and clearance of mycobacterial infection. J Immunol. 2002;168(9):4620–7.
14. Marino MW, Dunn A, Grail D, Inglese M, Noguchi Y, Richards E, et al. Characterization of tumor necrosis factor-deficient mice. Proc Natl Acad Sci U S A. 1997;94(15):8093–8.
15. Flynn JAL, Goldstein MM, Chan J, Triebold KJ, Pfeffer K, Lowenstein CJ, et al. Tumor necrosis factor-α is required in the protective immune response against mycobacterium tuberculosis in mice. Immunity. 1995;2(6):561–72.
16. Resende M, Cardoso MS, Fróis-Martins R, Borges M, Jordan MB, Castro AG, et al. TNF-mediated compensatory immunity to Mycobacterium avium in the absence of macrophage activation by IFN-γ. J Immunol. 2019;203(9):2451–8.
17. Zhou P, Miller G, Seder RA. Factors involved in regulating primary and secondary immunity to infection with Histoplasma capsulatum: TNF-alpha plays a critical role in maintaining secondary immunity in the absence of IFN-gamma. J Immunol. 1998;160(3):1359–68. http://www.ncbi.nlm.nih.gov/pubmed/9570555.
18. Mehrad B, Strieter RM, Standiford TJ. Role of TNF-alpha in pulmonary host defense in murine invasive aspergillosis. J Immunol. 1999;162(3):1633–40.
19. Huffnagle GB, Toews GB, Burdick MD, Boyd MB, McAllister KS, McDonald RA, et al. Afferent phase production of TNF-α is required for the development of protective T cell immunity to Cryptococcus neoformans. J Immunol. 1996;157(10):4529–36.
20. Lemos LLP, de Oliveira Costa J, Almeida AM, Junior HO, Barbosa MM, Kakehasi AM, et al. Treatment of psoriatic arthritis with anti-TNF agents: a systematic review and meta-analysis of efficacy, effectiveness and safety. Rheumatol Int. 2014;34:1345–60.

21. Ford AC, Sandborn WJ, Khan KJ, Hanauer SB, Talley NJ, Moayyedi P. Efficacy of biological therapies in inflammatory bowel disease: systematic review and meta-analysis. Am J Gastroenterol. 2011;106(4):644–59.
22. Oussalah A, Danese S, Peyrin-Biroulet L. Efficacy of TNF antagonists beyond one year in adult and pediatric inflammatory bowel diseases: a systematic review. Curr Drug Targets. 2010;11(2):156–75.
23. Yamauchi PS, Bissonnette R, Teixeira HD, Valdecantos WC. Systematic review of efficacy of anti-tumor necrosis factor (TNF) therapy in patients with psoriasis previously treated with a different anti-TNF agent. J Am Acad Dermatol. 2016;75(3):612–18.e6. https://doi.org/10.1016/j.jaad.2016.02.1221.
24. Kimball AB, Okun MM, Williams DA, Gottlieb AB, Papp KA, Zouboulis CC, et al. Two phase 3 trials of adalimumab for hidradenitis suppurativa. N Engl J Med. 2016;375(5):422–34.
25. Sheppard J, Joshi A, Betts KA, Hudgens S, Tari S, Chen N, et al. Effect of adalimumab on visual functioning in patients with noninfectious intermediate uveitis, posterior uveitis, and panuveitis in the VISUAL-1 and VISUAL-2 trials. JAMA Ophthalmol. 2017;135(6):511–8.
26. Tracey D, Klareskog L, Sasso EH, Salfeld JG, Tak PP. Tumor necrosis factor antagonist mechanisms of action: a comprehensive review. Pharmacol Ther. 2008;117(2):244–79.
27. Ueda N, Tsukamoto H, Mitoma H, Ayano M, Tanaka A, Ohta SI, et al. The cytotoxic effects of certolizumab pegol and golimumab mediated by transmembrane tumor necrosis factorα. Inflamm Bowel Dis. 2013;19(6):1224–31.
28. Horiuchi T, Mitoma H, Harashima SI, Tsukamoto H, Shimoda T. Transmembrane TNF-α: structure, function and interaction with anti-TNF agents. Rheumatology. 2010;49(7):1215–28.
29. Nesbitt A, Fossati G, Bergin M, Stephens P, Stephens S, Foulkes R, et al. Mechanism of action of certolizumab pegol (CDP870): in vitro comparison with other anti-tumor necrosis factor α agents. Inflamm Bowel Dis. 2007;13(11):1323–32.
30. Singh JA, Wells GA, Christensen R, Tanjong Ghogomu E, Maxwell LJ, Macdonald JK, et al. Adverse effects of biologics: a network meta-analysis and Cochrane overview. Cochrane Database Syst Rev. 2011;2011(2):CD008794.
31. Singh JA, Cameron C, Noorbaloochi S, Cullis T, Tucker M, Christensen R, et al. Risk of serious infection in biological treatment of patients with rheumatoid arthritis: a systematic review and meta-analysis. Lancet. 2015;386(9990):258–65.
32. Grijalva CG, Chen L, Delzell E, Baddley JW, Beukelman T, Winthrop KL, et al. Initiation of tumor necrosis factor-αantagonists and the risk of hospitalization for infection in patients with autoimmune diseases. JAMA. 2011;306(21):2331–9.
33. Minozzi S, Bonovas S, Lytras T, Pecoraro V, González-Lorenzo M, Bastiampillai AJ, et al. Risk of infections using anti-TNF agents in rheumatoid arthritis, psoriatic arthritis, and ankylosing spondylitis: a systematic review and meta-analysis. Expert Opin Drug Saf. 2016;15:11–34. [cited 2020 Oct 10]. https://www.tandfonline.com/doi/abs/10.1080/14740338.2016.1240783.
34. Kourbeti IS, Ziakas PD, Mylonakis E. Biologic therapies in rheumatoid arthritis and the risk of opportunistic infections: a meta-analysis. Clin Infect Dis. 2014;58(12):1649–57.
35. Galloway JB, Mercer LK, Moseley A, Dixon WG, Ustianowski AP, Helbert M, et al. Risk of skin and soft tissue infections (including shingles) in patients exposed to anti-tumour necrosis factor therapy: results from the British Society for Rheumatology Biologics Register. Ann Rheum Dis. 2013;72(2):229–34.
36. Van Dartel SAA, Fransen J, Kievit W, Flendrie M, Den Broeder AA, Visser H, et al. Difference in the risk of serious infections in patients with rheumatoid arthritis treated with adalimumab, infliximab and etanercept: results from the Dutch Rheumatoid Arthritis Monitoring (DREAM) registry. Ann Rheum Dis. 2013;72(6):895–900.
37. Doran MF, Crowson CS, Pond GR, O'Fallon WM, Gabriel SE. Frequency of infection in patients with rheumatoid arthritis compared with controls: a population-based study. Arthritis Rheum. 2002;46(9):2287–93.
38. Cao BL, Qasem A, Sharp RC, Abdelli LS, Naser SA. Systematic review and meta-analysis on the association of tuberculosis in Crohn's disease patients treated with tumor necrosis factor-α inhibitors (anti-TNFα). World J Gastroenterol. 2018;24(25):2764–75.

39. Ai JW, Zhang S, Ruan QL, Yu YQ, Zhang BY, Liu QH, et al. The risk of tuberculosis in patients with rheumatoid arthritis treated with tumor necrosis factor-α antagonist: a meta-analysis of both randomized controlled trials and registry/cohort studies. J Rheumatol. 2015;42(12):2229–37. [cited 2020 Oct 6]. https://pubmed.ncbi.nlm.nih.gov/26472414/.
40. Tubach F, Salmon D, Ravaud P, Allanore Y, Goupille P, Bréban M, et al. Risk of tuberculosis is higher with anti-tumor necrosis factor monoclonal antibody therapy than with soluble tumor necrosis factor receptor therapy: the three-year prospective French research axed on tolerance of biotherapies registry. Arthritis Rheum. 2009;60(7):1884–94. [cited 2020 Oct 10]. http://doi.wiley.com/10.1002/art.24632.
41. Zhang Z, Fan W, Yang G, Xu Z, Wang J, Cheng Q, et al. Risk of tuberculosis in patients treated with TNF-α antagonists: a systematic review and meta-analysis of randomised controlled trials. BMJ Open. 2017;7(3):e012567.
42. Winthrop KL, Chang E, Yamashita S, Iademarco MF, LoBue PA. Nontuberculous mycobacteria infections and anti-tumor necrosis factor-α therapy. Emerg Infect Dis. 2009;15(10):1556–61.
43. Winthrop KL, Baxter R, Liu L, Varley CD, Curtis JR, Baddley JW, et al. Mycobacterial diseases and antitumour necrosis factor therapy in USA. Ann Rheum Dis. 2013;72(1):37–42.
44. Toussi SS, Pan N, Walters HM, Walsh TJ. Infections in children and adolescents with juvenile idiopathic arthritis and inflammatory bowel disease treated with tumor necrosis factor-inhibitors: systematic review of the literature. Clin Infect Dis. 2013;57(9):1318–30.
45. Osterman MT, Sandborn WJ, Colombel JF, Peyrin-Biroulet L, Robinson AM, Zhou Q, et al. Crohn's disease activity and concomitant immunosuppressants affect the risk of serious and opportunistic infections in patients treated with adalimumab. Am J Gastroenterol. 2016;111(12):1806–15.
46. Strangfeld A, Eveslage M, Schneider M, Bergerhausen HJ, Klopsch T, Zink A, et al. Treatment benefit or survival of the fittest: what drives the time-dependent decrease in serious infection rates under TNF inhibition and what does this imply for the individual patient? Ann Rheum Dis. 2011;301(7):737–44.
47. Askling J, Fored CM, Brandt L, Baecklund E, Bertilsson L, Feltelius N, et al. Time-dependent increase in risk of hospitalisation with infection among Swedish RA patients treated with TNF antagonists. Ann Rheum Dis. 2007;66(10):1339–44.
48. Galloway JB, Hyrich KL, Mercer LK, Dixon WG, Fu B, Ustianowski AP, et al. Anti-TNF therapy is associated with an increased risk of serious infections in patients with rheumatoid arthritis especially in the first 6 months of treatment: updated results from the British Society for Rheumatology Biologics Register with special emph. Rheumatology. 2011;50(1):124–31.
49. Dommasch ED, Abuabara K, Shin DB, Nguyen J, Troxel AB, Gelfand JM. The risk of infection and malignancy with tumor necrosis factor antagonists in adults with psoriatic disease: a systematic review and meta-analysis of randomized controlled trials. J Am Acad Dermatol. 2011;64(6):1035–50.
50. Fouque-Aubert A, Jette-Paulin L, Combescure C, Basch A, Tebib J, Gossec L. Serious infections in patients with ankylosing spondylitis with and without TNF blockers: a systematic review and meta-analysis of randomised placebo-controlled trials. Ann Rheum Dis. 2010;69(10):1756–61.
51. Bonovas S, Fiorino G, Allocca M, Lytras T, Nikolopoulos GK, Peyrin-Biroulet L, et al. Biologic therapies and risk of infection and malignancy in patients with inflammatory bowel disease: a systematic review and network meta-analysis. Clin Gastroenterol Hepatol. 2016;14(10):1385–97.
52. Zhang D, Xiong B, Li X, Xu T, Yu M. Meta-analysis: serious adverse events in Crohn's disease patients treated with TNF-alpha inhibitors. Hepato-Gastroenterology. 2013;60(126):1333–42.
53. Galloway JB, Hyrich KL, Mercer LK, Dixon WG, Ustianowski AP, Helbert M, et al. Risk of septic arthritis in patients with rheumatoid arthritis and the effect of anti-TNF therapy: results from the British Society for Rheumatology Biologics Register. Ann Rheum Dis. 2011;70(10):1810–4.

54. Slifman NR, Gershon SK, Lee JH, Edwards ET, Braun MM. Listeria monocytogenes infection as a complication of treatment with tumor necrosis factor α-neutralizing agents. Arthritis Rheum. 2003;48(2):319–24.
55. Bodro M, Paterson DL. Listeriosis in patients receiving biologic therapies. Eur J Clin Microbiol Infect Dis. 2013;32(9):1225–30.
56. Peña-Sagredo JL, Hernández MV, Fernandez-Llanio N, Giménez-Ubeda E, Muñoz-Fernandez S, Ortiz A, et al. Listeria monocytogenes infection in patients with rheumatic diseases on TNF-alpha antagonist therapy: the Spanish Study Group experience. Clin Exp Rheumatol. 2008;26(5):854–9.
57. Lanternier F, Tubach F, Ravaud P, Salmon D, Dellamonica P, Bretagne S, et al. Incidence and risk factors of legionella pneumophila pneumonia during anti-tumor necrosis factor therapy: a prospective French study. Chest. 2013;144(3):990–8.
58. Kasahara S, Ando K, Saito K, Sekikawa K, Ito H, Ishikawa T, et al. Lack of tumor necrosis factor alpha induces impaired proliferation of hepatitis B virus-specific cytotoxic T lymphocytes. J Virol. 2003;77(4):2469–76.
59. Chyuan IT, Hsu PN. Tumor necrosis factor: the key to hepatitis B viral clearance. Cell Mol Immunol. 2018;15(8):731–3.
60. Terrault NA, Lok ASF, Mcmahon BJ, Chang K-M, Hwang JP, Jonas MM, et al. Update on prevention, diagnosis, and treatment of chronic hepatitis B: AASLD 2018 hepatitis B guidance American Association for the Study of Liver Diseases. Hepatology. 2018;67(4):1560–99.
61. Chung SJ, Kim JK, Park MC, Park YB, Lee SK. Reactivation of hepatitis B viral infection in inactive HBsAg carriers following anti-tumor necrosis factor-α therapy. J Rheumatol. 2009;36(11):2416–20.
62. Lan JL, Chen YM, Hsieh TY, Chen YH, Hsieh CW, Chen DY, et al. Kinetics of viral loads and risk of hepatitis B virus reactivation in hepatitis B core antibody-positive rheumatoid arthritis patients undergoing anti-tumour necrosis factor alpha therapy. Ann Rheum Dis. 2011;70(10):1719–25.
63. Pauly MP, Tucker LY, Szpakowski JL, Ready JB, Baer D, Hwang J, et al. Incidence of hepatitis B virus reactivation and hepatotoxicity in patients receiving long-term treatment with tumor necrosis factor antagonists. Clin Gastroenterol Hepatol. 2018;16(12):1964–73.
64. Lee YH, Bae SC, Song GG. Hepatitis B virus (HBV) reactivation in rheumatic patients with hepatitis core antigen (HBV occult carriers) undergoing anti-tumour necrosis factor therapy. Clin Exp Rheumatol. 2013;31(1):118–21.
65. Tamori A, Koike T, Goto H, Wakitani S, Tada M, Morikawa H, et al. Prospective study of reactivation of hepatitis B virus in patients with rheumatoid arthritis who received immunosuppressive therapy: evaluation of both HBsAg-positive and HBsAg-negative cohorts. J Gastroenterol. 2011;46(4):556–64.
66. Barone M, Notarnicola A, Lopalco G, Viggiani MT, Sebastiani F, Covelli M, et al. Safety of long-term biologic therapy in rheumatologic patients with a previously resolved hepatitis B viral infection. Hepatology. 2015;62(1):40–6.
67. Myint A, Tong MJ, Beaven SW. Reactivation of hepatitis B virus: a review of clinical guidelines. Clin Liver Dis. 2020;15(4):162–7.
68. Lopetuso LR, Mocci G, Marzo M, D'aversa F, Rapaccini GL, Guidi L, et al. Harmful effects and potential benefits of anti-tumor necrosis factor (TNF)-α on the liver. Int J Mol Sci. 2018;19(8):2199.
69. Iannone F, La Montagna G, Bagnato G, Gremese E, Giardina A, Lapadula G. Safety of etanercept and methotrexate in patients with rheumatoid arthritis and hepatitis C virus infection: a multicenter randomized clinical trial. J Rheumatol. 2014;41(2):286–92.
70. Pompili M, Biolato M, Miele L, Grieco A. Tumor necrosis factor-α inhibitors and chronic hepatitis C: a comprehensive literature review. World J Gastroenterol. 2013;19(44):7867–73.
71. Winthrop KL, Baddley JW, Chen L, Liu L, Grijalva CG, Delzell E, et al. Association between the initiation of anti-tumor necrosis factor therapy and the risk of herpes zoster. JAMA. 2013;309(9):887–95.

72. Strangfeld A, Listing J, Herzer P, Liebhaber A, Rockwitz K, Richter C, et al. Risk of herpes zoster in patients with rheumatoid arthritis treated with anti-TNF-α agents. JAMA. 2009;301(7):737–44.
73. Serac G, Tubach F, Mariette X, Salmon-Céron D, Ravaud P, Lioté F, et al. Risk of herpes zoster in patients receiving anti-TNF-α in the prospective French RATIO registry. J Invest Dermatol. 2012;132(3):726–9.
74. García-Doval I, Pérez-Zafrilla B, Descalzo MÁ, Roselló R, Hernández MV, Gómez-Reino JJ, et al. Incidence and risk of hospitalisation due to shingles and chickenpox in patients with rheumatic diseases treated with TNF antagonists. Ann Rheum Dis. 2010;69(10):1751–5.
75. Liao TL, Chen YM, Liu HJ, Chen DY. Risk and severity of herpes zoster in patients with rheumatoid arthritis receiving different immunosuppressive medications: a case-control study in Asia. BMJ Open. 2017;7(1):e014032.
76. Shalom G, Naldi L, Lebwohl M, Nikkels A, de Jong EMGJ, Fakharzadeh S, et al. Biological treatment for psoriasis and the risk of herpes zoster: results from the Psoriasis Longitudinal Assessment and Registry (PSOLAR). J Dermatolog Treat. 2019;30(6):534–9.
77. Lal H, Cunningham AL, Godeaux O, Chlibek R, Diez-Domingo J, Hwang S-J, et al. Efficacy of an adjuvanted herpes zoster subunit vaccine in older adults. N Engl J Med. 2015;372(22):2087–96.
78. Dagnew AF, Rausch D, Hervé C, Zahaf T, Levin MJ, Schuind A. Efficacy and serious adverse events profile of the adjuvanted recombinant zoster vaccine in adults with pre-existing potential immune-mediated diseases: a pooled post hoc analysis on two parallel randomized trials. Rheumatology. 2021;60:1226–33.
79. Dooling KL, Guo A, Patel M, Lee GM, Moore K, Belongia EA, et al. Recommendations of the Advisory Committee on Immunization Practices for use of herpes zoster vaccines. MMWR Morb Mortal Wkly Rep. 2018;67(3):103–8. [cited 2021 May 10]. http://www.cdc.gov/mmwr/volumes/67/wr/mm6703a5.htm?s_cid=mm6703a5_w.
80. Furer V, Rondaan C, Heijstek MW, Agmon-Levin N, Van Assen S, Bijl M, et al. 2019 update of EULAR recommendations for vaccination in adult patients with autoimmune inflammatory rheumatic diseases. Ann Rheum Dis. 2020;79(1):39–52.
81. Oxman MN, Levin MJ, Johnson GR, Schmader KE, Straus SE, Gelb LD, et al. A vaccine to prevent herpes zoster and postherpetic neuralgia in older adults. N Engl J Med. 2005;352(22):2271–84.
82. Schmader KE, Levin MJ, Gnann JW, McNeil SA, Vesikari T, Betts RF, et al. Efficacy, safety, and tolerability of herpes zoster vaccine in persons aged 50-59 years. Clin Infect Dis. 2012;54(7):922–8.
83. Filler SG, Yeaman MR, Sheppard DC. Tumor necrosis factor inhibition and invasive fungal infections. Clin Infect Dis. 2005;41(Suppl 3):S208–12.
84. Vergidis P, Avery RK, Wheat LJ, Dotson JL, Assi MA, Antoun SA, et al. Histoplasmosis complicating tumor necrosis factor-α blocker therapy: a retrospective analysis of 98 cases. Clin Infect Dis. 2015;61(3):409–17.
85. Wallis RS, Broder MS, Wong JY, Hanson ME, Beenhouwer DO. Granulomatous infectious diseases associated with tumor necrosis factor antagonists. Clin Infect Dis. 2004;38(9):1261–5.
86. Kaur N, Mahl TC. Pneumocystis jiroveci (carinii) pneumonia after infliximab therapy: a review of 84 cases. Dig Dis Sci. 2007;52(6):1481–4.
87. Harigai M, Koike R, Miyasaka N. Pneumocystis pneumonia associated with infliximab in Japan. N Engl J Med. 2007;357(18):1874–6.
88. Warris A, Bjørneklett A, Gaustad P. Invasive pulmonary aspergillosis associated with infliximab therapy. N Engl J Med. 2001;344(14):1099–100.
89. Baddley JW, Winthrop KL, Chen L, Liu L, Grijalva CG, Delzell E, et al. Non-viral opportunistic infections in new users of tumour necrosis factor inhibitor therapy: results of the SAfety assessment of biologic ThERapy (SABER) study. Ann Rheum Dis. 2014;73(11):1942–8.
90. Tsiodras S, Samonis G, Boumpas DT, Kontoyiannis DP. Fungal infections complicating tumor necrosis factor α blockade therapy. Mayo Clin Proc. 2008;83(2):181–94.

91. Wallis RS, Broder M, Wong J, Lee A, Hoq L. Reactivation of latent granulomatous infections by infliximab. Clin Infect Dis. 2005;41(Suppl 3):S194–8.
92. Bergstrom L, Yocum DE, Ampel NM, Villanueva I, Lisse J, Gluck O, et al. Increased risk of coccidioidomycosis in patients treated with tumor necrosis factor α antagonists. Arthritis Rheum. 2004;50(6):1956–66.
93. Taroumian S, Knowles SL, Lisse JR, Yanes J, Ampel NM, Vaz A, et al. Management of coccidioidomycosis in patients receiving biologic response modifiers or disease-modifying antirheumatic drugs. Arthritis Care Res. 2012;64(12):1903–9.
94. Olson TC, Bongartz T, Crowson CS, Roberts GD, Orenstein R, Matteson EL. Histoplasmosis infection in patients with rheumatoid arthritis, 1998-2009. BMC Infect Dis. 2011;11:145.
95. Takeuchi T, Tatsuki Y, Nogami Y, Ishiguro N, Tanaka Y, Yamanaka H, et al. Postmarketing surveillance of the safety profile of infliximab in 5000 Japanese patients with rheumatoid arthritis. Ann Rheum Dis. 2008;67(2):189–94.
96. Dixon WG, Watson K, Lunt M, Hyrich KL, Silman AJ, Symmons DPM. Rates of serious infection, including site-specific and bacterial intracellular infection, in rheumatoid arthritis patients receiving anti-tumor necrosis factor therapy: results from the British Society for Rheumatology Biologics Register. Arthritis Rheum. 2006;54(8):2368–76.
97. Louie GH, Wang Z, Ward MM. Trends in hospitalizations for Pneumocystis jiroveci pneumonia among patients with rheumatoid arthritis in the US: 1996-2007. Arthritis Care Res. 2010;62(12):3826–7.
98. Ferri C, Ferraccioli G, Ferrari D, Galeazzi M, Lapadula G, Montecucco C, et al. Safety of anti-tumor necrosis factor-α therapy in patients with rheumatoid arthritis and chronic hepatitis C virus infection. J Rheumatol. 2008;35(10):1944–9.

CD22, CD30, CD33, CD38, CD40, SLAMF-7 and CCR4

6

Lubos Drgona and Lucia Masarova

In this chapter, we describe observed infectious complications associated with the use of monoclonal antibodies (MoAb) against surface antigens CD22, CD30, CD33, CD38, CD40, SLAMF-7 (CD319), and CCR-4 predominantly in patients with hematologic malignancies. A summary of the infectious complications documented in randomized studies is presented in Table 6.1. Because of the shared presence of these antigens on various malignant cells and healthy immune system cells, infections associated with immunosuppression are often observed with these agents, and proper monitoring and prophylaxis are important aspects for their use in clinical practice. The overall risk of specific infections and proposed management is summarized in Table 6.2. We limit this chapter to unconjugated (or naked) and conjugated MoAb to toxins (antibody drug conjugates, ADC) as previously reviewed by the author [1]. ADC exploit the specific binding properties of MoAb for selective delivery of cytotoxic agents to tumor cells. There are three necessary components of ADC: the antibody, cytotoxic agent, and covalent linker [2]. This chapter does not cover bispecific MoAb (so called BiTEs) or chimeric antigen MoAb (CARTs), as they are analyzed in other chapters. The mechanisms of action of naked and conjugated targeted monoclonal antibodies revised in this chapter are schematically illustrated in Fig. 6.1.

L. Drgona (✉)
Department of Oncohematology, Comenius University and National Cancer Institute, Bratislava, Slovakia
e-mail: lubos.drgona@nou.sk

L. Masarova
Department of Leukemia, The University of Texas MD Anderson Cancer Center, Houston, TX, USA
e-mail: lmasarova@mdanderson.org

C. Cervera, J. M. Aguado (eds.), *Infectious Complications in Biologic and Targeted Therapies*, https://doi.org/10.1007/978-3-031-11363-5_6

Table 6.1 Summary of infectious complications in patients treated with agents targeting CD22, CD30, CD33, CD38, CD40, SLAMF7, and CCR4 (studies with control group)

Drug	Type of study [ref]	Treatment arms	No. of subjects	Rate of infections (drug vs. comparator)
Epratuzumab	Two phase 3 RCTs for SLE [6]	Epratuzumab (600 mg/m^2 weekly or 1200 mg/m^2 every 2 weeks) plus standard therapy vs. placebo plus standard therapy	1048 vs. 526	Overall infection: 52–61% vs. 60%; URTI: 12–15%vs. 11–14%; UTI: 10–14% vs. 11–18%; VZV: 1–4% vs. 2–3%
Inotuzumab ozogamicin	Phase 3 RCT for relapsed or refractory ALL [7]	Inotuzumab-ozogamicin vs. standard therapy	109 vs. 109	Febrile neutropenia (grade 3–4): 11% vs. 18%; pneumonia: 4% vs. 1%; sepsis: 2% vs. 5%; septic shock: 1% vs. 1%
Inotuzumab ozogamicin	Phase 2 study in newly diagnosed ALL in patients >60 years [9]	Standard therapy + inotuzumab ozogamicin vs. standard therapy	58 vs. 77	2 sepsis vs. 10 sepsis
Inotuzumab ozogamicin	Phase 3 RCT in relapsed or refractory ALL [8]	Inotuzumab-ozogamicin vs. standard therapy	164 vs. 143	Febrile neutropenia (all grades): 11.6% vs. 18.9%; sepsis 2.4% vs. 7.0%
Brentuximab vedotin	Phase 3 RCT for consolidation therapy after autologous HSCT in Hodgkin lymphoma [18, 66]	Brentuximab vs. placebo	167 vs. 160	Neutropenia:35% vs. 12%; URTI 26% vs. 23%; severe infection: 9% vs. 4%; VZV/HSV infection: 19 vs. 5 patients
Brentuximab vedotin	Phase 3 RCT in advanced stage Hodgkin lymphoma [16]	Brentuximab + chemotherapy vs. chemotherapy	664 vs. 670	Neutropenia (grade 3–4): 58% vs. 45%; febrile neutropenia: 9% vs. 4%
Brentuximab vedotin	Phase 3 RCT in CD30 + Peripheral T-cell lymphoma [17]	Brentuximab + chemotherapy vs. chemotherapy	226 vs. 226	Neutropenia: 35% vs. 34%; febrile neutropenia: 18% vs. 15%; infections grade 3–4: 19% vs. 14%
Gemtuzumab ozogamicin	RCTs for AML (pooled in: [1, 27])	Gemtuzumab + chemotherapy vs. chemotherapy	622 vs. 483	Serious infection (grade 3–4): 44% vs. 47%; febrile neutropenia:24% vs. 26%

Table 6.1 (continued)

Drug	Type of study [ref]	Treatment arms	No. of subjects	Rate of infections (drug vs. comparator)
Daratumumab	5 phase 3 RCTs in newly diagnosed or relapse/refractory myeloma [38]	Daratumumab + standard treatment vs. standard treatment	Total 3547	Infection (any grade): 58% vs. 48%; pneumonia (any grade): 12.6% vs. 7.7%; neutropenia (grade 3–4): RR 1.48(95% CI: 1.17–1.88, $p = 0.001$)
Isatuximab	2 RCTs in relapsed/refractory myeloma [42, 43]	Isatuximab + standard treatment vs. standard treatment	154 vs. 153; 179 vs. 123	URTI (any grade): 28% vs. 17%; URTI (grade 3–4): 3% vs. 1% and 32% vs. 28%)
Dacetuzumab	Phase 2 RCT in relapsed non-Hodgkin lymphoma [50]	Dacetuzumab + chemotherapy vs. placebo + chemotherapy	75 vs. 76	Neutropenia (grade 3–4): 33% vs. 24%; febrile neutropenia (grade 3–4): 16% vs. 9%
Eltuzumab	Phase 3 RCT in relapsed/refractory myeloma [56]	Elotuzumab + lenalidomide and dexamtehasone vs. lenalidomide and dexamethasone	321 vs. 325	Overall infection:81% vs. 74%; lymphopenia (grade 3–4): 77% vs. 49%; VZV: 4.1 vs. 2.2 per 100 pts-years
Elotuzumab	Phase 3 RCT in relapsed/refractory myeloma [57]	Elotuzumab + pomalidomide and dexamethasone vs. pomalidomide and dexamethasone	60 vs. 57	Overall infection (all grades): 65% vs. 65%; lymphopenia (grade 3–4): 8% vs. 2%; VZV infection (all grades): 5% vs. 2%
Mogamulizumab	Phase 2 RCT in adult T-cell leukemia/lymphoma [61]	Mogamulizumab + chemotherapy vs. chemotherapy	29 vs. 24	Overall infection: 66% vs. 67%; febrile neutropenia: 90% vs. 88%; lymphopenia (grade 3–4): 97% vs. 75%; CMV infection:14% vs. 0%
Mogamulizumab	Phase 3 RCT in relapsed cutaneous T-cell lymphoma [63]	Mogamulizumab vs. vorinostat	184 vs. 186	URTI (any grade): 10% vs. 5%; pneumonia: 6% vs. 3%; cellulitis: 4% vs. 5%

ALL acute lymphoblastic leukemia, *AML* acute myeloblastic leukemia, *CMV* cytomegalovirus, *HBV* hepatitis B virus, *HL* Hodgkin lymphoma, *HSCT* hematopoietic stem cell transplantation, *HSV* herpes simplex virus, *PjP Pneumocystis jirovecii* pneumonia; RCT, randomized clinical trial; RR, relative risk; SLE, systemic lupus erythematosus; URTI, upper respiratory tract infection; UTI, urinary tract infection; VZV, varicella zoster virus

Table 6.2 Summary of risk of infectious complications and suggested management strategies (adapted from [1, 64, 65])

Agent	Risk of neutropenia/ febrile neutropenia	Risk of HSV/ VZV infection /reactivation	Risk of HBV reactivation (if used without prophylaxis)	Risk of CMV infection	Risk of PjP infection	Other infections to be considered	Recommended prophylaxis
Epratuzumab	No/no	No	Low (<1%) to moderate (1–10%)	No	No	–	HBV prophylaxis or preemptive treatment in patients at risk
Inotuzumab ozogamicin	Yes/yes	No	Low (<1%) to moderate (1–10%)	No	Yes—in ALL patients with prolonged neutropenia	–	HBV prophylaxis or preemptive treatment in patients at risk
Brentuximab vedotin	Yes/yes (low)	Yes	Moderate (1–10%)	Yes	Yes—in HL patients after HSCT	PML	HSV/VZV prophylaxis in HL patients after HSCT; CMV monitoring; HBV prophylaxis or preemptive treatment in patients at risk
Gemtuzumab ozogamicin	Yes/yes	No	Low (<1%)	No	No	Prolonged neutropenia-related infections	Standard prophylaxis in AML patients during therapy
Daratumumab	Yes/yes	Yes	Moderate (1–10%)	No	No	–	HSV/VZV prophylaxis; HBV prophylaxis or preemptive treatment in patients at risk
Isatuximab	Yes/yes	Yes	Moderate (1–10%) to high (>10%)	No	No	–	HSV/VZV prophylaxis; HBV prophylaxis or preemptive treatment in patients at risk
Dacetuzumab	Yes/yes	Possible	Possible	Possible	Possible	–	According to individual risk

Elotuzumab	Yes/yes (low)	Yes	Possible	No	No	Lymphopenia-related infections	HSV/VZV prophylaxis; other prophylaxis according to individual risk
Mogamulizumab	Yes/yes	Yes	Moderate (1–10%) to high (>10%)	Yes	Possible	Lymphopenia-related infections	HSV/VZV prophylaxis; HBV prophylaxis or preemptive treatment in patients at risk, CMV monitoring; PjP prophylaxis

ALL acute lymphoblastic leukemia, *AML* acute myeloblastic leukemia, *CMV* cytomegalovirus, *HBV* hepatitis B virus, *HL* Hodgkin lymphoma, *HSCT* hematopoietic stem cell transplantation, *HSV* herpes simplex virus, *PjP Pneumocystis jirovecii* pneumonia, *PML* progressive multifocal leucoencephalopathy, *VZV* varicella zoster virus

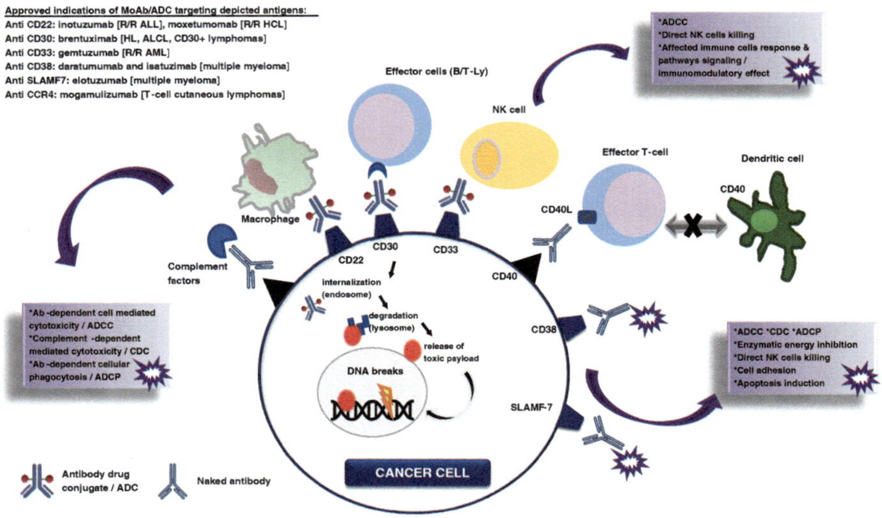

Fig. 6.1 Mechanism of action of naked and conjugated targeted monoclonal antibodies targeting CD22, CD30, CD33, CD38, CD40, SLAMF7, and CCR4. Antibodies can promote antitumor activity against cancer cells in a variety of ways: antibody-dependent cell-mediated cytotoxicity via recruitment of effector cells (ADCC), antibody-dependent cellular phagocytosis through macrophages or complement leading to cell lysis (ADCP), complement-mediated cytotoxicity (CDC), inhibition of enzymatic functions of cells via adenosine (ADP/NAD+), through NK cells with direct killing, antibody cross linking, alteration of effector cell response utilizing immunomodulating effect, via programmed cell death/induction of apoptosis. Most antibodies have multilevel activity (especially anti-CD38 and SLAMF-7). Anti-CD40 and SLAMF-7 antibodies also affect microenvironment and effective adhesion between myeloma cells or adhesion to bone marrow stroma (not shown in the figure). Major effect of ADC is to deliver toxic payload into nucleus leading to DNA disruption and subsequent cell death. *MoAb* monoclonal antibody, *ADC* antibody-drug conjugate, *R/R* relapsed/refractory, *ALL* acute lymphoid leukemia, *AML* acute myeloid leukemia, *HCL* hairy cell leukemia, *HL* Hodgkin lymphoma, *ALCL* anaplastic large cell lymphoma

CD22-Targeted Agents: Epratuzumab, Inotuzumab Ozogamicin, Moxetumomab Pasudotox

CD22 Antigen

CD22 antigen is a transmembrane glycoprotein expressed solely on mature B-cells including neoplastic blast cells (leukemia, lymphoma). Hematopoietic stem cells or other cell-lineages do not express CD22. CD22 receptor regulates B-cell functions and their responses to antigens via B-cell receptor activation and associated signaling pathways, serves as an adhesion molecule, plays important role in the migration of B-cells into gut lymphoid tissues and bone marrow, and as an important inhibitory receptor regulates induction of autoimmunity [3].

Mechanism of Action and Current Indications of Anti-CD22 Monoclonal Antibodies

The first fully humanized IgG1 MoAb targeting CD22 was epratuzumab. Upon administration and rapid internalization, epratuzumab causes phosphorylation of CD22 and downstream signaling molecules, but it does not block CD22 ligand binding, does not initiate CD22-mediated signal transduction or apoptosis, and does not demonstrate any direct cytotoxicity [4]. It has been studied for the treatment of non-Hodgkin lymphoma (NHL), acute lymphoblastic leukemia (ALL), and autoimmune Sjogren's syndrome and systemic lupus erythematosus (SLE). The drug does not hold any current approved indication.

Inotuzumab ozogamicin (inotuzumab) is a humanized anti-CD22 IgG4 ADC linked to a potent cytotoxin, calicheamicin, an antibiotic product of *Micromonospora echinospora calichensis*. Upon antibody binding to CD22 antigen on the B-cell surface, the complex is internalized via endocytosis; calicheamicin is released intracellularly and by causing DNA strand cleavage leads to cell apoptosis. Inotuzumab is used for the treatment of relapsed or refractory (R/R) adult precursor B-ALL and is under investigation for the treatment of B-ALL in pediatric patients. Off-label use was studied in aggressive and indolent NHLs.

Moxetumomab pasudotox is a recombinant, genetically fused immunotoxin, consisting of variable fragment of anti-CD22 MoAb and 38-kDa fragment of *Pseudomonas* exotoxin (PE38) as an innovative, linker-less ADC. Binding of this complex to the CD22 antigen leads to internalization and toxin release, which induce a cascade of apoptosis. It is approved for the treatment of R/R hairy cell leukemia. It has been evaluated for patients with NHL, ALL, and chronic lymphocytic leukemia (CLL), but further development for these indications was terminated.

Clinical Evidence

Clinical trials with epratuzumab, which was extensively evaluated in patients with autoimmune SLE and to a lesser extend in patients with R/R lymphoid malignancies, did not show an increased rate of infectious complications [5, 6].

Monotherapy with inotuzumab (vs. standard intensive chemotherapy) in the phase 3 randomized clinical trial (RCT) in patients with B-ALL showed similar rate of neutropenia, but lower rate of grade ≥3 febrile neutropenia (~15%) and overall infections [7]. Long-term follow-up of this study confirmed a high rate of neutropenia (~45%), but a lower rate of febrile neutropenia with inotuzumab in comparison with intense chemotherapy (27% vs. 54%, respectively) and no increased risk of invasive fungal infections [8]. In combination with low-intensity chemotherapy and/or CD19 MoAb blinatumumab, inotuzumab showed a lower risk of infection in older frail patients (including death due to sepsis) than standard intensive chemotherapy [9]. Therapy with inotuzumab, as opposed to intensive chemotherapy, was associated with higher incidence of febrile neutropenia only in patients with higher percentage of blasts (>90%) in bone marrow, whereas it remained high, irrespectively of blasts percent, with intensive chemotherapy. The grade of bone marrow leukemic involvement had no impact on the overall incidence of neutropenia and infections, including sepsis [10]. Children with R/R ALL treated with inotuzumab also had low rate of febrile neutropenia (12%) or overall infections (22% of grade ≥3) [11].

Moxetumomab pasudotox was the first recombinant antibody globally approved ADC for the treatment of R/R hairy cell leukemia. Pivotal phase 3 nonrandomized trial documented 16% grade ≥3 infections and 5% grade ≥3 febrile neutropenia [12].

Risk of Infections and Its Management

Administration of epratuzumab and inotuzumab is followed by a decrease of circulating and proliferating CD22+ B- cells for up to 12 months after the last dose. Long-term B- cell depletion was not documented after moxetumomab pasudotox. Therapy with these agents appear to cause neither significant decline of serum immunoglobulin levels nor significant increased risk of severe infections.

Similar mechanism of action to other targeted therapies focused on B-lymphocytes (like anti-CD20 MoAb, e.g., rituximab), and available clinical data may suggest the following conclusions and proposals for prevention:

- Generally, the risk of infections in patients treated with anti-CD22 agents is relatively low; usually the infection risk is determined by the underlying hematological malignancy, comorbid conditions, age, and concomitant therapy.
- Risk of infection should be individually evaluated in patients treated with anti-CD22 agents; universal antibacterial, antifungal (including anti-*Pneumocystis jirovecii*), or antiviral prophylaxis is not recommended, but prophylaxis should be individualized (e.g., patient with R/R ALL treated with inotuzumab with expected prolonged neutropenia).
- Given that anti-CD22 agents lead to depletion of all CD22+ B-lymphocytes, this therapy might be associated with reactivation of hepatitis B virus. Proper monitoring and prophylaxis is thus recommended in patients with hepatitis B surface antigen (HBsAg), and anti-HBc should be checked and confirmed by PCR DNA for HBV viral load; antiviral prophylaxis or therapy with tenofovir or entecavir-based regimens is recommended. Periodical monitoring of HBV DNA with preemptive antiviral treatment in patients who are HBsAg negative but anti-HBc-positive is also an alternative.

CD30-Targeted Agents: Brentuximab Vedotin

CD30 Antigen

CD30 is a 120-kDa transmembrane glycoprotein and a member of the tumor necrosis factor receptor superfamily. CD30 has a low level of expression in normal cells, mainly on subsets of activated T-cells (CD4 and CD8-positive) and B-cells, monocytes, and NK cells. Its ligand, CD30L, is more widely expressed on cells of the lymphoid and myeloid lineage. CD30 expression is also ubiquitously expressed on certain malignant cells, such as on Reed-Sternberg cells, the pathognomonic diagnostic cells for classical Hodgkin lymphoma (HL), and in anaplastic large cell lymphoma (ALCL). The full biological functions of CD30 on immune system are less understood than its role in tumorigenesis; but its complex effect involves downstream signaling via nuclear factor kappa B and mitogen-activated protein kinase/extracellular signal-regulated kinase pathways as well as regulation of the balance between Th1 and Th2 responses and generation of effector and memory T-cells [13].

Mechanism of Action and Current Indications for CD30 Monoclonal Antibodies

Brentuximab vedotin (brentuximab) is an ADC composed of a human/murine chimeric anti-CD30 IgG1 MoAb conjugated via a protease-cleavable linker with the microtubule disrupting agent monomethyl auristatin E (MMAE), a synthetic derivative of a natural cytostatic pseudopeptide originally isolated from the marine mollusk *Dorabella auricularia* [14]. Upon binding to CD30 on the surface of the T-lymphocyte, the drug is internalized by endocytosis and then the proteolytic enzymes cleave linkage and monomethyl auristatin A is released in the intracellular space, binds to tubulin, and by disruption on microtubules causes cell cycle arrest. The FDA (Federal Drug Administration) and EMA (European Medical Agency) approved brentuximab for the treatment of R/R HL, for consolidation therapy in patients with HL with high risk of relapse or progression after autologous stem cell transplantation, for newly diagnosed HL in combination with chemotherapy, and for CD30+ relapsed primary cutaneous ALCL or CD30+ mycosis fungoides.

Clinical Evidence

Monotherapy with brentuximab in patients with R/R HL and ALCL in phase 2 studies showed no specific infectious complications, and incidence of grade ≥3 neutropenia in 20–29% of participants [15]. The incidence of neutropenia was higher when brentuximab was administered in combination with chemotherapy. In phase 3 RCT comparing brentuximab + chemotherapy (AVD) to standard chemotherapy (ABVD) for the treatment of advanced stages HL, brentuximab was associated with higher risk of grade ≥3 neutropenia (58% vs. 45%, respectively) and with higher incidence of febrile neutropenia (9% vs. 4%, respectively) [16]. Phase 3 RCT, which compared brentuximab + chemotherapy (CHP) to standard chemotherapy (CHOP) in patients with untreated CD30+ peripheral T-cell lymphoma, showed similar rate of neutropenia between both arms (35% and 34%, respectively), which could have been reduced by the use of primary prophylaxis with granulocyte-colony stimulating factor (13% for both arms). The study also showed comparable rate of febrile neutropenia (18% vs. 15%) and grade ≥3 infections (19% vs. 14%) for brentuximab + CHP vs. CHOP, respectively [17]. Consolidation therapy with brentuximab in patients with high risk of relapse or progression of HL after autologous transplantation in a phase 3 RTC was associated with higher rate of neutropenia (35% vs. 12% in placebo arm, respectively) but only one case of febrile neutropenia. Treatment-related adverse events later reported by Nademanee [18] showed infections in 60% and 50% of patients treated with brentuximab vs. placebo, respectively (serious infections in 9% and 4%, respectively). Herpetic infections (VZV and HSV) were more frequent in brentuximab-treated patients than in the placebo arm (total 19 vs. 5 patients for brentuximab vs. placebo, respectively), but only once infection in each subgroup was of grade 3. VZV infections were also observed in patients on antiviral prophylaxis, but they occurred later when compared to patients without prophylaxis (median time to development of VZV from brentuximab was 200 days vs. 89 days with and without prophylaxis, respectively). Other opportunistic infections were not different between arms, and only one case of *Pneumocystis* pneumonia occurred in a patient noncompliant with recommended prophylaxis.

Severe CMV retinitis was observed after brentuximab treatment of CD30+ lymphomas. All cases were successfully treated with antivirals, but after brentuximab rechallenge, CMV infection relapsed, emphasizing the need of secondary CMV prophylaxis in case of continuation of brentuximab treatment [19]. CMV reactivation has been reported in 5 of 25 patients receiving brentuximab therapy for the relapse of HL after allogeneic hematopoietic transplantation, but only one patient presented with significant organ involvement [20]. The overall risk for CMV reactivation with brentuximab is considered low [21].

Progressive multifocal leukoencephalopathy (PML) is a rare but devastating neurological consequence of John Cunningham polyomavirus (JCV) infection in immunocompromised patients. PML after use of brentuximab has been reported in few case reports in patients with hematological malignancies. The duration of previous therapy before symptoms onset was shorter in cases of brentuximab-related PML (median of 6–9 weeks) than anti-CD20 MoAb-related PML (e.g., rituximab; median 63 weeks). The establishment of specific drug–disease causality is not easy, if even possible, because of disease-specific immune dysregulation in these patients and often sequential or concomitant use of various drugs. The exact role of brentuximab in the pathogenesis of PML is difficult to determine, but depletion of CD30-activated T-cells may reduce immune surveillance in central nervous system increasing the risk of PML [22]. A black box warning was inserted in the drug label in 2012.

There is a lack of clinical information regarding the risk of HBV reactivation in patients treated with brentuximab. However, the risk of HBV reactivation associated with brentuximab is estimated to be moderate (1 to <10%) taking other B-cell targeting agents as reference [23].

Risk of Infections and Its Management

The impact of brentuximab on immune system is poorly understood, but the effect on memory cells and impaired regulation of T/T-B cells is expected due to targeted antibody-dependent cell-mediated cytotoxicity (ADCC). Brentuximab also causes temporary neutropenia, which is especially important in patients with R/R disease and those after stem cell transplantation [21].

Recent knowledge and available clinical data offer the following suggestions and recommendations:

- The overall risk of infection in patients treated with brentuximab is similar to the risk in lymphoma patients per se. However, some increased risk may be possible in specific circumstances.
- Brentuximab-related neutropenia is a relatively common complication but carrying a relatively low risk of febrile neutropenia. Primary prophylaxis with G-CSF may be considered according to the patient's profile.
- No routine systemic antimicrobial prophylaxis is recommended; however, consider administration of anti-herpesvirus and anti-*Pneumocystis jirovecii* prophylaxis in patients receiving brentuximab for consolidation treatment after autologous hematopoietic stem cell transplantation.
- CMV monitoring is advisable in CMV seropositive patients during brentuximab therapy, especially in cases with symptoms compatible with CMV disease; in the case of previous CMV infection, secondary CMV prophylaxis is advisable if brentuximab is resumed.
- The risk of hepatitis B reactivation with brentuximab is moderate; screening for HBV is recommended before treatment in all patients with hematological malignancies; adequate management of HBsAg positive and anti-HBc positive is recommended, and these patients should receive appropriate prophylaxis.
- High alertness to PML is needed despite its rarity; the onset of neurological symptoms (except typical polyneuropathy) during brentuximab treatment should lead to drug discontinuation and appropriate diagnostic procedures.

CD33-Targeted Agents: Gemtuzumab Ozogamicin, Vadastuximab Talirine

CD33 Antigen

CD33 is a member of the sialic acid-binding immunoglobulin-like lectin (Siglec) family. While hematopoietic progenitor cells, myeloid cells, and monocytes (i.e., tissue macrophages, mast cells, and myeloid dendritic cells) express CD33, it has minor expression on granulocytes as well. CD33 antigen is expressed on the surface of leukemic blasts in more than 80% of cases of acute myeloid leukemia (AML) [24].

Mechanism of Action and Current Indications of Anti-CD33 Monoclonal Antibodies

Gemtuzumab ozogamicin (gemtuzumab) was the first to be approved by ADC for the use of patients with hematological malignancy. It is built with a humanized anti-CD33 immunoglobulin [Ig]G4 MoAb, a pH-sensitive hydrazone linker, and a calicheamicin derivative conjugated with the side chain reactive lysine residues of MoAb. The anti-CD33 antibody, lacking cytotoxic activity by itself, binds to the CD33 antigen, leading to internalization and release of the calicheamicin derivative into the leukemic cell. Initially, the drug was approved as a monotherapy for elderly patients with R/R AML. After subsequent studies in combination with chemotherapy, the drug showed excessive toxicity and was temporarily withdrawn from the market. Gemtuzumab was reapproved by the FDA and EMA after additional studies proved its efficacy and acceptable safety in 2017 and 2018. Currently, gemtuzumab is approved in newly diagnosed adult patients with CD33+ AML, in monotherapy for patients over the age of 2 with R/R CD33+ AML, and in combination with chemotherapy for CD33+ AML in 1 month or older pediatric patients (reviewed [25]). Gemtuzumab also showed promising results in patients with acute promyelocytic leukemia and is being used off-label for this indication. Among novel agents using conjugation with CD33 target, only vadastuximab talirine (SGN-CD33A) was evaluated in a phase 3 RCT. SGN-CD33A represents a novel anti-CD33 ADC conjugated to two molecules of pyrrolobenzodiazepine dimers via a protease-cleavable maleimidocaproyl-valinealanine dipeptide linker on engineered cysteine residues. This engineering technique creates a highly homogenous ADC with a controlled drug–antibody ratio, which should lead to greater stability in circulation and potentially lower off-target toxicity compared to gemtuzumab [26].

Clinical Evidence

Most clinical data on gemtuzumab come from combination studies where the agent was administered with approved anti-leukemic chemotherapies. Clinically relevant hematologic grade ≥3 adverse events in the early monotherapy trials included neutropenia and thrombocytopenia at rates of 34% and 22%, respectively. Subsequent monotherapy trials evidenced between 16% and 18% rates of febrile neutropenia and 35% and 39% rates of overall infections (reviewed [26]). Myelosuppression, notably persistent neutropenia and thrombocytopenia, remained the most common adverse event in all gemtuzumab clinical studies, including RCT. The incidence of grade ≥3 febrile neutropenia and infections ranged between 52–75% and 35–78%, respectively. Because gemtuzumab was used in combination with other antileukemic agents, the exact role of the agent in these side effects is hard to ascertain, but the duration of neutropenia, rate of infectious complications, febrile neutropenia and deaths due to infections were comparable across many clinical trials between patients treated with or without gemtuzumab [27]. The safety profile of gemtuzumab in pediatric patients did not differ from reports from adults [26, 28]. There were no specific infections reported, but one anecdotal case of PML was documented in a patient after allogeneic stem cell transplantation who was previously treated with gemtuzumab [29]. The novel CD33-targeted agent, SGN-CD33A, has available data from clinical trials in patients with R/R and newly diagnosed AML, including phase 3 RTC. Phase 1–2 studies showed acceptable mortality rates (<10%), but profound myelosuppression was observed in virtually all patients (with a median of occurrence between 6 and 10 weeks). A phase 3 RTC (CASCADE) compared a hypomethylating agent with or without SGN-CD33A in elderly patients with newly diagnosed AML and was prematurely terminated due to high mortality rate (including fatal infections) in the SGN-CD33A arm [30].

Risk of Infection and Its Management

As CD33 is widely expressed on bone marrow cells, the cytotoxic effect of CD33-targeted drugs leads to profound myelosuppression, including frequent severe neutropenia. The incidence of infections is closely related to the depth and length of neutropenia. The expected spectrum of infections is similar to that observed in the population of patients with AML, and appropriate preventive strategies need to be implemented throughout the entire induction and consolidation therapy.

Suggestions and recommendations:

- The specific risk of CD33-targeted agents on infection is not fully established, but available data evidenced the myelosuppressive effect of gemtuzumab and new members of this group.
- Due to the well-defined risk of infections in patients with AML on therapy, standard prophylactic strategies should be administered.

CD38-Targeted Agents: Daratumumab, Isatuximab

CD38 Antigens

The human CD38 antigen is a 46-kDa multifunctional transmembrane protein that is widely expressed early in the differentiation of CD34+ stem cells and mature immune cells, including activated T and B lymphocytes, granulocytes, monocytes, macrophages, and NK cells. CD38 is an immune-modulatory molecule; it plays an important role in the transduction of activating signals mediated by major receptor complexes in a wide variety of immune cells, especially regulatory B-cells and NK cells, regulates cell adhesion, including regulation of mesenchymal stromal or myeloid-derived suppressor cells, and plays a critical part in extracellular nucleotide homeostasis. Although CD38 is essential for an effective immune response, it might also enhance the immunosuppressive potential of regulatory lymphocytes [31]. Virtually all myeloma cells express high levels of CD38 on their surface, similar to normal plasma cells, but the expression on normal lymphoid or myeloid cells is low. Therefore, CD38 represents an attractive therapeutic target especially for multiple myeloma.

Mechanism of Action and Current Indications of Anti-CD38 Monoclonal Antibodies

Daratumumab is a fully human IgG1 kappa MoAb targeting CD38, leading to elimination of CD38+ malignant cells via different mechanisms, including complement-dependent cytotoxicity, ADCC, and antibody-dependent phagocytosis. Daratumumab is approved by the FDA and EMA for the treatment of R/R multiple myeloma in adult patients, either in monotherapy or in combination with bortezomib and dexamethasone or lenalidomide and dexamethasone, and for newly diagnosed multiple myeloma patients as part of multiple drug regimens (triplets or quadruplets).

Isatuximab is a chimeric mouse/human anti-CD38 IgG1 MoAb with different mechanisms of action as daratumumab; it mostly leads to ADCC and inhibition of ectoenzyme activity of CD38+ cells. It holds approval for R/R multiple myeloma in the combination with pomalidomide and dexamethasone, but multiple clinical studies evaluating its full efficacy are currently ongoing.

Clinical Evidence

Monotherapy with daratumumab in phase 2 studies was associated with low rate of grade ≥3 neutropenia (10%) and <1% rate of severe upper respiratory infections. As expected, its use in combination with other anti-myeloma agents showed higher incidence of infectious complications. Two pivotal studies with daratumumab in combination with doublets (dexamethasone and one other anti-myeloma agent) for the treatment of R/R disease showed comparable incidence of grade ≥3 infections in 20–30% of patients on therapy with and without daratumumab and similar rate of grade ≥3 pneumonia in 9% of patients (all arms). Neutropenia grade 3 or higher occurred in 13% and 52% and in 4% and 37% of patients treated with daratumumab versus the comparator arm, respectively. The rate of febrile neutropenia grade 3 or higher was relatively low, but slightly increased in the daratumumab arms (~6%) versus comparator arms (2–3%) [32, 33]. In patients with newly diagnosed myeloma, RCTs with daratumumab used in combination (doublets) showed that the incidence of neutropenia grade 3 or higher and infections grade 3 or higher was higher with daratumumab versus without it (up to 50% vs. ~35%, respectively, in the case of neutropenia; 32% vs. 23%, respectively, in the case of infections). Likewise, the rate of the pneumonia was higher with daratumumab (13% vs. 7% without it, respectively) [34]. Similarly, RTC with daratumumab added to triplets (dexamethasone, bortezomib, and melphalan) in newly diagnosed patients, evidenced higher incidence of infections grade 3 or higher (23.1% vs.14.7%) and severe pneumonia (11.3% vs. 4.0%, respectively) with daratumumab vs. without it [35], but the overall incidence of these complications did not differ from RTC where daratumumab was used in combinations with less agents (doublets). RTC using triplets with and without daratumumab in transplant-eligible patients showed again that daratumumab therapy had higher incidence of all infections (upper respiratory tract as the most common), and of neutropenia grade 3 or higher (~30% vs. 15% without daratumumab, respectively), but the incidence of severe, infections grade 3 or higher was comparable (~20% in all groups, grade 3 pneumonia in 4% vs. 2% of patients, respectively) [36, 37]. A meta-analysis of five phase 3 RCTs (including 3547 patients) evaluating the incidence of neutropenia, infection and pneumonia in patients with myeloma treated with daratumumab concluded that patients on daratumumab combination regimens experienced higher risk of all grades neutropenia with an RR of 1.48 (95% CI: 1.17–1.88; $p = 0.001$) [38]. The addition of daratumumab contributed to higher incidence of infections of all grades and of infections grade 3 or higher with RR of 1.27 (95% CI: 1.13–1.44; $p = 0.02$), including pneumonia grade 3 or higher (RR 2.07, 95% CI: 1.50–2.85, $p < 0.001$) in newly diagnosed patients with multiple myeloma [39].

Isatuximab was evaluated in phase 2 studies in patients with R/R multiple myeloma with a rate of pneumonia and sepsis of 6.3% and 5.2%, respectively, in patients on monotherapy, while pneumonia was documented in 9% of patients receiving isatuximab in combination (with doublets) [40, 41]. In two RCT evaluating isatuximab in combinations (with doublets), the rate of neutropenia grade 3 or higher was around 46% on isatuximab, and although the frequency of upper respiratory tract infections of any grade was higher with isatuximab compared to the control arm (28% vs. 17% [42], it was similar for upper respiratory infections grade 3 or higher (3% vs. 1% in one study [42] and 32% vs. 28% in other study [43]).

In general, patients with multiple myeloma have sevenfold increased risk of all infections, and up to tenfold higher risk of viral infections, especially by herpesviruses (VZV) [44]. The incidence of VZV in the pivotal studies of daratumumab in R/R myeloma ranged between 2% and 5%. This observation was subsequently confirmed in various retrospective studies, where most of the reported infections were viral, including herpesvirus reactivation, CMV retinitis, enterocolitis, CMV syndrome, and HSV encephalitis. Coinfections with bacterial and viral pathogens are not unusual in the real-life setting. Daratumumab is associated with moderate (<1% to <10%) reactivation risk of HBV [45].

Risk of Infection and Its Management

Anti-CD38 agents' targets deplete also normal CD38+ immune regulatory cells, including NK cells, skew the T-cell repertoire and promote T-cells expansion (e.g., oligoclonality of CD4+ and CD8+ T lymphocytes), which leads to an ineffective antiviral innate and adaptive immunity [46]. Studies have reported an increased risk of infections in multiple myeloma patients undergoing therapy with daratumumab, with a higher rate of infections in severely immunocompromised patients: those with R/R or progressive disease, and during and after stem cell transplantation. The infectious complications associated with isatuximab in combination with standard of care therapies demonstrated minimal increase of severe toxicity to the known safety profile of the individual agents.

Still, the cumulative effect of novel agents may play a role in an increased rate of specific infections when compared with conventional treatment. The risk of infectious complications in patients with multiple myeloma should be considered during the whole disease course and close attention shall be paid to those after multiple lines of therapies.

Suggestions and recommendations:

- Considering the drug-associated risk for anti-CD38 agents, both daratumumab and isatuximab carry low-level additive risk for overall infections. Notwithstanding, better identification of patients at risk is needed, and evaluating the immunological profile and subsets of functional immune cells could serve this purpose.
- Increased risk of viral infections, especially VZV, is present in patients with multiple myeloma treated with anti-CD38 agents. Previous or concurrent treatment with corticosteroids and proteasome inhibitors may further potentiate the risk. VZV and HSV prophylaxis is recommended in patients treated with daratumumab. Antiviral prophylaxis (acyclovir or valacyclovir) to prevent VZV reactivation should be initiated within 1 week after starting daratumumab and continued for 3 months following treatment. Anti-myeloma agents may pose an increased risk for CMV reactivation, but according to the available data there is no excess of CMV infections after therapy with daratumumab and isatuximab.
- Hepatitis B reactivation risk for daratumumab is moderate. Screening for HBV is recommended before treatment for all patients with hematological malignancies and should be done before the administration of daratumumab. Adequate management of HBsAg positive and anti-HBc positive patients is recommended.
- Seasonal influenza vaccination should be encouraged in patients treated with daratumumab.

CD40 Targeted Agents: Selicrelumab, Dacetuzumab, Lucatumumab

CD40 Antigen

CD40 is a cell surface molecule of the tumor necrosis factor receptor family. Under physiological conditions, CD40 is expressed on antigen-presenting cells, for example, myeloid and dendritic cells, and is responsible for their activation and proliferation (e.g., upregulation of costimulatory molecules [CD58, CD80/86, CD70] and downregulation of immunosuppressive molecules [PD-L1]). CD40 expression can also be found on platelets, fibroblasts, epithelial and endothelial cells, and hematopoietic progenitors. The natural ligand for CD40, (CD40L), is expressed on activated CD4+ T-cells, B cells, NK cells, and on memory CD8+ T cells. The interaction between CD40 and CD40L is critical for the regulation of immune responses including antigen-specific activation of naïve B and T cells, class switching and affinity maturation of immunoglobulins, secretion of cytokines, and development of memory cells [47]. CD40 expression was detected in various solid and hematologic malignancies (e.g., Hodgkin and non-Hodgkin lymphomas, Burkitt lymphoma, and multiple myeloma) altering immune systemic responses and allowing tumor cells escape [48].

Mechanism of Action, Approved Indications and Off-Labels Use of CD40 Monoclonal Antibodies

Few anti-CD40 MoAb were tested in patients with solid (selicrelumab) or hematologic malignancies (lucatumumab, dacetumumab), but none of these agents is currently approved or planned to enter phase 3 clinical trials. Lucatumumab and dacetumumab were evaluated in early phase studies for patients with R/R lymphomas, multiple myeloma and CLL, but further development was halted (reviewed [49]).

Clinical Evidence

Prolonged lymphocytopenia was observed after treatment with selicrelumab. During the phase 2 RCT of dacetuzumab + chemotherapy vs. chemotherapy alone in patients with R/R aggressive lymphoma, the rate of neutropenia and febrile neutropenia was higher in dacetuzumab (neutropenia grade 3 or higher of 33% vs. 24%, and febrile neutropenia of 16% vs. 9%, respectively) [50].

Risk of Infections and Its Management

The modest available data regarding the infection risk with the use of CD40-targeted agents does not allow to make firm conclusions. However, it is known that defected CD40 signaling (for instance inherited hyper-immunoglobulin M syndromes) leads to primary immune deficiency associated with high susceptibility to opportunistic infections, [51]. Theoretically, these syndromes (with their immune deficiency profile and spectrum of infections) could serve as a model to assess the risk in patients treated with CD40-targeted drugs.

Suggestions and recommendations:

- Therapy with CD40-targeted agents may be associated with an increased risk of neutropenia and infection.
- Extrapolating the data from inherited CD40 signaling deficiency syndromes (e.g., hyper-IgM syndrome), opportunistic infections such as *Pneumocystis jirovecii* pneumonia, CMV infection, invasive fungal infections, among others, should be expected. A prevention strategy (e.g., prophylaxis or preemptive therapy) is advised but, as there is scant data, individual risks need to be considered.

CD319 (SLAMF7) Agents: Elotuzumab

SLAMF7 (Previous CD139) Antigen

The glycoprotein signaling lymphocytic activation molecule (SLAMF7), previously known as cell-surface glycoprotein CD2 subset 1 or CD319, is a cell surface glycoprotein receptor and a member of the signaling lymphocyte activating molecular family. This receptor is highly expressed on plasma cells of all stages of differentiation, including malignant myeloma cells, and on NK cells. SLAMF7 is less expressed on CD8+ T lymphocytes, monocytes, and dendritic cells. The function of SLAMF7 is still not fully explained but it is suggested that it plays a role in NK cells activation and interaction between myeloma cells and their advantageous adhesion to bone marrow stromal cells. Soluble SLAMF7, sSLAMF7, further enhances the growth of myeloma cells via homophilic interaction with surface SLAMF7 and subsequent activation of the SHP-2 and ERK signaling pathways [52].

Mechanism of Action, Approved Indications, and Off-Label Use of Anti-CD139 Monoclonal Antibodies

Elotuzumab is a humanized IgG1 MoAb targeting SLAMF7. It binds to SLAMF7 receptor on the surface of plasma cells, tagging them for NK-plasma cell interaction and to SMAF7/CD16 receptors on NK cells, promoting their activation. This ADCC and NK-cell mediated cytotoxicity cause plasma cells death). Elotuzumab also suppresses sSLAMF7 and myeloma cell growth in vitro and in vivo through alteration of involved signaling pathways [52, 53]. Its efficacy in monotherapy is weak but increases significantly when used in combinations with standard anti-myeloma drugs, especially with immunomodulators. Elotuzumab is approved in combination with lenalidomide and dexamethasone or pomalidomide and dexamethasone for the therapy of R/R multiple myeloma. Ongoing clinical studies are investigating the position of elotuzumab in various clinical settings of patients with myeloma.

Clinical Evidence

Early phase 1 and 2 dose finding studies of elotuzumab in combination with other anti-myeloma agents reported lymphopenia/neutropenia grade 3 or higher, rates of upper respiratory tract infections, and febrile neutropenia/pneumonia at around 47%, 7%, and 14%, respectively [54, 55]. RCTs documented similar overall risk of infections) (adjusted for drug exposure) on elotuzumab combination with lenalidomide, dexamethasone or lenalidomide and dexamethasone alone (197 cases per 100 patient years in both groups). However, elotuzumab had higher incidence of VZV infections with respect to the comparator (4.1 vs. 2.2 cases per 100 patient-years, respectively), and lymphopenia grade 3 or higher (77% vs. 49%, respectively) [56]. Another phase 3 RCT evaluated elotuzumab with pomalidomide and dexamethasone versus pomalidomide and dexamethasone alone, and similarly showed comparable rate of infections: 65% of all grades in both groups, adjusted per 100 patient-years of 182 vs. 230 events with and without elotuzumab, respectively. VZV infection was reported in 5% of patients treated on elotuzumab combination arm and in 2% in the comparator arm (all grade 1 or 2). While neutropenia of grade 3 or higher was more common in the control group (27% vs. 13% in elotuzumab arm), lymphopenia was noticed more with elotuzumab (grade 3 or higher of 8% in elotuzumab arm vs. 2% in the control arm, respectively) [57].

Risk of Infections and Its Management

According to its mechanism of action, the expected on-target side effect of elotuzumab is lymphopenia. However, this has not translated into significantly increased risk of infections in clinical practice. RCTs have observed slightly higher incidence) of all reported infections, but the incidence of serious infections was similar or even lower with elotuzumab. VZV infections were documented at higher frequency with elotuzumab, likely linked to its lymphopenic potential. Based on the available data, the impact of elotuzumab on the risk of infections should be commensurate with other anti-myeloma drugs.

Suggestions and recommendations:

- Acyclovir or valacyclovir should be considered for anti VZV prophylaxis in seropositive patients.
- Lymphopenia is a relatively common adverse event during the treatment with elotuzumab and could increase the risk for opportunistic infections. Therefore, increased awareness is needed (monitoring of total lymphocyte count and subpopulations of lymphocytes should be considered).

CCR-4-Targeted Agents: Mogamulizumab

Chemokine Receptor 4, CCR-4

CCR-4 is one of the 18 known human chemokine receptors and plays an important role in T-cell's migration and homing to the skin. CCR-4 is normally expressed on regulatory T cells (T_{regs}) and is considered as dominant chemokine receptor on Th2 and cutaneous lymphocyte antigen-expressing skin-homing T-cells. T_{regs} are involved in the mechanism of cancer escape from host immunity. Depletion of non-malignant T_{regs} in patients who subsequently underwent allogeneic hematopoietic stem cell transplantation was associated with higher risk of graft versus host disease and non-relapse mortality [58]. CCR-4 expression is particularly high on malignant T-cells and in cutaneous T cell lymphomas. In adult T-cell leukemia/lymphoma (ATLL), high CCR-4 expression is common. In peripheral T-cell lymphoma (PTCL) and cutaneous T-cell lymphomas (CTCL), CCR-4 expression varies but positively correlates with advanced or R/R disease and with blood dissemination [59].

Mechanism of Action, Approved Indications, and Off-Label Use of CCR-4 Monoclonal Antibodies

Mogamulizumab is a first-in-class, recombinant defucosylated humanized IgG1 monoclonal antibody that targets CCR-4 and depletes CCR4-expressing cells by ADCC [60]. Mogamulizumab was initially approved in Japan for the treatment of patients with CCR4-positive ATLL and later for R/RPTCL and CTCL. FDA and EMA approved mogamulizumab in 2018 for patients with R/R mycosis fungoides or Sézary syndrome after at least one prior therapy. There are ongoing clinical trials in other subtypes of T-cell lymphomas, in solid cancer (monotherapy or in combination with, for example, checkpoint inhibitors), and in HTLV-1-associated diseases.

Clinical Evidence

There was no increased incidence of infectious complications in the initially conducted phase 2 studies with mogamulizumab. The use of primary anti-infectious prophylaxis in the initial single-arm study might had underestimated the real incidence of infections, but posterior studies did not use primary prophylaxis. Regarding hematological side effects that could impact the rate of infection, lymphopenia and neutropenia have been reported between 41–81% and around 40%, respectively. Slightly higher rate of CMV infection and CMV disease (pneumonia) were documented with mogamulizumab compared to control [61]. In the post-marketing surveillance study, CMV reactivation (viremia and/or disease) was shown to be the most common infection-related adverse event (rate of 8.3%) [62]. The results of the pivotal, phase 3 RTC in patients R/R CTCL treated with mogamulizumab or vorinostat have shown similar rate of infectious complications in both arms. The most common reported infections were upper respiratory tract and noticed in 10% and 5% of patients with mogamulizumab or vorinostat, respectively (all grade 1 and 2). The second most common infections were pneumonia (6% and 3%, respectively) and cellulitis (4% and 5%, respectively) [63]. Few case reports of HBV reactivation, fatal parainfluenza pneumonia, or disseminated mycobacterial infection have been reported with mogamulizumab.

Risk of Infection and Its Management

Targeting CCR-4 and depletion of CCR-4+ cells (T_{regs}) from T-lymphocyte population may be associated with a slightly increased risk of infection due to drug-induced lymphopenia. The contribution of CCR-4 blockade to this risk is hard to distinguish from the effect of other cytotoxic treatments and the intrinsic immune deficiency caused by T-cell lymphomas. The use of mogamulizumab in patients with autoimmune diseases is relatively contraindicated because of the increased risk of immune-mediated adverse events like myositis, myocarditis, pneumonitis, hepatitis, and hypothyroidism.

Suggestions and recommendations:

- Antiviral prophylaxis or preemptive approach should be used for prevention of CMV infection in CMV-seropositive patients.
- Screening for HBV infection should be performed before treatment and appropriate strategy (prophylaxis or close monitoring) should be considered for the individual patient according to local or international guidelines.
- Anti-herpesvirus and anti-pneumocystis prophylaxis is recommended in patients receiving mogamulizumab, reflecting the general experience in T-cell lymphoma patients.

References

1. Drgona L, Gudiol C, Lanini S, Salzberger B, Ippolito G, Mikulska M. ESCMID Study Group for Infections in Compromised Hosts (ESGICH) consensus document on the safety of targeted and biological therapies: an infectious diseases perspective (agents targeting lymphoid or myeloid cells surface antigens [II]: CD22, CD30, CD33, CD38, CD40, SLAMF-7 and CCR4). Clin Microbiol Infect. 2018;24(Suppl 2):S83–s94.
2. Abramson JS, Ghosh N, Smith SM. ADCs, BiTEs, CARs, and small molecules: a new era of targeted therapy in non-Hodgkin lymphoma. Am Soc Clin Oncol Educ Book. 2020;40:302–13.
3. Tedder TF, Poe JC, Haas KM. CD22: a multifunctional receptor that regulates B lymphocyte survival and signal transduction. Adv Immunol. 2005;88:1–50.
4. Carnahan J, Stein R, Qu Z, Hess K, Cesano A, Hansen HJ, et al. Epratuzumab, a CD22-targeting recombinant humanized antibody with a different mode of action from rituximab. Mol Immunol. 2007;44(6):1331–41.
5. Strauss SJ, Morschhauser F, Rech J, Repp R, Solal-Celigny P, Zinzani PL, et al. Multicenter phase II trial of immunotherapy with the humanized anti-CD22 antibody, epratuzumab, in combination with rituximab, in refractory or recurrent non-Hodgkin's lymphoma. J Clin Oncol. 2006;24(24):3880–6.
6. Clowse ME, Wallace DJ, Furie RA, Petri MA, Pike MC, Leszczyński P, et al. Efficacy and safety of epratuzumab in moderately to severely active systemic lupus erythematosus: results from two phase III randomized, double-blind, placebo-controlled trials. Arthritis Rheumatol. 2017;69(2):362–75.
7. Kantarjian HM, DeAngelo DJ, Stelljes M, Martinelli G, Liedtke M, Stock W, et al. Inotuzumab ozogamicin versus standard therapy for acute lymphoblastic leukemia. N Engl J Med. 2016;375(8):740–53.
8. Kantarjian HM, DeAngelo DJ, Stelljes M, Liedtke M, Stock W, Gökbuget N, et al. Inotuzumab ozogamicin versus standard of care in relapsed or refractory acute lymphoblastic leukemia: final report and long-term survival follow-up from the randomized, phase 3 INO-VATE study. Cancer. 2019;125(14):2474–87.
9. Jabbour EJ, DeAngelo DJ, Stelljes M, Stock W, Liedtke M, Gökbuget N, et al. Efficacy and safety analysis by age cohort of inotuzumab ozogamicin in patients with relapsed or refractory acute lymphoblastic leukemia enrolled in INO-VATE. Cancer. 2018;124(8):1722–32.
10. DeAngelo DJ, Advani AS, Marks DI, Stelljes M, Liedtke M, Stock W, et al. Inotuzumab ozogamicin for relapsed/refractory acute lymphoblastic leukemia: outcomes by disease burden. Blood Cancer J. 2020;10(8):81.
11. Bhojwani D, Sposto R, Shah NN, Rodriguez V, Yuan C, Stetler-Stevenson M, et al. Inotuzumab ozogamicin in pediatric patients with relapsed/refractory acute lymphoblastic leukemia. Leukemia. 2019;33(4):884–92.

12. Kreitman RJ, Dearden C, Zinzani PL, Delgado J, Karlin L, Robak T, et al. Moxetumomab pasudotox in relapsed/refractory hairy cell leukemia. Leukemia. 2018;32(8):1768–77.
13. Kennedy MK, Willis CR, Armitage RJ. Deciphering CD30 ligand biology and its role in humoral immunity. Immunology. 2006;118(2):143–52.
14. Brentuximab vedotin. Drugs R D. 2011;11(1):85–95.
15. Younes A, Gopal AK, Smith SE, Ansell SM, Rosenblatt JD, Savage KJ, et al. Results of a pivotal phase II study of brentuximab vedotin for patients with relapsed or refractory Hodgkin's lymphoma. J Clin Oncol. 2012;30(18):2183–9.
16. Connors JM, Jurczak W, Straus DJ, Ansell SM, Kim WS, Gallamini A, et al. Brentuximab vedotin with chemotherapy for stage III or IV Hodgkin's lymphoma. N Engl J Med. 2018;378(4):331–44.
17. Horwitz S, O'Connor OA, Pro B, Illidge T, Fanale M, Advani R, et al. Brentuximab vedotin with chemotherapy for CD30-positive peripheral T-cell lymphoma (ECHELON-2): a global, double-blind, randomised, phase 3 trial. Lancet. 2019;393(10168):229–40.
18. Nademanee A, Sureda A, Stiff P, Holowiecki J, Abidi M, Hunder N, et al. Safety analysis of brentuximab vedotin from the phase III AETHERA trial in Hodgkin lymphoma in the post-transplant consolidation setting. Biol Blood Marrow Transplant. 2018;24(11):2354–9.
19. Tudesq JJ, Vincent L, Lebrun J, Hicheri Y, Gabellier L, Busetto T, et al. Cytomegalovirus infection with retinitis after brentuximab vedotin treatment for CD30(+) lymphoma. Open Forum Infect Dis. 2017;4(2):ofx091.
20. Gopal AK, Ramchandren R, O'Connor OA, Berryman RB, Advani RH, Chen R, et al. Safety and efficacy of brentuximab vedotin for Hodgkin lymphoma recurring after allogeneic stem cell transplantation. Blood. 2012;120(3):560–8.
21. Maschmeyer G, De Greef J, Mellinghoff SC, Nosari A, Thiebaut-Bertrand A, Bergeron A, et al. Infections associated with immunotherapeutic and molecular targeted agents in hematology and oncology. A position paper by the European Conference on Infections in Leukemia (ECIL). Leukemia. 2019;33(4):844–62.
22. Multani A, Ho DY. JC polyomavirus infection potentiated by biologics. Infect Dis Clin North Am. 2020;34(2):359–88.
23. Mallet V, van Bömmel F, Doerig C, Pischke S, Hermine O, Locasciulli A, et al. Management of viral hepatitis in patients with haematological malignancy and in patients undergoing haemopoietic stem cell transplantation: recommendations of the 5th European Conference on Infections in Leukaemia (ECIL-5). Lancet Infect Dis. 2016;16(5):606–17.
24. Cao H, Crocker PR. Evolution of CD33-related siglecs: regulating host immune functions and escaping pathogen exploitation? Immunology. 2011;132(1):18–26.
25. Godwin CD, Gale RP, Walter RB. Gemtuzumab ozogamicin in acute myeloid leukemia. Leukemia. 2017;31(9):1855–68.
26. Wolska-Washer A, Robak T. Safety and tolerability of antibody-drug conjugates in cancer. Drug Saf. 2019;42(2):295–314.
27. Cortes JE, de Lima M, Dombret H, Estey EH, Giralt SA, Montesinos P, et al. Prevention, recognition, and management of adverse events associated with gemtuzumab ozogamicin use in acute myeloid leukemia. J Hematol Oncol. 2020;13(1):137.
28. Aplenc R, Alonzo TA, Gerbing RB, Lange BJ, Hurwitz CA, Wells RJ, et al. Safety and efficacy of gemtuzumab ozogamicin in combination with chemotherapy for pediatric acute myeloid leukemia: a report from the Children's Oncology Group. J Clin Oncol. 2008;26(14):2390–3295.
29. Fernández-Ruiz M, de la Serna J, Ruiz J, López-Medrano F. [Progressive multifocal leukoencephalopathy in a patient with acute myeloid leukaemia after allogeneic hematopoietic-cell transplantation]. Enferm Infecc Microbiol Clin. 2011;29(8):636–7.
30. Wang ES, Adés L, Fathi AT, Kreuzer KA, O'Meara MM, Liang S-Y, et al. CASCADE: a phase 3, randomized, double-blind study of vadastuximab talirine (33A) versus placebo in combination with azacitidine or decitabine in the treatment of older patients with newly diagnosed acute myeloid leukemia (AML). J Clin Oncol. 2017;35(15_suppl):TPS7066-TPS.

31. Morandi F, Airoldi I, Marimpietri D, Bracci C, Faini AC, Gramignoli R. CD38, a receptor with multifunctional activities: from modulatory functions on regulatory cell subsets and extracellular vesicles, to a target for therapeutic strategies. Cells. 2019;8(12):1527.
32. Dimopoulos MA, Oriol A, Nahi H, San-Miguel J, Bahlis NJ, Usmani SZ, et al. Daratumumab, lenalidomide, and dexamethasone for multiple myeloma. N Engl J Med. 2016;375(14):1319–31.
33. Palumbo A, Chanan-Khan A, Weisel K, Nooka AK, Masszi T, Beksac M, et al. Daratumumab, bortezomib, and dexamethasone for multiple myeloma. N Engl J Med. 2016;375(8):754–66.
34. Facon T, Kumar S, Plesner T, Orlowski RZ, Moreau P, Bahlis N, et al. Daratumumab plus lenalidomide and dexamethasone for untreated myeloma. N Engl J Med. 2019;380(22):2104–15.
35. Mateos MV, Dimopoulos MA, Cavo M, Suzuki K, Jakubowiak A, Knop S, et al. Daratumumab plus bortezomib, melphalan, and prednisone for untreated myeloma. N Engl J Med. 2018;378(6):518–28.
36. Voorhees PM, Kaufman JL, Laubach J, Sborov DW, Reeves B, Rodriguez C, et al. Daratumumab, lenalidomide, bortezomib, and dexamethasone for transplant-eligible newly diagnosed multiple myeloma: the GRIFFIN trial. Blood. 2020;136(8):936–45.
37. Moreau P, Attal M, Hulin C, Arnulf B, Belhadj K, Benboubker L, et al. Bortezomib, thalidomide, and dexamethasone with or without daratumumab before and after autologous stem-cell transplantation for newly diagnosed multiple myeloma (CASSIOPEIA): a randomised, open-label, phase 3 study. Lancet. 2019;394(10192):29–38.
38. Htut TWTZ, Sultan A, et al. Daratumumab-related hematological toxicities in patients with multiple myeloma: a combined analysis of five phase III randomized controlled trials. Blood. 2019;134(Suppl 1):3485.
39. Htut TWTA, Sultan A, et al. Updated meta-analysis of randomized controlled trials to evaluate the incidence of infection and pneumonia in patients with multiple myeloma treated with daratumumab. Blood. 2019;134(Suppl 1):4771.
40. Martin T, Baz R, Benson DM, Lendvai N, Wolf J, Munster P, et al. A phase 1b study of isatuximab plus lenalidomide and dexamethasone for relapsed/refractory multiple myeloma. Blood. 2017;129(25):3294–303.
41. Martin TRJ, Vij R, Cole C, et al. A dose finding phase II trial of isatuximab (SAR650984, anti-CD38 mAb) as a single agent in relapsed/refractory multiple myeloma. Blood. 2015;126:509.
42. Attal M, Richardson PG, Rajkumar SV, San-Miguel J, Beksac M, Spicka I, et al. Isatuximab plus pomalidomide and low-dose dexamethasone versus pomalidomide and low-dose dexamethasone in patients with relapsed and refractory multiple myeloma (ICARIA-MM): a randomised, multicentre, open-label, phase 3 study. Lancet. 2019;394(10214):2096–107.
43. Moreau P DM, Mikhael J, et al. Isatuximab plus carfilzomib and dexamethasone vs carfilzomib and dexamethasone in relapsed/refractory multiple myeloma (IKEMA): interim analysis of a phase 3, randomized, open-label study. European Hematologic Association Virtual. 2020;Abstract LB2603.
44. Blimark C, Holmberg E, Mellqvist UH, Landgren O, Björkholm M, Hultcrantz M, et al. Multiple myeloma and infections: a population-based study on 9253 multiple myeloma patients. Haematologica. 2015;100(1):107–13.
45. Kikuchi T, Kusumoto S, Tanaka Y, Oshima Y, Fujinami H, Suzuki T, et al. Hepatitis B virus reactivation in a myeloma patient with resolved infection who received daratumumab-containing salvage chemotherapy. J Clin Exp Hematopathol. 2020;60(2):51–4.
46. Johnsrud AJ, Johnsrud JJ, Susanibar SA, Kamimoto JJ, Kothari A, Burgess M, et al. Infectious and immunological sequelae of daratumumab in multiple myeloma. Br J Haematol. 2019;185(1):187–9.
47. Yellin MJ, Brett J, Baum D, Matsushima A, Szabolcs M, Stern D, et al. Functional interactions of T cells with endothelial cells: the role of CD40L-CD40-mediated signals. J Exp Med. 1995;182(6):1857–64.
48. Piechutta M, Berghoff AS. New emerging targets in cancer immunotherapy: the role of Cluster of Differentiation 40 (CD40/TNFR5). ESMO Open. 2019;4(Suppl 3):e000510.

49. Hassan SB, Sørensen JF, Olsen BN, Pedersen AE. Anti-CD40-mediated cancer immunotherapy: an update of recent and ongoing clinical trials. Immunopharmacol Immunotoxicol. 2014;36(2):96–104.
50. Fayad L, Ansell SM, Advani R, Coiffier B, Stuart R, Bartlett NL, et al. Dacetuzumab plus rituximab, ifosfamide, carboplatin and etoposide as salvage therapy for patients with diffuse large B-cell lymphoma relapsing after rituximab, cyclophosphamide, doxorubicin, vincristine and prednisolone: a randomized, double-blind, placebo-controlled phase 2b trial. Leuk Lymphoma. 2015;56(9):2569–78.
51. Davies EG, Thrasher AJ. Update on the hyper immunoglobulin M syndromes. Br J Haematol. 2010;149(2):167–80.
52. Kikuchi J, Hori M, Iha H, Toyama-Sorimachi N, Hagiwara S, Kuroda Y, et al. Soluble SLAMF7 promotes the growth of myeloma cells via homophilic interaction with surface SLAMF7. Leukemia. 2020;34(1):180–95.
53. Collins SM, Bakan CE, Swartzel GD, Hofmeister CC, Efebera YA, Kwon H, et al. Elotuzumab directly enhances NK cell cytotoxicity against myeloma via CS1 ligation: evidence for augmented NK cell function complementing ADCC. Cancer Immunol Immunother. 2013;62(12):1841–9.
54. Richardson PG, Jagannath S, Moreau P, Jakubowiak AJ, Raab MS, Facon T, et al. Elotuzumab in combination with lenalidomide and dexamethasone in patients with relapsed multiple myeloma: final phase 2 results from the randomised, open-label, phase 1b-2 dose-escalation study. Lancet Haematol. 2015;2(12):e516–27.
55. Mateos MV, Granell M, Oriol A, Martinez-Lopez J, Blade J, Hernandez MT, et al. Elotuzumab in combination with thalidomide and low-dose dexamethasone: a phase 2 single-arm safety study in patients with relapsed/refractory multiple myeloma. Br J Haematol. 2016;175(3):448–56.
56. Lonial S, Dimopoulos M, Palumbo A, White D, Grosicki S, Spicka I, et al. Elotuzumab therapy for relapsed or refractory multiple myeloma. N Engl J Med. 2015;373(7):621–31.
57. Dimopoulos MA, Dytfeld D, Grosicki S, Moreau P, Takezako N, Hori M, et al. Elotuzumab plus pomalidomide and dexamethasone for multiple myeloma. N Engl J Med. 2018;379(19):1811–22.
58. Fuji S, Inoue Y, Utsunomiya A, Moriuchi Y, Uchimaru K, Choi I, et al. Pretransplantation anti-CCR4 antibody mogamulizumab against adult T-cell leukemia/lymphoma is associated with significantly increased risks of severe and corticosteroid-refractory graft-versus-host disease, nonrelapse mortality, and overall mortality. J Clin Oncol. 2016;34(28):3426–33.
59. Blackmon AL, Pinter-Brown L. Spotlight on mogamulizumab-Kpkc for use in adults with relapsed or refractory mycosis fungoides or Sézary syndrome: efficacy, safety, and patient selection. Drug Des Devel Ther. 2020;14:3747–54.
60. Ni X, Jorgensen JL, Goswami M, Challagundla P, Decker WK, Kim YH, et al. Reduction of regulatory T cells by mogamulizumab, a defucosylated anti-CC chemokine receptor 4 antibody, in patients with aggressive/refractory mycosis fungoides and Sézary syndrome. Clin Cancer Res. 2015;21(2):274–85.
61. Ishida T, Jo T, Takemoto S, Suzushima H, Uozumi K, Yamamoto K, et al. Dose-intensified chemotherapy alone or in combination with mogamulizumab in newly diagnosed aggressive adult T-cell leukaemia-lymphoma: a randomized phase II study. Br J Haematol. 2015;169(5):672–82.
62. Ishitsuka K, Yurimoto S, Kawamura K, Tsuji Y, Iwabuchi M, Takahashi T, et al. Safety and efficacy of mogamulizumab in patients with adult T-cell leukemia-lymphoma in Japan: interim results of postmarketing all-case surveillance. Int J Hematol. 2017;106(4):522–32.
63. Kim YH, Bagot M, Pinter-Brown L, Rook AH, Porcu P, Horwitz SM, et al. Mogamulizumab versus vorinostat in previously treated cutaneous T-cell lymphoma (MAVORIC): an international, open-label, randomised, controlled phase 3 trial. Lancet Oncol. 2018;19(9):1192–204.
64. Ogawa E, Wei MT, Nguyen MH. Hepatitis B virus reactivation potentiated by biologics. Infect Dis Clin N Am. 2020;34(2):341–58.
65. Ho DY, Enriquez K, Multani A. Herpesvirus infections potentiated by biologics. Infect Dis Clin N Am. 2020;34(2):311–39.
66. Moskowitz CH, Nademanee A, Masszi T, et al; AETHERA Study Group. Brentuximab vedotin as consolidation therapy after autologous stem cell transplantation in patients with Hodgkin's lymphoma at risk of relapse or progression (AETHERA): a randomised, double-blind, placebo controlled, phase 3 trial. Lancet. 2015;385(9980):1853–862.

CD19, CD20 and CD52

7

Malgorzata Mikulska and Diana Averbuch

Introduction

Selective agents such as monoclonal antibodies (mAbs) targeting different surface proteins on lymphoid cells, mainly clusters of differentiation (CD), have been developed over the past three decades for the treatment of lymphoma, leukaemia and autoimmune diseases. In the setting of malignancy they have been mainly used in association with other chemotherapeutic agents, and subsequently also as monotherapy, particularly in case of salvage or maintenance treatment.

Rituximab, the first and the most widely used anti-CD20 antibody had initially been approved in 1998 for the treatment of diffused large B cell lymphoma, and over time the indications have expanded to other non-Hodgkin lymphomas (NHL), chronic lymphocytic leukaemia (CLL), rheumatoid arthritis (RA), granulomatosis with polyangiitis (GPA), microscopic polyangiitis and pemphigus vulgaris. Additionally, it has been widely used off-label in numerous autoimmune disorders such as multiple sclerosis (MS), idiopathic thrombocytopenic purpura, systemic lupus erythematosus (SLE) and autoimmune neuropathies. In the transplant setting it is used in graft versus host disease (GvHD) and pre-emptive treatment of post-transplant lymphoproliferative disorder (PTLD). From the point of view of

M. Mikulska (✉)
Division of Infectious Diseases, Department of Health Sciences (DISSAL), University of Genova, Genova, Italy

Ospedale Policlinico San Martino, Genova, Italy
e-mail: m.mikulska@unige.it

D. Averbuch
Faculty of Medicine, Hebrew University of Jerusalem, Pediatric Infectious Diseases Unit, Hadassah Medical Center, Jerusalem, Israel
e-mail: adiana@hadassah.org.il

C. Cervera, J. M. Aguado (eds.), *Infectious Complications in Biologic and Targeted Therapies*, https://doi.org/10.1007/978-3-031-11363-5_7

infectious complications, rituximab is an excellent example of how difficult it is to establish the general risk of infectious complications caused by a single targeted agent. Indeed, there are various reasons why such a widely used medication poses an enormous challenge, since numerous factors influence heavily the risk of infections [1, 2]. First, the underlying disease and consequent immune deficits, such as lymphocyte dysfunction in lymphoma or pre-existing hypogammaglobulinaemia (HGG) in CLL. Second, the concomitant and previous treatments, since clearly infections would be more frequent and more severe in a patient treated with combination chemotherapy for aggressive lymphoma compared to one receiving rituximab in monotherapy for an autoimmune disease. Finally, the total dose and the frequency of administration of anti- CD20 agents vary between the indications, and consequently this has an impact on the infectious risk.

Similar challenge can be noted with anti-CD52 treatment, since for all the aforementioned reasons, the rate of infectious complications vary significantly when this agent in used in haematological malignancies or transplant setting, compared to multiple sclerosis.

Also the management of infectious complications in patients treated with anti-CD19 agents has become more challenging since this drug class was repurposed. Initially anti-CD19 agents were used only in selected aggressive relapsed or refractory haematological malignancies such as acute lymphoblastic leukaemia (blinatumumab), but they were recently approved for use in the autoimmune setting as monotherapy for neuromyelitis optica (inebilizumab).

Anti-CD20 Agents

Available Agents and Their Main Indications

In addition to the first drug—rituximab (Mabthera®, Roche) and its biosimilars (the first approved in 2017), there are currently other agents approved (ofatumumab, ocrelizumab, obinutuzumab), including one conjugated with a radioactive isotope (^{90}Y-ibritumomab tiuxetan). Others are being developed in clinical trials (ublituximab), while some have been discontinued (Table 7.1).

Some anti-CD20 agents were approved for certain indications, while approval for the same indications has not been pursued for others. For example, the study of ocrelizumab in combination therapy for RA and proliferative lupus nephritis was terminated by the sponsor due to an increased incidence of serious infections.

Table 7.1 Characteristics of anti-CD20 agents

Agent	Type of antibody	Status of development (year of approval)	Approved indications	Off-label or experimental uses
Rituximab, Mabthera® and biosimilars	First-generation chimeric mAb	First approved, EMA and FDA (1998)	DLCBL, low-grade NHL or follicular lymphoma, CLL, RA, Wegener granulomatosis, microscopic polyangiitis	MS, GvHD, ITP, SLE, PTLD, autoimmune neuropathies or cytopenias, Rasmussen encephalitis, pemphigus vulgaris
^{90}Y-ibritumomab tiuxetan, Zevalin®	First-generation murine mAb conjugated with a radioactive isotope that kills both targeted and neighbouring cells	Approved (2002)	Follicular lymphoma, relapsed/refractory low-grade NHL or follicular lymphoma	No
Ocrelizumab, Ocrevus®	Second-generation humanized mAb	Approved, FDA (2017)	Relapsed or progressive MS	RA, SLE (trial discontinued in 2017 due to infections), autoimmune encephalitis, NHL
Ofatumumab, Arzerra®	Second-generation fully human mAb	Approved, EMA (2010), FDA (2009) for CLL, withdrawn EMA approval for CLL	CLL/indolent non-Hodgkin lymphoma	No
Ofatumumab, Kesimpta®		FDA (2020)	Relapsing forms of multiple sclerosis	No
Obinutuzumab, Gazyvaro®	Third-generation humanized mAb	Approved, EMA (2014), FDA (2013)	CLL, follicular lymphoma	Other lymphomas, kidney transplant desensitization, Waldenstrom macroglobulinemia, GvHD, hairy cell leukaemia, lupus nephritis

(continued)

Table 7.1 (continued)

Agent	Type of antibody	Status of development (year of approval)	Approved indications	Off-label or experimental uses
Ublituximab orphan EMA, not FDA	Third-generation fully human mAb	Phase 3 trials in CLL, NHL, relapsing remitting MS, neuromyelitis optica spectrum disorder	NA	–
Ocaratuzumab	Third-generation humanized mAb	Phase 1 and 2 trials in haematological malignancies; phase 3 in pemphigus	NA	–

First-generation: murine or chimeric (human-mouse) antibodies; Second-generation: humanized or fully human antibodies developed with the purpose of reducing immunogenicity and improving efficacy; Third-generation: antibodies with an engineered Fc region to boost antibody-dependent cell-mediated cytotoxicity (ADCC)

Mechanism of Action and the Pathogenesis of Increased Risk of Infectious Complications

These B-cell depleting agents act by inhibiting CD20 which is mainly expressed on both normal and malignant B-cells. CD20 expression begins at the pre-B phase and progressively increases in concentration until the mature stage, but it is not expressed by B-cell precursors or plasma cells. With prolonged use, however, the production of antibodies may be decreased leading to HGG, with the degree of HGG being directly associated with infection rates, although severe infections are generally infrequent.

Impairment of B-cell function is thought to be responsible for poor response to vaccination, particularly if including neoantigens (see section on Vaccination in Patients Receiving Anti-CD20, Anti-CD19 and Anti-CD52 Agents). This diminished response to vaccines could predispose to certain infections.

Additionally, some T-cells express CD20 (CD3+ CD20+ T-cells), which is the basis for the efficacy of these agents in diseases such as multiple sclerosis, when both CD20+ CD19+ B cells and CD20+ CD3+ T-cell are depleted under treatment [3].

Finally, anti-CD20 agents impact the immune response by modulating B/T-cell interactions rather than directly affecting humoral immunity. B-cell depletion exerts a deleterious impact on the induction, maintenance and activation of cell-mediated immunity, providing the rationale for treating rejection of a solid organ transplant and GvHD after allogeneic haematopoietic stem cell transplant (HSCT). The impact on these interactions might also explain the increased risk of opportunistic infections associated with impaired cellular immunity, which has been reported in certain cohorts; particularly if rituximab was used in association with other agents already affecting T-cell immunity, such as bendamustine [4].

The Rates of Infectious Complications in Patients Treated with Anti-CD20

The rate of infectious complications in patients treated with biological agents, such as anti-CD20 therapies, can be analysed based on the results from randomized controlled studies (RCT). These provide the advantage of a control group but might have the following limitations: (1) focusing mainly on efficacy and not on precise documentation of reported infectious complications, particularly if mild; (2) not being powered enough to detect rare infectious complications; (3) including only selected patients, with fewer comorbidities and less advanced disease; (4) not having a long enough follow-up to detect delayed infections.

It might be for these reasons that meta-analyses and pooled data analyses of rituximab in patients with lymphoma [5] and RA [6] did not show an increase in the incidence of infections compared to placebo. However, a large population study in patients with immune thrombocytopenia showed that the risk of serious infections (both viral and bacterial) was 2.6 times higher in subjects who received rituximab compared to those who did not, whereas such increase for corticosteroids was estimated as 3.8 times [7].

Similarly, in phase 3 RCTs in which ocrelizumab showed better efficacy than interferon (IFN)-β or placebo in the treatment of MS, infection rates were high in all arms: 71% ocrelizumab vs. 70% placebo; 57% and 60% in ocrelizumab vs. 54% and 53% in IFN-β, with upper respiratory tract infections and oral herpes simplex virus (HSV) more frequent in the ocrelizumab arms, but no differences in serious infections [8, 9]. In a systematic review of ocrelizumab for treatment of MS, including four RCTs, infection was the most common side effect (n = 1342, 39.2% of ocrelizumab-exposed patients) [10]. The rate was slightly increased compared to IFN-β: risk ratio (RR) of any infection 1.10; herpetic infection RR 1.75; respiratory tract infection RR = 1.42, with no increase in serious infections [10]. Long-term follow-up data from the trials reported an infection rate of 70 per 100 patient-years of exposure (the same as the placebo arm), with most infections being mild; the rate of severe infections was 2.74 per 100 patient-years, increasing to 4.13 when the open-label extension phase was also included [11]. No cases of progressive multifocal leukoencephalopathy (PML) were reported [11]. HBV-positive patients were excluded from these trials and therefore, in the drug label, the administration of ocrelizumab is contraindicated in patients with active HBV infection, while specialist evaluation is indicated for those with inactive infection.

The risk of infection seemed to be more pronounced when ocrelizumab was used in combination with other immunosuppressive agents, and for this reason clinical development of some trials was terminated by the sponsor [12, 13]. However, a meta-analysis of four RCTs in patients with RA treated with ocrelizumab and second-line therapy did not detect any increase in infectious complications, but infusion-related reactions were more frequent in the ocrelizumab arm [14].

There are more limited data available for ofatumumab, but the reported rates of any and severe infections were, respectively, 32% and 17% in a heavily pre-treated CLL population (including two cases of PML in patients previously treated with fludarabine, rituximab and alemtuzumab), and 32% and <1% in RA patients [15, 16]. When used as maintenance therapy in CLL patients, it resulted in a higher rate of progression-free survival, with a higher incidence of prolonged severe neutropenia and severe infections compared to placebo arm (5% vs. 2% and 13% vs. 8%, respectively) [17]. In a recent trial, MS patients treated with subcutaneous ofatumumab, had only a slightly higher rate of severe infectious complications than those treated with teriflunomide (2.5% and 1.8%) [18], while there was no difference in infectious complications in the ofatumumab arm compared to placebo [19].

Of note, in salvage treatment in patients with relapsed or refractory diffuse large B-cell lymphoma (DLBCL) after autologous stem-cell transplantation, there was no difference in the rate of infectious complications between chemotherapy containing ofatumumab or rituximab [20]. However, in a phase 3 open label trial assessing the efficacy and safety of ofatumumab as the sole maintenance agent versus observation in 477 patients with CLL, ofatumumab patients had improved progression-free survival, but infections (respiratory tract and herpes simplex virus) and neutropenia were more common [17].

Obinutuzumab is a third-generation anti-CD20 mAb designed to boost antibody-dependent cell-mediated cytotoxicity (ADCC) and to overcome mechanisms of rituximab resistance [21]. In pivotal trials of obinutuzumab in combination with chlorambucil for CLL, severe and life-threatening cytopenias were frequent, with both neutropenia (40% overall; 34% for grade 3 and 4) and thrombocytopenia (15% overall, 11% for grade 3–4) [22]. More recently, obinutuzumab has been studied in combination with venetoclax or Bruton-kinase inhibitors for CLL and as expected for the combination therapies (particularly containing venetoclax) and given the underlying disease, the rate of infectious complications was high, with 17.5% rate of grade 3–4 infections in obinutuzumab-venetoclax arm vs. 15% in obinutuzumab-chlorambucil arm and 7% rate of grade 3–4 pneumonia in obinutuzumab-ibrutinib arm vs. 4% in obinutuzumab-chlorambucil arm [23, 24].

In conclusion, infectious complications might be frequent in patients treated with anti-CD20 agents, particularly if used in combination and in haematological malignancies, but as long as they offer effective control of the underlying disease, appropriate management strategies should be put in place to mitigate this risk.

HBV Reactivation in Patients Treated with Anti-CD20 Agents

The studies included in the aforementioned meta-analyses did not specifically evaluate the most frequent infectious complication, i.e. HBV reactivation, but the role of rituximab in the reactivation of both chronic and resolved/occult HBV infection has been extensively documented [25–27], with 109 fatal cases documented in the Adverse Event reporting System [28]. In 2017 the risk of fatal HBV reactivation has been highlighted in cases of combined treatment with rituximab and bendamustine in lymphoma/CLL [29].

Although there are limited data on the risk of HBV reactivation with other anti-CD20 agents, it is plausible to assume a similar risk as with rituximab. Indeed, the risk of HBV reactivation, with an appropriate risk mitigation strategy, is mentioned in the drug label for all anti-CD20 agents. A single case of fulminant HBV infection was reported in a woman concomitantly treated with ofatumumab and methotrexate among 483 patients from three studies in rheumatoid arthritis [30].

Most of the data on the risk of HBV reactivation come from trials in lymphoma patients treated with combination chemotherapy containing rituximab.

For the purpose of managing the risk of HBV, three different populations should be considered:

1. Patients with chronic HBV hepatitis: increased ALT levels, presence of necroinflammation in liver; HBsAg positive, HBcAb positive, HBV-DNA positive (usually at >2000 UI), HBeAg positive or negative.
2. Patients with chronic HBV infection: normal ALT levels; HBsAg positive, HBcAb positive, HBV-DNA negative (or positive at low level, <2000 UI according to some definitions), usually HBeAg negative.
3. Patients with past (resolved) HBV infection: normal ALT levels; HBsAg negative, HBsAb positive or negative, HBcAb positive, HBV-DNA negative.

The main guidelines agree that patients in the first two categories should receive treatment (group 1) and treatment/prophylaxis of reactivation (group 2) with drugs that have a high barrier to inducing resistance, such as tenofovir (either tenofovir disoproxil fumarate[TFD] or tenofovir alafenamide [TAF]) or entecavir. In the second group, lamivudine use is discouraged since resistance is more likely to develop compared to TDF or ETV, and a breakthrough reactivation may occur, particularly in case of low-level viremia.

The length of antiviral administration in the first group is the same as it would be in the general population (frequently lifelong or until HBsAg seroconversion). In the second group, prophylaxis should be continued for at least 18 months after the last administration of anti-CD20 antibodies, and discontinued only if underlying disease is in remission. The monitoring of HBV-DNA and liver function tests every 3–6 months is recommended, and its usefulness is clear in case lamivudine is administered. With high barrier agents the risk of prophylaxis failure seems extremely low and less frequent monitoring might be sufficient. It is important that HBV-DNA be tested in case of any alanine transaminase (ALT) increase, and every 3 months after stopping the prophylaxis for at least 12 months, since many reactivations occur after discontinuation of antiviral prophylaxis.

In the third group, prophylaxis is generally recommended, and most of the guidelines recommend using, also in this setting, high barrier drugs, due to possible risk of breakthrough reactivation while receiving lamivudine. However, considering the absence of detectable HBV-DNA in these patients, the risk of developing resistance to lamivudine while on prophylaxis might be limited [31, 32]. Even if the use of high barrier drugs is expected to be more effective, and the price of TDF and entecavir has been significantly lowered in many parts of the world, it is correct to mention that only one randomized study reported superiority of high barrier drug (entecavir) over lamivudine in HBsAg positive lymphoma patients receiving rituximab-containing chemotherapy [33]. Moreover, in this pivotal trial, the rate of HBV reactivation was rather high for both drugs, but much higher for lamivudine (6.6% vs. 30%, respectively), while entecavir successfully reduced the rate of HBV-related hepatitis (0% vs. 13.3%) [33].

A recent study which reported data from patients with resolved hepatitis B and B-cell NHL treated with chemotherapy (mainly CHOP: cyclophosphamide, doxorubicin, vincristine and prednisone) which included obinutuzumab or rituximab, reported a 10.8% risk of HBV reactivation if prophylaxis was not administered [34]. The authors performed very stringent monitoring, with HBV-DNA tested monthly until 12 months after the last anti-CD20 administration, and defined reactivation as HBV-DNA ≥29 IU/mL. Among 326 patients with resolved HBV infection, 27 (8.2%) had HBV reactivation, occurring a median of 125 days after the first dose, with 36% of reactivations occurring after the end of chemotherapy. Among 94 patients who received prophylaxis (drug choice not pre-specified by study protocol), two developed HBV reactivation (one during lamivudine prophylaxis and one after stopping lamivudine). Very close HBV-DNA monitoring and rapid therapy might be the reason while HBV-related hepatitis did not develop in any of the patients. As expected, detectable HBV-DNA at baseline was strongly associated with an increased risk of reactivation [34]. Although chemotherapy was temporarily withdrawn in this study, other trials have shown that it might be safe to proceed with immunochemotherapy as long as rapid and effective pre-emptive high barrier treatment is provided [35, 36].

Other observational trials reported similarly low rate of breakthrough reactivation during lamivudine prophylaxis, supporting the benefit of its use if higher barrier drugs are unavailable or not cost-effective. For example, in a study of 85 HBsAg-negative, HBcAb-positive patients with NHL undergoing rituximab-based chemotherapy who received lamivudine prophylaxis for 18 months after the end of the chemotherapy, the HBV reactivation rate was 2% [37].

Overall, in this setting (patients with resolved HBV infection and lymphoma chemotherapy including anti-CD20 antibodies), prophylaxis is efficient in preventing HBV reactivation (the risk is particularly high in case of HBV-DNA positivity at baseline), and might prevent disruption of chemotherapy schedule. Close monitoring of HBV-DNA might still be needed during chemotherapy, particularly if lamivudine is used, but it is possible that with the use of high-barrier drugs, and if patient's compliance can be assured, such close monitoring might not be required. Close monitoring for reactivation is an alternative to prophylaxis in this setting, with pharmacological intervention only in case of reactivation. However, this strategy may pose problems depending on the logistics and availability of rapid molecular analyses [38]. The risk of HBV reactivation after the end of chemotherapy and after the end of prophylaxis is well recognized and monitoring for at least 12 months post-treatment is warranted in all patients. In the future, monitoring the surface antigen (HBsAg) in a highly sensitive assay instead of HBV-DNA might provide a less expensive and faster alternative [39].

Current European guidelines recommend that HBV-DNA-negative patients with resolved HBV infection (HBsAg-negative, HBcAb-positive) receive prophylaxis if the risk of HBV reactivation is >10% or undergo monitoring if the risk is <10% [32]. However, in the setting of autoimmune diseases, particularly if anti-CD20 agents are used in monotherapy, at lower doses than in haematology, and for an underlying disease that does not carry the risk of immune deficiency, the rate of HBV reactivation remains to be determined. For example, very low risk was reported in 38 patients with RA treated with rituximab (no cases of seroreversion to HBsAg, one case of HBV-DNA increase to 44 UI/mL) [40]. Consequently, the management strategy might differ in this setting, with cost-effectiveness of pharmacological prophylaxis, and the choice of agent, yet to be determined. In any case, regular HBV monitoring, with or without prophylaxis, is required during and after administration of anti-CD20, since reactivations might occur and require prompt treatment to prevent severe hepatitis [41].

Finally, anti-CD20 treatment should not be started in patients with active HBV infection, unless effective treatment has been provided and clinical and/or virological response is observed.

Other Infectious Complications

In addition to the well-established risk of HBV reactivation, exacerbation of hepatitis C virus (HCV), chronic hepatitis E virus (HEV) infection and severe enteroviral infections have all been reported in patients receiving rituximab therapy [42–46]. As have opportunistic infections resulting from impaired cell-mediated immunity such as PML or *Pneumocystis jirovecii* pneumonia (PJP) [47].

Similarly to patients with common variable immunodeficiency, severe enteroviral infections (non-polioviruses: coxsackieviruses, echoviruses and enteroviruses) may occur, such as fatal meningoencephalitis or fulminant hepatitis, and have been reported for rituximab [48], ocrelizumab [49] and obinutuzumab [45, 46]. These infections cannot be prevented, but awareness of this possibility should prompt rapid diagnostic tests with enterovirus-RNA assessment in blood, cerebrospinal fluid or tissue biopsy in case of suggestive clinical presentation. There is no specific antiviral treatment, but the use of IVIg has been proposed and reported to be effective in some cases, particularly in case of HGG [50, 51].

Pneumocystosis has been reported in haematology patients treated with rituximab-containing chemotherapy regimens. A meta-analysis of 11 cohort studies suggested that the use of rituximab-containing regimens in patients with lymphoma was associated with a significantly increased risk for PJP (with a risk ratio of 3.65), and that such risk was inversely associated with the receipt of anti-*Pneumocystis* prophylaxis [52]. However, a more recent single-centre study including 689 patients with B-cell lymphoma treated with R-CHOP (rituximab-CHOP) concluded that the cumulative incidence of PJP until 180 days after the last cycle of therapy was low (1.5%) [53], and below the conventional threshold (6%) for considering the use of prophylaxis [54]. The guidelines on PJP prophylaxis recognized an increased risk in with R-CHOP chemotherapy administered every 14 days, but not every 21 days [55]. In addition, safety analysis of post-marketing data showed a signal of increased frequency of opportunistic infections, including pneumocystosis in patients treated with bendamustine and rituximab. Additionally, high rates of cytomegalovirus (CMV) infection and varicella zoster virus (VZV) infection have been reported in patients treated with this combination, but the role of rituximab compared to bendamustine is difficult to assess. Based on these data, clinicians must always consider the concomitant therapies used with anti-CD20 agents to design the most suitable risk-management strategy.

Cases of PML associated with anti-CD20 agents have also been reported [56]. In some cases, the patients were treated with more than one biological agent (alemtuzumab, idelalisib, eculizumab, etc.). It has been recognized that rituximab confers an increased but unpredictable risk of PML [57].

Finally, it should be noted that the use of anti-CD20 monoclonal antibodies for chronic conditions (i.e. autoimmune diseases and indolent lymphomas) is increasing and, therefore, there is a need to establish best strategies for the management of late-onset complications among patients receiving multiple courses of treatment. Since many of these patients might be not eligible for standard RCTs, large population and open-label extension studies or adaptive trials may help to define such preventive approaches.

Hypogammaglobulinaemia and the Risk of Infections

CD20 is expressed on normal and malignant B-cells, but not on plasma cells. Therefore the use of anti-CD20 monoclonal antibodies does not immediately impair immunoglobulin production [58]. However, hypogammaglobulinaemia (HGG) may occur with increasing courses of therapy, particularly in haematology setting. Moreover, prolonged depletion of plasma cell precursors can reduce immunoglobulin levels and predispose for increased infection risks in some proportion of patients treated by B-cell targeted therapies for autoimmune rheumatic and neurological diseases [59–61].

A review of the literature published during the past 5 years (2016–2020) identified mainly uncontrolled studies reporting on treatment with rituximab. The rate of HGG differed between the studies and depended on the underlying disease, cut-off used to define HGG, pre-treatment levels, concomitant immune suppressive therapy and other factors (Table 7.2). HGG was defined using IgG cut-offs ranging from 4 to 8 g/L; and in children some studies used a cut-off of IgG <2 standard deviations for age.

In the largest cohort of 8633 patients with cancer (78%), autoimmune diseases (28%), haematological diseases (8%) or common variable immune deficiency (1%) receiving rituximab, only 25% had pre-treatment IgG levels known, and of those 48% had low IgG levels [62]. In this study, 23% of patients with mild and 21% of those with moderate HGG before rituximab treatment evolved to a more severe category after treatment [62].

Table 7.2 Summary of studies published during years 2016–2020 reporting on hypogammaglobulinaemia and/or infection rates in patients on rituximab therapy

Reference	Study design	Age group	Underlying disease	No. patients	Rate of low Ig levels	Definition of HGG	Infections rates
Malignancies							
De Angelis [65]	Retrospective single centre	Adults	NHL treated with CHOP/CVP or fludarabine ± RTX	266	RTX exposure was not associated with an increased risk of HGG	IgG < 6 g/L	Not reported specifically on RTX
Minard-Colin [63]	International, randomized controlled phase 3 trial	Children	High-risk, mature B-cell NHL stage III or IV or acute leukaemia	328	Low IgG: RTX vs. control: 70.3% vs. 46.8%, $p = 0.002$ (end of therapy); 55.9% vs. 25.4%, $p < 0.001$) (1 year after inclusion)	Less than the lower limit of the normal range	SI 18.5% RTX vs. 11.1% control ($p = 0.07$)
Chiou [64]	Retrospective single centre	Children	PTLD	17 RTX-treated vs. 11 non-RTX treated	Low IgG: 69% after 6 months ($p = 0.001$), 63% after 2 years ($p = 0.005$), 17% after 5 years ($p = 0.205$) in the RTX group, vs. none among none -RTX treated	<4 g/L	31.4/100 patient-years in RTX-treated patients, vs. 8.4/100 patient-years in non-RTX-treated patients ($p < 0.001$)
Autoimmune diseases							
Stabler [85]	Retrospective single centre	Adults	Autoimmune diseases	221	No data	<6 g/L	SI: 19% patients SI incidence 17.3 (1-year); 11.3 (2-year) per 100 person-years

(continued)

Table 7.2 (continued)

Reference	Study design	Age group	Underlying disease	No. patients	Rate of low Ig levels	Definition of HGG	Infections rates
Khojah [78]	Retrospective single centre	Children	Autoimmune conditions	63	Low IgG: 44% (61% within the first 6 months since therapy onset). 46% in SLE; 71% in autoimmune CNS disease; 60% in ANCA-associated vasculitis; 12% in the miscellaneous group ($p = 0.006$)	IgG <2 SD for age	11.1%
Thiel [79]	Retrospective single centre	Adults	Autoimmune diseases	120	Low IgG: GPA/MPA 31%, EGPA 36%, RA 9%, CTD 16% ($p = 0.01$) Low IgM: GPA/MPA 53%, EGPA 36%, RA 14%, CTD 5%	IgG <7 g/L; IgM <0.4 g/L	Not reported
Padoan [72]	Retrospective single centre	Adults	ANCA-associated vasculitis, CTD	68	15.8% low IgG, 41% low IgM, 10.2% low IgA	IgG <6 g/L; IgM <0.4 g/L; IgA <0.7 g/L	SI 7.4%, more frequently in those with IgG < 6 g/L (26.7% vs. 1.9%, $p = 0.007$)

Shah [83]	Retrospective single centre	Adults	ANCA-associated vasculitis	30	Low IgG 66%	IgG <7,5 g/L (severe ≤3,75 g/L)	57%; 13% requiring hospitalization Increased risk of infections requiring hospitalization with IgG level ≤3,75 g/L (OR 21 [95% confidence interval (CI) 1.1–404.1, $p = 0.04$]; and low IgA (OR 24.6 (95% CI 1.5–799.5, $p = 0.03$)
Cortazar [71]	Retrospective single centre	Adults	ANCA vasculitis	239	Low IgG 9% during induction 4.6% during maintenance	IgG <4 g/L	SI during induction 2.9 [95% CI, 1.2–6.0] per 10 patient years; during maintenance 0.85 [95% CI, 0.66–1.1] per 10 patient years; independently associated with an IgG level <4 g/L
Besada [70]	Retrospective, multicentre	Adults	GPA	29	45% (in 28% leading to RTX discontinuation)	IgG < 6 g/L	24% SI, 31% chronic infections
Besada [69]	Summary of studies	Adults	GPA	16 studies, 9–105 patients	Low IgG: Induction 0–27%; maintenance: 18% (2–45%)		SI: Induction 0–38% Maintenance 18% (11–33%)

(continued)

Table 7.2 (continued)

Reference	Study design	Age group	Underlying disease	No. patients	Rate of low Ig levels	Definition of HGG	Infections rates
Vollmer [84]	Retrospective multicentre	Adults	Multiple sclerosis and related disorders	1000	Low IgG 17.8 per 1000 person-years	<5 g/L	Infections requiring hospitalization: 6.5% (15.5% of them in patients with IgG <5 g/L)
Tallantyre [61]	Retrospective multicentre	Adults and children	Neuromyelitis optica spectrum disorders	50	Total HGG 64% (low IgG 38%, low IgM 56%, low IgA 18%)	IgG <6 g/L, IgM <0.4 g/L, IgA <0.8 g/L	SI 10%
Marcinno [89]	Retrospective single centre	Adults	Neuromyelitis optica spectrum disorders	15 vs. 6 healthy controls	Low IgG 73% (20% severe); Low IgA 40%; Low IgM 60% (13% severe)	IgG <7 g/L (severe <4 g/L); IgA (<0.7 g/L); IgM (<0.4 g/L, severe <0.2 g/L)	SI 13%
Evangelatos [75]	Retrospective multicentre	Adults	RA	83	43.4% any HGG, 31.3% low IgM, 24.1% low IgG (85% mild, 15% moderate no severe)	Mild (5–7 g/L), moderate (3–5 g/L) severe (<3 g/L)	No difference in the SI rate between patients with low or normal immunoglobulin levels
Md Yusof [82]	Retrospective single centre	Adults	RA, SLE, ANCA vasculitis, others	700	23%	IgM <0.5 g/L; IgA <0.8 g/L; IgG <6.0 g/L	SI: 21.3 per 100 person-years in low IgG acquired on RTX treatment, 9.8 per 100 person-years in normal IgG
Boleto [80]	Multicentre observational	Adults	RA	134	17.2% (2.7 events per 100 patients-years)	<6 g/L	SI: 9.7% of patients (1.5 events per 100 pt-years); 26.1% in patients with vs. 6.3% without severe HGG, $p = 0.033$

Reddy [73]	Retrospective single centre	Adults	SLE	57	21% low IgM 5% low IgG	<0.4 gm/L IgM <7 gm/L IgG	No increased infections risk
Aguiar [74]	Retrospective single centre	Mean age 26.39 ± 11.90 years	SLE	115	12.2% low IgG; 27.2% low IgM. Significant reduction of IgM ($p < 0.001$) and IgG ($p = 0.001$) levels. No difference in IgA	No definition	SI 11.3%
Haematological disorders							
Reboursiere [86]	Retrospective single centre	Mostly adult patients	ITP	35	44%; 2.9% severe	IgG <8 g/L; severe: IgG <5 g/L	SI: 6%
Deshayes [87]	Prospective multicentre	Adults	ITP	248	3.5% of 142 with known IgG levels	<5 g/L	23.8%; SI 8.5% (2/100 patient-years)
Levy [142]	32 studies summary	Adults and children	ITP	189	1.6%	<5 g/L	SI 1.6%
Ottaviano [77]	Multicentre Retrospective and prospective	Children	Autoimmune cytopenia	53	32% persistent low IgG	IgG <2 SD for age	12% infections requiring hospitalization; 15% recurrent respiratory infections

(continued)

Table 7.2 (continued)

Reference	Study design	Age group	Underlying disease	No. patients	Rate of low Ig levels	Definition of HGG	Infections rates
Nephrotic syndrome							
Colucci [68]	Single centre observational study	Children	Nephrotic syndrome frequently relapsing/ steroid-dependent. Control: 21 children with nephrotic syndrome treated with immune suppressive drugs	27	Cases vs. controls: Low IgG (41% vs. 65%), IgA (26% vs. 18%) or IgM (4% vs. 6%) (none significant) 15% RTX vs. 0% control severe low IgG; severe low IgA deficiency: 15% RTX vs. 0 controls	IgG <6 g/L (at baseline) or 7 g/L (at last follow-up); <160 mg/dL (severe) IgA <70 mg/dL, <10 mg/dL (severe), IgM <40 mg/dL	44%
Parmentier [66]	Retrospective multicentre	Children	Nephrotic syndrome steroid-dependent	107	29% of 86 with normal baseline IgG	IgG <2 SD for age	12.2% (28% of 46 children with HGG)
Marzuillo [67]	Retrospective single centre	Children	Nephrotic syndrome and normal pre-treatment IgG values	20	55% low IgG	Age-dependent norms	No SI
Others/mixed population							
Barmettler [62]	Retrospective Single centre	Adults	Cancer, autoimmune, CVID, haematological diseases	8633	19% of 342 with IgG levels checked	<6 g/L	SI increase since RTX from 17.2% to 21.7%; $p < 0.001$
Ebbo [143]	Retrospective multicentre	Adults	IgG4-related disease	33	9%	<5 g/L	SI: 12%; 12.1/100 patient years

SI severe infection, *HGG* hypogammaglobulinaemia, *RTX* rituximab, *NHL* non-Hodgkin lymphoma, *CHOP* cyclophosphamide, doxorubicin, vincristine and prednisone, *CVP* cyclophosphamide, vincristine, prednisone, *PTLD* post-transplant lymphoproliferative disorder, *SLE* Systemic lupus erythematosus, *CNS* central nervous system, *CVID* common variable immune deficiency, *GPA* granulomatosis with polyangiitis, *MPA* microscopic polyangiitis, *EGPA* eosinophilic granulomatosis with polyangiitis, *RA* rheumatoid arthritis, *CTD* connective tissue disease, *ANCA* anti-neutrophil cytoplasmic antibody, *ITP* immune thrombocytopenia

Variable rates were observed in patients with malignancies. In children with NHL or acute leukaemia the addition of six doses of rituximab to standard chemotherapy compared to standard chemotherapy alone resulted in significantly higher rates of HGG at the end of therapy (70.3% vs. 46.8%, $p = 0.002$) and at 1 year after inclusion (55.9% vs. 25.4%, $p < 0.001$) [63]. A significantly higher proportion of rituximab-treated children with PTLD developed HGG as compared to those who did not receive rituximab, with the difference persisting for 2 years (Table 7.2) [64]. On the contrary, rituximab exposure was not associated with an increased risk of HGG in 266 adults with NHL treated with CHOP/CVP (cyclophosphamide, vincristine, prednisone) or fludarabine [65].

Three studies (20–107 patients) reported high (29–55%) rates of HGG in children with nephrotic syndrome [66–68]. In one of them, 27 children with frequently relapsing/steroid-dependent nephrotic syndrome were treated with rituximab and compared to 21 controls under intense oral immunosuppression [68]. There was no significant difference between the rituximab-treated children and the controls in the frequency of low serum IgG (41% vs. 65%), IgA (26% vs. 18%) or IgM (4% vs. 6%) levels; however, the degree of HGG was different as 15% of rituximab-treated patients developed either severe IgG or IgA deficiency, compared to none of the controls.

A broad spectrum of HGG rates were reported in patients with autoimmune diseases (Table 7.2). A summary of 16 studies including 9–105 adult patients with GPA reported 0–27% HGG rate during remission induction; and 18% (2–45%) during maintenance rituximab therapy [69]. In one multicentre study of 29 patients with GPA, a third of patients discontinued rituximab therapy due to HGG [70]. Interestingly, the total number of doses did not linearly correlate with the decrease in the Ig levels in a retrospective single centre study of 239 adults with anti-neutrophil cytoplasmic antibodies (ANCA) vasculitis [71]. HGG occurred in 9% during induction phase, but only 4.6% of patients developed significant HGG with rituximab maintenance therapy (median of 2.4 years). IgG levels fell 52% per year during induction and 0.6% per year during maintenance. Of note, several studies in patients with different autoimmune diseases reported on higher rates, and deeper IgM decline as compared to that of IgG [61, 71–75]. IgA levels were less affected [61, 74, 76]. In one multicentre study, 43% of patients with RA developed HGG; of these patients 22.2% had a persistent decrease in two immunoglobulin subclasses; and all three classes were supressed in 11.1 [75].

In children, developing HGG on rituximab may be a sign of underlying primary immune deficiency (PID), as suggested by one paediatric study. In patients receiving rituximab for autoimmune cytopenias, with no prior diagnosis of PID, 17/53 (32%) developed HGG and of those, 9 (53%) were eventually diagnosed with a PID [77].

The majority of patients' Ig levels return to normal within 12 months after rituximab treatment but prolonged HGG can occur. In the study of 57 patients with SLE treated with rituximab and concomitant/sequential immunosuppressants, 21% had persistent IgM HGG (<0.4 g/L) and 5% had low IgG (<7 g/L) 12–144 months following rituximab therapy [73].

Several factors were associated with higher risk of HGG, among them are the following:

1. Demographic factors: younger age in children [66–68, 77];
2. Underlying diseases: the risk of persistent HGG was higher in patients with autoimmune haemolytic anaemia (AHA), and Evans syndrome (ES) (10/17; 59%) vs. immune thrombocytopenic purpura (ITP; 7/36; 19.4%) [77], in patients with autoimmune central nervous system (CNS) disease (8/14; 57%) and ANCA-associated vasculitis (3/10; 30%) vs. SLE (5/22 (22%) and miscellaneous autoimmune diseases (1/17; 6%) [78]; and in patients with ANCA-associated vasculitides (GPA; 17/55; 30.9% and eosinophilic granulomatosis with polyangiitis; 4/11; 36.4%) compared to those with RA (3/35; 8.6%) and connective tissue disease (3/19; 15.8%) [79]. These differences can be explained by higher probability of the underlying primary immune deficiency in patients with autoimmune cytopenia that was not yet diagnosed at the time of cytopenia detection; and higher rituximab exposure in patients with ANCA-associated vasculitis.
3. Concomitant immune suppression: cumulative cyclophosphamide dosage, daily prednisone intake >15 mg [72], not being on methotrexate [75, 80], therapy with mycophenolate mofetil compared with other immunosuppressants [73].
4. Low pre-treatment Ig levels [71–73, 75, 77, 80], long-lasting (>24 months) as compared to short lasting (<12 months) B-cell depletion [79].

HGG and the Risk of Infections

Iatrogenic HGG, similarly to what occurs in common variable immunodeficiency, typically results in a higher rate of infectious complications, and severe infections are infrequent but possible [62, 81].

Several studies reported on increased infection risk in patients treated with rituximab, especially those with low IgG or IgA levels, both at baseline and during treatment [64, 71, 72, 80, 82–84]. The most common infections being pneumonia, bacteraemia (including septic shock) and others [61, 65, 85–88]. On the contrary, low IgM levels were not associated with an increased infection risk [72, 82, 83].

Only some patients with HGG go on to develop infections. In a randomized control study the rate of severe infections was only mildly elevated in 164 rituximab + chemotherapy-treated children with malignancies as compared to 164 children treated with standard chemotherapy alone (18.5% vs. 11.1%, $p = 0.07$), despite a significantly higher proportion of HGG in the rituximab-treated patients [63]. Two studies in 15 and 50 adults with neuromyelitis optica spectrum disorders reported a 64–73% HGG rate, with 20% being severe in one of the studies [61, 89]; however, only 10–13% developed infections. Increased infection risk in patients treated with rituximab, as explained above, may be related to other factors, including presence of comorbidities (e.g. cancer, diabetes, chronic lung disease), previous and concomitant immune suppressive therapy (e.g. calcineurin inhibitors, steroids) and underlying disease characteristics (e.g. autoimmune CNS disease, primary immune deficiency, intestinal transplant and monomorphic disease in children with PTLD) [64, 68, 78, 82, 84, 85, 90].

Literature on other anti-CD20 agents is very scarce. None of the 50 adults with ITP who were treated with low dose veltuzumab developed HGG [91]. Another study of 14 children with nephrotic syndrome, who relapsed after rituximab and were treated with a sequential combination of obinutuzumab and daratumumab, reported a decrease in Ig levels in all patients, with complete absence of IgM in nine patients and IgA in three patients. IgG levels ranged from 2 to 6 g/L [92]. None of the patients developed severe infections.

In MS patients treated with ocrelizumab, the frequency of IgG, IgA and IgM levels below the lower limit of normal were 5%, 5% and 29%, compared to <1% before the ocrelizumab administration [11].

Hypogammaglobulinaemia (HGG) Management

Immunoglobulin replacement therapy (IgRT) was administered in 1–20% of rituximab-treated patients, mainly because of recurrent infections or decreased IgG levels [62, 63, 65, 71, 79, 83, 85, 93]. Among 4479 rituximab-treated patients, 4.5% of 3478 patients with cancer, 2.5% of 1241 patients with rheumatologic disorder and 9.7% of 340 patients with a hematologic disorder received IgRT. A higher cumulative dose of IgRT was associated with a reduced risk of serious infectious complications (HR, 0.98; 95% CI, 0.96–0.99; $p = 0.002$) [62]. Another indication for IgRT was an abnormal response to vaccines following rituximab therapy. Thirteen among 15 patients with NHL had an abnormal vaccine response to diphtheria, tetanus or *Streptococcus pneumoniae* vaccinations given 3–24 months after rituximab therapy; only seven of them had IgG levels less than 6 g/L and ten of them received IgRT [94].

UK recommendations for the management of secondary HGG due to B-cell depleting therapy in autoimmune rheumatic diseases were developed by the 17-member multidisciplinary taskforce committee and published in 2019 [60]. They recommended that Ig levels should be measured prior to starting therapy and repeated every 6–12 months for the duration of treatment and a minimum of 1 year after stopping treatment. The guidelines also state that HGG is not an absolute contraindication to continuing anti-CD20 agents since it can be transient and frequently asymptomatic. As far as IgRT is concerned, they recommended multidisciplinary evaluation, taking into consideration the combination of clinical manifestations (presence of serious, persistent, unusual or recurrent infections despite antibiotic prophylaxis), and laboratory parameters (the degree of HGG, especially IgG, and demonstration of impaired antibody responses to polysaccharide antigens). Asymptomatic HGG is not usually an indication for IgRT, unless IgG level is 3 g/L or lower (in that case immunological referral should be provided). A 3-month initial trial of antibiotic prophylaxis prior to initiating IgRT can be considered, although the strength of this recommendation is low. Finally, the decision to continue IgRT should be reviewed annually and based upon clinical and laboratory parameters, presence of adverse effects and potential risks including thromboembolism and haemolysis [60]. IgRT can be administered intravenously or subcutaneously, and the initial dose of 0.4 g/kg/month can be modified according to IgG levels and clinical results. The duration of IgRT should be based on clinical and laboratory evidence of immune recovery. Recovery of endogenous immunoglobulin production may occur over time, manifested by persistently raised IgG levels, as well as rising IgA levels, IgM levels and B cell numbers. Retrospective review of 16 patients with rituximab-treated autoimmune and IgRT due to recurrent infections revealed that two patients discontinued IgRT after 8 and 20 months due to recovered B-cells and Ig levels. The other 14 patients did not recover their cell counts after a mean of 45 months (range, 5 months to 12 years) [95]. Prolonged antibody deficiency following IgRT discontinuation should prompt investigation for PID [96].

In conclusion, HGG can complicate B-cell depleting therapy, affecting mainly IgM and IgG levels, and can be prolonged in some patients. It is more frequent in cases with lower pre-treatment IgG levels and concomitant therapies. While HGG is frequently asymptomatic, some proportion of patients can develop severe infections. There is limited data to support the use of antibiotic prophylaxis in patients with HGG, considering that continuous antibiotic pressure can lead to infections with resistant pathogens, and given that most respiratory infections are of viral origin and will not be prevented by antibiotic prophylaxis. Antibiotic treatment should be initiated rapidly if a bacterial infection is suspected and treatment and can limit subsequent morbidity and mortality. Additionally, IgRT should be considered in these patients, and if there is a resulting decrease in infections, its use should be annually reviewed until HGG has improved.

Neutropenia and the Risk of Infections

Neutropenia is a possible but rare side effect in anti-CD20 therapy. In case of radioisotope conjugated agents, immediate neutropenia can occur due to direct toxic effect, but these agents currently have very limited use.

Late onset neutropenia (LON), which is defined as developing >4 weeks after treatment, was reported to complicate over 5% of treatment episodes with rituximab. LON can occur also with other anti-CD20 agents and it appears to be under-recognized as a complication [97–101]. Interestingly, the rate of LON varies in different rheumatological diseases, being the highest in GPA and SLE patients (23% and 20%, respectively), and only 3% in RA patients, although the role of concomitant treatment with cyclophosphamide should be considered [102]. Most episodes seem asymptomatic and resolve over time; however, its incidence might be under-diagnosed due to confounding factors, and serious infectious complications are rare but possible [97]. The mechanism of LON is likely immune-mediated, with reported selective reduction in granulopoiesis and maturation arrest at the promyelocyte stage. The full impact of LON on the risk of infections remains unclear, although, together with low IgG levels, it is recognized as a predictor of increased risk of infectious complications in rheumatology patients [82, 101].

In conclusion, therapy with CD20-targeted agents is associated with at least a moderate increase in the risk of infection, particularly if used as part of combination regimen. Infection remains the most common non-haematological adverse effect of anti-CD20 monoclonal antibodies, including mainly respiratory tract infections and HBV reactivation. The consequences of the latter can be minimized with appropriate management strategy. The role of IgRT in cases of HGG is limited to patients with recurrent infections and severe HGG.

The main infectious complications in patients treated with anti-CD20 agents and the proposed management strategy are shown in Table 7.3.

Table 7.3 Main infectious complications in patients treated with anti-CD20 agents and the proposed management strategy

Infection	Management strategy	Comment
Chronic HBV infection or hepatitis **(HBsAg-positive)**	Treatment with high barrier drugs (tenofovir, entecavir)	HBV screening with HBsAg, HBsAb, HBcAb in all patients, HBV-DNA if HBcAb or HBsAg positive
HBV reactivation in resolved HBV infection **(HBsAg-negative, HBcAb-positive, HBsAb positive or negative)**	Pharmacological prophylaxis or in selected cases close monitoring of HBV-DNA followed by pre-emptive antiviral treatment with high barrier drugs	
Pneumocystis jirovecii pneumonia	Prophylaxis in case of certain combination treatment regimens	Increased risk reported only in patients receiving certain combination treatment regimens (R-CHOP 14, R-bendamustine, steroids)
Viral respiratory infections	Preventive measures (masks, vaccination of household contacts and healthcare workers for influenza) IgRT Patient vaccination before anti-CD20 therapy (influenza)	Reported increase in case of HGG
Severe enteroviral infections	Prompt diagnosis with enterovirus-RNA IVIg, particularly in case of HGG	
PML	Low threshold for clinical suspicion and prompt MRI evaluation	
VZV and HSV reactivation	Pharmacological prophylaxis with acyclovir or valacyclovir in case of certain combination treatment regimens Prompt intravenous treatment Household vaccination against VZV Patient vaccination against VZV at least 4 weeks before anti-CD20 treatment onset	
CMV reactivation	Regular CMV-DNA testing and pre-emptive therapy in case of some combination treatment regimens (e.g. R-bendamustine)	

CD19-Targeting Agents

Available Agents

Characteristics of anti-CD19 agents are reported in Table 7.4.

Blinatumomab (Blincyto®, Amgen) is a bispecific T-cell engager (BiTE) antibody construct designed to direct CD3-expressing cytotoxic T-cells to CD19-expressing B-cells [103]. It is approved by Food and Drug Administration (FDA) and European Medicine Agency (EMA) for the treatment of Philadelphia chromosome-negative relapsed or refractory B-cell precursor acute lymphoblastic leukaemia (ALL).

In 2017, blinatumomab was also approved by the FDA for Philadelphia chromosome-positive ALL. A single cycle of treatment consists of 4 weeks of continuous intravenous IV infusion followed by a 2-week treatment-free interval. A treatment course consists of up to a total of 5 cycles.

Inebilizumab (Uplizna® Viela Bio, previously known as MEDI-551, MedImmune) is a humanized, afucosylated IgG1 kappa monoclonal antibody that depletes CD19-expressing B-cells by means of antibody-dependent cell-mediated cytotoxicity (ADCC). It was approved in 2020 for neuromyelitis optica spectrum disorder [104], and it has also been studied in CLL, B-cell lymphoma, MS, systemic scleroderma and multiple myeloma.

Table 7.4 Characteristics of anti-CD19 agents

Agent	Mechanism of action	Year of first approval	Approved indications (year of first approval)	Off-label or experimental uses
Blinatumomab Blincyto®	Bispecific CD19-directed CD3+ T-cell engager causing CD19+ cell lysis	FDA 2014, EMA 2015	Ph-negative or Ph-positive CD19+ B-cell precursor ALL (relapsed or refractory or in first/second complete remission with minimal residual disease ≥0.1%)	DLBCL, NHL
Inebilizumab Uplizna®	Humanized anti-CD19 monoclonal antibody with antibody-dependent cell-mediated cytotoxicity (ADCC)	FDA 2020	NMOSD in AQP4-IgG positive antibodies	Kidney transplant desensitization, myasthenia gravis, IgG4-related disease, autoimmune encephalitis, diffuse large B-cell lymphoma, multiple sclerosis
Combotox	Immunotoxins targeting CD22 and CD19	–	NA	Phase 2 studies in ALL ongoing

AQP4-IgG immunoglobulin G autoantibodies against aquaporin-4, *NMOSD* neuromyelitis optica spectrum disease

Combotox, another anti-CD19 agent, is a 1:1 mixture of two immunotoxins (HD37-dgRTA and RFB4-dgRTA) obtained from coupling IgG1 monoclonal antibodies targeted against CD19 and CD22 and a deglycosylated ricin A chain (dgRTA, previously called dgA). CD19 is present on virtually every malignant lymphoblast in patients with B-lineage ALL, whereas the CD22 epitope is expressed on about 80% of the blast population. Therefore, B-cell ALL and B-cell lymphoma are the main therapeutic targets of combotox [105]. The dosage of combotox has not been standardized, and repeated cycles of treatment and escalation were permitted in the absence of grade 3–4 toxicity, or development of specific antibodies [105]. However, chimeric antigen receptor (CAR)-modified T-cells targeting CD19 have been introduced with much success, and are likely to replace immunotoxin combinations. CD19 is the most widely used target in CAR-T therapy; however, other CDs, including CD22, are also being studied. The review of infectious complications of CAR-T treatments is discussed in Chap. 17.

Mechanism of Action and the Risk of Infectious Complications

The expression of CD19 is almost exclusively restricted to B-cells. Its expression starts during early development stages of the cell, and continuous during many phases of the development of B cells, including plasma cells. Of note, CD19 is also present on the majority of B precursor ALL blasts, hence its main indication.

CD19-targeted agents deplete normal B-cells with the consequent reduction in IgG levels. In a phase 3 RCT HGG occurred in 6% of patients in the blinatumomab arm compared to 0.9% of those treated with conventional chemotherapy, while the rate of neutropenia was lower (38% versus 58%, respectively) [106]. The length of HGG is difficult to establish and may show a dose-dependent relationship, and since CD19, but not CD20, is expressed on plasmablasts, CD19-targeted agents are expected to induce a more profound decrease in serum immunoglobulin levels than CD20-targeted agents [107].

The risk of infections with the use of blinatumomab is significantly influenced by the underlying disease (ALL) or previous chemotherapies, but it might be lower compared to routinely used induction chemotherapy regimens. For example; 34% vs. 52% for FLAG regimen (fludarabine, high-dose cytosine arabinoside and granulocyte colony stimulating factors with or without anthracycline), although the frequency of upper respiratory tract infections and intravascular catheter-related bloodstream infections was higher (3–11%) among patients receiving blinatumomab [106, 108, 109]. The latter might be explained by blinatumomab's mode of administration requiring a continuous IV infusion for weeks. This complication is rarer in the case of inebilizumab which is administered by intermittent IV infusion. Cases of enteroviral encephalitis, pneumocystosis, PML, fungal, CMV and viral respiratory infections have also been reported for blinatumomab.

On the contrary, when inebilizumab was used in neuromyelitis optica or MS, there was no increase in the incidence of infectious complications, with urinary tract infection (UTI) being the most common infectious complication with a similar rate

(9–11%) in both arms in the phase 3 trial [104, 110]. However, considering the mechanism of action, the FDA label for inebilizumab carries warnings on the risk of HBV reactivation (prior screening is recommended, and it is contraindicated in patients with active HBV infection), HGG and TB reactivation (specialist consultation required for those with pre-existing low immunoglobulin levels, active or latent TB). Moreover, vaccination with live-attenuated vaccines is not recommended during or after treatment (until B-cell repletion). If live-attenuated vaccines are indicated, they should be administered at least 4 weeks prior to treatment onset. HGG is a well-recognized complication of treatment with blinatumomab, but reduction of IgG and IgM levels was also reported for inebilizumab, and treatment discontinuation has been suggested for those developing persistent HGG in this setting [104, 111]. Finally, the risk of late onset neutropenia has not yet been established for anti-CD19 agents, but at the end of the 6.5-month period in one RCT, the proportion of patients with any level of neutropenia was higher in the inebilizumab arm compared to placebo (12% vs. 4.2%) [112].

In conclusion, the rate of infectious complications with blinatumomab might be lower compared to standard chemotherapy, but it may be still increased, as is expected in the setting of relapsed or refractory ALL. The need for a continuous 4-week IV infusion is likely responsible for a non-negligible rate of catheter-associated infections, and careful management of intravenous lines is warranted. There is a high risk of HGG, and considering that many patients proceed to allogeneic stem cell transplant, which is also associated with HGG, IgRT should be considered. The rate of these complications is much lower in the case of inebilizumab used in NMO patients. For the management of infectious complications, the same considerations and strategies as for anti-CD20 agents should be used, in particular for the management of HBV infection, although there is limited data in the anti-CD19 setting specifically.

CD52-Targeting Agents

Available Agents

Alemtuzumab is a humanized IgG1 mAb that binds to CD52 and leads to the lysis of targeted cells by means of complement-dependent cytotoxicity and/or ADCC. There are currently two different alemtuzumab products being marketed: MabCampath® and Lemtrada® (Sanofi). In May 2001 alemtuzumab was approved by the FDA for the treatment of B-cell CLL in patients who have been treated with alkylating agents and have failed to respond to fludarabine therapy. This indication was approved by the EMA in 2001 and withdrawn for commercial reasons in 2011. MabCampath® is currently used in selected patients with CLL, GvHD, transplant conditioning regimens, or solid organ transplant patients through a patient access program. In 2013 alemtuzumab was EMA-approved (FDA in 2014), at a significantly lower dose, for the treatment of multiple sclerosis.

The standard dose of alemtuzumab for patients with B-cell CLL is 30 mg given intravenously three times weekly for up to 12 weeks (maximum dose of 1080 mg per year). Whereas for MS a two-cycle regimen of 12 mg daily for 5 days (total yearly dose of 60 mg) followed 12 months later by 12 mg daily for 3 days (total dose of 36 mg) is recommended. In renal transplant induction therapy a single dose of 30 mg is typically used.

Mechanism of Action and the Risk of Infectious Complications

CD52 is expressed on most mature lymphocytes (but not plasma cells), monocytes, macrophages, epithelial cells and thymocytes. Alemtuzumab induces severe depletion of peripheral blood lymphocytes (both T- and B-cells, and especially T CD4+), and this effect is more profound and long-lasting with repeated infusions. Considering the impact on the CD4+ T-cell subset, it is expected that patients will have an increased incidence of classic opportunistic infections (e.g. VZV, CMV, PJP and mycobacterial infections). Even with the lower doses of alemtuzumab used in multiple sclerosis, decreased CD4+ T-cell counts (<200 cells/μL) have been reported to persist months after the completion of therapy [113]; however the infectious risk was significantly lower.

Alemtuzumab has been tested in several phase 3 RCTs for B-cell CLL, induction therapy in kidney transplant recipients and MS. Additionally, there have been phase 2 trials in RA and other autoimmune conditions. The highest rates of infectious complications were found in patients with B-cell CLL and kidney transplant recipients, whereas the lowest were in MS [114–123].

Overall, alemtuzumab use in the haematology and transplant settings has been strongly associated with a significant risk of opportunistic infections such as: pneumocystosis, invasive aspergillosis, nocardiosis, PML, mycobacterial infections, CMV reactivations and CMV disease, listeriosis HBV reactivation, VZV and HSV infections. Different dosing regimens, disease-related immunosuppression and the prior or concomitant use of other immunosuppressive agents most likely account for these differences. In CLL patients, the risk of CMV reactivation (both asymptomatic and symptomatic) was significantly increased compared to the chlorambucil arm (51.7% vs. 7.4% and 15.4% vs. 0%, respectively) [114], while in solid organ transplant reciepients, the risk of CMV and any infection was similar compared to the basiliximab arm (approximatley 9.5% vs. 9.6% and 73% vs. 75%, respectively) [115, 116].

In MS studies, infections occurred more frequently with alemtuzumab use compared to interferon beta-1a treated patients (71% vs. 53%). These infections included various upper respiratory tract infections, urinary tract infections and herpetic infections (HSV 10% vs. 2%; VZV 5% vs. 1%). Serious infections were rare (3% vs. 1%), and the rate of infections in the alemtuzumab arm declined over the years of treatment [124]. While increased rates of HSV and VZV infections were found, the incidence of CMV infection was lower than 1 episode per

100 patient-years in pivotal trials, and few cases were reported in real life post-marketing experience. Therefore, according to the drug label, anti-herpes prophylaxis is mandatory during the first 2 months of treatment or until the CD4+ lymphocyte count is more than 200 cells/μL, whichever occurs later [125]. More recently, cases of listeriosis were reported in MS patients treated with alemtuzumab, and cotrimoxazole prophylaxis was even suggested [126–128]. However it should be kept in mind that, although much higher than in the general population, the rate of *Listeria* meningitis or bacteraemia was only 0.25% in the first month after each cycle of alemtuzumab administration, which is well below the established cut-off for cost effectiveness of cotrimoxazole prophylaxis for prevention of pneumocystosis in adult non-HIV patients (3.5–6%) and therefore its use is not recommended [54, 129]. However, all these data highlight the fact that the rate of infectious complications in MS patients treated with alemtuzumab is higher in real life than in pivotal trials, and most of the infections occurred in the first months after alemtuzumab administration, suggesting that physicians should be aware of these risks [126, 130]. Additionally, in the pivotal trials of alemtuzumab, neutropenia occurred in 20–25% of patients, with <2% developing severe neutropenia, but only one case of fatal neutropenia was reported [131, 132]. No cases of pneumocystosis were reported in this setting.

In conclusion, when alemtuzumab is administered in haematology or transplant settings, anti-HSV/VZV and anti-pneumocystis prophylaxis are recommended together with regular CMV-DNA monitoring. The duration of anti-pneumocystis prophylaxis upon discontinuation of alemtuzumab therapy is not well established, although it seems reasonable to continue its administration for at least 2–6 months or, alternatively, until the peripheral blood CD4+ T-cell count recovers to ≥200 cells/μL. In MS, anti-HSV/VZV prophylaxis is recommended, for at least 2 months or until the peripheral blood CD4+ T-cell count recovers to ≥200 cells/μL. In all patient populations, screening for past or current HBV infection, HCV infection and latent TB infection and should be performed. HBV should be managed with high barrier antiviral therapy in the case of HBsAg positivity, and prophylaxis or strict monitoring in case of HBsAg negative, HBcAb positive patients. Higher rates of human papilloma virus (HPV) infection were reported with alemtuzumab, thus pre-treatment vaccination and regular annual screening is warranted. Even though there are no RCTs supporting these recommendations (patients with HBV and HCV infection were excluded from MS trials), and such trials are unlikely to be performed since anti-CD52 agents are not often used, these strategies are reasonable given prolonged lymphopenia.

Finally, counselling on appropriate hygienic and food safety measures to reduce the risk of listeriosis or toxoplasmosis should be provided.

The overview of selected infectious complications and complications that might result in increased infection risk in patients treated with anti-CD20, CD19 and CD52 agents is provided in Table 7.5.

Table 7.5 The summary of selected infectious complications and complications that might result in increased infection risk in anti-CD20, CD19 and CD52 agents

Agent	Risk of HSV and VZV and anti-herpesvirus prophylaxis warranted	Risk of pneumocystosis and prophylaxis warranted	Risk of HBV reactivation and prophylaxis warranted for HBsAg+ and HBsAg− anti-HBc+	Risk of CMV infection and monitoring warranted	Other infections to be considered and comments	Risk of LON	Risk of HGG and IgRT warranted in selected patients
CD19-targeted agents							
Blinatumomab	Yes	ND but probably yes	Yes	No	CVC-associated BSI	ND (confounding factors)	Yes
Inebilizumab	No (at least not in NMO)	No	Probably yes Treatment for HBsAg+, monitoring for those only HBcAb+ might be acceptable	No	–	Yes	Probably yes, ND on IgRT

(continued)

Table 7.5 (continued)

Agent	Risk of HSV and VZV and anti-herpesvirus prophylaxis warranted	Risk of pneumocystosis and prophylaxis warranted	Risk of HBV reactivation and prophylaxis warranted for HBsAg+ and HBsAg− anti-HBc+	Risk of CMV infection and monitoring warranted	Other infections to be considered and comments	Risk of LON	Risk of HGG and IgRT warranted in selected patients
CD20-targeted agents							
Rituximab	No in monotherapy Yes in HM patients with certain concomitant therapies	No in monotherapy Yes in HM patients with certain concomitant therapies	Yes	No in monotherapy Yes in HM patients with certain concomitant therapies	Bacterial, mainly respiratory infections, PML, enteroviral infections	Yes	Yes/yes
Obinutuzumab		ND, consider depending on concomitant therapy	ND, probably yes	ND, symptom-based approach in HM	Enteroviral infections	Potentially yes	Yes/probably yes
Ofatumumab			Yes	No in monotherapy yes in HM patients with some concomitant therapies	Respiratory tract infections	Yes	Yes/yes
Ocrelizumab			ND, probably yes	No	PML (consider based on data with rituximab and previous treatment with natalizumab)	Yes	Yes/probably yes

CD52-targeted agents							
Alemtuzumab (MabCampath®)	Yes	Yes	Yes, prophylaxis	Yes	IFI, TB, BKV and JCV	Yes	No
Alemtuzumab (Lemtrada®)	Yes	No	Probably yes (monitoring for those only HBcAb+ might be acceptable)	No	HPV, TB, listeriosis, candidiasis	Potentially	No

CMV cytomegalovirus, *HBc* hepatitis B core antibody, *HBsAg* hepatitis B surface antigen, *HBV* hepatitis B virus, *HCV* hepatitis C virus, *HPV* human papillomavirus, *HSV* herpes simplex virus, *IFI* invasive fungal infection, *ND* no data available, *PML* progressive multifocal encephalopathy, *TB* active tuberculosis, *VZV* varicella-zoster virus

Vaccination in Patients Receiving Anti-CD20, Anti-CD19 and Anti-CD52 Agents

Vaccination is an important aspect of infection prevention in patients treated with immunosuppressive agents.

This is true particularly outside the setting of haematological malignancies, i.e. in autoimmune disorders, when treatment is prolonged and the patients carry out their everyday life in the community.

For safety reasons, live vaccines are contraindicated in patients receiving immunosuppressive agents, including anti-CD20, anti-CD19 and anti-CD52 agents. While no data for the latter two groups exist, live vaccines can be administered to patients at least 6 months after the last anti-CD20 treatment, as no safety issues are expected. Whether this is an optimal time point for maximum vaccine efficacy remains to be established [133]. Live attenuated Herpes Zoster vaccine is an exception and should be withheld at least 1 month following immunosuppressive therapy [134], although inactivated Herpes Zoster vaccine is currently preferred if available, due to its safety and efficacy [135]. Of note, an interval of 8 months is recommended between MMRV vaccination and the last IVIg administration, if IgRT (0.4 g/kg) was administered [136].

Indeed, while there are no safety concerns when using inactive vaccines in subjects receiving B or T cell depleting therapy, the question of obtaining a protective response is fundamental. In fact, impairment of B-cell function is thought to be accountable for poor response to vaccination, particularly if including neoantigens [137].

The effect of CD20-targeted therapy on vaccination has been recognized and much discussed in hematologic and rheumatologic settings [138, 139]. In patients with haematological malignancies receiving anti-CD20 therapy, the complete absence of serological response to influenza vaccination was reported by most of the studies, and this negative effect was present both during rituximab treatment and 6–10 months after the last administration (response rate between 0% and 29%) [139]. Among cancer patients, the response to two doses of ASO3-adjuvanted influenza vaccine was 28% in those with lymphoma, compared to 82% any in cancer patients, and rituximab treatment but not conventional chemotherapy was associated with lower response [140]. Therefore, current guidelines for haematology patients recommend waiting at least 6 months after the last dose of rituximab, before starting immunization programs, due to the extremely low chance of responding [139]. However, these data mainly come from lymphoma patients, in whom rituximab was used together with other chemotherapy. Therefore the negative effect of B cell-depleting agents might be more severe or pronounced compared to a setting where these agents are used as monotherapy.

Despite impaired responses reported for influenza, *Streptococcus pneumoniae* polysaccharide (PPSV23) and *Haemophilus influenzae* type b (Hib) conjugate vaccines, a prospective study in patients with ITP demonstrated that pneumococcal and Hib vaccines administered at least after 6 months from rituximab infusion had high efficacy in preventing mild and severe respiratory infections [7]. The negative effect of rituximab on vaccination was particularly evident for neoantigens and polysaccharide vaccines [137].

In a recent trial of patients with treatment-naïve MS who received the first dose of ocrelizumab, the response to immunization (including PPSV23 and influenza) was impaired but not abolished by the B cell-depleting treatment, and protective titres could be obtained in some subjects [141]. It remains unknown how the length of treatment with B-cell depleting agents affects the immunity, and in particular the probability of responding to vaccination.

Therefore, the optimal point for immunization would be before B-cell depleting therapy. Inactivated vaccines should be administered 2 or more weeks; and live vaccines should be administered 4 or more weeks before initiating such therapies [133]. While this might be feasible in autoimmune or rheumatological diseases, particularly in patients who have not received prior immunosuppressive therapy (live vaccines are contraindicated in case of any, not only B-cell or T-cell depleting agent), postponing treatment for at least 2 weeks after vaccination is rarely feasible in haematology and transplant settings.

References

1. Fernández-Ruiz M, Meije Y, Manuel O, Akan H, Carratalà J, Aguado JM, et al. ESCMID Study Group for Infections in Compromised Hosts (ESGICH) consensus document on the safety of targeted and biological therapies: an infectious diseases perspective (introduction). Clin Microbiol Infect. 2018;24(Suppl 2):S2–s9.
2. Mikulska M, Lanini S, Gudiol C, Drgona L, Ippolito G, Fernández-Ruiz M, et al. ESCMID Study Group for Infections in Compromised Hosts (ESGICH) consensus document on the safety of targeted and biological therapies: an infectious diseases perspective (agents targeting lymphoid cells surface antigens [I]: CD19, CD20 and CD52). Clin Microbiol Infect. 2018;24(Suppl 2):S71–s82.
3. Gingele S, Skripuletz T, Jacobs R. Role of CD20(+) T cells in multiple sclerosis: implications for treatment with ocrelizumab. Neural Regen Res. 2020;15(4):663–4.
4. Fung M, Jacobsen E, Freedman A, Prestes D, Farmakiotis D, Gu X, et al. Increased risk of infectious complications in older patients with indolent non-Hodgkin lymphoma exposed to bendamustine. Clin Infect Dis. 2019;68(2):247–55.
5. Lanini S, Molloy AC, Fine PE, Prentice AG, Ippolito G, Kibbler CC. Risk of infection in patients with lymphoma receiving rituximab: systematic review and meta-analysis. BMC Med. 2011;9:36.
6. van Vollenhoven RF, Fleischmann RM, Furst DE, Lacey S, Lehane PB. Longterm safety of rituximab: final report of the rheumatoid arthritis global clinical trial program over 11 years. J Rheumatol. 2015;42(10):1761–6.
7. Moulis G, Lapeyre-Mestre M, Palmaro A, Sailler L. Infections in non-splenectomized persistent or chronic primary immune thrombocytopenia adults: risk factors and vaccination effect. J Thromb Haemost. 2017;15(4):785–91.
8. Montalban X, Hauser SL, Kappos L, Arnold DL, Bar-Or A, Comi G, et al. Ocrelizumab versus placebo in primary progressive multiple sclerosis. N Engl J Med. 2017;376(3):209–20.
9. Hauser SL, Bar-Or A, Comi G, Giovannoni G, Hartung HP, Hemmer B, et al. Ocrelizumab versus interferon beta-1a in relapsing multiple sclerosis. N Engl J Med. 2017;376(3):221–34.
10. Ng HS, Rosenbult CL, Tremlett H. Safety profile of ocrelizumab for the treatment of multiple sclerosis: a systematic review. Expert Opin Drug Saf. 2020;19(9):1069–94.

11. Wolinsky JS, Arnold DL, Brochet B, Hartung HP, Montalban X, Naismith RT, et al. Long-term follow-up from the ORATORIO trial of ocrelizumab for primary progressive multiple sclerosis: a post-hoc analysis from the ongoing open-label extension of the randomised, placebo-controlled, phase 3 trial. Lancet Neurol. 2020;19(12):998–1009.
12. Mysler EF, Spindler AJ, Guzman R, Bijl M, Jayne D, Furie RA, et al. Efficacy and safety of ocrelizumab in active proliferative lupus nephritis: results from a randomized, double-blind, phase III study. Arthritis Rheum. 2013;65(9):2368–79.
13. Emery P, Rigby W, Tak PP, Dorner T, Olech E, Martin C, et al. Safety with ocrelizumab in rheumatoid arthritis: results from the ocrelizumab phase III program. PLoS One. 2014;9(2):e87379.
14. Abushouk AI, Ahmed H, Ismail A, Elmaraezy A, Badr AS, Gadelkarim M, et al. Safety and efficacy of ocrelizumab in rheumatoid arthritis patients with an inadequate response to methotrexate or tumor necrosis factor inhibitors: a systematic review and meta-analysis. Rheumatol Int. 2017;37(7):1053–64.
15. Moreno C, Montillo M, Panayiotidis P, Dimou M, Bloor A, Dupuis J, et al. Ofatumumab in poor-prognosis chronic lymphocytic leukemia: a phase IV, non-interventional, observational study from the European Research Initiative on Chronic Lymphocytic Leukemia. Haematologica. 2015;100(4):511–6.
16. Taylor PC, Quattrocchi E, Mallett S, Kurrasch R, Petersen J, Chang DJ. Ofatumumab, a fully human anti-CD20 monoclonal antibody, in biological-naive, rheumatoid arthritis patients with an inadequate response to methotrexate: a randomised, double-blind, placebo-controlled clinical trial. Ann Rheum Dis. 2011;70(12):2119.
17. van Oers MH, Kuliczkowski K, Smolej L, Petrini M, Offner F, Grosicki S, et al. Ofatumumab maintenance versus observation in relapsed chronic lymphocytic leukaemia (PROLONG): an open-label, multicentre, randomised phase 3 study. Lancet Oncol. 2015;16(13):1370–9.
18. Hauser SL, Bar-Or A, Cohen JA, Comi G, Correale J, Coyle PK, et al. Ofatumumab versus Teriflunomide in Multiple Sclerosis. N Engl J Med. 2020;383(6):546–57.
19. Bar-Or A, Grove RA, Austin DJ, Tolson JM, VanMeter SA, Lewis EW, et al. Subcutaneous ofatumumab in patients with relapsing-remitting multiple sclerosis. Neurology. 2018;90(20):e1805.
20. van Imhoff GW, McMillan A, Matasar MJ, Radford J, Ardeshna KM, Kuliczkowski K, et al. Ofatumumab versus rituximab salvage chemoimmunotherapy in relapsed or refractory diffuse large B-cell lymphoma: the ORCHARRD study. J Clin Oncol. 2016;35(5):544–51.
21. Freeman CL, Sehn LH. A tale of two antibodies: obinutuzumab versus rituximab. Br J Haematol. 2018;182(1):29–45.
22. Evans SS, Clemmons AB. Obinutuzumab: a novel anti-CD20 monoclonal antibody for chronic lymphocytic leukemia. J Adv Pract Oncol. 2015;6(4):370–4.
23. Fischer K, Al-Sawaf O, Bahlo J, Fink AM, Tandon M, Dixon M, et al. Venetoclax and obinutuzumab in patients with CLL and coexisting conditions. N Engl J Med. 2019;380(23):2225–36.
24. Moreno C, Greil R, Demirkan F, Tedeschi A, Anz B, Larratt L, et al. Ibrutinib plus obinutuzumab versus chlorambucil plus obinutuzumab in first-line treatment of chronic lymphocytic leukaemia (iLLUMINATE): a multicentre, randomised, open-label, phase 3 trial. Lancet Oncol. 2019;20(1):43–56.
25. Evens AM, Jovanovic BD, Su YC, Raisch DW, Ganger D, Belknap SM, et al. Rituximab-associated hepatitis B virus (HBV) reactivation in lymphoproliferative diseases: meta-analysis and examination of FDA safety reports. Ann Oncol. 2011;22(5):1170–80.
26. Mozessohn L, Chan KK, Feld JJ, Hicks LK. Hepatitis B reactivation in HBsAg-negative/HBcAb-positive patients receiving rituximab for lymphoma: a meta-analysis. J Viral Hepat. 2015;22(10):842–9.
27. Ziakas PD, Karsaliakos P, Mylonakis E. Effect of prophylactic lamivudine for chemotherapy-associated hepatitis B reactivation in lymphoma: a meta-analysis of published clinical trials and a decision tree addressing prolonged prophylaxis and maintenance. Haematologica. 2009;94(7):998–1005.

28. Martin ST, Cardwell SM, Nailor MD, Gabardi S. Hepatitis B reactivation and rituximab: a new boxed warning and considerations for solid organ transplantation. Am J Transplant. 2014;14(4):788–96.
29. UK drug safety update. 2017. https://www.gov.uk/drug-safety-update/bendamustine-levact-increased-mortality-observed-in-recent-clinical-studies-in-off-label-use-monitor-for-opportunistic-infections-hepatitis-b-reactivation.
30. Quattrocchi E, Østergaard M, Taylor PC, van Vollenhoven RF, Chu M, Mallett S, et al. Safety of repeated open-label treatment courses of intravenous ofatumumab, a human anti-CD20 monoclonal antibody, in rheumatoid arthritis: results from three clinical trials. PLoS One. 2016;11(6):e0157961.
31. Nicolini LA, Zappulo E, Viscoli C, Mikulska M. Management of chronic viral hepatitis in the hematological patient. Expert Rev Anti-Infect Ther. 2018;16(3):227–41.
32. EASL. 2017 Clinical practice guidelines on the management of hepatitis B virus infection. J Hepatol. 2017;67(2):370–98.
33. Huang H, Li X, Zhu J, Ye S, Zhang H, Wang W, et al. Entecavir vs lamivudine for prevention of hepatitis B virus reactivation among patients with untreated diffuse large B-cell lymphoma receiving R-CHOP chemotherapy: a randomized clinical trial. JAMA. 2014;312(23):2521–30.
34. Kusumoto S, Arcaini L, Hong X, Jin J, Kim WS, Kwong YL, et al. Risk of HBV reactivation in patients with B-cell lymphomas receiving obinutuzumab or rituximab immunochemotherapy. Blood. 2019;133(2):137–46.
35. Seto WK, Chan TS, Hwang YY, Wong DK, Fung J, Liu KS, et al. Hepatitis B reactivation in patients with previous hepatitis B virus exposure undergoing rituximab-containing chemotherapy for lymphoma: a prospective study. J Clin Oncol. 2014;32(33):3736–43.
36. Kusumoto S, Tanaka Y, Suzuki R, Watanabe T, Nakata M, Takasaki H, et al. Monitoring of hepatitis B virus (HBV) DNA and risk of HBV reactivation in B-cell lymphoma: a prospective observational study. Clin Infect Dis. 2015;61(5):719–29.
37. Loglio A, Viganò M, Grossi G, Labanca S, Goldaniga M, Pompa A, et al. Lamivudine prophylaxis prevents hepatitis B virus reactivation in anti-HBc positive patients under rituximab for non-Hodgkin lymphoma. Dig Liver Dis. 2019;51(3):419–24.
38. Seto WK, Chan TS, Hwang YY, Mak LY, Wong DK, Fung J, et al. Monitoring and treatment of patients undergoing immunotherapy with anti-CD20 who are exposed to HBV. Clin Gastroenterol Hepatol. 2019;17(7):1410–2.
39. Kusumoto S, Tanaka Y, Suzuki R, Watanabe T, Nakata M, Sakai R, et al. Ultra-high sensitivity HBsAg assay can diagnose HBV reactivation following rituximab-based therapy in patients with lymphoma. J Hepatol. 2020;73(2):285–93.
40. Varisco V, Viganò M, Batticciotto A, Lampertico P, Marchesoni A, Gibertini P, et al. Low risk of hepatitis B virus reactivation in HBsAg-negative/anti-HBc-positive carriers receiving rituximab for rheumatoid arthritis: a retrospective multicenter Italian study. J Rheumatol. 2016;43(5):869–74.
41. Ciardi MR, Iannetta M, Zingaropoli MA, Salpini R, Aragri M, Annecca R, et al. Reactivation of hepatitis B virus with immune-escape mutations after ocrelizumab treatment for multiple sclerosis. Open Forum Infect Dis. 2018;6(1):ofy356.
42. Marignani M, Mangone M, Cox MC, Angeletti S, Veggia B, Ferrari A, et al. HCV-positive status and hepatitis flares in patients with B-cell non-Hodgkin's lymphoma treated with rituximab-containing regimens. Dig Liver Dis. 2011;43(2):139–42.
43. Fraticelli P, Bagnarelli P, Tarantino G, Martino GP, Benfaremo D, Nobili L, et al. Chronic hepatitis E in a patient treated with rituximab and mycophenolate mofetil for Sjogren's syndrome. Rheumatology (Oxford). 2016;55(12):2275–7.
44. Kassab S, Saghi T, Boyer A, Lafon ME, Gruson D, Lina B, et al. Fatal case of enterovirus 71 infection and rituximab therapy, France, 2012. Emerg Infect Dis. 2013;19(8):1345–7.
45. Dendle C, Gilbertson M, Korman TM, Golder V, Morand E, Opat S. Disseminated enteroviral infection associated with obinutuzumab. Emerg Infect Dis. 2015;21(9):1661–3.

46. Eyckmans T, Wollants E, Janssens A, Schoemans H, Lagrou K, Wauters J, et al. Coxsackievirus A16 encephalitis during obinutuzumab therapy, Belgium, 2013. Emerg Infect Dis. 2014;20(5):913–5.
47. Kelesidis T, Daikos G, Boumpas D, Tsiodras S. Does rituximab increase the incidence of infectious complications? A narrative review. Int J Infect Dis. 2011;15(1):e2–e16.
48. Palacios T, Bartelt L, Scheld W, Lopes MB, Kelting SM, Holland S, et al. Fatal Coxsackie meningoencephalitis in a patient with B-cell lymphopenia and hypogammaglobulinemia following rituximab therapy. Ann Allergy Asthma Immunol. 2015;115(2):148–50.
49. Nicolini LA, Canepa P, Caligiuri P, Mikulska M, Novi G, Viscoli C, et al. Fulminant hepatitis associated with echovirus 25 during treatment with ocrelizumab for multiple sclerosis. JAMA Neurol. 2019;76(7):866–7.
50. Higer M, Cana D, Podlech J, Schadmand-Fischer S, Schwarting A, Teschner D, et al. Life-threatening disseminated enterovirus infection during combined rituximab and ibrutinib maintenance treatment for mantle cell lymphoma: a case report. J Med Case Rep. 2020;14(1):135.
51. Abzug MJ. The enteroviruses: problems in need of treatments. J Infect. 2014;68(Suppl 1):S108–14.
52. Jiang X, Mei X, Feng D, Wang X. Prophylaxis and treatment of Pneumocystis jiroveci pneumonia in lymphoma patients subjected to rituximab-contained therapy: a systemic review and meta-analysis. PLoS One. 2015;10(4):e0122171.
53. Barreto JN, Ice LL, Thompson CA, Tosh PK, Osmon DR, Dierkhising RA, et al. Low incidence of pneumocystis pneumonia utilizing PCR-based diagnosis in patients with B-cell lymphoma receiving rituximab-containing combination chemotherapy. Am J Hematol. 2016;91(11):1113–7.
54. Stern A, Green H, Paul M, Vidal L, Leibovici L. Prophylaxis for Pneumocystis pneumonia (PCP) in non-HIV immunocompromised patients. Cochrane Database Syst Rev. 2014;2014(10):Cd005590.
55. Maertens J, Cesaro S, Maschmeyer G, Einsele H, Donnelly JP, Alanio A, et al. ECIL guidelines for preventing Pneumocystis jirovecii pneumonia in patients with haematological malignancies and stem cell transplant recipients. J Antimicrob Chemother. 2016;71(9):2397–404.
56. Carson KR, Evens AM, Richey EA, Habermann TM, Focosi D, Seymour JF, et al. Progressive multifocal leukoencephalopathy after rituximab therapy in HIV-negative patients: a report of 57 cases from the Research on Adverse Drug Events and Reports project. Blood. 2009;113(20):4834–40.
57. Chahin S, Berger JR. A risk classification for immunosuppressive treatment-associated progressive multifocal leukoencephalopathy. J Neurovirol. 2015;21(6):623–31.
58. Singh V, Gupta D, Almasan A. Development of novel anti-Cd20 monoclonal antibodies and modulation in Cd20 levels on cell surface: looking to improve immunotherapy response. J Cancer Sci Ther. 2015;7(11):347–58.
59. Marco H, Smith RM, Jones RB, Guerry MJ, Catapano F, Burns S, et al. The effect of rituximab therapy on immunoglobulin levels in patients with multisystem autoimmune disease. BMC Musculoskelet Disord. 2014;15:178.
60. Wijetilleka S, Mukhtyar C, Jayne D, Ala A, Bright P, Chinoy H, et al. Immunoglobulin replacement for secondary immunodeficiency after B-cell targeted therapies in autoimmune rheumatic disease: systematic literature review. Autoimmun Rev. 2019;18(5):535–41.
61. Tallantyre EC, Whittam DH, Jolles S, Paling D, Constantinesecu C, Robertson NP, et al. Secondary antibody deficiency: a complication of anti-CD20 therapy for neuroinflammation. J Neurol. 2018;265(5):1115–22.
62. Barmettler S, Ong MS, Farmer JR, Choi H, Walter J. Association of immunoglobulin levels, infectious risk, and mortality with rituximab and hypogammaglobulinemia. JAMA Netw Open. 2018;1(7):e184169.
63. Minard-Colin V, Auperin A, Pillon M, Burke GAA, Barkauskas DA, Wheatley K, et al. Rituximab for high-risk, mature B-cell non-Hodgkin's lymphoma in children. N Engl J Med. 2020;382(23):2207–19.

64. Chiou FK, Beath SV, Patel M, Gupte GL. Hypogammaglobulinemia and bacterial infections following pediatric post-transplant lymphoproliferative disorder in the rituximab era. Pediatr Transplant. 2019;23(6):e13519.
65. De Angelis F, Tosti ME, Capria S, Russo E, D'Elia GM, Annechini G, et al. Risk of secondary hypogammaglobulinaemia after rituximab and fludarabine in indolent non-Hodgkin lymphomas: a retrospective cohort study. Leuk Res. 2015;39(12):1382–8.
66. Parmentier C, Delbet JD, Decramer S, Boyer O, Hogan J, Ulinski T. Immunoglobulin serum levels in rituximab-treated patients with steroid-dependent nephrotic syndrome. Pediatr Nephrol. 2020;35(3):455–62.
67. Marzuillo P, Guarino S, Esposito T, Di Sessa A, Orsini SI, Capalbo D, et al. Rituximab-induced IgG hypogammaglobulinemia in children with nephrotic syndrome and normal pre-treatment IgG values. World J Clin Cases. 2019;7(9):1021–7.
68. Colucci M, Carsetti R, Serafinelli J, Rocca S, Massella L, Gargiulo A, et al. Prolonged impairment of immunological memory after anti-CD20 treatment in pediatric idiopathic nephrotic syndrome. Front Immunol. 2019;10:1653.
69. Besada E. Low immunoglobulin levels increase the risk of severe hypogammaglobulinemia in granulomatosis with polyangiitis patients receiving rituximab. BMC Musculoskelet Disord. 2016;17:6.
70. Besada E. Risk factors and adverse events poorly predict infections and hypogammaglobulinemia in granulomatosis with polyangiitis patients receiving rituximab. Autoimmune Dis. 2016;2016:8095695.
71. Cortazar FB, Pendergraft WF III, Wenger J, Owens CT, Laliberte K, Niles JL. Effect of continuous B cell depletion with rituximab on pathogenic autoantibodies and total IgG levels in antineutrophil cytoplasmic antibody-associated vasculitis. Arthritis Rheumatol. 2017;69(5):1045–53.
72. Padoan R, Felicetti M, Gatto M, Polito P, Doria A, Schiavon F. Rituximab-associated hypogammaglobulinaemia in ANCA-associated vasculitis and connective tissue diseases: a longitudinal observational study. Clin Exp Rheumatol. 2020;38 Suppl 124(2):188–94.
73. Reddy V, Martinez L, Isenberg DA, Leandro MJ, Cambridge G. Pragmatic treatment of patients with systemic lupus erythematosus with rituximab: long-term effects on serum immunoglobulins. Arthritis Care Res. 2017;69(6):857–66.
74. Aguiar R, Araujo C, Martins-Coelho G, Isenberg D. Use of rituximab in systemic lupus erythematosus: a single center experience over 14 years. Arthritis Care Res. 2017;69(2):257–62.
75. Evangelatos G, Fragoulis GE, Klavdianou K, Moschopoulou M, Vassilopoulos D, Iliopoulos A. Hypogammaglobulinemia after rituximab for rheumatoid arthritis is not rare and is related with good response: 13 years real-life experience. Rheumatology (Oxford). 2020;60(5):2375–82.
76. Pranzatelli MR, Tate ED, McGee NR, MacArthur CA. Evaluation of responsiveness to reduced-dose rituximab in corticotropin/intravenous immunoglobulin/rituximab combination immunotherapy for opsoclonus-myoclonus syndrome. Pediatr Neurol. 2018;85:71–5.
77. Ottaviano G, Marinoni M, Graziani S, Sibson K, Barzaghi F, Bertolini P, et al. Rituximab unveils hypogammaglobulinemia and immunodeficiency in children with autoimmune cytopenia. J Allergy Clin Immunol Pract. 2020;8(1):273–82.
78. Khojah AM, Miller ML, Klein-Gitelman MS, Curran ML, Hans V, Pachman LM, et al. Rituximab-associated Hypogammaglobulinemia in pediatric patients with autoimmune diseases. Pediatr Rheumatol Online J. 2019;17(1):61.
79. Thiel J, Rizzi M, Engesser M, Dufner AK, Troilo A, Lorenzetti R, et al. B cell repopulation kinetics after rituximab treatment in ANCA-associated vasculitides compared to rheumatoid arthritis, and connective tissue diseases: a longitudinal observational study on 120 patients. Arthritis Res Ther. 2017;19(1):101.
80. Boleto G, Avouac J, Wipff J, Forien M, Dougados M, Roux C, et al. Predictors of hypogammaglobulinemia during rituximab maintenance therapy in rheumatoid arthritis: a 12-year longitudinal multi-center study. Semin Arthritis Rheum. 2018;48(2):149–54.

81. Kado R, Sanders G, McCune WJ. Diagnostic and therapeutic considerations in patients with hypogammaglobulinemia after rituximab therapy. Curr Opin Rheumatol. 2017;29(3):228–33.
82. Md Yusof MY, Vital EM, McElvenny DM, Hensor EMA, Das S, Dass S, et al. Predicting severe infection and effects of hypogammaglobulinemia during therapy with rituximab in rheumatic and musculoskeletal diseases. Arthritis Rheumatol. 2019;71(11):1812–23.
83. Shah S, Jaggi K, Greenberg K, Geetha D. Immunoglobulin levels and infection risk with rituximab induction for anti-neutrophil cytoplasmic antibody-associated vasculitis. Clin Kidney J. 2017;10(4):470–4.
84. Vollmer BL, Wallach AI, Corboy JR, Dubovskaya K, Alvarez E, Kister I. Serious safety events in rituximab-treated multiple sclerosis and related disorders. Ann Clin Transl Neurol. 2020;7(9):1477–87.
85. Stabler S, Giovannelli J, Launay D, Cotteau-Leroy A, Heusele M, Lefevre G, et al. Serious infectious events and immunoglobulin replacement therapy in patients with autoimmune diseases receiving rituximab: a retrospective cohort study. Clin Infect Dis. 2020;72(5):727–37.
86. Reboursiere E, Fouques H, Maigne G, Johnson H, Chantepie S, Gac AC, et al. Rituximab salvage therapy in adults with immune thrombocytopenia: retrospective study on efficacy and safety profiles. Int J Hematol. 2016;104(1):85–91.
87. Deshayes S, Khellaf M, Zarour A, Layese R, Fain O, Terriou L, et al. Long-term safety and efficacy of rituximab in 248 adults with immune thrombocytopenia: results at 5 years from the French prospective registry ITP-ritux. Am J Hematol. 2019;94(12):1314–24.
88. Karim MY. Increased awareness of hypogammaglobulinemia after B cell-targeted therapy: comment on the article by Md Yusof et al. Arthritis Rheumatol. 2020;72(7):1230–1.
89. Marcinno A, Marnetto F, Valentino P, Martire S, Balbo A, Drago A, et al. Rituximab-induced hypogammaglobulinemia in patients with neuromyelitis optica spectrum disorders. Neurol Neuroimmunol Neuroinflamm. 2018;5(6):e498.
90. Kavcic M, Fisher BT, Seif AE, Li Y, Huang YS, Walker D, et al. Leveraging administrative data to monitor rituximab use in 2875 patients at 42 freestanding children's hospitals across the United States. J Pediatr. 2013;162(6):1252–8.e1.
91. Liebman HA, Saleh MN, Bussel JB, Negrea OG, Horne H, Wegener WA, et al. Comparison of two dosing schedules for subcutaneous injections of low-dose anti-CD20 veltuzumab in relapsed immune thrombocytopenia. Haematologica. 2016;101(11):1327–32.
92. Dossier C, Prim B, Moreau C, Kwon T, Maisin A, Nathanson S, et al. A global antiB cell strategy combining obinutuzumab and daratumumab in severe pediatric nephrotic syndrome. Pediatr Nephrol. 2020;36(5):1175–82.
93. Kant S, Azar A, Gapud EJ, Antiochos B, Manno R, Seo P, et al. Subcutaneous immunoglobulin for antibody deficiency in antineutrophil cytoplasmic antibody (ANCA)-associated vasculitis. Cureus. 2019;11(12):e6367.
94. Mustafa SS, Jamshed S, Vadamalai K, Ramsey A. The use of 20% subcutaneous immunoglobulin replacement therapy in patients with B cell non-Hodgkin lymphoma with humoral immune dysfunction after treatment with rituximab. Clin Lymphoma Myeloma Leuk. 2020;20(9):e590–e6.
95. Barmettler S, Price C. Continuing IgG replacement therapy for hypogammaglobulinemia after rituximab—for how long? J Allergy Clin Immunol. 2015;136(5):1407–9.
96. Patel V, Cowan J. Discontinuation of immunoglobulin replacement therapy in patients with secondary antibody deficiency. Expert Rev Clin Immunol. 2020;16(7):711–6.
97. Zonozi R, Wallace ZS, Laliberte K, Huizenga NR, Rosenthal JM, Rhee EP, et al. Incidence, clinical features, and outcomes of late-onset neutropenia from rituximab for autoimmune disease. Arthritis Rheumatol. 2020;73(2):347–54.
98. Zanetta C, Robotti M, Nozzolillo A, Sangalli F, Liberatore G, Nobile-Orazio E, et al. Late onset absolute neutropenia associated with ocrelizumab treatment in multiple sclerosis: a case report and review of the literature. J Neurol Sci. 2020;409.
99. Emmanouilides C, Witzig TE, Wiseman GA, Gordon LI, Wang H, Schilder R, et al. Safety and efficacy of yttrium-90 ibritumomab tiuxetan in older patients with non-Hodgkin's lymphoma. Cancer Biother Radiopharm. 2007;22(5):684–91.

100. Shah S, Kavadichanda CG, Belani P, Ganesh RN, Negi VS. Early onset neutropenia and thrombocytopenia following rituximab in lupus nephritis. Int J Rheum Dis. 2019;22(5):946–50.
101. Monaco WE, Jones JD, Rigby WF. Rituximab associated late-onset neutropenia—a rheumatology case series and review of the literature. Clin Rheumatol. 2016;35(10):2457–62.
102. Tesfa D, Ajeganova S, Hägglund H, Sander B, Fadeel B, Hafström I, et al. Late-onset neutropenia following rituximab therapy in rheumatic diseases: association with B lymphocyte depletion and infections. Arthritis Rheum. 2011;63(8):2209–14.
103. Hladnik L, Augustin K, DeFrates S. Advancements in therapy for acute lymphoblastic leukemia: blinatumomab. J Adv Pract Oncol. 2016;7(1):76–82.
104. Cree BAC, Bennett JL, Kim HJ, Weinshenker BG, Pittock SJ, Wingerchuk DM, et al. Inebilizumab for the treatment of neuromyelitis optica spectrum disorder (N-MOmentum): a double-blind, randomised placebo-controlled phase 2/3 trial. Lancet. 2019;394(10206):1352–63.
105. Schindler J, Gajavelli S, Ravandi F, Shen Y, Parekh S, Braunchweig I, et al. A phase I study of a combination of anti-CD19 and anti-CD22 immunotoxins (Combotox) in adult patients with refractory B-lineage acute lymphoblastic leukaemia. Br J Haematol. 2011;154(4):471–6.
106. Kantarjian H, Stein A, Gokbuget N, Fielding AK, Schuh AC, Ribera JM, et al. Blinatumomab versus chemotherapy for advanced acute lymphoblastic leukemia. N Engl J Med. 2017;376(9):836–47.
107. Zugmaier G, Topp MS, Alekar S, Viardot A, Horst HA, Neumann S, et al. Long-term follow-up of serum immunoglobulin levels in blinatumomab-treated patients with minimal residual disease-positive B-precursor acute lymphoblastic leukemia. Blood Cancer J. 2014;4:244.
108. Kantarjian HM, Stein AS, Bargou RC, Grande Garcia C, Larson RA, Stelljes M, et al. Blinatumomab treatment of older adults with relapsed/refractory B-precursor acute lymphoblastic leukemia: results from 2 phase 2 studies. Cancer. 2016;122(14):2178–85.
109. Martinelli G, Boissel N, Chevallier P, Ottmann O, Gokbuget N, Topp MS, et al. Complete hematologic and molecular response in adult patients with relapsed/refractory Philadelphia chromosome-positive B-precursor acute lymphoblastic leukemia following treatment with blinatumomab: results from a phase II, single-arm, multicenter study. J Clin Oncol. 2017;35(16):1795–802.
110. Agius MA, Klodowska-Duda G, Maciejowski M, Potemkowski A, Li J, Patra K, et al. Safety and tolerability of inebilizumab (MEDI-551), an anti-CD19 monoclonal antibody, in patients with relapsing forms of multiple sclerosis: results from a phase 1 randomised, placebo-controlled, escalating intravenous and subcutaneous dose study. Mult Scler. 2019;25(2):235–45.
111. UPLIZNA. FDA. Highlights of prescribing information. 2020.
112. Frampton JE. Inebilizumab: first approval. Drugs. 2020;80(12):1259–64.
113. Hill-Cawthorne GA, Button T, Tuohy O, Jones JL, May K, Somerfield J, et al. Long term lymphocyte reconstitution after alemtuzumab treatment of multiple sclerosis. J Neurol Neurosurg Psychiatry. 2012;83(3):298–304.
114. Skoetz N, Bauer K, Elter T, Monsef I, Roloff V, Hallek M, et al. Alemtuzumab for patients with chronic lymphocytic leukaemia. Cochrane Database Syst Rev. 2012;2012(2):CD008078.
115. Hanaway MJ, Woodle ES, Mulgaonkar S, Peddi VR, Kaufman DB, First MR, et al. Alemtuzumab induction in renal transplantation. N Engl J Med. 2011;364:1909–19.
116. Haynes R, Harden P, Judge P, Blackwell L, Emberson J, Landray MJ, et al. Alemtuzumab-based induction treatment versus basiliximab-based induction treatment in kidney transplantation (the 3C study): a randomised trial. Lancet. 2014;384(9955):1684–90.
117. Cohen JA, Coles AJ, Arnold DL, Confavreux C, Fox EJ, Hartung H-P, et al. Alemtuzumab versus interferon beta 1a as first-line treatment for patients with relapsing-remitting multiple sclerosis: a randomised controlled phase 3 trial. Lancet. 2012;380(1819–28):1819–28.
118. Coles AJ, Compston DA, Selmaj KW, Lake SL, Moran S, Margolin DH, et al. Alemtuzumab vs. interferon beta-1a in early multiple sclerosis. N Engl J Med. 2008;359(17):1786–801.

119. Coles AJ, Twyman CL, Arnold DL, Cohen JA, Confavreux C, Fox EJ, et al. Alemtuzumab for patients with relapsing multiple sclerosis after disease-modifying therapy: a randomised controlled phase 3 trial. Lancet. 2012;380(9856):1829–39.
120. Abad S, Gyan E, Moachon L, Bouscary D, Sicard D, Dreyfus F, et al. Tuberculosis due to Mycobacterium bovis after alemtuzumab administration. Clin Infect Dis. 2003;37(2):e27–8.
121. Cheung WW, Tse E, Leung AY, Yuen KY, Kwong YL. Regular virologic surveillance showed very frequent cytomegalovirus reactivation in patients treated with alemtuzumab. Am J Hematol. 2007;82(2):108–11.
122. Malek SK, Obmann MA, Gotoff RA, Foltzer MA, Hartle JE, Potdar S. Campath-1H induction and the incidence of infectious complications in adult renal transplantation. Transplantation. 2006;81(1):17–20.
123. Thursky KA, Worth LJ, Seymour JF, Miles Prince H, Slavin MA. Spectrum of infection, risk and recommendations for prophylaxis and screening among patients with lymphoproliferative disorders treated with alemtuzumab*. Br J Haematol. 2006;132(1):3–12.
124. Wray S, Havrdova E, Snydman DR, Arnold DL, Cohen JA, Coles AJ, et al. Infection risk with alemtuzumab decreases over time: pooled analysis of 6-year data from the CAMMS223, CARE-MS I, and CARE-MS II studies and the CAMMS03409 extension study. Mult Scler J. 2018;25(12):1605–17.
125. Lemtrada. FDA. Highlights of prescribing information. 2019.
126. Holmøy T, Fevang B, Olsen DB, Spigset O, Bø L. Adverse events with fatal outcome associated with alemtuzumab treatment in multiple sclerosis. BMC Res Notes. 2019;12(1):497.
127. Holmøy T, von der Lippe H, Leegaard TM. Listeria monocytogenes infection associated with alemtuzumab—a case for better preventive strategies. BMC Neurol. 2017;17(1):65.
128. Coles A, Roberston N, Al-Araji A, Waller B, Brenner B, Mclean B, et al. Association of British neurologist 2017. Guidance on the prevention of Listeria infection after alemtuzumab treatment of multiple sclerosis. 2017. https://imagevault.nhi.no/publishedmedia/ndzf3wdzn-nrt2lnnbp0b/Guidance_on_the_prevention_of_Listeria_infection_after_alemtuzumab_treatment_of_multiple_sclerosis.pdf.
129. Green H, Paul M, Vidal L, Leibovici L. Prophylaxis of Pneumocystis pneumonia in immunocompromised non-HIV-infected patients: systematic review and meta-analysis of randomized controlled trials. Mayo Clin Proc. 2007;82(9):1052–9.
130. Buonomo AR, Zappulo E, Viceconte G, Scotto R, Borgia G, Gentile I. Risk of opportunistic infections in patients treated with alemtuzumab for multiple sclerosis. Expert Opin Drug Saf. 2018;17(7):709–17.
131. Baker D, Giovannoni G, Schmierer K. Marked neutropenia: significant but rare in people with multiple sclerosis after alemtuzumab treatment. Mult Scler Relat Disord. 2017;18:181–3.
132. Yiannopoulou KG, Papadimitriou D, Anastasiou AI, Siakantaris M. Neutropenia with fatal outcome in a multiple sclerosis patient 23 days after alemtuzumab infusion. Mult Scler Relat Disord. 2018;23:15–6.
133. Rubin LG, Levin MJ, Ljungman P, Davies EG, Avery R, Tomblyn M, et al. 2013 IDSA clinical practice guideline for vaccination of the immunocompromised host. Clin Infect Dis. 2014;58(3):309–18.
134. Harpaz R, Ortega-Sanchez IR, Seward JF. Prevention of herpes zoster: recommendations of the Advisory Committee on Immunization Practices (ACIP). MMWR Recomm Rep. 2008;57(Rr-5):1–30; quiz CE2–4.
135. Dooling KL, Guo A, Patel M, Lee GM, Moore K, Belongia EA, et al. Recommendations of the Advisory Committee on Immunization Practices for use of herpes zoster vaccines. MMWR Morb Mortal Wkly Rep. 2018;67(3):103–8.
136. Ezeanolue E, Harriman K, Hunter P, Kroger A, Pellegrini C. General best practice guidelines for immunization. Best practices guidance of the Advisory Committee on Immunization Practices (ACIP). www.cdc.gov/vaccines/hcp/acip-recs/generalrecs/downloads/general-recs.pdf. Accessed 10 Feb 2021.

137. Bingham CO III, Looney RJ, Deodhar A, Halsey N, Greenwald M, Codding C, et al. Immunization responses in rheumatoid arthritis patients treated with rituximab: results from a controlled clinical trial. Arthritis Rheum. 2010;62(1):64–74.
138. Friedman MA, Winthrop KL. Vaccines and disease-modifying antirheumatic drugs: practical implications for the rheumatologist. Rheum Dis Clin North Am. 2017;43(1):1–13.
139. Mikulska M, Cesaro S, de Lavallade H, Di Blasi R, Einarsdottir S, Gallo G, et al. Vaccination of patients with haematological malignancies who did not have transplantations: guidelines from the 2017 European Conference on Infections in Leukaemia (ECIL 7). Lancet Infect Dis. 2019;19(6):e188–e99.
140. Hottinger AF, George A-CC, Bel M, Favet L, Combescure C, Meier S, et al. A prospective study of the factors shaping antibody responses to the AS03-adjuvanted influenza A/H1N1 vaccine in cancer outpatients. Oncologist. 2012;17(3):436–45.
141. Bar-Or A, Calkwood JC, Chognot C, Evershed J, Fox EJ, Herman A, et al. Effect of ocrelizumab on vaccine responses in patients with multiple sclerosis: the VELOCE study. Neurology. 2020;95(14):e1999–2008.
142. Levy R, Mahevas M, Galicier L, Boutboul D, Moroch J, Loustau V, et al. Profound symptomatic hypogammaglobulinemia: a rare late complication after rituximab treatment for immune thrombocytopenia. Report of 3 cases and systematic review of the literature. Autoimmun Rev. 2014;13(10):1055–63.
143. Ebbo M, Grados A, Samson M, Groh M, Loundou A, Rigolet A, et al. Long-term efficacy and safety of rituximab in IgG4-related disease: data from a French nationwide study of thirty-three patients. PLoS One. 2017;12(9):e0183844.

Cell-Surface Receptors: EGFR- and VEGFR-Targeted Agents

8

Juan Aguilar-Company and Isabel Ruiz-Camps

Introduction

In this chapter, we analyze the risk of infection associated with the use of antineoplastic agents targeting cell surface receptors and associated pathways. Specifically, this chapter focuses on drugs acting on the epidermal growth factor receptor (EGFR) and the vascular endothelial growth factor (VEGF)-related pathways.

It should be noted that these agents act on pathways also present in normal, healthy cells. Therefore, susceptibility to infections may be altered in heterogeneous ways [1, 2]. Additionally, in an individual patient, underlying diseases and previous or concomitant treatments (such as chemotherapy or corticosteroids) will also influence the risk of infection. Relevant studies addressing infection-related complications associated with a specific agent or group of agents are shown in Table 8.1. In view of the limited data published so far for some of these drugs, clinical reviews, expert recommendations, and scientific society guidelines are the only available source of information [3, 4].

The provided recommendations are open for modification based on ongoing and future clinical observations. Increased awareness by clinicians and constant reporting are required to identify infections related to the use of these agents.

J. Aguilar-Company (✉)
Oncology Department, Vall d'Hebron Hospital Universitari, Barcelona, Spain

Infectious Diseases Department, Vall d'Hebron Hospital Universitari, Barcelona, Spain

I. Ruiz-Camps
Infectious Diseases Department, Vall d'Hebron Hospital Universitari, Barcelona, Spain

C. Cervera, J. M. Aguado (eds.), *Infectious Complications in Biologic and Targeted Therapies*, https://doi.org/10.1007/978-3-031-11363-5_8

Table 8.1 Studies reporting infections associated with EGFR and VEGF/VEGFR-targeted therapies

Study	Agents studied	Type of study	Highlights
Funakoshi et al. [76]	Anti-EGFR mAbs	Meta-analysis of clinical trials	Increased risk of severe infections (RR 1.34, 95%CI 1.33–1.66, $p < 0.001$) and of fever and neutropenia (RR 1.27, 95%CI, 1.09–1.48, $p = 0.002$)
Qi et al. [77]	Anti-EGFR mAbs	Meta-analysis of clinical trials	RR of severe infections 1.49, 95%CI 1.1–1.62, $p = 0.003$
Wang et al. [88]	Anti-EGFR TKIs	Meta-analysis of clinical trials	OR of all-grade infections 1.48 (95%CI: 1.12–1.96, $p = 0.006$) No differences in severe infections
Guerriero et al. [80] Ricci et al. [81]	Cetuximab	Case reports	*Staphylococcus aureus* skin abscesses complicating severe papulopustular rash
Grenader et al. [89] Li et al. [90]	Erlotinib	Case reports	*Staphylococcus aureus* bacteremia complicating severe papulopustular rash
Eilers et al. [78]	EGFR and HER2 inhibitors	Retrospective study of patients evaluated in a dermatological clinic	83 of 221 patients classified as having any type of bacterial, viral, or fungal skin infection
Lord et al. [79]	Cetuximab	Case series of patients treated with cetuximab and radiotherapy for HNSCC	10 of 14 patients presented skin superinfection with *Staphylococcus aureus*
Schutz et al. [93]	Bevacizumab	Meta-analysis of clinical trials	Increased risks of all-grade (RR = 1.15, 95%CI 1.01–1.30, $p = 0.033$) and high-grade (RR = 1.08, 95%CI 1.02–1.13, $p = 0.005$) neutropenia, and febrile neutropenia (RR = 1.31, 95%CI 1.08–1.58, $p = 0.006$)
Qi et al. [94]	Bevacizumab	Meta-analysis of clinical trials	Increased risk of all-grade (RR = 1.45, 95%CI 1.27–1.66, $p < 0.001$) and high-grade (RR = 1.59, 95%CI 1.42–1.79, $p < 0.001$) infection, and of fistulae/abscesses (RR = 2.13, 95%CI 1.06–4.27, $p = 0.033$)
Zhang et al. [95]	Aflibercept	Meta-analysis of clinical trials	Increased risk of high grade (RR = 1.87, 95% CI 1.52, 2.30, $p < 0.001$) and fatal (OR = 2.16, 95%CI 1.14–4.11, $p = 0.018$) infections
Schutz et al. [96]	Sorafenib	Meta-analysis of clinical trials	Increased risk of all-grade (RR = 1.69, 95%CI 1.33–2.17) and high-grade (RR = 1.61, 95%CI 1.02–2.57) neutropenia and high-grade lymphopenia (RR = 1.84, 95%CI 1.22–2.78)
Schutz et al. [97]	Sorafenib, sunitinib, and pazopanib	Meta-analysis of clinical trials	Only 3 fatal infections among 4679 patients from 10 studies, no other infectious events reported
Chamilos et al. [98]	Sorafenib	Case series and literature review	5 cases of invasive fungal infection in patients treated with sorafenib

EGFR epidermal growth factor receptor, *HNSCC* head and neck squamous cell cancer, *mAbs* monoclonal antibodies, *TKIs* tyrosine kinase inhibitors

Agents Targeting EGFR

EGFR, also known as ErbB-1 or human epidermal growth factor receptor 1 (HER1), is a transmembrane glycoprotein comprising an extracellular domain, with binding sites for its ligands, and a cytoplasmic domain with tyrosine kinase (TK) activity. EGFR is one of the four proteins in the ErbB (or HER) family of receptor TKs, also including ErbB2/HER2, ErbB3/HER3, and ErbB4/HER4. These receptors initiate intracellular signaling pathways including Ras/MAPK and Ras/PI3K/Akt/mTOR, which are linked to cell proliferation, differentiation, and survival. ErbB family receptors play a crucial role in many types of cancer [5, 6]. Pharmacological inhibition of ErbB receptors, particularly EGFR or HER2, alone or in combination with chemotherapy or other targeted therapies, has been shown to be effective in the treatment of several types of cancer (Table 8.2).

Table 8.2 EGFR and VEGF/VEGFR-targeted agents and approved indications

Drug	Approved indication	Clinical trial
Cetuximab	Metastatic colorectal cancer (RAS-wild type, alone or in combination with chemotherapy)	COIN [7] CRYSTAL [8] CA225-025 [9]
	Metastatic colorectal cancer (BRAF-mutated, in combination with encorafenib)	BEACON [10]
	Locoregional head and neck squamous cell carcinoma (in combination with radiotherapy)	BONNER [11]
	Recurrent locoregional or metastatic head and neck squamous cell carcinoma (in combination with cisplatin and 5-fluouracil)	EXTREME [12]
Panitumumab	Colorectal cancer (RAS wild-type, alone or in combination with chemotherapy)	PRIME [13] 20050181 [14] NCT00113763 [15]
Gefitinib	Metastatic non-small cell lung cancer (NSCLC) harboring EGFR exon 19 deletions or exon 21 (L858R) substitution mutations	IPASS [16] IFUM [17]
Erlotinib	Metastatic NSCLC harboring EGFR exon 19 deletions or exon 21 (L858R) substitution mutations	EURTAC [18] NCT00036647 [19] OPTIMAL [20]
	Locally advanced, unresectable or metastatic pancreatic cancer, in combination with gemcitabine	NCIC CTG PA.3 [21]
Afatinib	Metastatic NSCLC harboring EGFR exon 19 deletions or exon 21 (L858R) substitution mutations	LUX-Lung 3, LUX-Lung 6 [22]
Dacomitinib	Metastatic NSCLC harboring EGFR exon 19 deletions or exon 21 (L858R) substitution mutations	ARCHER 1009 [23] ARCHER 1050 [24]
Osimertinib	Metastatic NSCLC harboring EGFR T790M resistance mutation First-line treatment in patients with NSCLC harboring EGFR exon 19 deletions or exon 21 (L858R) substitution mutations	AUREA3 [25] FLAURA [26]

(continued)

Table 8.2 (continued)

Drug	Approved indication	Clinical trial
Bevacizumab	Metastatic colorectal cancer, in combination with chemotherapy	AVF2107, NO16966, ARTIST, AVF0780, AVF2192, AGITG MAX, E3200 [27]
	Metastatic non-squamous NSCLC, in combination with chemotherapy	AVAiL [28] BO17704 [29]
	Metastatic breast cancer, in combination with chemotherapy	NCT00028990 [30] RIBBON-1 [31]
	Advanced/metastatic RCC, in combination with interferon-a 2a	BO17705 [32]
	Glioblastoma multiforme in combination with chemotherapy	NCT00345163 [33]
	Ovarian, fallopian tube or primary peritoneal cancer, various regimes	GOG-0218 [34] AURELIA [35] OCEANS [36] GOG-0213
	Advanced cervical cancer, various regimes	GOG-0240 [37]
	HCC, in combination with atezolizumab	IMbrave150 [38]
Aflibercept	Metastatic colorectal cancer, in combination with FOLFIRI	VELOUR [39]
Ramucirumab	Gastric cancer, alone or in combination with paclitaxel	REGARD [40] RAINBOW [41]
	Colorectal cancer	RAISE [42]
	NSCLC, various regimes	RELAY [43] REVEL [44]
	HCC	REACH-2 [45]
Sorafenib	HCC	SHARP [46]
	RCC	TARGET [47]
	Differentiated thyroid cancer	DECISION [48]
Pazopanib	RCC	VEG105192 [49]
	Soft tissue sarcoma	PALETTE [50]
Axitinib	RCC, alone or in combination with checkpoint inhibitors	JAVELIN Renal 101 [51] KEYNOTE-426 [51] NCT00678392 [52]
Cabozantinib	RCC	METEOR [53] CABOSUN [54]
	HCC	CELESTIAL [55]
	Medullary thyroid cancer	EXAM [56]
Regorafenib	CRC	CORRECT [57]
	GIST	GRID [58]
	HCC	RESORCE [59]
Sunitinib	Gastrointestinal stromal tumors	NCT00075218 [60]
	RCC	NCT00083889 [61]
	Neuroendocrine pancreatic cancer	NCT00428597 [62]
Lenvatinib	RCC	NCT01136733 [63]
	HCC	REFLECT [64]
	Differentiated thyroid cancer	SELECT [65]
Vandetanib	Medullary thyroid cancer	NCT00410761 [66]

GIST gastrointestinal stromal tumor, *HCC* hepatocellular carcinoma, *NSCLC* non-small cell lung cancer, *RCC* renal cell carcinoma

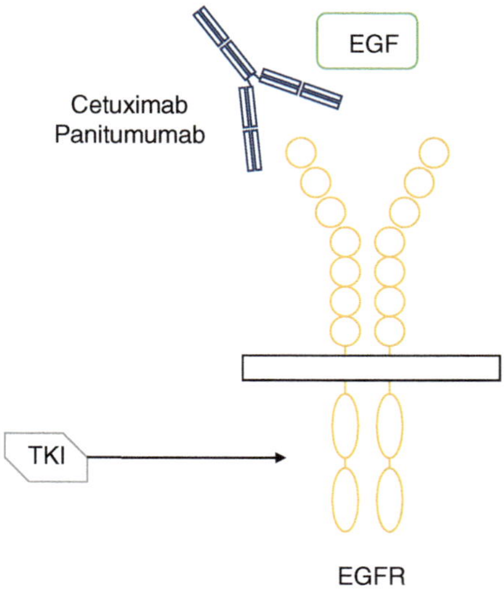

Fig. 8.1 Structure and mode of action of EGFR-targeted agents

Agents targeting EGFR (Fig. 8.1) can be classified as:

- Monoclonal antibodies (mAbs): These agents bind to the extracellular component of the EGFR and prevent epidermal growth factor from binding to its receptor, impeding its activation. They are administered intravenously.
- TK inhibitors (TKIs): These drugs bind to the intracellular TK domain of the EGFR blocking its activity. They are administered orally, due to their high oral bioavailability.

mAbs Against EGFR

Mechanism of Action

Two mAbs targeting EGFR are currently approved: cetuximab (Erbitux®, Merck/Eli Lilly), which is a murine-human chimeric IgG1 mAb, and panitumumab (Vectibix®, Amgen), a fully human IgG2 mAb. Cetuximab induces EGFR internalization and degradation once bound to the external domain of EGFR. Panitumumab, a fully humanized antibody that does not trigger antibody-dependent cell-mediated cytotoxicity and shows a lower risk of hypersensitivity reactions, was developed more recently [67].

Approved Indications

These agents are approved for patients with RAS wild-type metastatic colorectal cancer, either in combination with chemotherapy as first- or second-line treatment or as single agents after failure of oxaliplatin- and irinotecan-based regimens [7–9, 13–15, 68, 69]. Additionally, cetuximab has been more recently approved in combination with encorafenib for the treatment of BRAF-mutated colorectal cancer [10]. Cetuximab, in combination with radiation, is also approved for the treatment of patients with locally advanced head and neck squamous cell carcinoma (HNSCC) [11, 70] and in combination with platinum and fluorouracil chemotherapy as first-line therapy for recurrent or metastatic HNSCC [12].

Expected Impact on Susceptibility to Infection

Basic research suggests that modification of EGFR pathways might influence the risk of infection. Heparin-binding epidermal growth factor (EGF)-like growth factors (HB-EGF) play an important role in regulating the proliferation of hematopoietic maturing cells. The biologic effects of HB-EGF are exerted through EGFR, as demonstrated after the blockade of its activity by anti-EGFR mAbs [1]. Thus, cetuximab and panitumumab might affect the proliferation of neutrophils and lead to neutropenia. Two meta-analyses of randomized controlled trials (RCTs) showed a higher risk of neutropenia in patients treated with cetuximab compared to control arms [71, 72]. EGF is also involved in tumor necrosis factor α-induced respiratory burst and phagocytic activity through the EGFR TK pathway [73]. Downregulation of EGFR-dependent signaling in non-tumor tissues may also impair normal immune innate immunity function [74]. Toll-like receptors (TLRs) constitute an important class of sensors that detect highly conserved microbial motifs (pathogen-associated molecular patterns) and activate cellular responses. TLR-3 function has been found to depend on EGFR activation and Scr binding [2]. Dysregulated EGFR function in normal respiratory epithelium and dendritic cells may also contribute to the risk of infection.

Most patients treated with EGFR mAbs agents experience dermatologic toxicity, generally in the form of papulopustular rash, xerosis, and paronychia. EGFR is instrumental in maintaining epidermal homeostasis through regulation of keratinocyte proliferation, differentiation, migration, and survival. Therefore, EGFR-targeted therapies lead to strong dysregulation in the keratinocyte cycle and strong inflammatory responses. Such skin toxicity occurs in up to 75% of patients in a dose-dependent fashion after 1–2 weeks of therapy. The eruption consists of folliculocentric pruritic papules that evolve into pustules, mostly distributed in head, neck, trunk, and proximal upper extremities). Microorganisms do not appear to contribute to the pathogenesis of EGFR-targeted agent-induced rash in the earlier phases, as the initial pustule is sterile. Nevertheless, secondary infection of the affected skin with bacteria, dermatophytes, or viruses may follow [75].

Available Clinical Data

Two meta-analyses have evaluated the risk of high-grade infections (grade 3 or higher according to the Common Terminology Criteria for Adverse Events, with febrile neutropenia classified as high-grade infection) associated with the use of cetuximab or panitumumab [76, 77]. Both included phase 2 and 3 RCTs published before 2014. In these meta-analyses, treatment with anti-EGFR mAbs was associated with an increase in the incidence of high-grade infection, with relative risks of 1.34 (95%CI, 1.1–1.62, $p < 0.001$) and 1.49 (95%CI, 1.1–1.62, $p = 0.003$), respectively. Interestingly, in subgroup analysis, such increased risk was limited to specific tumor types (colorectal carcinoma, non-small cell lung carcinoma [NSCLC] and HNSCC) and to cases in which anti-EGFR mAbs were used in conjunction with cisplatin or irinotecan. Unfortunately, detailed data on specific infection types or causative microorganisms were lacking in the studies, as most of these events were simply categorized as severe infection, fever, and neutropenia, pneumonia, or sepsis.

Skin and soft tissue infections complicating papulopustular rash induced by EGFR-targeted therapy have been reported in the literature as case reports and retrospective case series. Of note, some of them included complicated forms due to *Staphylococcus aureus*, such as impetiginized dermatitis superinfection [78, 79] or skin abscesses requiring surgical management [80, 81]. Two meta-analyses of RCTs and nonrandomized intervention studies evaluating the efficacy of oral tetracyclines (doxycycline of minocycline) for the prevention of papulopustular rash showed significant benefit in terms of reduced incidence of moderate to severe forms [82, 83]. Topical corticosteroids and antibiotics (e.g., clindamycin) have been also used as prophylaxis or treatment, although its efficacy has not been adequately evaluated. The use of systemic antibiotic therapy is recommended in cases of severe rash or impetiginized dermatitis.

Conclusions and Suggested Prevention Strategies

- In view of available data, therapy with EGFR-targeted mAbs is associated with a meaningful increase in the risk of infection, an increased risk of drug-induced neutropenia, and secondary infection in cases of severe cutaneous adverse events. In order to reduce the length of drug-induced neutropenia, the use of G-CSF may be considered in cases of delayed recovery of absolute neutrophil counts.
- No clear benefit is expected from the universal use of antiviral, antifungal, or anti-*Pneumocystis* prophylaxis for patients receiving such therapy, although an individualized infection risk assessment seems advisable.
- Prevention of the development of papulopustular rash in patients receiving anti-EGFR mAbs should be based on low-potency topical steroids combined with moisturizer and sunscreen for the first 6 weeks of therapy. On the basis of results from RCTs, the administration of systemic antibiotics (doxycycline 100 mg every 12 h or minocycline 100 mg daily) for the first 6–8 weeks is also recommended. The clinician must be aware of the risk of secondary infections.

EGFR-Targeted TKIs

Mechanism of Action

The implication of the ErbB family of receptors in oncogenesis has been previously discussed. The mechanisms by which the EGFR signaling pathway becomes oncogenic are numerous and often specific for each type of cancer. In NSCLC, mutations in the intracellular TK domain of EGFR enhance ligand-inducing autophosphorylation and confer increased sensitivity to specific TKIs [84]. The discovery of these activating mutations in the TK domain of the EGFR gene has represented a major step forward in the design of personalized therapeutic approaches in patients with NSCLC. The most common oncogenic mutations are deletions in exon 19 (present in 45–50% of cases) and a point mutation (L858R) in exon 21 (35–45% of cases). The estimated frequency of EGFR mutations is approximately 15% and is more prevalent in certain subgroups, such as women, patients with an Asian background, never-smokers, and those with adenocarcinoma histology [85].

Approved Indications

First-generation EGFR TKIs include gefitinib (Iressa®, AstraZeneca) [16, 17] and erlotinib (Tarceva®, Roche) [18–20]. Both agents act by reversible (noncovalent) binding to the TK domain of EGFR. Second generation of irreversible EGFR inhibitors comprises afatinib (Giotrif®, Boehringer Ingelheim) [22, 86] and dacomitinib (Vizimtro®, Pfizer) [23, 24]. These agents confer remarkable improvements in response rates and progression-free survival compared to conventional chemotherapy across several RCTs. Thus, gefitinib, erlotinib, afatinib, and dacomitinib have been approved by the FDA and EMA as first-line therapies for the treatment of patients with advanced NSCLC harboring EGFR-sensitizing mutations. Finally, erlotinib is also approved in combination with gemcitabine for the treatment of metastatic pancreatic cancer [21].

Unfortunately, the acquisition of resistance mutations in the EGFR gene to first- and second-generation TKIs is a common phenomenon, prompting the development of more potent targeted agents. The EGFR T790M mutation has been identified as the most common acquired resistance mechanism. This newer generation of TKIs includes osimertinib (Tagrisso®, AstraZeneca) and the HER2 inhibitors lapatinib (Tyverb®, Novartis Pharmaceuticals) and neratinib (Nerlynx®, Puma Biotechnology). Osimertinib is a potent, irreversible third-generation EGFR TKI active against the T790M EGFR resistance mutation. It shows central nervous system penetration, with cases reported of sustained tumor regression in brain metastases. The FDA and EMA approved its use for patients with locally advanced or metastatic NSCLC harboring the T790M mutation and for its use as first-line therapy [25, 26].

Expected Impact on Infection Risk

As previously commented, basic research suggests that EGFR may play a role in innate immunity and in skin and airway normal function. EGFR TKIs exhibit an acceptable safety profile, with most adverse events consisting of rash, paronychia, diarrhea, hepatotoxicity, and, less frequently, interstitial lung disease and pneumonitis.

Available Clinical Data

Pivotal studies comparing EGFR TKIs with chemotherapy in NSCLC showed a clearly reduced rate of neutropenia [16, 18, 20, 21, 25]. In meta-analysis of four RCTs including 1929 patients with NSCLC, participants receiving conventional chemotherapy experienced significantly higher rates of neutropenia than those receiving gefitinib. As example, the occurrence of all-grade and grade 3 or higher neutropenia was much less common in the gefitinib arms (7% vs. 84% and 3% vs. 69%, respectively) [87]. A meta-analysis of trials evaluating the risk of infection associated with erlotinib and gefitinib given for NSCLC has also been published, including a total of 25 RCTs with 13,436 patients. These trials evaluated erlotinib as single agent compared to placebo, as single agent compared to chemotherapy, or given together with chemotherapy compared to chemotherapy and placebo. The odds ratio of all-grade infections was 1.48 (95%CI: 1.12–1.96, $p = 0.006$), but an association with high-grade infections or fatal infections was not shown. The addition of EGFR TKIs to chemotherapy showed a tendency to increase the risk of infections in comparison with chemotherapy alone (OR 1.24, 95%CI: 0.75–3.05, $p = 0.39$) [88]. As with the use of anti-EGFR mAbs, cutaneous adverse events, most notably papulopustular rash and paronychia, are frequent in patients treated with EGFR TKIs. Impetiginized dermatitis may also be present [78, 89, 90]; previously exposed management strategies also apply to EGFR TKIs [75, 91].

Taken together, these data suggest treatment with EGFR TKIs seems to be safe in terms of infectious complications.

Conclusions and Suggested Prevention Strategies

- In view of available data, therapy with EGFR TKIs is not associated with a meaningful increase in the risk of infection.
- No clear benefit is expected from the universal use of antiviral, antifungal, or anti-*Pneumocystis* prophylaxis for patients receiving such therapy, although an individualized infection risk assessment seems advisable.

- Papulopustular rash and paronychia constitute frequent adverse events and should be managed with topical steroids, tetracyclines, and topical antibiotics according to guidelines and center experience. Secondary infections complicating cutaneous adverse events have been described.

Agents Targeting VEGF/VEGF Receptor (VEGFR)

Angiogenesis, the formation of new capillary blood vessels from the preexisting vasculature, constitutes a key process in tumor progression by mediating invasion and metastasis of cancer cells. A complex network of multiple proangiogenic signaling molecules, such as VEGF, platelet-derived growth factor (PDGF), fibroblast growth factor (FGF), or placental growth factor (PlGF) families and their respective receptors, stimulate intracellular signaling pathways that trigger formation of new blood vessels, tumor growth, and metastatic spread [92]. Inhibition of the VEGF family members and their corresponding receptors and downstream signaling pathways has become an attractive therapeutic target that has demonstrated improved outcomes across several tumor types (Tables 8.2). As for EGFR inhibitors, two types of agents can be defined (Fig. 8.2):

- Intravenous drugs targeting VEGF/VEGFR (the mAbs bevacizumab and ramucirumab and the soluble VEGFR aflibercept).
- TKIs targeting VEGFR as well as other angiogenic pathways. They are administered orally, due to their high oral bioavailability.

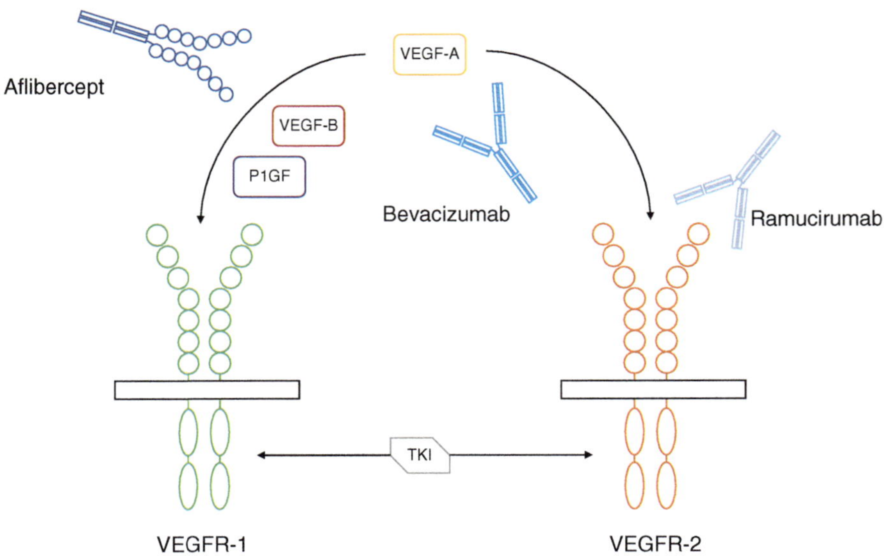

Fig. 8.2 Structure and mode of action of VEGF/VEGFR-targeted agents

Intravenous Agents Targeting VEGF/VEGFR

Mechanism of Action

Among the different angiogenic molecules, VEGF-A represents a dominant promoter that stimulates the endothelial cell proliferation and migration, ultimately leading to the formation of new blood vessels. Accordingly, increased VEGF mRNA expression has been demonstrated in many human tumors, including lung, breast, gastrointestinal tract, renal cell, and ovarian carcinomas. VEGF-A acts via two TK receptors: VEGFR-1 and VEGFR-2, which are present on the surface of endothelial cells. However, VEGF-B and PlGF bind only to VEGFR-1.

Approved Indications

Bevacizumab (Avastin®, Roche) was the first antiangiogenic drug to be approved in 2004 as an antitumoral agent. It is a humanized IgG1 mAb that targets VEGF-A and prevents binding to VEGFR-1 and VEGFR-2 on the surface of endothelial cells. Bevacizumab is approved, in combination with fluoropyrimidine-based therapy, for the treatment of metastatic colorectal cancer [27], in combination with platinum-based chemotherapy for non-squamous NSCLC [28, 29] and in combination with paclitaxel or capecitabine for metastatic breast cancer [30, 31], although this indication was removed by the FDA due to safety concerns. Further indications include renal cell carcinoma (RCC) in combination with interferon-α-2a [32], glioblastoma multiforme [33], ovarian carcinoma [34–36, 99], cervical carcinoma [37], and hepatocellular carcinoma (HCC) [38].

Aflibercept (Zaltrap®, Sanofi-Aventis) is a recombinant fusion protein composed of the ligand-binding domains of the extracellular portions of VEGFR-1 and VEGFR-2 linked to the fragment crystallizable (Fc) portion of human IgG1, which acts as a soluble decoy receptor, inhibiting the binding of VEGF-A, VEGF-B, and PlGF to VEGFR. It is currently approved in combination with chemotherapy for patients with metastatic colorectal cancer [39].

Ramucirumab is a direct VEGFR-2 antagonist that binds with high affinity to the extracellular domain of VEGFR-2 and blocks the binding of natural ligands. Current indications include gastric cancer [40, 41], colorectal cancer [42], NSCLC [43, 44], and HCC [45].

Expected Impact on Susceptibility to Infection

VEGF-related pathways also play a role in the immune system. The blockade of the biologic functions of VEGF can delay leukocyte recovery after concomitant conventional cytotoxic chemotherapy, thereby increasing the incidence and severity of resulting neutropenia [100]. Bevacizumab may modulate intracellular T-cell immunity within the tumor microenvironment and eventually T-cell proliferation, migration, and activation [101]. In addition, the occurrence of gastrointestinal perforation (potentially leading to secondary peritonitis or bacteremia) is a well-established complication of VEGF-targeted agents, with a pooled incidence of 0.9% (and a related mortality of 21.7%) in a meta-analysis of bevacizumab trials [102]. Similar figures have been reported for aflibercept [77]. This complication is more common among patients with colorectal carcinoma and RCC, as well as in those with previous diverticulitis or peptic ulcer disease, receipt of local radiotherapy, or recent surgical or endoscopic procedures. The physiologic proangiogenic role of VEGF in non-tumor tissues also explains the increased risk of delayed postoperative wound healing and postoperative complications (including surgical site infection) observed with anti-VEGF therapies, particularly among patients with colorectal carcinoma [103].

Available Clinical Data

Data derived from a large number of RCTs allows to delineate the clinical impact of bevacizumab on infection susceptibility. An increased incidence of neutropenia was demonstrated in a meta-analysis including 15,263 patients; the risk of febrile neutropenia was also increased compared to control arms (RR = 1.31, 95%CI 1.08–1.58) [93]. A large meta-analysis pooling data from 41 RCTs and more than 30,000 patients with various cancer types (mostly colorectal carcinoma) concluded that the use of bevacizumab significantly increased the incidence of all-grade (RR = 1.45, 95%CI 1.27–1.66) and serious (RR = 1.59, 95%CI 1.42–1.79) infection. The pooled incidences for all-grade, severe, and fatal infections were 7.8%, 3.0%, and 0.9%, respectively. In subgroup analyses, the association between bevacizumab therapy and infection was modulated by the use of concomitant therapies (i.e., taxanes, capecitabine, gemcitabine, or oxaliplatin) and related with NSCLC, colorectal carcinoma, breast cancer, and gastric cancer. Although detailed information on infectious syndromes was not available for most trials, the infection risk related to bevacizumab seemed to be limited to febrile neutropenia, fistulae, or abscesses and pneumonia, but not sepsis or colitis [94]. There are anecdotal reports of infectious complications associated with bevacizumab, for example, *Bacteroides fragilis* sepsis [104]; however, the contributing role of previous or concomitant cytotoxic therapies is difficult to discern. One study suggested an increased risk of complications associated with implantable central venous access ports, such as infection or wound dehiscence [105]. A meta-analysis that included 4310 patients treated with aflibercept reported an increased risk of serious (RR = 1.87, 95%CI 1.52–2.30) and fatal (OR = 2.16, 95%CI 1.14–4.11) infections [95]. As for ramucirumab, two of the pivotal trials reported a higher risk of neutropenia but similar rates of febrile neutropenia [41, 42] and one reported a higher incidence of febrile neutropenia [44].

Conclusions and Suggested Prevention Strategies

- In view of available data, therapy with intravenous antiangiogenic agents is associated with a meaningful increase in the risk of infection, drug-induced neutropenia, and febrile neutropenia. In order to reduce the length of drug-induced neutropenia, the use of G-CSF may be considered in cases of delayed recovery of absolute neutrophil counts.
- Clinicians caring for patients receiving such therapy should be aware of the increased risk of gastrointestinal perforation (potentially resulting in secondary peritonitis and bacteremia), particularly in the presence of predisposing conditions such as colorectal carcinoma, previous diverticulitis or local radiotherapy, or recent surgical or endoscopic procedures, as well as wound healing complications.
- No clear benefit is expected from the universal use of antiviral, antifungal, or anti-*Pneumocystis* prophylaxis for patients receiving these agents, although an individualized infection risk assessment seems advisable.

TKIs Targeting VEGFR

Mechanism of Action, Approved Indications, and Off-Label Use

Various agents targeting VEGFR, or specifically its intracellular TK domain (as well as those of other angiogenic signaling pathways), have been developed in an attempt to improve antitumor efficacy and overcome resistance to VEGF blockade alone [106]. Sorafenib (Nexavar®, Bayer), sunitinib (Sutent®, Pfizer), axitinib (Inlyta®, Pfizer), and pazopanib (Votrient®, Novartis Pharmaceuticals) are small-molecule TKIs that target the VEGF pathway, either alone or in combination with a number of other pathways such as PDGF, c-Kit, BRAF, or FLT3 (the so-called multikinase inhibitors). Regorafenib (Stivarga®, Bayer), vandetanib (Caprelsa®, AstraZeneca), and cabozantinib (Cabometyx® in tablets or Cometriq® in capsules, Ipsen Pharma) are potent TKIs targeted not only against VEGFR and previously mentioned pathways but also against the RET receptor and angiopoietin-1 receptor.

Expected Impact on Susceptibility to Infection

As previously suggested for VEGF-targeted agents, the blockade of VEGF signaling pathway through the inhibition of the TK receptor activity seems to modulate T-cell functionality within the tumor microenvironment [107], among other complex intratumoral immune environment modifications. Therapy with sunitinib and sorafenib has been found to inhibit activation, proliferation, and cytokine production in peripheral blood T cells [108, 109]; nevertheless, in a study including 43 patients, no infections were recorded despite changes in circulating lymphocytes [110]. These subtle changes in host immunity seem unlikely to exert a negative impact on host immunity.

As this group contains multiple agents, tolerability is diverse, drug- and dose-dependent. Most common adverse events include hypertension, diarrhea, fatigue, and skin rash, but not infectious events. Stomatitis and hand-foot syndrome are other frequently observed toxicities. In general terms, adverse events profile of multi-targeted TKIs appears to be worse than that of agents selectively targeting only the VEGF pathway.

Available Clinical Data

Although the pooled incidence of all-grade neutropenia with sorafenib therapy was reported to reach 18% in a meta-analysis including 3221 patients, high-grade neutropenia was rare (5%) [96]. A meta-analysis of fatal adverse events in RCC trials with sorafenib, sunitinib, and pazopanib identified only three episodes of fatal sepsis among 4679 patients, with no other references to neutropenia or other infection-related adverse events [97]. Of note, five cases of invasive fungal infection have been reported in patients treated with sorafenib. Some of the patients had additional risk factors; downregulation of ERK pathway has been proposed, among others, as a possible underlying mechanism [98]. Overall, these results suggest that the use of these TKIs, either multitargeted or selective for the VEGFR pathway, is not associated with a meaningful increase in the risk of infection.

Conclusions and Suggested Prevention Strategies

- In view of available data, therapy with VEGFR TKIs does not increase the risk of infection.
- No clear benefit is expected from the universal use of antiviral, antifungal, or anti-*Pneumocystis* prophylaxis for patients receiving these agents, although an individualized infection risk assessment seems advisable.

References

1. Krampera M, Pasini A, Rigo A, Scupoli MT, Tecchio C, Malpeli G, et al. HB-EGF/HER-1 signaling in bone marrow mesenchymal stem cells: inducing cell expansion and reversibly preventing multilineage differentiation. Blood. 2005;106:59–66.
2. Yamashita M, Chattopadhyay S, Fensterl V, Saikia P, Wetzel JL, Sen GC. Epidermal growth factor receptor is essential for toll-like receptor 3 signaling. Sci Signal. 2012;5:50.
3. Reinwald M, Boch T, Hofmann WK, Buchheidt D. Risk of infectious complications in hemato-oncological patients treated with kinase inhibitors. Biomark Insights. 2015;103:55–68.
4. Aguilar-Company J, Fernández-Ruiz M, García-Campelo R, Garrido-Castro AC, Ruiz-Camps I. ESCMID Study Group for infections in compromised hosts (ESGICH) consensus document on the safety of targeted and biological therapies: an infectious diseases perspective (cell surface receptors and associated signaling pathways). Clin Microbiol Infect. 2018;24:S41–52.

5. Sharma SV, Bell DW, Settleman J, Haber DA. Epidermal growth factor receptor mutations in lung cancer. Nat Rev Cancer. 2007;7:169–81.
6. Hynes NE, Lane HA. ERBB receptors and cancer: the complexity of targeted inhibitors. Nat Rev Cancer. 2005;5:341–54.
7. Maughan TS, Adams RA, Smith CG, Meade AM, Seymour MT, Wilson RH, et al. Addition of cetuximab to oxaliplatin-based first-line combination chemotherapy for treatment of advanced colorectal cancer: results of the randomised phase 3 MRC COIN trial. Lancet. 2011;377:2103–14.
8. Van Cutsem E, Köhne C-H, Hitre E, Zaluski J, Chang Chien C-R, Makhson A, et al. Cetuximab and chemotherapy as initial treatment for metastatic colorectal cancer. N Engl J Med. 2009;360:1408–17.
9. Jonker DJ, O'Callaghan CJ, Karapetis CS, Zalcberg JR, Tu D, Au H-J, et al. Cetuximab for the treatment of colorectal cancer. N Engl J Med. 2007;357:2040–8.
10. Kopetz S, Grothey A, Yaeger R, Van Cutsem E, Desai J, Yoshino T, et al. Encorafenib, binimetinib, and cetuximab in BRAF V600E–mutated colorectal cancer. N Engl J Med. 2019;381:1632–43.
11. Bonner J, Harari PM, Giralt J, Azarnia N, Shin DM, Cohen RB, et al. Radiotherapy plus cetuximab for squamous-cell carcinoma of the head and neck. N Engl J Med. 2006;354:567–78.
12. Vermorken JB, Mesia R, Rivera F, Remenar E, Kawecki A, Rottey S, et al. Platinum-based chemotherapy plus cetuximab in head and neck cancer. N Engl J Med. 2008;359:1116–27.
13. Douillard JY, Siena S, Cassidy J, Tabernero J, Burkes R, Barugel M, et al. Final results from PRIME: randomized phase III study of panitumumab with FOLFOX4 for first-line treatment of metastatic colorectal cancer. Ann Oncol. 2014;25:1346–55.
14. Peeters M, Price TJ, Cervantes A, Sobrero AF, Ducreux M, Hotko Y, et al. Final results from a randomized phase 3 study of FOLFIRI ± panitumumab for second-line treatment of metastatic colorectal cancer. Ann Oncol. 2014;25:107–16.
15. Van-Cutsem E, Peeters M, Siena S, Humblet Y, Hendlisz A, Neyns B, et al. Open-label phase III Trial of panitumumab plus best supportive care compared with best supportive care alone in patients with chemotherapy-refractory metastatic colorectal cancer. J Clin Oncol. 2010;25:1658–64.
16. Fukuoka M, Wu Y-L, Thongprasert S, Sunpaweravong P, Leong S-S, Sriuranpong V, et al. Biomarker analyses and final overall survival results from a phase III, randomized, open-label, first-line study of gefitinib versus carboplatin/paclitaxel in clinically selected patients with advanced non–small-cell lung cancer in Asia (IPASS). J Clin Oncol. 2011;29:2866–74.
17. Douillard J-Y, Ostoros G, Cobo M, Ciuleanu T, McCormack R, Webster A, et al. First-line gefitinib in Caucasian EGFR mutation-positive NSCLC patients: a phase-IV, open-label, single-arm study. Br J Cancer. 2014;110:55–62.
18. Rosell R, Carcereny E, Gervais R, Vergnenegre A, Massuti B, Felip E, et al. Erlotinib versus standard chemotherapy as first-line treatment for European patients with advanced EGFR mutation-positive non-small-cell lung cancer (EURTAC): a multicentre, open-label, randomised phase 3 trial. Lancet Oncol. 2012;13:239–46.
19. Shepherd FA, Rodrigues Pereira J, Ciuleanu T, Tan EH, Hirsh V, Thongprasert S, et al. Erlotinib in previously treated non-small-cell lung cancer. N Engl J Med. 2005;353:123–32.
20. Zhou C, Wu Y-L, Chen G, Feng J, Liu X-Q, Wang C, et al. Erlotinib versus chemotherapy as first-line treatment for patients with advanced EGFR mutation-positive non-small-cell lung cancer (OPTIMAL, CTONG-0802): a multicentre, open-label, randomised, phase 3 study. Lancet Oncol. 2011;12:735–42.
21. Moore MJ, Goldstein D, Hamm J, Figer A, Hecht JR, Gallinger S, et al. Erlotinib plus gemcitabine compared with gemcitabine alone in patients with advanced pancreatic cancer: a phase III trial of the National Cancer Institute of Canada Clinical Trials Group. J Clin Oncol. 2007;25:1960–6.
22. Yang JC-H, Wu Y-L, Schuler M, Sebastian M, Popat S, Yamamoto N, et al. Afatinib versus cisplatin-based chemotherapy for EGFR mutation-positive lung adenocarcinoma (LUX-Lung

3 and LUX-Lung 6): analysis of overall survival data from two randomised, phase 3 trials. Lancet Oncol. 2015;16:141–51.
23. Ramalingam SS, Jänne PA, Mok T, O'Byrne K, Boyer MJ, Von Pawel J, et al. Dacomitinib versus erlotinib in patients with advanced-stage, previously treated non-small-cell lung cancer (ARCHER 1009): a randomised, double-blind, phase 3 trial. Lancet Oncol. 2014;15:1369–78.
24. Wu Y-L, Cheng Y, Zhou X, Lee KH, Nakagawa K, Niho S, et al. Dacomitinib versus gefitinib as first-line treatment for patients with EGFR-mutation-positive non-small-cell lung cancer (ARCHER 1050): a randomised, open-label, phase 3 trial. Lancet Oncol. 2017;18:1454–66.
25. Mok TS, Wu Y-L, Ahn M-J, Garassino MC, Kim HR, Ramalingam SS, et al. Osimertinib or platinum–pemetrexed in EGFR T790M–positive lung cancer. N Engl J Med. 2017;376:629–40.
26. Soria J-C, Ohe Y, Vansteenkiste J, Reungwetwattana T, Chewaskulyong B, Lee KH, et al. Osimertinib in untreated EGFR -mutated advanced non–small-cell lung cancer. N Engl J Med. 2018;378:113–25.
27. Hurwitz HI, Tebbutt NC, Kabbinavar F, Giantonio BJ, Guan Z-Z, Mitchell L, et al. Efficacy and safety of bevacizumab in metastatic colorectal cancer: pooled analysis from seven randomized controlled trials. Oncologist. 2013;18:1004–12.
28. Reck M, von Pawel J, Zatloukal P, Ramlau R, Gorbounova V, Hirsh V, et al. Overall survival with cisplatin–gemcitabine and bevacizumab or placebo as first-line therapy for nonsquamous non-small-cell lung cancer: results from a randomised phase III trial (AVAiL). Ann Oncol. 2010;21:1804–9.
29. Sandler A, Gray R, Perry MC, Brahmer J, Schiller JH, Dowlati A, et al. Paclitaxel–carboplatin alone or with bevacizumab for non-small-cell lung cancer. N Engl J Med. 2006;355:2542–50.
30. Miller K, Wang M, Gralow J, Dickler M, Cobleigh M, Perez EA, et al. Paclitaxel plus bevacizumab versus paclitaxel alone for metastatic breast cancer. N Engl J Med. 2007;357:2666–76.
31. Robert NJ, Diéras V, Glaspy J, Brufsky AM, Bondarenko I, Lipatov ON, et al. RIBBON-1: randomized, double-blind, placebo-controlled, phase III Trial of chemotherapy with or without bevacizumab for first-line treatment of human epidermal growth factor receptor 2-negative, locally recurrent or metastatic breast cancer. J Clin Oncol. 2011;29:1252–60.
32. Escudier B, Bellmunt J, Négrier S, Bajetta E, Melichar B, Bracarda S, et al. Phase III trial of bevacizumab plus interferon Alfa-2a in patients with metastatic renal cell carcinoma (AVOREN): final analysis of overall survival. J Clin Oncol. 2010;28:2144–50.
33. Friedman HS, Prados MD, Wen PY, Mikkelsen T, Schiff D, Abrey LE, et al. Bevacizumab alone and in combination with irinotecan in recurrent glioblastoma. J Clin Oncol. 2009;27:4733–40.
34. Burger RA, Brady MF, Bookman MA, Fleming GF, Monk BJ, Huang H, et al. Incorporation of bevacizumab in the primary treatment of ovarian cancer. N Engl J Med. 2011;365:2473–83.
35. Pujade-Lauraine E, Hilpert F, Weber B, Reuss A, Poveda A, Kristensen G, et al. Bevacizumab combined with chemotherapy for platinum-resistant recurrent ovarian cancer: the AURELIA open-label randomized phase III trial. J Clin Oncol. 2014;32:1302–8.
36. Aghajanian C, Blank SV, Goff BA, Judson PL, Teneriello MG, Husain A, et al. OCEANS: a randomized, double-blind, placebo-controlled phase III trial of chemotherapy with or without bevacizumab in patients with platinum-sensitive recurrent epithelial ovarian, primary peritoneal, or fallopian tube cancer. J Clin Oncol. 2012;30:2039–45.
37. Tewari KS, Sill MW, Penson RT, Huang H, Ramondetta LM, Landrum LM, et al. Bevacizumab for advanced cervical cancer: final overall survival and adverse event analysis of a randomised, controlled, open-label, phase 3 trial (Gynecologic Oncology Group 240). Lancet. 2017;390:1654–63.
38. Finn RS, Qin S, Ikeda M, Galle PR, Ducreux M, Kim T-Y, et al. Atezolizumab plus bevacizumab in unresectable hepatocellular carcinoma. N Engl J Med. 2020;382:1894–905.
39. Van Cutsem E, Tabernero J, Lakomy R, Prenen H, Prausová J, Macarulla T, et al. Addition of aflibercept to fluorouracil, leucovorin, and irinotecan improves survival in a phase III randomized trial in patients with metastatic colorectal cancer previously treated with an oxaliplatin-based regimen. J Clin Oncol. 2012;30:3499–506.

40. Fuchs CS, Tomasek J, Yong CJ, Dumitru F, Passalacqua R, Goswami C, et al. Ramucirumab monotherapy for previously treated advanced gastric or gastro-oesophageal junction adenocarcinoma (REGARD): an international, randomised, multicentre, placebo-controlled, phase 3 trial. Lancet. 2014;383:31–9.
41. Wilke H, Muro K, Van Cutsem E, Oh S-C, Bodoky G, Shimada Y, et al. Ramucirumab plus paclitaxel versus placebo plus paclitaxel in patients with previously treated advanced gastric or gastro-oesophageal junction adenocarcinoma (RAINBOW): a double-blind, randomised phase 3 trial. Lancet Oncol. 2014;15:1224–35.
42. Tabernero J, Yoshino T, Cohn AL, Obermannova R, Bodoky G, Garcia-Carbonero R, et al. Ramucirumab versus placebo in combination with second-line FOLFIRI in patients with metastatic colorectal carcinoma that progressed during or after first-line therapy with bevacizumab, oxaliplatin, and a fluoropyrimidine (RAISE): a randomised, double-blin. Lancet Oncol. 2015;16:499–508.
43. Nakagawa K, Garon EB, Seto T, Nishio M, Ponce Aix S, Paz-Ares L, et al. Ramucirumab plus erlotinib in patients with untreated, EGFR-mutated, advanced non-small-cell lung cancer (RELAY): a randomised, double-blind, placebo-controlled, phase 3 trial. Lancet Oncol. 2019;20:1655–69.
44. Garon EB, Ciuleanu T-E, Arrieta O, Prabhash K, Syrigos KN, Goksel T, et al. Ramucirumab plus docetaxel versus placebo plus docetaxel for second-line treatment of stage IV non-small-cell lung cancer after disease progression on platinum-based therapy (REVEL): a multicentre, double-blind, randomised phase 3 trial. Lancet. 2014;384:665–73.
45. Zhu AX, Kang Y-K, Yen C-J, Finn RS, Galle PR, Llovet JM, et al. Ramucirumab after sorafenib in patients with advanced hepatocellular carcinoma and increased α-fetoprotein concentrations (REACH-2): a randomised, double-blind, placebo-controlled, phase 3 trial. Lancet Oncol. 2019;20:282–96.
46. Llovet JM, Ricci S, Mazzaferro V, Hilgard P, Gane E, Blanc J-F, et al. Sorafenib in advanced hepatocellular carcinoma. N Engl J Med. 2008;359:378–90.
47. Escudier B, Eisen T, Stadler WM, Szczylik C, Oudard S, Siebels M, et al. Sorafenib in advanced clear-cell renal-cell carcinoma. N Engl J Med. 2007;356:125–34.
48. Brose MS, Nutting CM, Jarzab B, Elisei R, Siena S, Bastholt L, et al. Sorafenib in radioactive iodine-refractory, locally advanced or metastatic differentiated thyroid cancer: a randomised, double-blind, phase 3 trial. Lancet. 2014;384:319–28.
49. Sternberg CN, Hawkins RE, Wagstaff J, Salman P, Mardiak J, Barrios CH, et al. A randomised, double-blind phase III study of pazopanib in patients with advanced and/or metastatic renal cell carcinoma: final overall survival results and safety update. Eur J Cancer. 2013;49:1287–96.
50. van der Graaf WT, Blay J-Y, Chawla SP, Kim D-W, Bui-Nguyen B, Casali PG, et al. Pazopanib for metastatic soft-tissue sarcoma (PALETTE): a randomised, double-blind, placebo-controlled phase 3 trial. Lancet. 2012;379:1879–86.
51. Motzer RJ, Penkov K, Haanen J, Rini BI, Albiges L, Campbell MT, et al. Avelumab plus axitinib versus sunitinib for advanced renal-cell carcinoma. N Engl J Med. 2019;380:1116–27.
52. Motzer RJ, Escudier B, Tomczak P, Hutson TE, Michaelson MD, Negrier S, et al. Axitinib versus sorafenib as second-line treatment for advanced renal cell carcinoma: overall survival analysis and updated results from a randomised phase 3 trial. Lancet Oncol. 2013;14:552–62.
53. Choueiri TK, Escudier B, Powles T, Tannir NM, Mainwaring PN, Rini BI, et al. Cabozantinib versus everolimus in advanced renal cell carcinoma (METEOR): final results from a randomised, open-label, phase 3 trial. Lancet Oncol. 2016;17:917–27.
54. Choueiri TK, Hessel C, Halabi S, Sanford B, Michaelson MD, Hahn O, et al. Cabozantinib versus sunitinib as initial therapy for metastatic renal cell carcinoma of intermediate or poor risk (Alliance A031203 CABOSUN randomised trial): progression-free survival by independent review and overall survival update. Eur J Cancer. 2018;94:115–25.
55. Abou-Alfa GK, Meyer T, Cheng A-L, El-Khoueiry AB, Rimassa L, Ryoo B-Y, et al. Cabozantinib in patients with advanced and progressing hepatocellular carcinoma. N Engl J Med. 2018;379:54–63.

56. Elisei R, Schlumberger MJ, Müller SP, Schöffski P, Brose MS, Shah MH, et al. Cabozantinib in progressive medullary thyroid cancer. J Clin Oncol. 2013;31:3639–46.
57. Grothey A, Cutsem E, Sobrero A, Siena S, Falcone A, Ychou M, et al. Regorafenib monotherapy for previously treated metastatic colorectal cancer (CORRECT): an international, multicentre, randomised, placebo-controlled, phase 3 trial. Lancet. 2013;381:303–12.
58. Demetri GD, Reichardt P, Kang Y-K, Blay J-Y, Rutkowski P, Gelderblom H, et al. Efficacy and safety of regorafenib for advanced gastrointestinal stromal tumours after failure of imatinib and sunitinib (GRID): an international, multicentre, randomised, placebo-controlled, phase 3 trial. Lancet. 2013;381:295–302.
59. Bruix J, Qin S, Merle P, Granito A, Huang Y-H, Bodoky G, et al. Regorafenib for patients with hepatocellular carcinoma who progressed on sorafenib treatment (RESORCE): a randomised, double-blind, placebo-controlled, phase 3 trial. Lancet. 2017;389:56–66.
60. Demetri GD, van Oosterom AT, Garrett CR, Blackstein ME, Shah MH, Verweij J, et al. Efficacy and safety of sunitinib in patients with advanced gastrointestinal stromal tumour after failure of imatinib: a randomised controlled trial. Lancet. 2006;368:1329–38.
61. Motzer RJ, Hutson TE, Tomczak P, Michaelson MD, Bukowski RM, Rixe O, et al. Sunitinib versus interferon alfa in metastatic renal-cell carcinoma. N Engl J Med. 2007;356:115–24.
62. Raymond E, Dahan L, Raoul J-L, Bang Y-J, Borbath I, Lombard-Bohas C, et al. Sunitinib malate for the treatment of pancreatic neuroendocrine tumors. N Engl J Med. 2011;364:501–13.
63. Motzer RJ, Hutson TE, Glen H, Michaelson MD, Molina A, Eisen T, et al. Lenvatinib, everolimus, and the combination in patients with metastatic renal cell carcinoma: a randomised, phase 2, open-label, multicentre trial. Lancet Oncol. 2015;16:1473–82.
64. Cheng A-L, Finn RS, Qin S, Han K-H, Ikeda K, Piscaglia F, et al. Phase III trial of lenvatinib (LEN) vs sorafenib (SOR) in first-line treatment of patients (pts) with unresectable hepatocellular carcinoma (uHCC). J Clin Oncol. 2017;35:4001.
65. Schlumberger M, Tahara M, Wirth LJ, Robinson B, Brose MS, Elisei R, et al. Lenvatinib versus placebo in radioiodine-refractory thyroid cancer. N Engl J Med. 2015;372:621–30.
66. Wells SA, Robinson BG, Gagel RF, Dralle H, Fagin JA, Santoro M, et al. Vandetanib in patients with locally advanced or metastatic medullary thyroid cancer: a randomized, double-blind phase III trial. J Clin Oncol. 2012;30:134–41.
67. Xie YH, Chen YX, Fang JY. Comprehensive review of targeted therapy for colorectal cancer. Signal Transduct Target Ther. 2020;5:116.
68. Cunningham D, Humblet Y, Siena S, Khayat D, Bleiberg H, Santoro A, et al. Cetuximab monotherapy and cetuximab plus irinotecan in irinotecan-refractory metastatic colorectal cancer. N Engl J Med. 2004;351:337–45.
69. Hecht JR, Patnaik A, Berlin J, Venook A, Malik I, Tchekmedyian S, et al. Panitumumab monotherapy in patients with previously treated metastatic colorectal cancer. Cancer. 2007;110:980–8.
70. Bonner JA, Harari PM, Giralt J, Cohen RB, Jones CU, Sur RK, et al. Radiotherapy plus cetuximab for locoregionally advanced head and neck cancer: 5-year survival data from a phase 3 randomised trial, and relation between cetuximab-induced rash and survival. Lancet Oncol. 2010;11:21–8.
71. Cui R, Chu L, Liu Z-Q, Xiao Y-Y, Zhu X-L, Chen Y-J, et al. Hematologic toxicity assessment in solid tumor patients treated with cetuximab: a pooled analysis of 18 randomized controlled trials. Int J Cancer. 2016;138:2771–3.
72. Wang L, Chen Y-Z, Shi D, Shi X-Y, Zou Z, Zhao J-H. Incidence and risk of severe neutropenia in advanced cancer patients treated with cetuximab. Drugs R D. 2011;11:317–26.
73. Hardbower DM, Singh K, Asim M, Verriere TG, Olivares-Villagómez D, Barry DP, et al. EGFR regulates macrophage activation and function in bacterial infection. J Clin Invest. 2016;126:3296–312.
74. Burgel P-R, Nadel JA. Epidermal growth factor receptor-mediated innate immune responses and their roles in airway diseases. Eur Respir J. 2008;32:1068–81.

75. Lacouture ME, Anadkat MJ, Bensadoun R-J, Bryce J, Chan A, Epstein JB, et al. Clinical practice guidelines for the prevention and treatment of EGFR inhibitor-associated dermatologic toxicities. Support Care Cancer. 2011;19:1079–95.
76. Funakoshi T, Suzuki M, Tamura K. Infectious complications in cancer patients treated with anti-EGFR monoclonal antibodies cetuximab and panitumumab: a systematic review and meta-analysis. Cancer Treat Rev. 2014;40:1221–9.
77. Qi W-X, Fu S, Zhang Q, Guo X-M. Incidence and risk of severe infections associated with anti-epidermal growth factor receptor monoclonal antibodies in cancer patients: a systematic review and meta-analysis. BMC Med. 2014;12:203.
78. Eilers RE, Gandhi M, Patel JD, Mulcahy MF, Agulnik M, Hensing T, et al. Dermatologic infections in cancer patients treated with epidermal growth factor receptor inhibitor therapy. J Natl Cancer Inst. 2010;102:47–53.
79. Lord HK, Junor E, Ironside J. Cetuximab is effective, but more toxic than reported in the bonner trial. Clin Oncol. 2008;20:96.
80. Guerriero C, Ricci F, Paradisi A, Fossati B, Valentini V, Pacelli F, et al. Subcutaneous abscess as a side-effect of cetuximab therapy. Eur J Dermatol. 2011;21:277–8.
81. Ricci F, Guerriero C, Paradisi A, Fossati B, Miccichè F, Valentini V, et al. Multiple abscesses in a patient treated with cetuximab. Eur J Dermatol. 2013;23:103–4.
82. Bachet J-B, Peuvrel L, Bachmeyer C, Reguiai Z, Gourraud PA, Bouché O, et al. Folliculitis induced by EGFR inhibitors, preventive and curative efficacy of tetracyclines in the management and incidence rates according to the type of EGFR inhibitor administered: a systematic literature review. Oncologist. 2012;17:555–68.
83. Petrelli F, Borgonovo K, Cabiddu M, Coinu A, Ghilardi M, Lonati V, et al. Antibiotic prophylaxis for skin toxicity induced by antiepidermal growth factor receptor agents: a systematic review and meta-analysis. Br J Dermatol. 2016;175:1166–74.
84. Lynch TJ, Bell DW, Sordella R, Gurubhagavatula S, Okimoto RA, Brannigan BW, et al. Activating mutations in the epidermal growth factor receptor underlying responsiveness of non-small-cell lung cancer to gefitinib. N Engl J Med. 2004;350:2129–39.
85. Rosell R, Moran T, Queralt C, Porta R, Cardenal F, Camps C, et al. Screening for epidermal growth factor receptor mutations in lung cancer. N Engl J Med. 2009;361:958–67.
86. Soria J-C, Felip E, Cobo M, Lu S, Syrigos K, Lee KH, et al. Afatinib versus erlotinib as second-line treatment of patients with advanced squamous cell carcinoma of the lung (LUX-Lung 8): an open-label randomised controlled phase 3 trial. Lancet Oncol. 2015;16:897–907.
87. Ku GY, Haaland BA, de Lima Lopes G. Gefitinib vs. chemotherapy as first-line therapy in advanced non-small cell lung cancer: meta-analysis of phase III trials. Lung Cancer. 2011;74:469–73.
88. Wang Y, Wang M, Wang Q, Geng Z, Sun M. Incidence and risk of infections associated with EGFR-TKIs in advanced non-small-cell lung cancer: a systematic review and meta-analysis of randomized controlled trials. Oncotarget. 2017;8:29406–15.
89. Grenader T, Gipps M, Goldberg A. Staphylococcus aureus bacteremia secondary to severe erlotinib skin toxicity. Clin Lung Cancer. 2008;9:59–60.
90. Li J, Peccerillo J, Kaley K, Saif MW. Staphylococcus aureus bacteremia related with erlotinib skin toxicity in a patient with pancreatic cancer. JOP. 2009;10:338–40.
91. Melosky B, Leighl NB, Rothenstein J, Sangha R, Stewart D, Papp K. Management of EGFR TKI–induced dermatologic adverse events. Curr Oncol. 2015;22:123.
92. Hicklin DJ, Ellis LM. Role of the vascular endothelial growth factor pathway in tumor growth and angiogenesis. J Clin Oncol. 2005;23:1011–27.
93. Schutz FAB, Jardim DLF, Je Y, Choueiri TK. Haematologic toxicities associated with the addition of bevacizumab in cancer patients. Eur J Cancer. 2011;47:1161–74.
94. Qi W-X, Fu S, Zhang Q, Guo X-M. Bevacizumab increases the risk of infections in cancer patients: a systematic review and pooled analysis of 41 randomized controlled trials. Crit Rev Oncol Hematol. 2015;94:323–36.

95. Zhang X, Ran Y, Shao Y, Wang K, Zhu Y. Incidence and risk of severe infections associated with aflibercept in cancer patients: a systematic review and meta-analysis. Br J Clin Pharmacol. 2016;81:33–40.
96. Schutz FAB, Je Y, Choueiri TK. Hematologic toxicities in cancer patients treated with the multi-tyrosine kinase sorafenib: a meta-analysis of clinical trials. Crit Rev Oncol Hematol. 2011;80:291–300.
97. Schutz FAB, Je Y, Richards CJ, Choueiri TK. Meta-analysis of randomized controlled trials for the incidence and risk of treatment-related mortality in patients with cancer treated with vascular endothelial growth factor tyrosine kinase inhibitors. J Clin Oncol. 2012;30:871–7.
98. Chamilos G, Lionakis MS, Kontoyiannis DP. Reply to Bazaz and Denning. Clin Infect Dis. 2018;67:157–9.
99. Coleman RL, Brady MF, Herzog TJ, Sabbatini P, Armstrong DK, Walker JL, et al. Bevacizumab and paclitaxel–carboplatin chemotherapy and secondary cytoreduction in recurrent, platinum-sensitive ovarian cancer (NRG Oncology/Gynecologic Oncology Group study GOG-0213): a multicentre, open-label, randomised, phase 3 trial. Lancet Oncol. 2017;18:779–91.
100. Novitskiy SV, Csiki I, Huang Y, Johnson DH, Harth EM, Carbone DP, et al. Anti-vascular endothelial growth factor treatment in combination with chemotherapy delays hematopoietic recovery due to decreased proliferation of bone marrow hematopoietic progenitor cells. J Thorac Oncol. 2010;5:1410–5.
101. Kaur S, Chang T, Singh SP, Lim L, Mannan P, Garfield SH, et al. CD47 signaling regulates the immunosuppressive activity of VEGF in T cells. J Immunol. 2014;193:3914–24.
102. Hapani S, Chu D, Wu S. Risk of gastrointestinal perforation in patients with cancer treated with bevacizumab: a meta-analysis. Lancet Oncol. 2009;10:559–68.
103. Zhang H, Huang Z, Zou X, Liu T. Bevacizumab and wound-healing complications: a systematic review and meta-analysis of randomized controlled trials. Oncotarget. 2016;7:82473–81.
104. Lieuw-a-Fa M, Peringa J, Leeksma O, Terpstra W. Sepsis from liver abscesses in metastatic colorectal carcinoma after chemoimmunotherapy. J Clin Oncol. 2008;26:1381–2.
105. Berardi R, Rinaldi S, Santini D, Vincenzi B, Giampieri R, Maccaroni E, et al. Increased rates of local complication of central venous catheters in the targeted anticancer therapy era: a 2-year retrospective analysis. Support Care Cancer. 2015;23:1295–302.
106. Zhao Y, Adjei AA. Targeting angiogenesis in cancer therapy: moving beyond vascular endothelial growth factor. Oncologist. 2015;20:660–73.
107. Santoni M, Berardi R, Amantini C, Burattini L, Santini D, Santoni G, et al. Role of natural and adaptive immunity in renal cell carcinoma response to VEGFR-TKIs and mTOR inhibitor. Int J Cancer. 2014;134:2772–7.
108. Gu Y, Zhao W, Meng F, Qu B, Zhu X, Sun Y, et al. Sunitinib impairs the proliferation and function of human peripheral T cell and prevents T-cell-mediated immune response in mice. Clin Immunol. 2010;135:55–62.
109. Zhao W, Gu YH, Song R, Qu BQ, Xu Q. Sorafenib inhibits activation of human peripheral blood T cells by targeting LCK phosphorylation. Leukemia. 2008;22:1226–33.
110. Powles T, Chowdhury S, Bower M, Saunders N, Lim L, Shamash J, et al. The effect of sunitinib on immune subsets in metastatic clear cell renal cancer. Urol Int. 2011;86:53–9.

Interleukin-1 Targeted Agents

9

Mosaab Alam, Allison Mah, and Sara Belga

Introduction

Interleukin-1 (IL-1) was initially discovered in the mid-1980s under various names such as leukocyte endogenous mediator, endogenous pyrogen, and osteoclast-activating factor [1], indicating multiple biological functions attributed to this cytokine. In the past two decades, several other IL-1 members were identified. Currently, 11 family members of IL-1 cytokines and 10 IL-1 receptors (IL-R) have been identified [2]. This review will focus mainly on IL-1α and IL-1β since these represent the best studied cytokines [3].

IL-1α and IL-1β are two cytokines that have similar biological activities [1]. Once they bind to their receptors, they trigger a cascade of inflammatory mediators such as chemokine and cytokine production, neutrophil activation, and the appearance of fever [2]. IL-1α is found in epithelial cells and mucosal membranes throughout the body [4]. IL-1β is predominantly found in innate immune cells such as monocytes and tissue macrophages [1, 5]. IL-1β is secreted systemically, while IL-1α is activated locally in the cell membrane [1]. In the setting of inflammation, IL-1α migrates toward the cell surface activating adjacent cells by binding with IL-1R [6, 7]. During ischemia and cell death, IL-1α and its precursor are released from cells inducing sterile inflammation of neutrophilic predominance [8–10]. This generates tissue destruction at the site of injury [4]. Once IL-1α binds to its receptors on resident macrophages, IL-1β precursor is synthesized by them. The IL-1β precursor is then activated by the pro-inflammatory protease caspase-1 [4, 5]. Activation of IL-1β is stimulated by several additional factors including microbial

M. Alam · A. Mah · S. Belga (✉)
Department of Medicine, University of British Columbia, Vancouver, BC, Canada

Division of Infectious Diseases, University of British Columbia, Vancouver, BC, Canada
e-mail: sara.belga@ubc.ca

C. Cervera, J. M. Aguado (eds.), *Infectious Complications in Biologic and Targeted Therapies*, https://doi.org/10.1007/978-3-031-11363-5_9

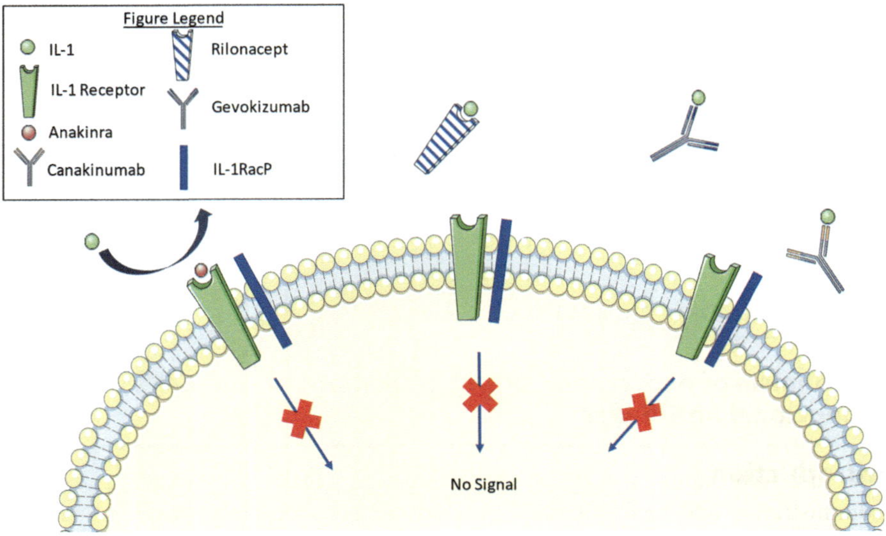

Fig. 9.1 Structure and function of each IL-1-targeted agent and its mechanism of action on IL-1 and IL-1R

products, tumor necrosis factor (TNF), and IL-1β itself [4]. The active IL-1β binds to endothelial receptors, promoting monocyte migration and opening of endothelial intracellular junctions resulting in capillary leak [4]. IL-1Ra is an inhibitory cytokine of the IL-1 family as it binds to IL-1R but does not induce an intracellular pro-inflammatory response [11].

Inhibition of the IL-1 pathway (Fig. 9.1) has been the target of treatments for several inflammatory conditions such as rheumatoid arthritis (RA) [12], juvenile idiopathic arthritis (JIA) [13, 14], adult-onset Still's disease (AOSD) [13], autoinflammatory syndromes including cryopyrin-associated periodic fever syndrome (CAPS) [15], TNF-associated periodic syndrome (TRAPS) [16], familial Mediterranean fever (FMF) [15], and mevalonate kinase deficiency (hyper-IgD syndrome) [15, 17]. IL-1 agents are also used off label for the treatment of gout [18–21], refractory pericarditis [22], Bechet's disease [23, 24], pyoderma gangrenosum [25], and neutrophilic dermatosis (Sweet's syndrome) [26].

Available IL-1-Targeting Agents

Anakinra is a recombinant IL-1Ra approved by the American Food and Drug administration (FDA) in 2001 [4]. It is similar to the structure of the natural IL-1Ra but differs by an extra methionine residue manufactured from *Escherichia coli* [3]. Anakinra is approved for treatment of RA, JIA, AOSD, and CAPS [2, 3]. Canakinumab is a fully human IL-1β antagonist that blocks IL-1β's interaction with IL-1R. It is approved for treatment of CAPS, TRAPS, mevalonate kinase deficiency, and AOSD [2]. Rilonacept is a soluble decoy receptor that binds to IL-1 thereby inhibiting the binding of IL-1 to IL-1R. Rilonacept is currently approved for CAPS [2]. Similar to canakinumab, gevokizumab is a potent humanized IL-1β antagonist that has not yet been FDA approved [2, 3].

Infectious Complications of Interleukin-1 (IL-1)-Targeted Agents

Anakinra

Tables 9.1 and 9.2 summarize the risk of infection reported in clinical trials and the described infections for each drug, respectively. A meta-analysis of seven randomized controlled trials (RCTs) and three extension studies demonstrated no increased risk of infections when anakinra was compared to placebo, with a pooled relative

Table 9.1 Summary of risk of infections associated with IL-1-targeted agents

Reference (year)	Study design, No. of patients indication	Agent	Study duration	Risk of infections
Nikfar et al. (2018) [12]	Meta-analysis of 7 RCTs and 3 extension studies (4706 patients); RA	Anakinra	24–52 weeks	No difference of infectious risk between anakinra and placebo (Pooled RR 1.06; CI 0.94–1.20)
Cohen et al. (2002) [27]	Placebo-controlled RCT; 419 patients; RA	Anakinra	24 weeks	Similar risk of infections: 22% in placebo vs. 24% in anakinra. No reported serious infections
Nuki et al. (2002) [28]	Placebo-controlled RCT; 472 patients; RA	Anakinra	76 weeks	No risk of serious infection associated with anakinra, 0.91–1.1 events per 100 patient-years for anakinra vs. 1.4 events per 100 patient-years for placebo
Fleishmann et al. (2003) [29]	Placebo-controlled RCT; 1,414 patients; RA	Anakinra	26 weeks	Serious infections for anakinra 2.1% vs. 0.4% for placebo
Fleishmann et al. (2006) [30]	6 months placebo-controlled RCT followed by an open-label cohort; 1346 patients; RA	Anakinra	3 years	Increased incidence of serious infections with anakinra, EAE 5.37 for anakinra vs. 1.65 for placebo per 100 patient-years; three opportunistic infections in the anakinra group (nontuberculous mycobacteria, histoplasmosis, and esophageal candidiasis)
Schiff et al. (2004) [31]	Placebo-controlled RCT; 1,414 patients; RA	Anakinra	26 weeks	Slight increase in risk of serious infections in high-risk patients (at least one comorbidity) 2.5% for anakinra vs. 1.1% for placebo

(continued)

Table 9.1 (continued)

Reference (year)	Study design, No. of patients indication	Agent	Study duration	Risk of infections
Ridker et al. (2017) [32]	Placebo-controlled RCT; 10,061 patients; acute myocardial infarction	Canakinumab	48 months	Increased incidence of fatal infection or sepsis, 0.31 events per 100 patients-years for canakinumab vs. 0.18 events per 100 patient-years for placebo
Schlesinger et al. (2011) [18]	Double-blind controlled trial comparing canakinumab vs. colchicine; 432 patients; gout	Canakinumab	24 weeks	Increased risk of infection 18% for canakinumab vs. 12% for colchicine. 6 serious infections (pneumonia, sepsis, gangrene, erysipelas, tonsilitis, ear infection)
Schlesinger et al. (2012) [19]	Double-blind controlled trial comparing canakinumab to triamcinolone; 456 patients; gout	Canakinumab	24 weeks	Increased incidence of infection 20% for canakinumab vs. 12% for triamcinolone. Four serious infections (jaw abscess, arm abscess, pneumonia, and gastroenteritis)
Ruperto et al. (2012) [33]	Placebo-controlled RCT followed by an open-label phase; 177 patients; sJIA	Canakinumab	4 weeks (RCT) 2 years (open label)	Similar rates of infection in RCT; one varicella case for canakinumab and one gastroenteritis for placebo. 4% rates of infections in each group in the open-label phase
Ruperto et al. (2018) [34]	5-year long-term extension phase of previous study; 75 patients; sJIA	Canakinumab	5 years	Incidence of serious infection 10.28 per 100 patients-years, four notable infections (toxoplasmosis, CMV infection, *Salmonella* gastroenteritis, and adenovirus infection)
De Benedetti (2018) [15]	Placebo-controlled RCT (16 weeks) followed by secondary randomization (40 weeks); 63 crFMF, 72 MKD, 46 TRAPS patients	Canakinumab	40 weeks	Ten serious infections in the treatment group vs. 2 in placebo group; 7.4 events per 100 patient-years in open-label phase
Sundy et al. (2014) [35]	Placebo-controlled RCT; 1,315 patients; gout	Rilonacept	20 weeks	Similar incidence of serious infections 0.5% for rilonacept vs. 0.9% for placebo
Klein et al. (2020) [22]	Placebo-controlled RCT; 86 patients; recurrent pericarditis	Rilonacept	24 weeks	URTI (23%) for rilonacept vs. 0% for placebo; all infections were reported as mild or moderate; no reported serious infections

Table 9.1 (continued)

Reference (year)	Study design, No. of patients indication	Agent	Study duration	Risk of infections
Hoffman et al. (2008) [36]	Placebo-controlled RCT; 44 patients; CAPS	Rilonacept	24 weeks	Incidence of infection 48% for rilonacept vs. 17% for placebo, mild to moderate URTI being most common (26%) for rilonacept; one case of severe bronchitis reported
Hoffman et al. (2012) [37]	Open-label trial; CAPS	Rilonacept	72 weeks	Two severe infections (pneumococcal meningitis and tooth abscess), one death from pneumococcal meningitis
Ilowite et al. (2014) [38]	Placebo-controlled RCT followed by open-label phase; 71 patients; sJIA	Rilonacept	24 weeks to 2 years	Similar rates of infections between rilonacept and placebo (16% and 20% respectively). Four serious infections for rilonacept (varicella, viral URTI, *Salmonella* gastroenteritis, streptococcal pharyngitis)
Tugal-Tutkun et al. (2018) [39]	Placebo-controlled RCT followed by open-label extension phase; 83 patients; Bechet's uveitis	Gevokizumab	28 to 420 days	Similar risk of infections between gevokizumab and placebo. No opportunistic infections reported

EAE exposure-adjusted event, *CAPS* cryopyrin-associated periodic syndrome, *RA* rheumatoid arthritis, *sJIA* systemic juvenile idiopathic arthritis, *URTI* upper respiratory tract infection

Table 9.2 Summary of described infections associated with IL-1-targeted agents

Agent	Bacterial and viral infections	Fungal and parasitic infections
Anakinra	*Common infections* URTI [40], pneumonia [29, 30], cellulitis [29, 30], UTI [40] *Rare infections* Pulmonary TB [41], TB myositis [42], NTM infection [30], varicella [43], CMV hepatitis [44]	Esophageal candidiasis [30], histoplasmosis [30], visceral leishmaniasis [43]
Canakinumab	*Common infections* Pneumonia [18, 32, 34], cellulitis [32], UTI [32], gastroenteritis [34] *Rare infections* Erysipelas [18], gangrene [18], sepsis [18], tonsilitis [18], subcutaneous abscess [34], streptococcal tonsilitis [34], salmonella gastroenteritis [34], CMV [34], varicella [34], adenovirus [34], TB [32]	Toxoplasmosis [34]

(continued)

Table 9.2 (continued)

Agent	Bacterial and viral infections	Fungal and parasitic infections
Rilonacept	*Common infections* URTI [22, 37] *Rare infections* Severe bronchitis [36], Pneumococcal meningitis [37], tooth abscess [37], Streptococcal pharyngitis [38], Salmonella gastroenteritis [38], Varicella [38]	None reported
Gevokizumab	*Common infections* Nasopharyngitis [39], URTI [39] *Rare infections* None reported	None reported

CMV cytomegalovirus, *NTM* nontuberculous mycobacteria, *TB* tuberculosis, *URTI* upper respiratory tract infection, *UTI* urinary tract infection

risk (RR) of 1.06 (CI 0.94–1.20) [12]. Multiple placebo-controlled RCTs have evaluated long-term safety of anakinra in RA [27–30]. Cohen et al. evaluated the efficacy and safety of anakinra for 24 weeks and demonstrated no serious infections in both groups assigned to methotrexate (MTX) and placebo vs. MTX and anakinra [27]. Similarly, Nuki et al. demonstrated no increased risk of infection with anakinra compared to placebo on evaluation of almost 500 patients with RA for a total period of 76 weeks, with an incidence rate (IR) of 0.91, 1.0, 1.1, and 1.4 events per 100 patient-years for the 30 mg, 75 mg, and 150 mg of anakinra and the placebo groups, respectively [28]. Schiff et al. conducted a post hoc analysis of an RCT, comparing safety of anakinra versus placebo in patients with RA and coexisting comorbidities [31]. Comorbidities were defined as having had at least one cardiovascular, pulmonary, or central nervous system events; infection; renal insufficiency; diabetes; or malignancy [31]. The incidence of serious infections was similar between high-risk patients receiving anakinra (2.5%), compared to all the patients receiving anakinra in the study (2.1%) [31].

Another meta-analysis included 74 RCTs evaluating the safety of multiple interleukin (IL) inhibitors, of which 8 RCTs evaluated anakinra [45]. After stratifying risk for serious infections for each IL inhibitor, an increased odd of serious infection was associated with anakinra compared to placebo (odds ratio 2.67; CI 1.03–6.90). Fleishmann et al. evaluated the safety of anakinra compared to placebo in an RCT, followed by an open-label extension trial for 3 years [29, 30]. A total of 1414 patients were recruited. Serious infections (defined as infections requiring hospitalization and the use of intravenous antibiotics) were observed in 23 patients in the anakinra group (2.1%) vs. only one patient in the placebo group (0.4%); $P = 0.068$ [29]. Pneumonia was the most common serious infection followed by cellulitis, in ten patients and three patients, respectively [29]. Five patients had underlying chronic pulmonary disease and three patients had a history of prior pneumonia [29]. Additionally, out of three patients with cellulitis, two had underlying diabetes and one had a toe ulcer at baseline. Of note, none of these serious infections were fatal.

However, 6 out of 23 patients permanently discontinued anakinra due to infection [29]. Organisms isolated in pneumonia and

cellulitis cases were *Streptococcus pneumoniae* and *Staphylococcus aureus*, respectively. None of the patients developed tuberculosis (TB) or opportunistic infections [29]. The 3-year open-label extension trial that included 1346 patients reported a higher incidence of serious infections with anakinra compared to placebo, with adjusted event rates of 5.37 vs. 1.65 per 100 patient-years, respectively [30]. Pneumonia was again the most common infection (1.50 events per 100 patient-years), followed by cellulitis (1.20 events per 100 patient-years). Rates of infections were significantly lower in patients who did not receive corticosteroids at baseline (2.87 events per 100 patient-years), with an incidence rate of pneumonia of 0.96 events per 100 patient-years and of cellulitis of 0.21 events per 100 patient-years [30]. Overall, the event rate of serious infections was consistently low throughout the entire treatment period [30].

Many of the autoinflammatory conditions for which anti-IL-1 therapy has been studied affect children [3].

In an observational study of 18 patients, the use of anakinra in neonatal-onset multisystem inflammatory disease (NOMID) was assessed. Fifteen patients had upper respiratory tract infections (URTI), and two patients had urinary tract infections (UTI). None of the infections required drug discontinuation [40]. A similar cohort evaluated the use of anakinra for 5 years and found similar results, with URTI being the most common infection [46]. The only two serious infections reported were wound infections, and none of these required drug discontinuation [46].

Although many studies demonstrated no increased risk of infection, some studies did find an increased rate of infection in patients treated with anakinra. Nevertheless, the majority of infections reported were not serious, suggesting an overall good safety profile of anakinra [31].

Canakinumab

Two RCTs assessed the safety and efficacy of canakinumab in gout [18, 19]. Schlesinger et al. evaluated the efficacy and safety of canakinumab vs. daily colchicine in 432 patients [18]. Overall, the incidence of infections was slightly increased with canakinumab use compared to colchicine (18% vs. 12%, respectively) [18]. Additionally, six serious infections (pneumonia, erysipelas, gangrene, sepsis, tonsilitis, and ear infection) were reported in canakinumab vs. none reported in the colchicine group. Similarly, a 12-week RCT followed by a 12-week double blind extension study, β-RELIEVED and β-RELIEVED-II, denoted increased risk of infections in patients receiving canakinumab compared to placebo (20% vs. 12%, respectively), mostly reported as mild infections [19]. Four serious infections occurred in the canakinumab group (1.8%)—jaw abscess, arm abscess, pneumonia, and gastroenteritis—all requiring hospitalization, and three requiring antibiotic therapy [19].

More recently, the CANTOS trial, a placebo-controlled RCT that recruited more than 10,000 patients, evaluated canakinumab use in the treatment of atherosclerosis. In contrast to other trials studying biologic therapies, CANTOS provided the opportunity to observe the risk of infections in patients who have no prior or current history of autoimmune disease and/or receipt of immunosuppression [32]. Infection rates of canakinumab vs. placebo were similar, 3.14 vs. 2.86 events per 100 patient-years, respectively, ($P = 0.14$) [32]. However, fatal infections or sepsis were higher in the canakinumab group vs. placebo, with an IR of 0.31 vs. 0.18 per 100 patient-years, respectively ($P = 0.02$) [32]. Individuals who had fatal infections were more likely to be older and have diabetes [32].

In the pediatric age group, a canakinumab placebo-controlled RCT of sJIA followed by an open-label extension phase [33, 34] demonstrated no differences in the incidence of infections at 29 days [33]. Similarly, serious infections were similar between the two groups in the open-label phase, with 4% in each group [33]. Patients from this study were able to enter an open-label long-term extension phase for 5 years [34]. Serious infections occurred at an incidence rate (IR) of 10.28 per 100 patient-years. The most common infection was gastroenteritis (1.05 per 100 patient-years), followed by pneumonia (0.84 per 100 patient-years) [34]. Other infections included varicella, septic shock, subcutaneous abscess, and streptococcal tonsilitis, all with equivalent rates of 0.42 per 1000 patient-years [34]. In autoinflammatory diseases, a three-part double-blind, placebo-controlled, randomized withdrawal study of patients ($n = 35$) with CAPS demonstrated an increased risk of infection in patients receiving canakinumab compared to placebo (12 vs. 9 patients; $P = 0.03$) [47].

Rilonacept

Rilonacept has been studied for the treatment of gout, pericarditis, and autoinflammatory disorders.

In the RESURGE study, a multicenter placebo-controlled trial that evaluated 1315 patients with gout for a period of 20 weeks, the incidence of serious infections was similar between rilonacept and placebo groups, 0.5% and 0.9%, respectively [35].

Recently, the RHAPSODY trial recruited 86 patients with recurrent pericarditis in a placebo-controlled RCT [22]. Rilonacept demonstrated a significantly lower recurrence of pericarditis. Infections were more frequent in the rilonacept group (23%) compared to placebo (0%). However, all infections were mild to moderate URTI, which did not require drug discontinuation [22].

In autoinflammatory conditions, Hoffman et al. conducted a placebo-controlled RCT on 44 patients with CAPS [36]. Overall, the incidence of infections was more frequent in the rilonacept arm compared to placebo (48% vs. 17%, respectively) with URTI being the most common infection, reported in 26% for rilonacept and 4% for placebo. One case of severe bronchitis was reported with rilonacept, but there have been no reports of opportunistic infections associated with this agent [36]. In addition to the 44 patients recruited in the Hoffman et al. RCT, an additional 57 patients entered the open-label phase (101 patients total) [37]. Two severe infections (pneumococcal meningitis and tooth abscess) were reported in the open-label phase [37]. Additionally, one death from pneumococcal meningitis was reported in a 71-year-old female patient with a history of recurrent skin infections [37]. The investigator deemed this infection to be unrelated to rilonacept therapy [37]. A placebo-controlled RCT of sJIA patients demonstrated similar rates of infections between rilonacept and placebo (46% and 61%, respectively) [38]. Four serious infections were reported in the rilonacept group (varicella, viral URTI, Salmonella gastroenteritis, streptococcal pharyngitis) [38].

Gevokizumab

Given that this monoclonal antibody is not yet approved, there is limited data of its safety and risk of infections. Cavelti-Weder et al. evaluated the efficacy and safety of gevokizumab in patients with type 2 diabetes in a dose-escalation RCT [48]. Gevokizumab was administered either as a single dose intravenously (0.01–3.0 mg/kg) or as single or multiple subcutaneous doses (0.03–0.3 mg/kg). No serious infectious adverse events were observed at any dose of gevokizumab [48]. More recently, Tugal-Tutkun et al. performed a placebo-controlled RCT followed by an open-label extension phase that evaluated the use of gevokizumab in Bechet's uveitis [39]. This study evaluated 83 patients for a total duration of 420 days. Infections were similar between placebo and gevokizumab (46% vs. 51%, respectively); most common infections were nasopharyngitis and URTI [39]. Positive interferon-gamma released assay (IGRA) was reported in two patients in the gevokizumab group. Both patients received prophylactic TB therapy with either isoniazid or rifampin, with no reported cases of active TB [39].

Tuberculosis

There is scarce and weak evidence regarding the risk of TB with anakinra use. Two cases of pulmonary TB and TB pyomyositis have been reported in association with combined anakinra and corticosteroid use for treatment of RA [41, 42]. Additionally, data from a Canadian RA registry that included over 110,000 patients showed no statistically significant increased risk of TB in patients receiving anakinra, with an adjusted rate ratio (ARR) 1.3 events per 1000 patient-years (CI 0.8–2.1) [49].

Only six cases of TB were confirmed in individuals treated with canakinumab, all reported in the CANTOS trial. The same rate of TB was reported in both arm of the trial (0.06% each), five of those cases occurred in India and one case in Taiwan [32]. It is important to recognize that most RCTs evaluating IL-1-targeted therapies to date have taken place in low TB prevalence areas [3].

Opportunistic Infections

Opportunistic infections have only been reported in four patients with RA receiving anakinra, one case of nontuberculous mycobacteria infection in a patient receiving concomitant prednisone and MTX, one case of esophageal candidiasis in a patient with cirrhosis and on concomitant prednisone, and one case of histoplasmosis [30]. Additionally, one case of CMV hepatitis has been reported in a patient with JIA treated with anakinra [44]. In an observational cohort of 35 patients with systemic juvenile idiopathic arthritis (sJIA) and AOSD, one case of visceral leishmaniasis and two cases of varicella were identified [43]. Visceral leishmaniasis occurred 6 months after anakinra therapy in a child with sJIA. Of note, the child lived in an endemic area, in France, prior to starting therapy [43].

Four cases of opportunistic infections were identified with canakinumab use for sJIA including toxoplasmosis, CMV infection, Salmonella gastroenteritis, and adenovirus infection [34].

Conclusions

IL-1 inhibition has emerged as an important therapy for many patient groups over the last two decades. These biologic agents have been demonstrated to be generally safe, and although there may be an increased risk of infection, when infections do occur, these appear to be mostly mild to moderate in severity with the most common infections being URTIs, pneumonia, and cellulitis. The risk of severe infections associated with anti-IL-1 therapy may be increased in older patients with comorbidities, particularly with canakinumab, but more data is needed. Rare cases of TB and other opportunistic infections have been reported in association with IL-1 therapy, but the exact contribution of the IL-1 therapy to the development of these infections remains unclear.

Acknowledgment Figure created with support from Servier medical art (https://smart.servier.com/).

Conflicts of Interest The authors have no conflicts of interest to declare regarding the publication of this manuscript.

References

1. Sims JE, Smith DE. The IL-1 family: regulators of immunity. Nat Rev Immunol. 2010;10(2):89–102.
2. Davis JS, Ferreira D, Paige E, Gedye C, Boyle M. Infectious complications of biological and small molecule targeted immunomodulatory therapies. Clin Microbiol Rev. 2020;33(3):e00035–19.
3. Winthrop KL, Mariette X, Silva JT, Benamu E, Calabrese LH, Dumusc A, et al. ESCMID Study Group for Infections in Compromised Hosts (ESGICH) Consensus Document on the

safety of targeted and biological therapies: an infectious diseases perspective (Soluble immune effector molecules [II]: agents targeting interleukins, immunoglobulins and complement factors). Clin Microbiol Infect. 2018;24:21–40.

4. Dinarello CA, Simon A, van der Meer JWM. Treating inflammation by blocking interleukin-1 in a broad spectrum of diseases. Nat Rev Drug Discov. 2012;11(8):633–52.
5. Lopez-Castejon G, Brough D. Understanding the mechanism of IL-1β secretion. Cytokine Growth Factor Rev. 2011;22(4):189–95.
6. Kaplanski G, Farnarier C, Kaplanski S, Porat R, Shapiro L, Bongrand P, et al. Interleukin-1 induces interleukin-8 secretion from endothelial cells by a juxtacrine mechanism. Blood. 1994;84(12):4242–8.
7. Kurt-Jones EA, Beller DI, Mizel SB, Unanue ER. Identification of a membrane-associated interleukin 1 in macrophages. Proc Natl Acad Sci U S A. 1985;82(4):1204–8.
8. Chen CJ, Kono H, Golenbock D, Reed G, Akira S, Rock KL. Identification of a key pathway required for the sterile inflammatory response triggered by dying cells. Nat Med. 2007;13(7):851–6.
9. Cohen I, Rider P, Carmi Y, Braiman A, Dotan S, White MR, et al. Differential release of chromatin-bound IL-1α discriminates between necrotic and apoptotic cell death by the ability to induce sterile inflammation. Proc Natl Acad Sci. 2010;107(6):2574–9.
10. Rider P, Carmi Y, Guttman O, Braiman A, Cohen I, Voronov E, et al. IL-1α and IL-1β recruit different myeloid cells and promote different stages of sterile inflammation. J Immunol. 2011;187(9):4835–43.
11. Arend WP, Malyak M, Guthridge CJ, Gabay C. Interleukin-1 receptor antagonist: role in biology. Annu Rev Immunol. 1998;16:27–55.
12. Nikfar S, Saiyarsarai P, Tigabu BM, Abdollahi M. Efficacy and safety of interleukin-1 antagonists in rheumatoid arthritis: a systematic review and meta-analysis. Rheumatol Int. 2018;38(8):1363–83.
13. Feist E, Quartier P, Fautrel B, Schneider R, Sfriso P, Efthimiou P, et al. Efficacy and safety of canakinumab in patients with Still's disease: exposure-response analysis of pooled systemic juvenile idiopathic arthritis data by age groups. Clin Exp Rheumatol. 2018;36(4):668–75.
14. Horneff G, Schulz AC, Klotsche J, Hospach A, Minden K, Foeldvari I, et al. Experience with etanercept, tocilizumab and interleukin-1 inhibitors in systemic onset juvenile idiopathic arthritis patients from the BIKER registry. Arthritis Res Ther. 2017;19(1):256.
15. De Benedetti F, Gattorno M, Anton J, Ben-Chetrit E, Frenkel J, Hoffman HM, et al. Canakinumab for the treatment of autoinflammatory recurrent fever syndromes. N Engl J Med. 2018;378(20):1908–19.
16. Gentileschi S, Rigante D, Vitale A, Sota J, Frediani B, Galeazzi M, et al. Efficacy and safety of anakinra in tumor necrosis factor receptor-associated periodic syndrome (TRAPS) complicated by severe renal failure: a report after long-term follow-up and review of the literature. Clin Rheumatol. 2017;36(7):1687–90.
17. van der Hilst JCH, Bodar EJ, Barron KS, Frenkel J, Drenth JPH, van der Meer JWM, et al. Long-term follow-up, clinical features, and quality of life in a series of 103 patients with hyperimmunoglobulinemia D syndrome. Medicine. 2008;87(6):301–10.
18. Schlesinger N, Mysler E, Lin H-Y, De Meulemeester M, Rovensky J, Arulmani U, et al. Canakinumab reduces the risk of acute gouty arthritis flares during initiation of allopurinol treatment: results of a double-blind, randomised study. Ann Rheum Dis. 2011;70(7):1264–71.
19. Schlesinger N, Alten RE, Bardin T, Schumacher HR, Bloch M, Gimona A, et al. Canakinumab for acute gouty arthritis in patients with limited treatment options: results from two randomised, multicentre, active-controlled, double-blind trials and their initial extensions. Ann Rheum Dis. 2012;71(11):1839–48.
20. Thueringer JT, Doll NK, Gertner E. Anakinra for the treatment of acute severe gout in critically ill patients. Semin Arthritis Rheum. 2015;45(1):81–5.
21. Tran AP, Edelman J. Interleukin-1 inhibition by anakinra in refractory chronic tophaceous gout. Int J Rheum Dis. 2011;14(3):e33–7.

22. Klein AL, Imazio M, Cremer P, Brucato A, Abbate A, Fang F, et al. Phase 3 trial of interleukin-1 trap rilonacept in recurrent pericarditis. N Engl J Med. 2020;384:31–41.
23. Cantarini L, Talarico R, Generali E, Emmi G, Lopalco G, Costa L, et al. Safety profile of biologic agents for Behçet's disease in a multicenter observational cohort study. Int J Rheum Dis. 2017;20(1):103–8.
24. Fabiani C, Vitale A, Emmi G, Lopalco G, Vannozzi L, Guerriero S, et al. Interleukin (IL)-1 inhibition with anakinra and canakinumab in Behçet's disease-related uveitis: a multicenter retrospective observational study. Clin Rheumatol. 2017;36(1):191–7.
25. Acquitter M, Plantin P, Kupfer I, Auvinet H, Marhadour T. Anakinra improves pyoderma gangrenosum in psoriatic arthritis: a case report. Ann Intern Med. 2015;163(1):70–1.
26. Kluger N, Gil-Bistes D, Guillot B, Bessis D. Efficacy of anti-interleukin-1 receptor antagonist anakinra (Kineret®) in a case of refractory Sweet's syndrome. Dermatology. 2011;222(2):123–7.
27. Cohen S, Hurd E, Cush J, Schiff M, Weinblatt ME, Moreland LW, et al. Treatment of rheumatoid arthritis with anakinra, a recombinant human interleukin-1 receptor antagonist, in combination with methotrexate: Results of a twenty-four-week, multicenter, randomized, double-blind, placebo-controlled trial. Arthritis Rheum. 2002;46(3):614–24.
28. Nuki G, Bresnihan B, Bear MB, McCabe D. Long-term safety and maintenance of clinical improvement following treatment with anakinra (recombinant human interleukin-1 receptor antagonist) in patients with rheumatoid arthritis: Extension phase of a randomized, double-blind, placebo-controlled trial. Arthritis Rheum. 2002;46(11):2838–46.
29. Fleischmann RM, Schechtman J, Bennett R, Handel ML, Burmester GR, Tesser J, et al. Anakinra, a recombinant human interleukin-1 receptor antagonist (r-metHuIL-1ra), in patients with rheumatoid arthritis: a large, international, multicenter, placebo-controlled trial. Arthritis Rheum. 2003;48(4):927–34.
30. Fleischmann RM, Tesser J, Schiff MH, Schechtman J, Burmester GR, Bennett R, et al. Safety of extended treatment with anakinra in patients with rheumatoid arthritis. Ann Rheum Dis. 2006;65(8):1006–12.
31. Schiff MH, DiVittorio G, Tesser J, Fleischmann R, Schechtman J, Hartman S, et al. The safety of anakinra in high-risk patients with active rheumatoid arthritis: six-month observations of patients with comorbid conditions. Arthritis Rheum. 2004;50(6):1752–60.
32. Ridker PM, Everett BM, Thuren T, MacFadyen JG, Chang WH, Ballantyne C, et al. Antiinflammatory therapy with canakinumab for atherosclerotic disease. N Engl J Med. 2017;377(12):1119–31.
33. Ruperto N, Brunner HI, Quartier P, Constantin T, Wulffraat N, Horneff G, et al. Two randomized trials of canakinumab in systemic juvenile idiopathic arthritis. N Engl J Med. 2012;367(25):2396–406.
34. Ruperto N, Brunner HI, Quartier P, Constantin T, Wulffraat NM, Horneff G, et al. Canakinumab in patients with systemic juvenile idiopathic arthritis and active systemic features: results from the 5-year long-term extension of the phase III pivotal trials. Ann Rheum Dis. 2018;77(12):1710–9.
35. Sundy JS, Schumacher HR, Kivitz A, Weinstein SP, Wu R, King-Davis S, et al. Rilonacept for gout flare prevention in patients receiving uric acid-lowering therapy: results of RESURGE, a phase III, international safety study. J Rheumatol. 2014;41(8):1703–11.
36. Hoffman HM, Throne ML, Amar NJ, Sebai M, Kivitz AJ, Kavanaugh A, et al. Efficacy and safety of rilonacept (interleukin-1 trap) in patients with cryopyrin-associated periodic syndromes: results from two sequential placebo-controlled studies. Arthritis Rheum. 2008;58(8):2443–52.
37. Hoffman HM, Throne ML, Amar NJ, Cartwright RC, Kivitz AJ, Soo Y, et al. Long-term efficacy and safety profile of rilonacept in the treatment of cryopryin-associated periodic syndromes: results of a 72-week open-label extension study. Clin Ther. 2012;34(10):2091–103.
38. Ilowite NT, Prather K, Lokhnygina Y, Schanberg LE, Elder M, Milojevic D, et al. Randomized, double-blind, placebo-controlled trial of the efficacy and safety of rilonacept in the treatment of systemic juvenile idiopathic arthritis. Arthritis Rheumatol. 2014;66(9):2570–9.

39. Tugal-Tutkun I, Pavesio C, De Cordoue A, Bernard-Poenaru O, Gül A. Use of gevokizumab in patients with Behçet's disease uveitis: an international, randomized, double-masked, placebo-controlled study and open-label extension study. Ocul Immunol Inflamm. 2018;26(7):1023–33.
40. Goldbach-Mansky R, Dailey NJ, Canna SW, Gelabert A, Jones J, Rubin BI, et al. Neonatal-onset multisystem inflammatory disease responsive to interleukin-1β inhibition. N Engl J Med. 2006;355(6):581–92.
41. Settas LD, Tsimirikas G, Vosvotekas G, Triantafyllidou E, Nicolaides P. Reactivation of pulmonary tuberculosis in a patient with rheumatoid arthritis during treatment with IL-1 receptor antagonists (anakinra). J Clin Rheumatol. 2007;13(4):219–20.
42. Migkos MP, Somarakis GA, Markatseli TE, Matthaiou M, Kosta P, Voulgari PV, et al. Tuberculous pyomyositis in a rheumatoid arthritis patient treated with anakinra. Clin Exp Rheumatol. 2015;33(5):734–6.
43. Lequerré T, Quartier P, Rosellini D, Alaoui F, De Bandt M, Mejjad O, et al. Interleukin-1 receptor antagonist (anakinra) treatment in patients with systemic-onset juvenile idiopathic arthritis or adult onset still disease: preliminary experience in France. Ann Rheum Dis. 2008;67(3):302–8.
44. Ilowite N, Porras O, Reiff A, Rudge S, Punaro M, Martin A, et al. Anakinra in the treatment of polyarticular-course juvenile rheumatoid arthritis: safety and preliminary efficacy results of a randomized multicenter study. Clin Rheumatol. 2009;28(2):129–37.
45. Bilal J, Berlinberg A, Riaz IB, Faridi W, Bhattacharjee S, Ortega G, et al. Risk of infections and cancer in patients with rheumatologic diseases receiving interleukin inhibitors: a systematic review and meta-analysis. JAMA Netw Open. 2019;2(10):e1913102.
46. Sibley CH, Plass N, Snow J, Wiggs EA, Brewer CC, King KA, et al. Sustained response and prevention of damage progression in patients with neonatal-onset multisystem inflammatory disease treated with anakinra: a cohort study to determine three- and five-year outcomes. Arthritis Rheum. 2012;64(7):2375–86.
47. Lachmann HJ, Kone-Paut I, Kuemmerle-Deschner JB, Leslie KS, Hachulla E, Quartier P, et al. Use of canakinumab in the cryopyrin-associated periodic syndrome. N Engl J Med. 2009;360(23):2416–25.
48. Cavelti-Weder C, Babians-Brunner A, Keller C, Stahel MA, Kurz-Levin M, Zayed H, et al. Effects of gevokizumab on glycemia and inflammatory markers in type 2 diabetes. Diabetes Care. 2012;35(8):1654–62.
49. Brassard P, Kezouh A, Suissa S. Antirheumatic drugs and the risk of tuberculosis. Clin Infect Dis. 2006;43(6):717–22.

Interleukin-6 Targeted Agents

10

Matteo Rinaldi, Giuseppe Ferraro,
and Maddalena Giannella

Introduction

Interleukin-6 (IL-6) is best known for its pro-inflammatory effects. However, this pleomorphic cytokine also has anti-inflammatory, pro-resolution, and regenerative properties; it is important for pathogen clearance and triggers the release of acute-phase proteins via the liver. Anti-inflammatory and antibacterial activities of IL-6 are mediated by classical signaling, whereas pro-inflammatory effects are mediated by trans-signaling. Monoclonal antibodies against IL-6R, such as tocilizumab, do not discriminate between classical signaling and trans-signaling, blocking both pathways. An increased incidence of bacterial infections has been observed in patients treated with monoclonal antibodies against IL-6R, particularly in those who are receiving concomitant corticosteroids. In this chapter, the mechanism of action and the incidence and types of infections reported in patients receiving IL-6 blocking agents are reviewed.

M. Rinaldi · G. Ferraro
Infectious Diseases Unit, IRCCS Azienda Ospedaliero-Universitaria di Bologna, Policlinico di Sant'Orsola, Bologna, Italy

M. Giannella (✉)
Infectious Diseases Unit, IRCCS Azienda Ospedaliero-Universitaria di Bologna, Policlinico di Sant'Orsola, Bologna, Italy

Department of Medical and Surgical Sciences, Alma Mater Studiorum University of Bologna, Bologna, Italy
e-mail: maddalena.giannella@unibo.it

C. Cervera, J. M. Aguado (eds.), *Infectious Complications in Biologic and Targeted Therapies*, https://doi.org/10.1007/978-3-031-11363-5_10

Mechanism of Action and Expected Impact on Infection Risk

Interleukine-6 (IL-6) is a pleomorphic pro-inflammatory cytokine linked to immune regulation, acute phase response, and hematopoiesis [1, 2]. Its activity is expressed throughout the membrane-bound and the soluble IL-6 receptor (IL6-R). The membrane-bound form or "*classical*-signaling" pathway is mainly expressed in hepatocytes and hematopoietic cells, and it interacts with a second protein, gp130, resulting in a functional receptor complex that may trigger the downstream signaling cascade. The soluble form of IL-6R is involved in the "*trans*-signaling" pathway, and it is able to potentially activate all nucleated cells, as gp130 is present ubiquitously (see Fig. 10.1). Notably, the membrane-bound pathway is related to tissue regeneration and protects from bacterial infection, whereas the soluble receptor is linked to pro-inflammatory activity [3]. IL-6 dysregulation has been linked to several autoimmune disorders, such as rheumatoid arthritis (RA), vasculitis, and inflammatory bowel disease [2, 4].

To date, two agents targeting IL-6 and/or its receptor have been approved for different immune disorders: tocilizumab (TCZ) and siltuximab.

TCZ is a humanized IgG1 monoclonal antibody that inactivates both the membrane-bound and soluble forms of IL6-R. It is approved for RA, polyarticular or systemic juvenile idiopathic arthritis and, recently, for giant cell arteritis [1, 5]. Recently, the role of TCZ in both prevention and treatment of graft vs. host disease (GVHD) has been investigated [6, 7]. The drug can be administered through intravenous infusion or subcutaneous injection, and the duration of treatment depends on

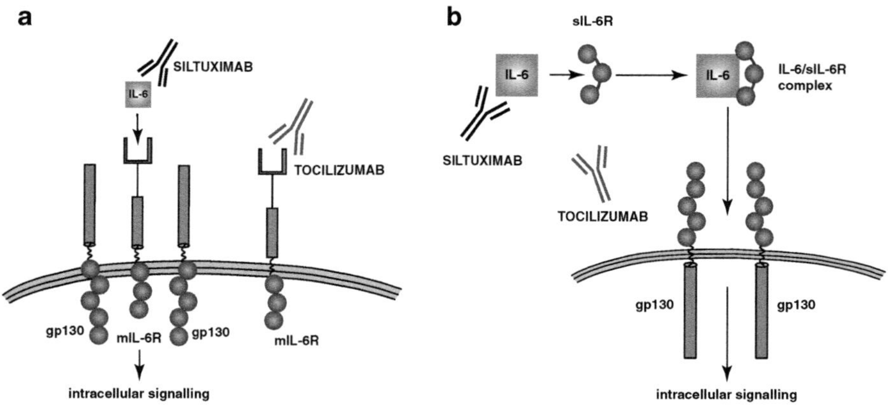

Fig. 10.1 Signaling pathways of IL-6 and activity of IL6-targeted agents. (**a**) *cis*-signaling expressed through the membrane-bound IL6-receptor (mIL-6R). Once IL-6 binds to mIL-6R it interacts with gp130, forming a receptor complex and triggering the intracellular signaling. (**b**) *trans*-signaling, IL6 interacts with the soluble form of the receptor (sIL-6R), produced by the cleavage of mIL-6R, resulting in a functional complex (IL-6/sIL-6R). This complex interacts with gp130, preceding the intracellular cascade. Tocilizumab interacts with both mIL-6R and sIL-6R, while siltuximab binds directly IL-6. The final effect of both drugs is the prevention of the downstream intracellular signaling

the patient's response. Of concern, the effects of TCZ cannot be reversed after administration, and at high serum concentrations, it has a terminal half-life of approximately 16 days. Although its half-life does not necessarily preclude its use, the impossibility of eliminating the drug may be problematic in patients more prone to sudden fluctuation of their disease.

Siltuximab consists of a human-murine IgG1 monoclonal antibody able to bind and inactivate circulating IL-6. It has been approved for the treatment of multicentric Castleman's disease [8]. In addition, different agents targeting IL-6 or its receptor are under clinical development, such as sirukumab and olokizumab for the treatment of RA. Recently, a novel agent called sarilumab has been approved from FDA for moderate to severe RA. Clazakizumab reached promising results in a double-blind, phase 2, randomized clinical trial in psoriatic arthritis patients [9]. In addition, a novel gp130 fusion protein called olamkicept that only binds the complex IL-6/soluble IL6R is under evaluation in a phase 2 trial in patients with active inflammatory bowel disease (ClinicalTrials.gov Identifier: NCT03235752).

Because of their activity, these agents show a prompt action in decreasing inflammatory markers, such as C-reactive protein. Indeed, their immunomodulatory effect may result in severe and potentially life-threatening bacterial infections characterized by significant discrepancy in both clinic and laboratory markers [10, 11]. Previous researchers have shown that IL-6 has a key role in supporting immunocompetent responses to all types of infections, especially bacterial [12].

Available Clinical Data

Most data about the infection risk associated with IL-6 inhibitors come from studies on patients treated with TCZ for rheumatoid arthritis (RA). In several randomized controlled trials (RCT), the occurrence of severe infections was generally assessed as a secondary outcome among safety issues (see Table 10.1). Severe infections were generally defined as events resulting in hospitalization or death. To note, in most studies, there was no predefined protocol for systematic search or surveillance for infectious complications. In addition, it is worth mentioning that the infection risk in RA is complex and likely multifactorial. High disease activity, multimorbidity, treatment/disease-related immunosuppression, and polypharmacy all likely contribute.

Data from RCTs including patients with moderate to severe RA show different infection incidence rates, varying from 1.53 (0.57–4.08) serious infections per 100 patient-years in naive patients up to 9.98 (4.99–19.96) in patients already treated with TNF inhibitors [19, 23]. The hypothesis is that cumulative and longer immunosuppression could lead to an increased risk of severe infection. Notably, the median age and the comorbidities of patients enrolled in RCT are usually lower than that of real-life cohorts.

Real-life studies exhibit even higher percentages. Indeed, an open-label real-life study conducted in Germany including 850 patients treated with TCZ for active rheumatoid arthritis found a rate of serious infection of 5.3%, with a rate of 4.4

Table 10.1 Principal studies evaluating the incidence rate of severe infections in patients treated with TCZ for autoimmune disorders

Author, study, year, reference	Study design	Indication for TCZ	Study duration	Patients (Total)	TCZ dose	Control group (N, type)	Prior treatment	N of SI/arm	Incidence rate (95%CI)
Kremer (LITHE), 2011 [13]	Phase III RCT	RA	1 year	1196	4 mg/kg 8 mg/kg	393, placebo	MTX	12/399 14/398	3.7 (2.1–6.52) 4 (2.37–6.75)
Gabay (ADACTA), 2013 [14]	Phase IV RCT	RA	24 weeks	326	8 mg/kg	163, Adalimumab	MTX	6/163	6.52 (2.93–14.51)
Genovese (TOWARD), 2008 [15]	Phase III RCT	RA	24 weeks	1220	8 mg/kg	415, placebo	DMARD	22/805	5.9 (3.88–8.96)
Maini (CHARISMA), 2006 [16]	Phase II RCT	RA	20 weeks	359	2 mg/kg 8 mg/kg	49, MTX	MTX	4/53 3/50	19.87 (7.46–52.94) 15.79 (5.09–48.96)
Fleischmann LITHE, 2013 [17]	Phase III RCT	RA	2 years	1196	4 mg/kg 8 mg/kg	392, placebo-MTX	MTX	16/597 40/983	3.1 (1.9–5.06) 3 (2.2–4.09)
Smolen (OPTION), 2008 [18]	Phase III RCT	RA	24 weeks	623	4 mg/kg 8 mg/kg	204, placebo	MTX	3/214 6/205	3.05 (0.98–9.46) 6.05 (2.72–13.47)
Jones (AMBITION), 2010 [19]	Phase III RCT	RA	24 weeks	673	8 mg/kg	284, MTX 101, placebo	MTX-naive	4/288	1.53 (0.57–4.08)
Yazici (ROSE), 2012 [20]	Phase III RCT	RA	24 weeks	619	8 mg/kg	207, placebo	DMARD	10/412	7.87 (4.23–14.63)
Nishimoto (SAMURAI), 2007 [21]	Phase III RCT	RA	1 year	306	8 mg/kg	148, DMARDs	DMARD	12/158	7.64 (4.34–13.45)
Nishimoto (SATORI), 2009 [22]	Phase III RCT	RA	24 weeks	127	8 mg/kg	66, MTX	MTX	2/61	7.17 (1.79–28.68)
Emery (RADIATE), 2008 [23]	Phase III RCT	RA	24 weeks	499	4 mg/kg 8 mg/kg	160, placebo	TNFi	3/163 8/175	5.72 (1.84–17.74) 9.98 (4.99–19.96)
Burmester (TAMARA), 2011 [24]	Phase III OL study	RA	24 weeks	286	8 mg/kg	/	DMARD	9/286	6.74 (3.51–12.95)
Nishimoto (STREAM), 2009 [25]	OL	RA	5 years	143	8 mg/kg	/	DMARD	25/143	5.7 (3.85–8.44)

TCZ tocilizumab, *SI* severe infections, *CI* confidence interval, *DMARD* disease-modifying antirheumatic drug, *MTX* methotrexate, *OL* open label, *RCT* randomized controlled trial, *TNFi* tumor necrosis factor inhibitor events per 100 patient-years over 52 weeks of follow-up [26]. An extremely large Japanese post-marketing surveillance cohort of patients treated with TCZ for the same indication reached nine events per 100 patient-years [27]. Finally, in a US cohort, the rate of severe infections requiring hospitalization attested up to 14.9 events per 100 patient-years [28]. As already stated, the higher median age and the higher rate of previous treatments with anti-TNF agents could account for the difference in infection incidence rates reported in RCTs and in observational studies.

Even the dose of TCZ administered seems to play a role in increasing the risk of infection. A phase III randomized controlled trial evaluating the clinical response of TCZ administered at different doses showed a risk of severe infections of 5.72 (1.84–17.74) with TCZ 4 mg/kg, but this risk was nearly doubled (9.98, 4.99–19.96) for the dosage of 8 mg/kg [23]. A meta-analysis conducted by Shiff et al. including eight different studies (of them, five phase III trials) exhibited a similar rate of serious infection in control group and TCZ 4 mg/Kg group, attesting both at 3.5 per 100 patient-years. In addition, serious infections increased at 4.9/100 patient-years if TCZ was administered at 8 mg/kg [29]. However, the authors found that older age, high body mass index, and previous administration of a TNF inhibitor were associated with infection development, regardless of the treatment group. This latter aspect has been confirmed in other larger studies evaluating patients previously exposed to anti-TNF agents [23, 30].

A systematic review published in 2015 compared the clinical impact of disease-modifying antirheumatic drugs (DMARDs) on infections development [31]. TCZ was associated with an incidence rate of serious infections of 5.45 per 100 patient-years, a risk even higher if compared to other immunomodulant agents such as rituximab (see Table 10.2).

A randomized, double-blind, phase III trial comparing sarilumab vs. adalimumab showed similar rates of infections (28.8% in sarilumab group vs. 27.7% in adalimumab group) and serious infections (1.1% in both groups) [32]. Recently, a large cohort study of 16074 patients receiving TCZ was propensity score-matched to a cohort of 33,109 patients treated with TNF inhibitors, focusing on the risk of serious infections [33]. The authors found that the risk of severe infections was similar between the two groups; however, TCZ was found to be associated with an increased risk of skin and soft tissue infections (HR 2.38, 95% CI 1.47–3.86) and serious infections including bacterial, viral, and opportunistic agents (HR 1.19, 95% CI 1.03–1.33) if compared to TNF-α inhibitors.

Although specific sites of infection were rarely reported in previous studies, severe infections consisted mainly in lower respiratory tract infections, followed by

Table 10.2 Rates of severe infections per 100 patient-years observed in different studies

Drug	Number of patients enrolled	Rates of severe infections (95%CI)
Abatacept	5953	3.04 (2.49–3.72)
Rituximab	2926	3.72 (2.99–4.62)
Tocilizumab	5547	5.45 (4.26–6.96)
Infliximab	4592	6.11 (5.24–7.12)
Etanercept	7141	4.06 (3.26–5.08)
Adalimumab	6570	5.04 (3.80–6.69)

urinary tract infections, cellulitis, and primary bloodstream infections that required hospital admission and systemic antibiotic therapy [23, 29].

Even though patients exposed to IL6-targeting agents may be at increased risk of opportunistic infections, few studies evaluated this aspect. The previously mentioned meta-analysis showed an absolute number of 22 opportunistic infections, with a rate of 0.23 events per 100 patient-years [29]. Fourteen of these infections were considered serious events. Of interest, eight cases were *Mycobacterium tuberculosis* reactivation, followed by *P. jirovecii* infection, cryptococcosis, and *Mycobacterium avium* infection. Similarly, a post-marketing study in Japan found a rate of pulmonary tuberculosis reactivation of 0.05%, similar to other anti-TNF-α agents [27]. However, the authors reported an increased risk of nontuberculous mycobacteria and *P. jirovecii* infections, accounting for 0.22% and 0.16%, respectively. Even varicella-zoster virus (VZV) reactivation during TCZ administration has been observed, but its incidence is comparable to other biological agents. A retrospective study from the USA showed an incidence of VZV reactivation of 4.3% during TCZ treatment, a rate consistently lower if compared with the occurrence of VZV reactivation during rituximab, reaching up to 19.4% [34]. However, absolute incidence rate per 100 patient-years was similar in both groups (2.15 TCZ vs. 2.27 rituximab). Little is known about hepatitis B virus (HBV) reactivation in patients treated with TCZ. Although data are restricted to case reports, mainly because HBc-positive patients were excluded from randomized trials, HBV reactivation is a possible event, usually with self-limited viremia and without clinical implications [35, 36]. A retrospective study of 152 patients treated with DMARDs (25 of them receiving TCZ) recorded an overall HBV reactivation of 4.6%, and the absence of anti-HBs was found to be a risk factor for reactivation [37]. These findings suggest to perform a microbiological work-up before starting a IL6 or a IL6-R-targeted agent, including screening for latent tuberculosis infection and serological status for HBV, in order to prevent reactivations [38, 39].

More recently, IL-6 inhibitors have been employed in mild to critically ill patients with COVID-19 diagnosis with controversial results in terms of overall mortality. To date, seven randomized controlled trials have been published including a total of 3204 patients treated with IL-6 inhibitors vs. 2982 receiving placebo and/or best available treatment [40, 41] (see Table 10.3). The overall rate of infection among the two groups was of 4.7% and 3.7% with a median follow-up duration of 28 days. No study had a predefined protocol for the active search of infection complications. It is worth mentioning that the RECOVERY study accounts for more than half of patients treated with TCZ in published RCTs. Patients enrolled in this study presented with a mild to moderate COVID-19; thus, they were generally at low risk of superinfection; indeed the infection rate was very low in both treatment and control arms [46]. Differently, in RCT studies focusing on patients with critical disease, the infection rates were higher in both treatment and control arms [44].

Real-life experiences drew a very different picture [47–50] (see Table 10.3). Reviewing four observational studies including a total of 257 patients treated with IL-6 inhibitors and 471 controls, the rates of infections were 42% vs. 19.3% with a

Table 10.3 Reported cases of infectious complications in patients treated with tocilizumab for COVID-19

Reference	Study type	Numbers of patients included in treatment and in control group	Setting (i.e., moderate severe or critical COVID-19)	Numbers of infections in treatment arm and in control group or risk estimation (i.e., RR, RD, etc.)	Type of infections reported in treatment arm (i.e., bacterial, fungal, viral, opportunistic etc.)	Follow-up duration (days)	Systematic search for superinfection
Stone, 2020 [42]	RCT, multicenter USA	161 vs. 82	Moderate disease	13 (8.1%) vs. 14 (17.1%) RR 0.47 [0.23–0.95]	Not reported	28 days	No
Salvarani, 2021 [43]	RCT, multicenter Italy	60 vs. 66	Mild disease	1 (0.6%) vs. 4 (6.1%) RR 0.26 [0.03–2.28]	Bacterial	30 days	No
Hermine, 2021 [40]	RCT, multicenter France	64 vs. 67	Mild to moderate disease	2 (1.2%) vs. 13 (19.4%) RR 0.16 [0.04–0.70]	Bacterial	28 days	No
Rosas, 2021 [44]	RCT, international	295 vs. 143	Critical disease	113 (38.3%) vs. 58 (40.5%) RR 0.95 [0.75–1.22]	112 bacterial, 1 fungal	28 days	No
Salama, 2020 [41]	RCT, international	249 vs. 128	Mild to moderate disease	19 (7.6) vs. 21 (16.4%) RR 0.91 [0.51–1.64]	Not reported	28 days	No
Gordon, 2021 [45]	RCT, international	353 vs. 402	Critical disease	1 vs. not reported	Bacterial	21 days	No
Recovery Collaborative Group, 2021 [46]	RCT, UK	2022 vs. 2094	Mild to moderate	3 vs. not reported	Bacterial	28 days	No
Somers, 2020 [47]	Observational controlled study, USA	78 vs. 76	Critical disease	42 (54%) vs. 20 (26%) p-value <0.001	Bacterial and fungal	28 days	No
Kimmig, 2021 [48]	Observational study, USA	54 vs. 57	Critical disease	29 (53.7%) vs. 16 (28.1%) p-value 0.029	26 bacterial, 3 fungal	Not reported	No
Falcone et al., 2021 [49]	Observational study, Italy	51 vs. 264	Mild to severe disease	20 (29%) vs. 49 (18.5%) OR 5.09 [2.2–11.8]	Bacterial and fungal	30 days	No
Pettit, 2020 [50]	Observational study, USA	74 vs. 74	Moderate to severe disease	17 (23%) vs. 6 (8%) p-value 0.013	1 bacterial, 2 fungal	58 days	No

statistically significant association with the exposure to IL-6 inhibitors in all studies, even after adjustment for confounding factors [49].

Most infections consisted of bloodstream infections due to bacterial agents, with few cases of candidemia, only one opportunistic infection was reported in a patient with CMV syndrome and high levels of CMV DNA on blood sample.

Conclusions and Suggested Prevention Strategies

Current evidence on the infection risk associated with the use of IL-6- or IL-6R-targeted agents consists mostly of studies including patients treated with tocilizumab for a chronic autoimmune condition such as RA. On the other hand, during the COVID-19 pandemic, a huge amount of data on these agents has been obtained from its use in hospitalized patients for COVID-19. The incidence of severe (secondary) infections in observational studies was higher than that observed in randomized controlled trials for both conditions. For patients with RA, such incidence seems to be similar or slightly higher than that associated with the use of other DMARDs, in particular anti-TNF-α agents. However, a systematic active search or surveillance screening for infectious disease during or after tocilizumab treatment has not yet been performed. The concomitant or prior use of immunosuppressive drugs and the severity of the underlying condition are other confounding factors hampering a real estimation of the infection risk in patients treated with IL-6 inhibitors.

In general, it seems advisable to implement the prevention strategies suggested for patients receiving anti-TNF-α therapy, including screening for latent tuberculosis and chronic HBV infection (followed by appropriate prophylaxis or therapy if needed). However, the performance of these assays was challenging during COVID-19 surges. Age-appropriate inactivated vaccination (i.e., trivalent inactivated influenza, pneumococcal or Hib vaccines) has been also suggested in patients with chronic diseases treated with IL-6 inhibitors.

References

1. Calabrese LH, Rose-John S. IL-6 biology: implications for clinical targeting in rheumatic disease. Nat Rev Rheumatol. 2014;10(12):720–7.
2. Ishihara K, Hirano T. IL-6 in autoimmune disease and chronic inflammatory proliferative disease. Cytokine Growth Factor Rev. 2002;13(4-5):357–68.
3. Scheller J, Chalaris A, Schmidt-Arras D, Rose-John S. The pro- and anti-inflammatory properties of the cytokine interleukin-6. Biochim Biophys Acta. 2011;1813(5):878–88.
4. Hirano T. Interleukin 6 in autoimmune and inflammatory diseases: a personal memoir. Proc Jpn Acad Ser B Phys Biol Sci. 2010;86(7):717–30.
5. Walker UA. Trial of tocilizumab in giant-cell arteritis. N Engl J Med. 2017;377(15):1493.
6. Kennedy GA, Tey SK, Buizen L, Varelias A, Gartlan KH, Curley C, et al. A phase 3 double-blind study of the addition of tocilizumab vs placebo to cyclosporin/methotrexate GVHD prophylaxis. Blood. 2021;137(14):1970–9.

7. Melgarejo-Ortuño A, Escudero-Vilaplana V, Revuelta-Herrero JL, Bailen R, Collado-Borrell R, Gomez-Centurión I, et al. Tocilizumab as salvage treatment of refractory pulmonary acute graft-versus-host disease. J Oncol Pharm Pract. 2021;27(3):751–5.
8. van Rhee F, Wong RS, Munshi N, Rossi JF, Ke XY, Fosså A, et al. Siltuximab for multicentric Castleman's disease: a randomised, double-blind, placebo-controlled trial. Lancet Oncol. 2014;15(9):966–74.
9. Mease PJ, Gottlieb AB, Berman A, Drescher E, Xing J, Wong R, et al. The efficacy and safety of clazakizumab, an anti-interleukin-6 monoclonal antibody, in a phase IIb study of adults with active psoriatic arthritis. Arthritis Rheumatol. 2016;68(9):2163–73.
10. Rose-John S, Winthrop K, Calabrese L. The role of IL-6 in host defence against infections: immunobiology and clinical implications. Nat Rev Rheumatol. 2017;13(7):399–409.
11. Jones G, Ding C. Tocilizumab: a review of its safety and efficacy in rheumatoid arthritis. Clin Med Insights Arthritis Musculoskelet Disord. 2010;3:81–9.
12. Hunter CA, Jones SA. IL-6 as a keystone cytokine in health and disease. Nat Immunol. 2015;16(5):448–57.
13. Kremer JM, Blanco R, Brzosko M, Burgos-Vargas R, Halland AM, Vernon E, et al. Tocilizumab inhibits structural joint damage in rheumatoid arthritis patients with inadequate responses to methotrexate: results from the double-blind treatment phase of a randomized placebo-controlled trial of tocilizumab safety and prevention of structural joint damage at one year. Arthritis Rheum. 2011;63(3):609–21.
14. Gabay C, Emery P, van Vollenhoven R, Dikranian A, Alten R, Pavelka K, et al. Tocilizumab monotherapy versus adalimumab monotherapy for treatment of rheumatoid arthritis (ADACTA): a randomised, double-blind, controlled phase 4 trial. Lancet. 2013;381(9877):1541–50.
15. Genovese MC, McKay JD, Nasonov EL, Mysler EF, da Silva NA, Alecock E, et al. Interleukin-6 receptor inhibition with tocilizumab reduces disease activity in rheumatoid arthritis with inadequate response to disease-modifying antirheumatic drugs: the tocilizumab in combination with traditional disease-modifying antirheumatic drug therapy study. Arthritis Rheum. 2008;58(10):2968–80.
16. Maini RN, Taylor PC, Szechinski J, Pavelka K, Bröll J, Balint G, et al. Double-blind randomized controlled clinical trial of the interleukin-6 receptor antagonist, tocilizumab, in European patients with rheumatoid arthritis who had an incomplete response to methotrexate. Arthritis Rheum. 2006;54(9):2817–29.
17. Fleischmann RM, Halland AM, Brzosko M, Burgos-Vargas R, Mela C, Vernon E, et al. Tocilizumab inhibits structural joint damage and improves physical function in patients with rheumatoid arthritis and inadequate responses to methotrexate: LITHE study 2-year results. J Rheumatol. 2013;40(2):113–26.
18. Smolen JS, Beaulieu A, Rubbert-Roth A, Ramos-Remus C, Rovensky J, Alecock E, et al. Effect of interleukin-6 receptor inhibition with tocilizumab in patients with rheumatoid arthritis (OPTION study): a double-blind, placebo-controlled, randomised trial. Lancet. 2008;371(9617):987–97.
19. Jones G, Sebba A, Gu J, Lowenstein MB, Calvo A, Gomez-Reino JJ, et al. Comparison of tocilizumab monotherapy versus methotrexate monotherapy in patients with moderate to severe rheumatoid arthritis: the AMBITION study. Ann Rheum Dis. 2010;69(1):88–96.
20. Yazici Y, Curtis JR, Ince A, Baraf H, Malamet RL, Teng LL, et al. Efficacy of tocilizumab in patients with moderate to severe active rheumatoid arthritis and a previous inadequate response to disease-modifying antirheumatic drugs: the ROSE study. Ann Rheum Dis. 2012;71(2):198–205.
21. Nishimoto N, Hashimoto J, Miyasaka N, Yamamoto K, Kawai S, Takeuchi T, et al. Study of active controlled monotherapy used for rheumatoid arthritis, an IL-6 inhibitor (SAMURAI): evidence of clinical and radiographic benefit from an X-ray reader-blinded randomised controlled trial of tocilizumab. Ann Rheum Dis. 2007;66(9):1162–7.
22. Nishimoto N, Miyasaka N, Yamamoto K, Kawai S, Takeuchi T, Azuma J, et al. Study of active controlled tocilizumab monotherapy for rheumatoid arthritis patients with an inadequate

response to methotrexate (SATORI): significant reduction in disease activity and serum vascular endothelial growth factor by IL-6 receptor inhibition therapy. Mod Rheumatol. 2009;19(1):12–9.
23. Emery P, Keystone E, Tony HP, Cantagrel A, van Vollenhoven R, Sanchez A, et al. IL-6 receptor inhibition with tocilizumab improves treatment outcomes in patients with rheumatoid arthritis refractory to anti-tumour necrosis factor biologicals: results from a 24-week multicentre randomised placebo-controlled trial. Ann Rheum Dis. 2008;67(11):1516–23.
24. Burmester GR, Feist E, Kellner H, Braun J, Iking-Konert C, Rubbert-Roth A. Effectiveness and safety of the interleukin 6-receptor antagonist tocilizumab after 4 and 24 weeks in patients with active rheumatoid arthritis: the first phase IIIb real-life study (TAMARA). Ann Rheum Dis. 2011;70(5):755–9.
25. Nishimoto N, Miyasaka N, Yamamoto K, Kawai S, Takeuchi T, Azuma J. Long-term safety and efficacy of tocilizumab, an anti-IL-6 receptor monoclonal antibody, in monotherapy, in patients with rheumatoid arthritis (the STREAM study): evidence of safety and efficacy in a 5-year extension study. Ann Rheum Dis. 2009;68(10):1580–4.
26. Iking-Konert C, von Hinüber U, Richter C, Schwenke H, Gürtler I, Kästner P, et al. ROUTINE-a prospective, multicentre, non-interventional, observational study to evaluate the safety and effectiveness of intravenous tocilizumab for the treatment of active rheumatoid arthritis in daily practice in Germany. Rheumatology. 2016;55(4):624–35.
27. Koike T, Harigai M, Inokuma S, Ishiguro N, Ryu J, Takeuchi T, et al. Effectiveness and safety of tocilizumab: postmarketing surveillance of 7901 patients with rheumatoid arthritis in Japan. J Rheumatol. 2014;41(1):15–23.
28. Yun H, Xie F, Delzell E, Chen L, Levitan EB, Lewis JD, et al. Risk of hospitalised infection in rheumatoid arthritis patients receiving biologics following a previous infection while on treatment with anti-TNF therapy. Ann Rheum Dis. 2015;74(6):1065–71.
29. Schiff MH, Kremer JM, Jahreis A, Vernon E, Isaacs JD, van Vollenhoven RF. Integrated safety in tocilizumab clinical trials. Arthritis Res Ther. 2011;13(5):R141.
30. Bykerk VP, Ostör AJ, Alvaro-Gracia J, Pavelka K, Ivorra JA, Graninger W, et al. Tocilizumab in patients with active rheumatoid arthritis and inadequate responses to DMARDs and/or TNF inhibitors: a large, open-label study close to clinical practice. Ann Rheum Dis. 2012;71(12):1950–4.
31. Strand V, Ahadieh S, French J, Geier J, Krishnaswami S, Menon S, et al. Systematic review and meta-analysis of serious infections with tofacitinib and biologic disease-modifying antirheumatic drug treatment in rheumatoid arthritis clinical trials. Arthritis Res Ther. 2015;17:362.
32. Burmester GR, Lin Y, Patel R, van Adelsberg J, Mangan EK, Graham NM, et al. Efficacy and safety of sarilumab monotherapy versus adalimumab monotherapy for the treatment of patients with active rheumatoid arthritis (MONARCH): a randomised, double-blind, parallel-group phase III trial. Ann Rheum Dis. 2017;76(5):840–7.
33. Pawar A, Desai RJ, Solomon DH, Santiago Ortiz AJ, Gale S, Bao M, et al. Risk of serious infections in tocilizumab versus other biologic drugs in patients with rheumatoid arthritis: a multidatabase cohort study. Ann Rheum Dis. 2019;78(4):456–64.
34. Yun H, Xie F, Delzell E, Chen L, Levitan EB, Lewis JD, et al. Risks of herpes zoster in patients with rheumatoid arthritis according to biologic disease-modifying therapy. Arthritis Care Res. 2015;67(5):731–6.
35. Nakamura J, Nagashima T, Nagatani K, Yoshio T, Iwamoto M, Minota S. Reactivation of hepatitis B virus in rheumatoid arthritis patients treated with biological disease-modifying antirheumatic drugs. Int J Rheum Dis. 2016;19(5):470–5.
36. Barone M, Notarnicola A, Lopalco G, Viggiani MT, Sebastiani F, Covelli M, et al. Safety of long-term biologic therapy in rheumatologic patients with a previously resolved hepatitis B viral infection. Hepatology. 2015;62(1):40–6.
37. Watanabe T, Fukae J, Fukaya S, Sawamukai N, Isobe M, Matsuhashi M, et al. Incidence and risk factors for reactivation from resolved hepatitis B virus in rheumatoid arthritis patients treated with biological disease-modifying antirheumatic drugs. Int J Rheum Dis. 2019;22(4):574–82.

38. Winthrop KL, Mariette X, Silva JT, Benamu E, Calabrese LH, Dumusc A, et al. ESCMID Study Group for Infections in Compromised Hosts (ESGICH) Consensus Document on the safety of targeted and biological therapies: an infectious diseases perspective (soluble immune effector molecules [II]: agents targeting interleukins, immunoglobulins and complement factors). Clin Microbiol Infect. 2018;24(Suppl 2):S21–40.
39. Carmona L, Gómez-Reino JJ, Rodríguez-Valverde V, Montero D, Pascual-Gómez E, Mola EM, et al. Effectiveness of recommendations to prevent reactivation of latent tuberculosis infection in patients treated with tumor necrosis factor antagonists. Arthritis Rheum. 2005;52(6):1766–72.
40. Hermine O, Mariette X, Tharaux PL, Resche-Rigon M, Porcher R, Ravaud P, et al. Effect of tocilizumab vs usual care in adults hospitalized With COVID-19 and moderate or severe pneumonia: a randomized clinical trial. JAMA Intern Med. 2021;181(1):32–40.
41. Salama C, Han J, Yau L, Reiss WG, Kramer B, Neidhart JD, et al. Tocilizumab in patients hospitalized with covid-19 pneumonia. N Engl J Med. 2021;384(1):20–30.
42. Stone JH, Frigault MJ, Serling-Boyd NJ, Fernandes AD, Harvey L, Foulkes AS, et al. Efficacy of tocilizumab in patients hospitalized with Covid-19. N Engl J Med. 2020;383(24):2333–44.
43. Salvarani C, Dolci G, Massari M, Merlo DF, Cavuto S, Savoldi L, et al. Effect of tocilizumab vs standard care on clinical worsening in patients hospitalized with COVID-19 pneumonia: a randomized clinical trial. JAMA Intern Med. 2021;181(1):24–31.
44. Rosas IO, Bräu N, Waters M, Go RC, Hunter BD, Bhagani S, et al. Tocilizumab in hospitalized patients with severe covid-19 pneumonia. N Engl J Med. 2021;384(16):1503–16.
45. Gordon AC, Mouncey PR, Al-Beidh F, Rowan KM, Nichol AD, Arabi YM, et al. Interleukin-6 receptor antagonists in critically ill patients with covid-19. N Engl J Med. 2021;384(16):1491–502.
46. Group RC. Tocilizumab in patients admitted to hospital with COVID-19 (RECOVERY): a randomised, controlled, open-label, platform trial. Lancet. 2021;397(10285):1637–45.
47. Somers EC, Eschenauer GA, Troost JP, Golob JL, Gandhi TN, Wang L, et al. Tocilizumab for treatment of mechanically ventilated patients with COVID-19. Clin Infect Dis. 2020;73(2):e445–54.
48. Kimmig LM, Wu D, Gold M, Pettit NN, Pitrak D, Mueller J, et al. IL6 inhibition in critically ill COVID-19 patients is associated with increased secondary infections. medRxiv. 2020.
49. Falcone M, Tiseo G, Giordano C, Leonildi A, Menichini M, Vecchione A, et al. Predictors of hospital-acquired bacterial and fungal superinfections in COVID-19: a prospective observational study. J Antimicrob Chemother. 2021;76(4):1078–84.
50. Pettit NN, Nguyen CT, Mutlu GM, Wu D, Kimmig L, Pitrak D, et al. Late onset infectious complications and safety of tocilizumab in the management of COVID-19. J Med Virol. 2021;93(3):1459–64.

Interleukin-12 and -23 Targeted Agents

11

Mario Fernández-Ruiz

Introduction: The Role of IL-12 and IL-23 in Immunity and Disease

Interleukin (IL)-12 and IL-23 are two structurally related proinflammatory cytokines that play a central role in regulating T-cell immune responses. The IL-12 family of cytokines—which includes IL-12, IL-23, IL-27, and IL-35—is produced by dendritic cells (DCs), monocytes, macrophages, and B cells in response to microbial pathogens [1]. From a structural point of view, chain sharing is a key feature of the IL-12 cytokine and cytokine receptor families. Indeed, IL-12 is a heterodimeric cytokine composed of two covalently linked glycosylated subunits (p35 and p40, also known as α- and β-chains, respectively), which combine to form the biologically active IL-12p70. The p40 subunit (encoded by the *IL12B* gene) is shared by IL-23, where it forms a heterodimer with another partner p19 [2]. The p19 subunit exhibits an overall sequence identity of ~40% with IL-12p35 [3]. The identical p40 subunit of both cytokines binds to IL-12 receptor β1 subunit (IL-12Rβ1), whereas IL-12p35 and IL-23p19 bind to IL-12Rβ2 and IL-23R, respectively. Upon receptor binding, the intracellular signaling pathway involves Janus kinase-2 (JAK-2) and tyrosine kinase-2 (TYK-2) and leads to the activation of the transcription factor signal transducer and activator of transcription-4 (STAT-4) [4].

The IL-12 cytokine family is instrumental in modulating the behavior of multiple T-cell populations. IL-12 promotes the differentiation of *naïve* CD4+ T lymphocytes to Th1 cells and creates a positive feedback by inducing interferon (IFN)-γ production by T cells, which primes in turn additional antigen-presenting cells for IL-12 production [5]. In addition, IL-12 enhances the release of IFN-γ by natural killer cells [1]. On the other hand, IL-23 contributes to the maintenance and

M. Fernández-Ruiz (✉)
Unit of Infectious Diseases, Hospital Universitario "12 de Octubre", Instituto de Investigación Hospital "12 de Octubre" (imas12), Madrid, Spain

Department of Medicine, School of Medicine, Universidad Complutense, Madrid, Spain

C. Cervera, J. M. Aguado (eds.), *Infectious Complications in Biologic and Targeted Therapies*, https://doi.org/10.1007/978-3-031-11363-5_11

expansion of Th17 cells upon activation by IL-6 and transforming growth factor-β and favors the acquisition of their pathogenic phenotype [6]. It also participates in neutrophil recruitment and Th2 cytokine production [7].

The pathogenesis of psoriasis involves the activation of abnormal Th1 and Th17 cell responses in the skin and the subsequent release of an array of cytokines such as the tumor necrosis factor (TNF)-α, IFN-γ, IL-17, or IL-22. It has been shown that IL-12 and IL-23 mRNA is overexpressed in psoriatic lesions [8], and polymorphisms in genes encoding for both cytokines and their receptors modulate the risk of psoriasis [9]. Much of the role initially attributed to IL-12 in psoriasis pathogenesis [10] has been shown to be played by the IL-23 secreted by dermal DCs, which triggers IL-17-producing Th17 clonal expansion and drives the upregulation of psoriasis-related genes by epidermal keratinocytes. This process ultimately leads to dysregulated keratinocyte differentiation and hyperproliferation and epidermal thickening [11].

Animal models, population genetics, and observational studies support the importance of IL-12 and IL-23 in the regulation of gut mucosal inflammation. In view of its role in the differentiation and expansion of Th1 and Th17 cell responses, the IL-12/IL-23 axis has been proposed as one of the mechanistic pathways involved in inflammatory bowel disease (IBD), although activities previously ascribed to IL-12 seems to be actually mediated by IL-23 [12]. Both IL-12 and IL-23 mRNAs are upregulated in the inflamed mucosa of patients with Crohn's disease (CD) and ulcerative colitis (UC) [13]. Increasing evidence shows a relevant role for Th17 cells in intestinal inflammation, with genome-wide association studies reporting an association between polymorphisms in the gene encoding for IL-23R and the incidence of IBD [14]. It has been also demonstrated that IL-23 is mainly produced by CD14+ intestinal macrophages, which act as key players in the perpetuation of gut inflammation (particularly in CD patients that are resistant to TNF-α blockers) [15].

IL-12 and IL-23 as Therapeutic Targets

Given the central involvement as key drivers of inflammation of IL-12 and IL-23 in the pathogenesis of psoriasis and IBD, various monoclonal antibodies (mAbs) targeting either the shared p40 subunit or the IL-23-specific p19 subunit have been added over the past years to the therapeutic armamentarium (Table 11.1). Ustekinumab was the first anti-IL-12/23p40 mAb approved by the Food and Drug Administration (FDA) in September 2009 for the treatment of moderate to severe plaque psoriasis in adults and subsequently for active psoriatic arthritis (September 2013) and moderately to severely active CD in patients who have previously failed or are intolerant to corticosteroids or immunomodulators, including anti-TNF-α agents (September 2016). The application for a marketing authorization in the USA and Europe for a second anti-IL-12/23p40 mAb—briakinumab—was withdrawn by the manufacturer in 2011 on the grounds of safety signals observed in clinical trials, including a possible increased risk of major cardiovascular adverse events (MACE), serious infections, and malignancies [16]. Guselkumab and tildrakizumab, two

Table 11.1 Summary of IL-12/23-targeted agents

Agent	Mechanism of action	Indications (agency, year of approval)	Dosing regimens
Ustekinumab (Stelara®)	Fully human IgG1 κ mAb targeting IL-12/23p40 subunit	Moderate to severe plaque psoriasis (FDA and EMA, 2009) Active PsA (FDA and EMA, 2013) Moderately to severely active CD (FDA and EMA, 2016) Moderately to severely active UC (FDA and EMA, 2019) Pediatric (≥12 years) moderate to severe plaque psoriasis (EMA and FDA, 2017)	*Psoriasis and PsA:* 45–90 mg SC initially and 4 weeks later, followed by 45–90 mg SC every 12 weeks[a] *CD and UC*: 260–520 mg IV initially, followed by 90 mg SC every 8 weeks[b]
Briakinumab (Ozespa®)	Fully human IgG1 λ mAb targeting IL-12/23p40 subunit	Not approved (marketing authorization request withdrawn in 2011)	200 mg SC initially and 4 weeks later, followed by 100 mg SC every 4–12 weeks[c]
Guselkumab (Tremfya®)	Fully human IgG1 λ mAb targeting IL-23p19 subunit	Moderate to severe plaque psoriasis (FDA and EMA, 2017) Active PsA (FDA and EMA, 2020)	100 mg SC initially and 4 weeks later, and every 8 weeks thereafter
Tildrakizumab (Ilumetri®)	Humanized IgG1 κ mAb targeting IL-23p19 subunit	Moderate to severe plaque psoriasis (FDA and EMA, 2019)	100 mg SC initially and 4 weeks later, and every 12 weeks thereafter
Risankizumab (Skyrizi®)	Humanized IgG1 κ mAb targeting IL-23p19 subunit	Moderate to severe plaque psoriasis (FDA and EMA, 2019) Active PsA (EMA, 2021)	150 mg SC initially and 4 weeks later, and every 12 weeks thereafter

CD Crohn's disease, *EMA* European Medicines Agency, *FDA* Food and Drug Administration, *IL* interleukin, *IV* intravenously, *mAb* monoclonal antibody, *PsA* psoriatic arthritis, *SC* subcutaneously, *UC* ulcerative colitis

[a]Weight-based induction and maintenance dosing: 45 mg if body weight ≤100 kg and 90 mg if >100 kg

[b]Weight-based induction dosing: 260 mg if body weight <260 mg, 390 mg if 55–85 Kg, and 520 mg if >85 kg

[c]Different dosing regimens were evaluated in phase III trials

anti-IL-23p19 mAbs, were FDA-approved for the treatment of plaque psoriasis in 2017 and 2018, respectively, whereas a third member of this family—risankizumab—granted approval in US and European markets in 2019. In addition, guselkumab has been recently cleared by the FDA and the European Medicines Agency for use in active psoriatic arthritis. Finally, ustekinumab and guselkumab are being currently tested for a large number of skin (e.g., pityriasis rubra pilaris or hidradenitis suppurativa) and autoimmune conditions (e.g., systemic lupus erythematosus [SLE], giant cell arteritis or primary biliary cirrhosis, among others).

In line with other biological agents reviewed in the present book, some cautions should be considered when interpreting, in terms of infectious complications, safety data derived from the pivotal randomized clinical trials (RCTs) that led to the approval of anti-IL-12/23p40 and anti-IL-23p19 mAbs [17]. First, phase II and III trials are not powered to detect uncommon albeit potentially severe adverse events (AEs). Since psoriasis, psoriatic arthritis, and CD are chronic conditions that often require ongoing treatment, the assessment of long-term safety upon cumulative IL-12/23 blockade—beyond the usual follow-up duration in most trials—becomes of the utmost importance. In addition, trial exclusion criteria are often applied to patients with increased baseline risk of infectious complications. For instance, eligible patients with a history of recurrent mucocutaneous candidiasis or testing positive for human immunodeficiency virus (HIV), hepatitis B virus (HBV), or hepatitis C virus (HCV) were excluded from the clinical development programs. Risk minimization strategies applied are crucial for the correct interpretation of data regarding the incidence of active tuberculosis (TB), as systematic screening for latent TB infection (LTBI) was mandatory at entry to every trial regardless of the expected risk of reactivation according to the mode of action of the agent. The background TB prevalence should be also kept in mind, since most studies were performed in low-prevalence countries. Finally, definitions used for the different types of infection (serious, opportunistic) were not homogeneous across studies nor was the level of detail in the reporting of the event (i.e., clinical syndrome or causative agent) [18].

Overall and Serious Infections

IL-12-Targeted Agents

No relevant safety concerns emerged from pivotal RCTs included in the clinical development programs of ustekinumab for psoriasis, psoriatic arthritis, and IBD [19–21], and the incidence of serious AEs was generally comparable between experimental and control groups. For instance, 22–31% of psoriasis patients treated with ustekinumab at different doses (45 or 90 mg) in two phase III trials had any type of infection as compared to 20–27% of those receiving placebo. Serious infections were reported by 0–0.8% versus 0.4–0.5%, respectively [22, 23]. Nasopharyngitis and upper respiratory tract infection were the most common events [24]. Similar findings were reported from phase III trials for psoriatic arthritis [25], with 27.1% and 24.0% of ustekinumab- and placebo-treated patients experiencing any infection (mild to moderate in severity) through week 16 [26]. An integrated safety data analysis from phase II/III trials combined across approved indications assessed the occurrence of infection between ustekinumab- and placebo-treated patients through 4521 and 674 patient-years (PYs), respectively. Of note, one third of the participants received ustekinumab for more than 1 year. The observed rates for overall and serious infection were comparable between the ustekinumab (138.1 and 3.3 events per 100 PYs) and placebo groups (135.8 and 2.9 per 100 PYs, respectively). As expected considering the differences in disease burden and background therapies, the incidence of infection was higher among patients with CD than psoriasis or psoriatic arthritis although was comparable between the ustekinumab and placebo groups within each indication. On the other hand, the incidence was not meaningfully increased in patients who did versus those who did not receive methotrexate or corticosteroids at baseline [21].

The favorable safety profile observed in RCTs has been largely confirmed in real-world experiences. A population-based cohort study based on two US claims databases investigated the risk of serious infection requiring hospitalization in patients with psoriasis or psoriatic arthritis on ustekinumab or other biological therapies. The adjusted incidence rates among ustekinumab initiators ranged from 0.59 to 0.95 events per 100 PYs, resulting in a lower risk than TNF-α- or IL-17-targeted agents. Sepsis, cellulitis, and pneumonia were the most common types of infection [27]. These findings are consistent with other post-marketing studies [28–30]. For instance, in a retrospective cohort of commercially insured US psoriasis patients (with 11,560 treatment episodes followed up for a median of 0.6 years), the propensity score-adjusted risk of serious infection for ustekinumab was similar to anti-IL-17 agents but, again, significantly lower when new anti-TNF-α agents users served as reference (hazard ratio [HR]: 0.59; 95% confidence interval [CI]: 0.39–0.90). It should be noted that the previous treatment history of the patient influences the infection risk, since rates differed between biologic *naïve* and biologic-experienced ustekinumab initiators (0.9 and 1.7 per 100 PYs, respectively) [28]. A sensibly higher incidence of serious infection has been reported for CD patients (6.4 events per 100 PYs) [31], which may be explained by the heterogeneity across studies in outcome definitions or previous exposure to TNF-α blockers, as well as by the differences between psoriasis and IBD in the baseline infection risk. As for non-approved indications, an open-label extension (OLE) study evaluated the safety through 2 years of ustekinumab added to background therapies in patients with active SLE. Most of the participants were concurrently receiving systemic corticosteroids or an antimetabolite drug (azathioprine, mycophenolate mofetil, or methotrexate). Overall, two thirds of the patients allocated to the ustekinumab arm developed one or more episodes of infection (versus 47.6% in the placebo arm). Most of these events were mild in severity (respiratory and urinary tract infections), although there were nine cases of serious infection requiring hospitalization among ustekinumab-treated patients (9.7%) [32].

As mentioned above and in contrast to ustekinumab, safety concerns were raised already in the clinical development program for briakinumab. For instance, the rate of serious infectious events in a phase III psoriasis trial was 2.9% in the briakinumab arm as compared to 0.7% in the etanercept arm and 1.5% in the placebo arm [33]. In another trial comparing briakinumab with methotrexate, the incidence of serious infections through week 52 of therapy was also higher in the experimental than in the control group (4.1 versus 2.7 events per 100 PYs, respectively) [34]. Most importantly, an increased risk of MACEs was observed with briakinumab, particularly during the initial treatment-induction phase and in patients with elevated baseline cardiovascular risk. This finding was suggested to be related with a paradoxical increase of the proatherogenic IL-12 leading to atherosclerotic plaque destabilization [35, 36]. Conflicting results on this associated have been reported for ustekinumab [37, 38].

IL-23-Targeted Agents

With regard to anti-IL-23p19 agents, data from pivotal RCTs show that guselkumab, tildrakizumab, and risankizumab have a favorable risk-benefit profile in patients with moderate to severe psoriasis, with no significant safety concerns observed to date [39]. Similarly to ustekinumab trials, the most commonly reported AEs were nasopharyngitis and upper respiratory tract infections. A pooled analysis of two phase III RCTs with more than 1800 patients compared the long-term safety of adalimumab—an anti-TNF-α mAb—with that of guselkumab. The overall incidence for any infection in the guselkumab groups through weeks 52 and 100 was 100.47 and 81.74 events per 100 PYs, whereas the corresponding figures for serious infection fell to 1.22 and 1.06, respectively. Of note, the incidence of serious infection was more common, while participants were receiving adalimumab (1.79 per 100 PYs) before crossover to guselkumab [40]. On the other hand, a meta-analysis comprising 1,533 and 710 psoriasis patients receiving risankizumab and standard care, respectively, reported a nearly 50% increase in the risk of infection with risankizumab (odds ratio [OR]: 1.44; 95% CI: 1.13–1.83) as compared to control group, although most of these events were mild to moderate and did not lead to treatment discontinuation [41]. In fact, a recent network meta-analysis concluded that the three anti-IL-23p19 mAbs exhibited the lowest rates of toxicity leading to treatment discontinuation as compared to ustekinumab or anti-TNF-α agents [42]. Another meta-analysis comparing the safety of IL-17- and IL-23-targeted agents in the treatment of psoriasis (21 RCTs with 14,935 patients) found a lower overall incidence of AEs for anti-IL-23p19 mAbs, with tildrakizumab at a 200-mg dose being associated with the lowest relative risk (RR) compared to placebo (0.88; 95% CI: 0.78–0.99). The risk of serious AEs, however, was comparable between both types of therapy [43]. It should be noted that real-world data for anti-IL-23p19 mAbs are still emerging, although available studies have no revealed new safety signals [44, 45].

Tuberculosis

Derived from its role in Th1 differentiation, IL-12 is instrumental in the initiation and maintenance of acquired immunity against *Mycobacterium tuberculosis* [46], including induction of IFN-γ synthesis [47], successful granuloma formation [48], and maturation of the Th1 IFN-γ-producing T-cell phenotype [49]. This involvement is clearly demonstrated by a rare condition known as Mendelian susceptibility to mycobacterial disease (MSMD), which is characterized by the development of severe disease due to low virulence environmental mycobacteria, *M. bovis* or bacille Calmette-Guérin (BCG), as well as *M. tuberculosis*, *Salmonella* spp., and other intracellular pathogens [50]. Patients with MSMD exhibit inherited defects in some element of the IL-12/IL-23/IFN-γ axis, being autosomal recessive (AR) IL-12Rβ1 deficiency the most common form [51]. Since IL-12Rβ1 dimerizes with either IL-12Rβ2 to form the IL-12 receptor or with IL-23R to form the IL-23 receptor

[52], the uncommon AR complete deficiency of the p40 subunit shared by both cytokines manifests as a clinical phenocopy of IL-12Rβ1 deficiency [53]. Mutations in other genes (such as *IFNGR1*, *IFNGR2*, *STAT1*, *NEMO*, or *TYK2*) have been also identified in MSMD patients, the products of which are involved in IFN-γ-mediated immunity [54, 55]. Beyond the MSDM condition, mutations in the *IL12RB1* gene can also underlie monogenic TB in families with no history of infection due to environmental mycobacteria [56, 57].

Based on this biological rationale, it would be expected that the use of the anti-IL-12/23p40 therapies would lead to an increased risk of LTBI reactivation and active TB. Indeed, a case of TB diagnosed at approximately 3 months from the first dose of ustekinumab was anecdotally reported in a 65-year-old Taiwanese patient recruited in a phase III trial for psoriasis in the setting of a false negative screening for LTBI [58]. The recurrence of peripheral lymph node TB 8 months following the discontinuation of ustekinumab [59] or the development of peritoneal TB despite the previous receipt of LTBI treatment [60] has been also described, as well as a soft tissue infection due to *M. abscessus* in a CD patient with repeated exposure to soil microorganisms [61].

Nevertheless, data coming from both pivotal RCTs, OLE studies, and post-marketing surveillance programs suggest that the incidence of TB in patients receiving ustekinumab is actually low, provided that adequate screening for (and treatment of) LTBI is timely implemented. This highlights that the impact of a given biological agent of the host's susceptibility to infection should not be mechanistically inferred from the analogous inborn error of immunity [17]. Only one case of active TB was observed in the pooled analysis of five phase III trials conducted in North America, Europe, and Asia and comprising 3177 patients (cumulative incidence of 0.03%) [62]. A nationwide database analysis from South Korea—an intermediate-incidence country—found three cases of active TB among more than 2800 patients that received ustekinumab for a mean period of 691.1 days. The standardized incidence ratio using the general population as reference was 0.76 (95% CI: 0.59–2.02), indicating no increased risk of developing TB associated with IL-12/23 blockade [63]. Similar experiences have been reported from Taiwan—in which no cases of TB were observed among 27 patients diagnosed with LTBI either at baseline or during the serial testing with an IFN-γ release assay (IGRA) regardless of whether a 9-month course of isoniazid (INH) was completed or not—[64], Japan [65], and Spain [66]. Finally, a multicenter, longitudinal, psoriasis-based registry carried out at 93 institutions recruited more than 3400 ustekinumab-treated patients (totaling 5923 PYs). Again, no TB cases were reported, thus confirming a low risk of LTBI reactivation related to anti-IL-12/23 mAbs in the setting of contemporary risk-minimization practices [30]. Interestingly, the incidence of active TB across phase II/III RCTs for IBD, ankylosing spondylitis, rheumatoid arthritis, psoriasis, and psoriatic arthritis was significantly lower among patients treated with ustekinumab than those receiving anti-TNF-α therapies, with incidence rates estimated at 0.02 (95% CI: 0.00–0.06) and 0.28 (95% CI: 0.21–0.37) cases per 100 PYs, respectively [67].

In comparison to IL-12, IL-23 appears to be less relevant in mounting and maintaining effective immune responses against *M. tuberculosis*. As stated above, IL-23 is an important driver of Th17 differentiation and survival [68] and an upstream regulator of IL-17 and IL-22 synthesis [69]. Both IL-17—with its different family members—and IL-22 are the major effector cytokines of Th17 cells and contribute to the rapid response to pathogens, by recruiting neutrophils to the site of infection and by inducing the production of antimicrobial peptides (such as REG proteins or lipocalin-2). In addition, IL-17 and IL-22 contribute to maintain mucosal barrier immunity [70]. Despite in vivo models showing the involvement of IL-17 in mature granuloma formation in mycobacteria-infected lungs [71, 72], data coming from clinical trials [73–75] and observational experiences [76] has not revealed an increased incidence of active TB associated with the use of the anti-IL-17 agents secukinumab, ixekizumab, and brodalumab. In addition, no reversal effect of secukinumab on *M. tuberculosis* dormancy was observed in vitro [77]. In light of this evidence, it is not expected that blocking the upstream cytokine IL-23 would result in a meaningful increased risk of LTBI reactivation. No episodes of active TB were reported through 1 year of therapy in a pooled analysis of two phase III RCTs evaluating the safety of guselkumab for psoriatic arthritis [78]. In the same line, there were no cases of TB through 3 years of guselkumab therapy in the pivotal trials for psoriasis either [79]. Finally, a phase II OLE study of risankizumab for moderate to severe CD revealed no cases of TB after a median duration of treatment of 33 months, despite the fact that most patients had been previously exposed to TNF-α blockers or were receiving corticosteroids [80].

The systematic screening for LTBI prior to the initiation of therapy—followed by the prompt administration of appropriate treatment as required—are the mainstays for the prevention of active TB in patients receiving biological agents. On the basis of the experience gained from TNF-α-targeted agents, such strategy was mandatory in all the trials performed in the clinical development program of IL-12/23 blockers, despite differences in the theoretical risk of progression to active TB associated with each therapeutic family. This circumstance should be borne in mind when interpreting the results derived from safety data analysis based on RCTs. The aforementioned analysis of phase III RCTs of ustekinumab at different dosage for plaque psoriasis regimens analyzed the safety of INH for the treatment of LTBI, diagnosed by means of a positive tuberculin skin test (TST) or IGRA at the baseline evaluation. As per study protocol, all participants with newly identified LTBI were scheduled to receive INH for at least 6 months, and those who were unable to complete the required course of treatment had to be discontinued from the study. Overall, 167 patients with LTBI (5.3% of the trial populations) were treated with INH. As expected, this group experienced a higher frequency of liver function test abnormalities (viz., elevated ALT values) compared to non-INH-treated participants (9.4–17.9% versus 1.2–6.5%, respectively, across different trials). The rate of study agent discontinuation due to INH toxicity, however, was low (3.0%) and comparable between ustekinumab and control groups through weeks 12 and 28 [62]. Similar results have been recently reported for patients recruited in the guselkumab trials [81].

In conclusion, and despite the theoretical risk of LTBI reactivation related to IL-12—and to a much lesser extent IL-23—blockade, available evidence shows that the incidence of active TB among patients treated with ustekinumab, guselkumab, risankizumab, or tildrakizumab is not meaningfully increased. The interpretation of these studies, however, is conditioned by the widespread implementation of pre-treatment LTBI screening. The risk of TB, in any case, would be lower than that well-established for TNF-α blockers [82]. Finally, it should be noted that current guidelines supported by scientific societies recommend systematic screening for LTBI before initiating any biological therapy for the treatment of psoriasis [83, 84] or IBD [85, 86], with no agent-specific strategies across different therapeutic families.

Other Opportunistic Infections

The favorable safety profile reported for IL-12/23-targeted agents is extensible to opportunistic infections (OIs) other than TB. No episodes qualifying for the definition of OI were reported from phase II/III RTCs of guselkumab [87, 88] or risankizumab [89], whereas the corresponding figures for briakinumab (0.7 events per 100 PYs) [34] or ustekinumab (0.58 events per 100 PYs) [90] were low. A theoretical concern lies on the involvement of IL-23 in the differentiation, expansion, and functionality of Th17 cells, which play a central role in the host defense against *Candida* spp. [91]. Indeed, patients with autosomal dominant chronic mucocutaneous candidiasis—a primary immunodeficiency characterized by the susceptibility to infection of the skin, nails, and mucous membranes by *Candida* and dermatophytes—may show a functional impairment in the IL-12/23 pathway [92]. Nevertheless, clinical experience has not confirmed the potential for this AE. There were only two cases of fungal esophagitis and one oral candidiasis among 65 CD patients included in an OLE study of risankizumab (1.8 events per 100 PYs) [80]. The occurrence of cutaneous or oral candidiasis across psoriasis trials of tildrakizumab (0.2 and 0.7 events per 100 PYs in the 100-mg and 200-mg groups, respectively) [93] or risankizumab (0.6 events per 100 PYs) [94] was also uncommon. The risk of superficial or esophageal candidiasis, therefore, is clearly lower compared to IL-17 blockers [95]. This different was highlighted by a combined analysis of different safety drug databases, a population-based drug prescriptions registry, and a single-center psoriasis cohort, with estimated RRs of 10.20, 2.03, and 1.76 for anti-IL-17/IL-17R, anti-TNF-α, and anti-IL-12/23 agents, respectively [96]. Finally, no cases of invasive fungal infection were found in a systematic review of anti-IL-12/23p40 or anti-IL-23p19 mAbs for psoriasis [97].

Regarding herpes zoster (HZ), some case reports early suggested a potential risk of severe forms with multidermatomal involvement upon the initiation of ustekinumab [98]. This association has not been eventually confirmed. A systematic review and meta-analysis of RCTs and observational studies assessed the incidence of HZ in patients with psoriasis or psoriatic arthritis treated with different biological agents. The use of ustekinumab was not found to increase the risk as compared to nonbiological therapies (OR, 2.20; 95% CI, 0.89–5.44), which was in contrast with the significant association observed for TNF-α blockers (OR, 1.50; 95% CI, 1.11–2.02) [99]. Other meta-analyses [100] and population-based studies [27] found no differences between ustekinumab and TNF-α- or IL-17-targeted agents. The incidence of HZ in the pooled analysis of phase II/III RCTs performed in the more heavily immunosuppressed population of IBD patients was estimated at 1.04 events per 100 PYs, which was similar to that observed in the control arms (1.34 per 100 PYs) [90]. In the same line, the reported incidence among psoriasis patients on tildrakizumab for up to 148 weeks was as low as 0.05 events per 100 PYs [101].

Episodes of OI due to other herpesviruses are anecdotal, including the development of facial herpes simplex virus infection in a psoriasis patient on guselkumab therapy (with the most recent dose being given 5 weeks ago) that had just received the first injection of the BNT162b2 mRNA vaccine for coronavirus disease 2019 (COVID-19) [102], or varicella-zoster virus (VZV) meningitis in a 77-year-old woman patient 8 weeks after initiation of ustekinumab [103]. There have been some cases of cytomegalovirus colitis in IBD patients recruited in ustekinumab trials, although all of them occurred at least 4 months after therapy discontinuation and while the patients were receiving concomitant immunosuppressive therapies, thus questioning the potential causal relationship [90, 104]. *Listeria* meningitis, disseminated histoplasmosis, and cryptosporidiosis have been occasionally reported with the use of ustekinumab in patients with IBD [90].

Viral Hepatitis

Hepatitis B Virus

Since IL-12 plays a role in achieving a sustained control of HBV replication, there is a theoretical risk of viral reactivation associated with the use of IL-12/23-targeted agents. The antiviral effect of IL-12 appears to be mainly driven by its ability to induce IFN-γ production and HBV-specific central memory CD8+ T-cell responses [105, 106]. The administration of recombinant IL-12, in fact, has been shown to increase the odds of HBV DNA clearance [107]. As expected, patients with documented active HBV infection were excluded from pivotal RCTs evaluating the safety and efficacy of ustekinumab for psoriasis [22, 23, 108], psoriatic arthritis [25], or IBD [109, 110]. A retrospective study from Taiwan that included 14 patients with psoriasis and chronic HBV infection—most of them with positive hepatitis B surface antigen (HBsAg)—treated with at least two doses of ustekinumab found two episodes (14.3%) of mild HBV reactivation that were not associated with liver enzyme abnormalities. Of note, both patients were not receiving entecavir. In addition, no cases of viral reactivation were observed in the three patients with occult HBV infection (HBsAg-negative, anti-HBV core [HBc]-positive) despite the lack of antiviral prophylaxis [111]. These results were confirmed in a larger psoriasis cohort treated with ustekinumab and followed up for 24 months, with annual rates for HBV reactivation of 17.4% and 1.5% among inactive carriers (HBsAg/

anti-HBc-positive with baseline HBV DNA levels <2000 IU/mL and normal liver tests) and patients with occult HBV infection, respectively. There were no cases of severe hepatitis or liver failure [112].

The contribution of IL-23 to the host's response against HBV is less clear, although it seems to promote liver inflammation, tissue damage, and hepatocellular carcinoma development among chronically infected patients [113, 114]. It has been reported the successful use of guselkumab in a patient with palmoplantar psoriasis, positive anti-HBc antibody, and negative HBsAg, without evidence of viral reactivation or impairment of liver function tests over 1-year course of treatment [115]. A similarly favorable safety profile was also observed in a HBsAg/anti-HBc-positive pediatric patient with detectable HBV DNA at baseline that received a 12-week guselkumab regimen on entecavir prophylaxis [116].

Hepatitis C Virus

In the same line of HBV, IL-12 enhances cytotoxic T-cell responses against HCV and contributes to the clearance of acute HCV infection [117, 118]. Available data concerning the safety of IL-12/23 blockers in the setting of HCV infection, however, is much limited. Beyond single cases in which no unfavorable outcomes were reported [119, 120], a small series found a mild to moderate increase in the HCV viral load in three out of four psoriasis patients treated with ustekinumab for a mean of 8 months, although only one of them fulfilled the criterion of HCV reactivation after 1 month of therapy [111]. In a second series comprising four HCV patients treated with ustekinumab for 12–17 months, one of them experienced a slight increase in viral load, whereas AST and ALT levels increased in another case [121]. It should be noted, however, that most of these experiences were prior to the widespread use of direct-acting antiviral agents, which have substantially changed to the natural history of hepatitis C.

Recommendations for Infection Risk Management

Taking into account the evidence summarized in the previous lines, it can be concluded that the administration of IL-12/23-targeted agents does not entail a meaningful increase in the risk of infectious complications among patients with psoriasis, psoriatic arthritis, or IBD. Therefore, the ESCMID Study Group for Infections in Compromised Hosts (ESGICH) Consensus Document did not recommend the use of antibacterial, antiviral, or antifungal prophylaxis during the course of anti-IL12/23 therapies [122]. Guidelines endorsed by the American Academy of Dermatology states that the initiation of therapy in psoriasis patients with active infection should be done in consultation with an infectious disease specialist [83]. In that scenario, it would be reasonable to balance the expected benefit derived from IL-12/23 blockade on the underlying condition against the risk entailed by an ongoing disseminated bacterial infection (i.e., sepsis) or the availability of active antimicrobial agents [123].

Due to the theoretical risk of progression to active TB, particularly for anti-IL-12/23p40 mAbs, screening for LTBI should be systematically performed at the pretreatment evaluation, followed by appropriate therapy if needed with a 6- to 9-month course of INH or an equivalent regimen (e.g., rifampicin for 4 months [124] or weekly INH and rifapentine for 3 months [125]). Such an approach should be also extended to patients with a past history of active TB in whom an adequate course of treatment cannot be confirmed. These recommendations are supported by clinical guidelines regarding the use of biological agents in patients with psoriasis [83, 84] or IBD [85, 86] and are also included in the corresponding prescribing information. The screening for LTBI may be based on IGRA—either in enzyme-linked immunosorbent assay (QuantiFERON-TB® in different versions, Qiagen, Hilden, Germany) or enzyme-linked immunospot formats (T-SPOT®.TB, Oxford Immunotec, Oxford, United Kingdom)—or TST, with the former having the advantages of better reproducibility and specificity. Moreover, TST results may be difficult to interpret in psoriasis patients [126]. In the absence of specific recommendations, it seems reasonable to apply the usual practice with TNF-α blockers and postpone the initiation of the anti-IL-12/23 agent until at least 1 month of LTBI therapy has been completed [82]. If the patient has active TB, the anti-IL-12/23 agent must be postponed for a longer period, ideally until the completion of anti-TB therapy (or at least once sterilization of sputum cultures and clinical improvement have been achieved).

In addition to LTBI, screening for HIV, HBV, and HCV infection should be also included in the baseline evaluation. Patients living with HIV and with no recent history of OI may receive anti-IL-12/23 therapies, provided that they are also receiving highly active antiretroviral therapy and have achieved undetectable viral load and normalized CD4+ T-cell count [83]. Patients testing positive for HBV or HCV may benefit from an initial consultation with a hepatologist. Antiviral prophylaxis with a high genetic barrier agent (such as entecavir) should be considered in HBsAg-positive patients for preventing HBV reactivation. On the other hand, there is insufficient evidence to recommend periodic screening for reactivation of occult HBV infection among HBsAg-negative anti-HBc-positive patients [122].

Finally, age-appropriate inactivated vaccination (i.e., seasonal trivalent influenza vaccine [TIV], HZ subunit vaccine, mRNA-based COVID-19 vaccine, or pneumococcal and *Haemophilus influenzae* type b conjugate vaccines) should be administered. The response rate to the 23-valent polysaccharide pneumococcal vaccine (at least a twofold increase in antibody levels for ≥7 serotypes) was comparable between psoriasis patients treated or not treated with ustekinumab (96.6% and 92.6%, respectively) [127]. In another study, the seroprotection rates against A/H2N3 and B influenza vaccine strains following TIV were similar between CD patients receiving ustekinumab and healthy controls, with a numerically lower rate against A/H1N1 (78.6% versus 90.0%, respectively) [128]. As stated in the prescribing information, live-virus vaccines (i.e., VZV or measles-mumps-rubella) are contraindicated in patients receiving anti-IL-12/23 mAbs, particularly in the presence of concomitant immunosuppression, and the BCG vaccine should not be given for 1 year prior to initiation of therapy or following its discontinuation [122].

References

1. Vignali DA, Kuchroo VK. IL-12 family cytokines: immunological playmakers. Nat Immunol. 2012;13:722–8.
2. Lupardus PJ, Garcia KC. The structure of interleukin-23 reveals the molecular basis of p40 subunit sharing with interleukin-12. J Mol Biol. 2008;382:931–41.
3. Oppmann B, Lesley R, Blom B, Timans JC, Xu Y, Hunte B, et al. Novel p19 protein engages IL-12p40 to form a cytokine, IL-23, with biological activities similar as well as distinct from IL-12. Immunity. 2000;13:715–25.
4. Watford WT, Hissong BD, Bream JH, Kanno Y, Muul L, O'Shea JJ. Signaling by IL-12 and IL-23 and the immunoregulatory roles of STAT4. Immunol Rev. 2004;202:139–56.
5. Trinchieri G. Interleukin-12 and the regulation of innate resistance and adaptive immunity. Nat Rev Immunol. 2003;3:133–46.
6. Aggarwal S, Ghilardi N, Xie MH, de Sauvage FJ, Gurney AL. Interleukin-23 promotes a distinct CD4 T cell activation state characterized by the production of interleukin-17. J Biol Chem. 2003;278:1910–4.
7. Gaffen SL, Jain R, Garg AV, Cua DJ. The IL-23-IL-17 immune axis: from mechanisms to therapeutic testing. Nat Rev Immunol. 2014;14:585–600.
8. Torti DC, Feldman SR. Interleukin-12, interleukin-23, and psoriasis: current prospects. J Am Acad Dermatol. 2007;57:1059–68.
9. Cargill M, Schrodi SJ, Chang M, Garcia VE, Brandon R, Callis KP, et al. A large-scale genetic association study confirms IL12B and leads to the identification of IL23R as psoriasis-risk genes. Am J Hum Genet. 2007;80:273–90.
10. Shaker OG, Moustafa W, Essmat S, Abdel-Halim M, El-Komy M. The role of interleukin-12 in the pathogenesis of psoriasis. Clin Biochem. 2006;39:119–25.
11. Chan TC, Hawkes JE, Krueger JG. Interleukin 23 in the skin: role in psoriasis pathogenesis and selective interleukin 23 blockade as treatment. Ther Adv Chronic Dis. 2018;9:111–9.
12. Kashani A, Schwartz DA. The expanding role of anti-IL-12 and/or anti-IL-23 antibodies in the treatment of inflammatory bowel disease. Gastroenterol Hepatol. 2019;15:255–65.
13. Nemeth ZH, Bogdanovski DA, Barratt-Stopper P, Paglinco SR, Antonioli L, Rolandelli RH. Crohn's disease and ulcerative colitis show unique cytokine profiles. Cureus. 2017;9:e1177.
14. Kobayashi T, Okamoto S, Hisamatsu T, Kamada N, Chinen H, Saito R, et al. IL23 differentially regulates the Th1/Th17 balance in ulcerative colitis and Crohn's disease. Gut. 2008;57:1682–9.
15. Schmitt H, Neurath MF, Atreya R. Role of the IL23/IL17 pathway in Crohn's disease. Front Immunol. 2021;12:622934.
16. Langley RG, Papp K, Gottlieb AB, Krueger GG, Gordon KB, Williams D, et al. Safety results from a pooled analysis of randomized, controlled phase II and III clinical trials and interim data from an open-label extension trial of the interleukin-12/23 monoclonal antibody, briakinumab, in moderate to severe psoriasis. J Eur Acad Dermatol Venereol. 2013;27:1252–61.
17. Fernandez-Ruiz M, Meije Y, Manuel O, Akan H, Carratala J, Aguado JM, et al. ESCMID Study Group for infections in compromised hosts (ESGICH) consensus document on the safety of targeted and biological therapies: an infectious diseases perspective (introduction). Clin Microbiol Infect. 2018;24(2):2–9.
18. Winthrop KL, Novosad SA, Baddley JW, Calabrese L, Chiller T, Polgreen P, et al. Opportunistic infections and biologic therapies in immune-mediated inflammatory diseases: consensus recommendations for infection reporting during clinical trials and postmarketing surveillance. Ann Rheum Dis. 2015;74:2107–16.
19. Meng Y, Dongmei L, Yanbin P, Jinju F, Meile T, Binzhu L, et al. Systematic review and meta-analysis of ustekinumab for moderate to severe psoriasis. Clin Exp Dermatol. 2014;39:696–707.

20. Kawalec P, Mocko P, Malinowska-Lipien I, Brzostek T. Efficacy and safety of ustekinumab in the induction therapy of TNF-alpha-refractory Crohn's disease patients: a systematic review and meta-analysis. J Comp Eff Res. 2017;6:601–12.
21. Ghosh S, Gensler LS, Yang Z, Gasink C, Chakravarty SD, Farahi K, et al. Ustekinumab safety in psoriasis, psoriatic arthritis, and Crohn's disease: an integrated analysis of phase II/III clinical development programs. Drug Saf. 2019;42:751–68.
22. Leonardi CL, Kimball AB, Papp KA, Yeilding N, Guzzo C, Wang Y, et al. Efficacy and safety of ustekinumab, a human interleukin-12/23 monoclonal antibody, in patients with psoriasis: 76-week results from a randomised, double-blind, placebo-controlled trial (PHOENIX 1). Lancet. 2008;371:1665–74.
23. Papp KA, Langley RG, Lebwohl M, Krueger GG, Szapary P, Yeilding N, et al. Efficacy and safety of ustekinumab, a human interleukin-12/23 monoclonal antibody, in patients with psoriasis: 52-week results from a randomised, double-blind, placebo-controlled trial (PHOENIX 2). Lancet. 2008;371:1675–84.
24. Croxtall JD. Ustekinumab: a review of its use in the management of moderate to severe plaque psoriasis. Drugs. 2011;71:1733–53.
25. McInnes IB, Kavanaugh A, Gottlieb AB, Puig L, Rahman P, Ritchlin C, et al. Efficacy and safety of ustekinumab in patients with active psoriatic arthritis: 1 year results of the phase 3, multicentre, double-blind, placebo-controlled PSUMMIT 1 trial. Lancet. 2013;382:780–9.
26. Ritchlin C, Rahman P, Kavanaugh A, McInnes IB, Puig L, Li S, et al. Efficacy and safety of the anti-IL-12/23 p40 monoclonal antibody, ustekinumab, in patients with active psoriatic arthritis despite conventional non-biological and biological anti-tumour necrosis factor therapy: 6-month and 1-year results of the phase 3, multicentre, double-blind, placebo-controlled, randomised PSUMMIT 2 trial. Ann Rheum Dis. 2014;73:990–9.
27. Jin Y, Lee H, Lee MP, Landon JE, Merola JF, Desai RJ, et al. Risk of hospitalized serious infection after initiating ustekinumab or other biologics for psoriasis or psoriatic arthritis. Arthritis Care Res. 2021. https://doi.org/10.1002/acr.24630.
28. Li X, Andersen KM, Chang HY, Curtis JR, Alexander GC. Comparative risk of serious infections among real-world users of biologics for psoriasis or psoriatic arthritis. Ann Rheum Dis. 2020;79:285–91.
29. Dommasch ED, Kim SC, Lee MP, Gagne JJ. Risk of serious infection in patients receiving systemic medications for the treatment of psoriasis. JAMA Dermatol. 2019;155:1142.
30. Kalb RE, Fiorentino DF, Lebwohl MG, Toole J, Poulin Y, Cohen AD, et al. Risk of serious infection with biologic and systemic treatment of psoriasis: results from the psoriasis longitudinal assessment and registry (PSOLAR). JAMA Dermatol. 2015;151:961–9.
31. Macaluso FS, Maida M, Ventimiglia M, Cottone M, Orlando A. Effectiveness and safety of Ustekinumab for the treatment of Crohn's disease in real-life experiences: a meta-analysis of observational studies. Expert Opin Biol Ther. 2020;20:193–203.
32. van Vollenhoven RF, Hahn BH, Tsokos GC, Lipsky P, Gordon RM, Fei K, et al. Efficacy and safety of ustekinumab in patients with active systemic lupus erythematosus: results through 2 years of an open-label extension in a phase 2 study. J Rheumatol. 2021;49(4):380–7. https://doi.org/10.3899/jrheum.210805.
33. Gottlieb AB, Leonardi C, Kerdel F, Mehlis S, Olds M, Williams DA. Efficacy and safety of briakinumab vs. etanercept and placebo in patients with moderate to severe chronic plaque psoriasis. Br J Dermatol. 2011;165:652–60.
34. Reich K, Langley RG, Papp KA, Ortonne JP, Unnebrink K, Kaul M, et al. A 52-week trial comparing briakinumab with methotrexate in patients with psoriasis. N Engl J Med. 2011;365:1586–96.
35. Tzellos T, Kyrgidis A, Trigoni A, Zouboulis CC. Association of ustekinumab and briakinumab with major adverse cardiovascular events: an appraisal of meta-analyses and industry sponsored pooled analyses to date. Dermato-Endocrinology. 2012;4:320–3.
36. Tzellos T, Kyrgidis A, Zouboulis CC. Re-evaluation of the risk for major adverse cardiovascular events in patients treated with anti-IL-12/23 biological agents for chronic plaque

psoriasis: a meta-analysis of randomized controlled trials. J Eur Acad Dermatol Venereol. 2013;27:622–7.
37. Lee MP, Desai RJ, Jin Y, Brill G, Ogdie A, Kim SC. Association of ustekinumab vs TNF inhibitor therapy with risk of atrial fibrillation and cardiovascular events in patients with psoriasis or psoriatic arthritis. JAMA Dermatol. 2019;155:700–7.
38. Poizeau F, Nowak E, Kerbrat S, Le Nautout B, Droitcourt C, Drici MD, et al. Association between early severe cardiovascular events and the initiation of treatment with the anti-interleukin 12/23p40 antibody ustekinumab. JAMA Dermatol. 2020;156:1208–15.
39. Crowley JJ, Warren RB, Cather JC. Safety of selective IL-23p19 inhibitors for the treatment of psoriasis. J Eur Acad Dermatol Venereol. 2019;33:1676–84.
40. Reich K, Papp KA, Armstrong AW, Wasfi Y, Li S, Shen YK, et al. Safety of guselkumab in patients with moderate-to-severe psoriasis treated through 100 weeks: a pooled analysis from the randomized VOYAGE 1 and VOYAGE 2 studies. Br J Dermat. 2019;180:1039–49.
41. Singh S, Singh S, Thangaswamy A, Thangaraju P, Varthya SB. Efficacy and safety of risankizumab in moderate to severe psoriasis: a systematic review and meta-analysis. Dermatol Ther. 2021;34:e14487. https://doi.org/10.1111/dth.14487.
42. Shear NH, Betts KA, Soliman AM, Joshi A, Wang Y, Zhao J, et al. Comparative safety and benefit-risk profile of biologics and oral treatment for moderate-to-severe plaque psoriasis: a network meta-analysis of clinical trial data. JAMA Dermatol. 2021;85:572–81.
43. Cui L, Chen R, Subedi S, Yu Q, Gong Y, Chen Z, et al. Efficacy and safety of biologics targeting IL-17 and IL-23 in the treatment of moderate-to-severe plaque psoriasis: a systematic review and meta-analysis of randomized controlled trials. Int Immunopharmacol. 2018;62:46–58.
44. Malara G, Trifiro C, Bartolotta A, Giofre C, D'Arrigo G, Testa A, et al. Real-world effectiveness and safety of Guselkumab for the treatment of psoriasis: a 6-month prospective study in a series of psoriatic patients. Eur Rev Med Pharmacol Sci. 2021;25:406–12.
45. Gerdes S, Bräu B, Hoffmann M, Korge B, Mortazawi D, Wiemers F, et al. Real-world effectiveness of guselkumab in patients with psoriasis: health-related quality of life and efficacy data from the noninterventional, prospective, German multicenter PERSIST trial. J Dermatol. 2021;48:1854–62.
46. Cooper AM, Solache A, Khader SA. Interleukin-12 and tuberculosis: an old story revisited. Curr Opin Immunol. 2007;19:441–7.
47. Cooper AM, Magram J, Ferrante J, Orme IM. Interleukin 12 (IL-12) is crucial to the development of protective immunity in mice intravenously infected with mycobacterium tuberculosis. J Exp Med. 1997;186:39–45.
48. Cooper AM, Roberts AD, Rhoades ER, Callahan JE, Getzy DM, Orme IM. The role of interleukin-12 in acquired immunity to Mycobacterium tuberculosis infection. Immunology. 1995;84:423–32.
49. Wu CY, Warrier RR, Carvajal DM, Chua AO, Minetti LJ, Chizzonite R, et al. Biological function and distribution of human interleukin-12 receptor beta chain. Eur J Immunol. 1996;26:345–50.
50. Casanova JL, Abel L. Genetic dissection of immunity to mycobacteria: the human model. Annu Rev Immunol. 2002;20:581–620.
51. Bustamante J, Boisson-Dupuis S, Abel L, Casanova JL. Mendelian susceptibility to mycobacterial disease: genetic, immunological, and clinical features of inborn errors of IFN-gamma immunity. Semin Immunol. 2014;26:454–70.
52. van de Vosse E, Haverkamp MH, Ramirez-Alejo N, Martinez-Gallo M, Blancas-Galicia L, Metin A, et al. IL-12Rbeta1 deficiency: mutation update and description of the IL12RB1 variation database. Hum Mutat. 2013;34:1329–39.
53. Prando C, Samarina A, Bustamante J, Boisson-Dupuis S, Cobat A, Picard C, et al. Inherited IL-12p40 deficiency: genetic, immunologic, and clinical features of 49 patients from 30 kindreds. Medicine. 2013;92:109–22.
54. Doffinger R, Altare F, Casanova JL. Genetic heterogeneity of Mendelian susceptibility to mycobacterial infection. Microbes Infect. 2000;2:1553–7.

55. Bustamante J. Mendelian susceptibility to mycobacterial disease: recent discoveries. Hum Genet. 2020;139:993–1000.
56. Tabarsi P, Marjani M, Mansouri N, Farnia P, Boisson-Dupuis S, Bustamante J, et al. Lethal tuberculosis in a previously healthy adult with IL-12 receptor deficiency. J Clin Immunol. 2011;31:537–9.
57. Altare F, Ensser A, Breiman A, Reichenbach J, Baghdadi JE, Fischer A, et al. Interleukin-12 receptor beta1 deficiency in a patient with abdominal tuberculosis. J Infect Dis. 2001;184:231–6.
58. Tsai TF, Chiu HY, Song M, Chan D. A case of latent tuberculosis reactivation in a patient treated with ustekinumab without concomitant isoniazid chemoprophylaxis in the PEARL trial. Br J Dermatol. 2013;168:444–6.
59. Sanchez-Moya AI, Dauden E. Peripheral lymph node recurrence of tuberculosis after ustekinumab treatment. Arch Dermatol. 2012;148:1332–3.
60. Lynch M, Roche L, Horgan M, Ahmad K, Hackett C, Ramsay B. Peritoneal tuberculosis in the setting of ustekinumab treatment for psoriasis. JAAD Case Rep. 2017;3:230–2.
61. Shim HH, Cai SCS, Chan W, Low JGH, Tan HH, Ling KL. *Mycobacterium abscessus* infection during ustekinumab treatment in Crohn's disease: a case report and review of the literature. J Crohn's Colitis. 2018;12:1505–7.
62. Tsai TF, Ho V, Song M, Szapary P, Kato T, Wasfi Y, et al. The safety of ustekinumab treatment in patients with moderate-to-severe psoriasis and latent tuberculosis infection. Br J Dermatol. 2012;167:1145–52.
63. Cho SI, Kang S, Kim YE, Lee JY, Jo SJ. Ustekinumab does not increase tuberculosis risk: results from a national database in South Korea. J Am Acad Dermatol. 2020;82:1243–5.
64. Hsiao CY, Chiu HY, Wang TS, Tsai TF. Serial QuantiFERON-TB gold testing in patients with psoriasis treated with ustekinumab. PLoS One. 2017;12:e0184178.
65. Kaneko S, Tsuruta N, Yamaguchi K, Miyagi T, Takahashi K, Higashi Y, et al. Mycobacterium tuberculosis infection in psoriatic patients treated with biologics: Real-world data from 18 Japanese facilities. J Dermatol. 2020;47:128–32.
66. Salguero Fernandez I, Gil MH, Sanz MS, Gullon GR. An analysis of drug survival, effectiveness, and safety in moderate to severe psoriasis treated with ustekinumab: an observational study of 69 patients in routine clinical practice. Actas Dermosifiliogr. 2019;110:244–6.
67. Loftus EV, Sloan S, Ramachandran P, Yang Z, Guo CY, Gasink C. Comparison of rates of active tuberculosis infection in the phase 2 and 3 clinical trial programs for anti-IL12/23 and anti-TNFs. Gastroenterology. 2017;152(5):596.
68. Di Cesare A, Di Meglio P, Nestle FO. The IL-23/Th17 axis in the immunopathogenesis of psoriasis. J Invest Dermatol. 2009;129:1339–50.
69. Gasse P, Riteau N, Vacher R, Michel ML, Fautrel A, di Padova F, et al. IL-1 and IL-23 mediate early IL-17A production in pulmonary inflammation leading to late fibrosis. PLoS One. 2011;6:e23185.
70. Valeri M, Raffatellu M. Cytokines IL-17 and IL-22 in the host response to infection. Pathol Dis. 2016;74:111. https://doi.org/10.1093/femspd/ftw111.
71. Okamoto Yoshida Y, Umemura M, Yahagi A, O'Brien RL, Ikuta K, Kishihara K, et al. Essential role of IL-17A in the formation of a mycobacterial infection-induced granuloma in the lung. J Immunol. 2010;184:4414–22.
72. Umemura M, Yahagi A, Hamada S, Begum MD, Watanabe H, Kawakami K, et al. IL-17-mediated regulation of innate and acquired immune response against pulmonary mycobacterium Bovis Bacille Calmette-Guérin infection. J Immunol. 2007;178:3786–96.
73. Fowler E, Ghamrawi RI, Ghiam N, Liao W, Wu JJ. Risk of tuberculosis reactivation during interleukin-17 inhibitor therapy for psoriasis: a systematic review. J Eur Acad Dermatol Venereol. 2020;34:1449–56.
74. Elewski BE, Baddley JW, Deodhar AA, Magrey M, Rich PA, Soriano ER, et al. Association of secukinumab treatment with tuberculosis reactivation in patients with psoriasis, psoriatic arthritis, or ankylosing spondylitis. JAMA Dermatol. 2021;157:43–51.

75. van de Kerkhof PC, Griffiths CE, Reich K, Leonardi CL, Blauvelt A, Tsai TF, et al. Secukinumab long-term safety experience: a pooled analysis of 10 phase II and III clinical studies in patients with moderate to severe plaque psoriasis. JAMA Dermatol. 2016;75(83-98):e4.
76. Ribero S, Licciardello M, Quaglino P, Dapavo P. Efficacy and safety of secukinumab in patients with plaque psoriasis and latent tuberculosis. Case Rep Dermatol. 2019;11:23–8.
77. Kammüller M, Tsai T-F, Griffiths CE, Kapoor N, Kolattukudy PE, Brees D, et al. Inhibition of IL-17A by secukinumab shows no evidence of increased Mycobacterium tuberculosis infections. Clin Transl Immunol. 2017;6:e152.
78. Rahman P, Ritchlin CT, Helliwell PS, Boehncke WH, Mease PJ, Gottlieb AB, et al. Pooled safety results through 1 year of 2 phase III trials of guselkumab in patients with psoriatic arthritis. J Rheumatol. 2021;48:1815–23.
79. Reich K, Griffiths CEM, Gordon KB, Papp KA, Song M, Randazzo B, et al. Maintenance of clinical response and consistent safety profile with up to 3 years of continuous treatment with guselkumab: results from the VOYAGE 1 and VOYAGE 2 trials. J Am Acad Dermatol. 2020;82:936–45.
80. Ferrante M, Feagan BG, Panes J, Baert F, Louis E, Dewit O, et al. Long-term safety and efficacy of risankizumab treatment in patients with Crohn's disease: results from the phase 2 open-label extension study. J Crohns Colitis. 2021;15:2001–10.
81. Puig L, Tsai TF, Bhutani T, Uy J, Ramachandran P, Song M, et al. Safety in moderate-to-severe plaque psoriasis patients with latent tuberculosis treated with guselkumab and anti-tuberculosis treatments concomitantly: results from pooled phase 3 VOYAGE 1 & VOYAGE 2 trials. J Eur Acad Dermatol Venereol. 2020;34:1744–9.
82. Fernandez-Ruiz M, Aguado JM. Risk of infection associated with anti-TNF-alpha therapy. Expert Rev Anti-Infect Ther. 2018;16:939–56.
83. Menter A, Strober BE, Kaplan DH, Kivelevitch D, Prater EF, Stoff B, et al. Joint AAD-NPF guidelines of care for the management and treatment of psoriasis with biologics. J Am Acad Dermatol. 2019;80:1029–72.
84. Smith CH, Yiu ZZN, Bale T, Burden AD, Coates LC, Edwards W, et al. British Association of Dermatologists guidelines for biologic therapy for psoriasis 2020: a rapid update. Br J Dermatol. 2020;183:628–37.
85. Lamb CA, Kennedy NA, Raine T, Hendy PA, Smith PJ, Limdi JK, et al. British Society of Gastroenterology consensus guidelines on the management of inflammatory bowel disease in adults. Gut. 2019;68:106.
86. Mir Viladrich I, Dauden Tello E, Solano-Lopez G, Lopez Longo FJ, Taxonera Samso C, Sanchez Martinez P, et al. Consensus document on prevention and treatment of tuberculosis in patients for biological treatment. Arch Bronconeumol. 2016;52:36–45.
87. McInnes IB, Rahman P, Gottlieb AB, Hsia EC, Kollmeier AP, Chakravarty SD, et al. Efficacy and safety of Guselkumab, an interleukin-23p19-specific monoclonal antibody, through one year in biologic-naive patients with psoriatic arthritis. Arthritis Rheumatol. 2021;73:604–16.
88. Ritchlin CT, Helliwell PS, Boehncke WH, Soriano ER, Hsia EC, Kollmeier AP, et al. Guselkumab, an inhibitor of the IL-23p19 subunit, provides sustained improvement in signs and symptoms of active psoriatic arthritis: 1 year results of a phase III randomised study of patients who were biologic-naive or TNFalpha inhibitor-experienced. RMD Open. 2021;7(1):e001457. https://doi.org/10.1136/rmdopen-2020-001457.
89. Ostor A, Van den Bosch F, Papp K, Asnal C, Blanco R, Aelion J, et al. Efficacy and safety of risankizumab for active psoriatic arthritis: 24-week results from the randomised, double-blind, phase 3 KEEPsAKE 2 trial. Ann Rheum Dis. 2021;80:138–9.
90. Sandborn WJ, Feagan BG, Danese S, O'Brien CD, Ott E, Marano C, et al. Safety of ustekinumab in inflammatory bowel disease: pooled safety analysis of results from phase 2/3 studies. Inflamm Bowel Dis. 2021;27:994–1007.
91. Kagami S, Rizzo HL, Kurtz SE, Miller LS, Blauvelt A. IL-23 and IL-17A, but not IL-12 and IL-22, are required for optimal skin host defense against Candida albicans. J Immunol. 2010;185:5453–62.

92. van de Veerdonk FL, Plantinga TS, Hoischen A, Smeekens SP, Joosten LA, Gilissen C, et al. STAT1 mutations in autosomal dominant chronic mucocutaneous candidiasis. N Engl J Med. 2011;365:54–61.
93. Blauvelt A, Reich K, Papp KA, Kimball AB, Gooderham M, Tyring SK, et al. Safety of tildrakizumab for moderate-to-severe plaque psoriasis: pooled analysis of three randomized controlled trials. Br J Dermatol. 2018;179:615–22.
94. Gordon KB, Lebwohl M, Papp KA, Bachelez H, Wu JJ, Langley RG, et al. Long-term safety of risankizumab from 17 clinical trials in patients with moderate-to-severe plaque psoriasis. Br J Dermatol. 2021;186(3):466–75. https://doi.org/10.1111/bjd.20818.
95. Bilal J, Berlinberg A, Bhattacharjee S, Trost J, Riaz IB, Kurtzman DJB. A systematic review and meta-analysis of the efficacy and safety of the interleukin (IL)-12/23 and IL-17 inhibitors ustekinumab, secukinumab, ixekizumab, brodalumab, guselkumab and tildrakizumab for the treatment of moderate to severe plaque psoriasis. J Dermatolog Treat. 2018;29:569–78.
96. Davidson L, van den Reek J, Bruno M, van Hunsel F, Herings RMC, Matzaraki V, et al. Risk of candidiasis associated with interleukin-17 inhibitors: a real-world observational study of multiple independent sources. Lancet Reg Health Eur. 2022;13:100266.
97. Lee MP, Wu KK, Lee EB, Wu JJ. Risk for deep fungal infections during IL-17 and IL-23 inhibitor therapy for psoriasis. Cutis. 2020;106:199–205.
98. Failla V, Nikkels AF. Ustekinumab and herpes zoster. Dermatology. 2011;222:119–22.
99. Zou A, Chen Y, Shi N, Ye Y. Risk of herpes zoster associated with biological therapies for psoriasis and psoriatic arthritis: a systematic review and meta-analysis. Medicine. 2021;100:e27368.
100. Tang Z, Shen M, Chen X. Risk of herpes zoster among psoriasis patients taking biologics: A network meta-analysis of cohort studies. Front Med. 2021;8:665559. https://doi.org/10.3389/fmed.2021.665559.
101. Reich K, Warren RB, Iversen L, Puig L, Pau-Charles I, Igarashi A, et al. Long-term efficacy and safety of tildrakizumab for moderate-to-severe psoriasis: pooled analyses of two randomized phase III clinical trials (reSURFACE 1 and reSURFACE 2) through 148 weeks. Br J Dermatol. 2020;182:605–17.
102. Kluger N, Klimenko T, Bosonnet S. Herpes simplex, herpes zoster and periorbital erythema flares after SARS-CoV-2 vaccination: 4 cases. Ann Dermatol Venereol. 2021;149(1):58–60.
103. Stollberger C, Finsterer J. Varicella zoster virus meningitis under ustekinumab because of plaque psoriasis. J Dermatol. 2017;44:703–5.
104. Sandborn WJ, Rutgeerts P, Gasink C, Jacobstein D, Zou B, Johanns J, et al. Long-term efficacy and safety of ustekinumab for Crohn's disease through the second year of therapy. Aliment Pharmacol Ther. 2018;48:65–77.
105. Cavanaugh VJ, Guidotti LG, Chisari FV. Interleukin-12 inhibits hepatitis B virus replication in transgenic mice. J Virol. 1997;71:3236–43.
106. Xiong SQ, Lin BL, Gao X, Tang H, Wu CY. IL-12 promotes HBV-specific central memory CD8+ T cell responses by PBMCs from chronic hepatitis B virus carriers. Int Immunopharmacol. 2007;7:578–87.
107. Carreno V, Zeuzem S, Hopf U, Marcellin P, Cooksley WG, Fevery J, et al. A phase I/II study of recombinant human interleukin-12 in patients with chronic hepatitis B. J Hepatol. 2000;32:317–24.
108. Landells I, Marano C, Hsu MC, Li S, Zhu Y, Eichenfield LF, et al. Ustekinumab in adolescent patients age 12 to 17 years with moderate-to-severe plaque psoriasis: results of the randomized phase 3 CADMUS study. J Am Acad Dermatol. 2015;73:594–603.
109. Feagan BG, Sandborn WJ, Gasink C, Jacobstein D, Lang Y, Friedman JR, et al. Ustekinumab as induction and maintenance therapy for Crohn's disease. N Engl J Med. 2016;375:1946–60.
110. Sands BE, Sandborn WJ, Panaccione R, O'Brien CD, Zhang H, Johanns J, et al. Ustekinumab as induction and maintenance therapy for ulcerative colitis. N Engl J Med. 2019;381:1201–14.
111. Chiu HY, Chen CH, Wu MS, Cheng YP, Tsai TF. The safety profile of ustekinumab in the treatment of patients with psoriasis and concurrent hepatitis B or C. Br J Dermatol. 2013;169:1295–303.

112. Ting SW, Chen YC, Huang YH. Risk of Hepatitis B reactivation in patients with psoriasis on ustekinumab. Clin Drug Investig. 2018;38:873–80.
113. Xia L, Tian D, Huang W, Zhu H, Wang J, Zhang Y, et al. Upregulation of IL-23 expression in patients with chronic hepatitis B is mediated by the HBx/ERK/NF-kappaB pathway. J Immunol. 2012;188:753–64.
114. Zang M, Li Y, He H, Ding H, Chen K, Du J, et al. IL-23 production of liver inflammatory macrophages to damaged hepatocytes promotes hepatocellular carcinoma development after chronic hepatitis B virus infection. Biochim Biophys Acta Mol basis Dis. 2018;1864:3759–70.
115. Duncan JR, Orlowski TJ, Elewski BE. Safety of guselkumab in hepatitis B virus infection. Dermatol Online J. 2019;25:37–9. https://doi.org/10.1016/j.jdcr.2020.12.006.
116. Song EJ, Whitman P, Samsel J. The use of ustekinumab and guselkumab in a pediatric psoriasis patient with active hepatitis B infection. JAAD Case Rep. 2021;8:37–9.
117. Lechner F, Wong DK, Dunbar PR, Chapman R, Chung RT, Dohrenwend P, et al. Analysis of successful immune responses in persons infected with hepatitis C virus. J Exp Med. 2000;191:1499–512.
118. Zeuzem S, Carreno V. Interleukin-12 in the treatment of chronic hepatitis B and C. Antivir Res. 2001;52:181–8.
119. Abuchar A, Vitiello M, Kerdel FA. Psoriasis treated with ustekinumab in a patient with hepatitis C. Int J Dermatol. 2013;52:381–2.
120. Malara G, Lo M. Ustekinumab treatment in psoriatic patient suffering from chronic hepatitis C. J Am Acad Dermatol. 2012;4(1):2016.
121. Navarro R, Vilarrasa E, Herranz P, Puig L, Bordas X, Carrascosa JM, et al. Safety and effectiveness of ustekinumab and antitumour necrosis factor therapy in patients with psoriasis and chronic viral hepatitis B or C: a retrospective, multicentre study in a clinical setting. Br J Dermatol. 2013;168:609–16.
122. Winthrop KL, Mariette X, Silva JT, Benamu E, Calabrese LH, Dumusc A, et al. ESCMID Study Group for Infections in Compromised Hosts (ESGICH) Consensus Document on the safety of targeted and biological therapies: an infectious diseases perspective (soluble immune effector molecules [II]: agents targeting interleukins, immunoglobulins and complement factors). Clin Microbiol Infect. 2018;24(2):21–40.
123. Noreña I, Fernandez-Ruiz M, Aguado JM. Is there a real risk of bacterial infection in patients receiving targeted and biological therapies? Enferm Infecc Microbiol Clin 2020. https://doi.org/10.1016/j.eimc.2020.10.019.
124. Menzies D, Adjobimey M, Ruslami R, Trajman A, Sow O, Kim H, et al. Four months of rifampin or nine months of isoniazid for latent tuberculosis in adults. N Engl J Med. 2018;379:440–53.
125. Sterling TR, Villarino ME, Borisov AS, Shang N, Gordin F, Bliven-Sizemore E, et al. Three months of rifapentine and isoniazid for latent tuberculosis infection. N Engl J Med. 2011;365:2155–66.
126. Tsiouri G, Gaitanis G, Kiorpelidou D, Dionysiou A, Efthymiou A, Daskalopoulos G, et al. Tuberculin skin test overestimates tuberculosis hypersensitivity in adult patients with psoriasis. Dermatology. 2009;219:119–25.
127. Brodmerkel C, Wadman E, Langley RG, Papp KA, Bourcier M, Poulin Y, et al. Immune response to pneumococcus and tetanus toxoid in patients with moderate-to-severe psoriasis following long-term ustekinumab use. J Drugs Dermatol. 2013;12:1122–9.
128. Doornekamp L, Goetgebuer RL, Schmitz KS, Goeijenbier M, van der Woude CJ, Fouchier R, et al. High immunogenicity to influenza vaccination in Crohn's disease patients treated with Ustekinumab. Vaccine. 2020;8:455. https://doi.org/10.3390/vaccines8030455.

Sphingosine-1 Phosphate Receptor Modulators

12

Sabina Herrera and Marta Bodro

Biologic/Immune-Targeted Agent

Sphingolipids have roles in the regulation of cell growth, death, senescence, adhesion, migration, inflammation, angiogenesis, and intracellular trafficking. Ceramide, sphingosine, sphingosine-1-phosphate (S1P), ceramide-1-phosphate, and lyso-sphingomyelin are some examples of sphingolipids. Sphingosine is a sphingolipid and a key component of a complex lipid metabolism that is continuously forming and degrading bioactive metabolites. It is also the biosynthetic substrate for a number of diverse sphingolipids. A balance exists between sphingolipid synthesis and degradation that determines the concentration of lipids in different cellular compartments [1], and it is of extreme importance to regulate the traffic of leukocytes among other functions.

Leukocyte migration across vessels into peripheral and lymphoid tissues is essential for host defense. Leukocytes are specialized in sensing different signals from the environment, so they can be directed. These extracellular signals must be transmitted across the leukocyte's cytoplasmic membrane, enabling several intracellular signaling cascades to activate cell movement. The composition of the membrane, proteins, and sphingolipids primarily is therefore extremely important for this process to be successful. Mislocalization of membrane proteins is known to deleteriously affect cellular functions that may cause a variety of diseases [2].

Sphingosine is phosphorylated by type 1 and 2 sphingosine kinases to form sphingosin-1-phosphate. S1P strongly influences cell survival and plays a significant role in chemotaxis, angiogenesis, vascular maturation, receptor-specific regulation endothelial barrier integrity, and vascular permeability. S1P has a very special role in innate and adaptive immunity, including regulation of immune responses, immunosurveillance, leukocyte differentiation, and lymphocyte trafficking by

S. Herrera · M. Bodro (✉)
Infectious Diseases Department, Hospital Clínic de Barcelona, Catalonia, Spain
e-mail: sherrera@clinic.cat; mbodro@clinic.cat

C. Cervera, J. M. Aguado (eds.), *Infectious Complications in Biologic and Targeted Therapies*, https://doi.org/10.1007/978-3-031-11363-5_12

binding to one of five known G protein-coupled receptors (GPCRs) [3]. G protein-coupled receptors (GPCRs) constitute the largest superfamily of receptors for signaling molecules and ligands and currently comprise hundreds of receptors. They have seven transmembrane domains. Many ligands, such as hormones, neurotransmitters, and very small molecules to large proteins can bind and activate GPCRs, leading to a multitude of physiological processes [4].

The sphingosine-1-phosphate receptor 1 (S1P1) also known as endothelial differentiation gene 1 (EDG1) is of prime importance for the activation of the immune system as it regulates the differentiation, egress, and migration of macrophages, mast cells, natural killer cells, dendritic cells, neutrophils, and hematopoietic precursors. Differentiation, recirculation, and trafficking of T and B lymphocytes are the foundation for the development of autoimmune diseases such as multiple sclerosis and make S1P1 a target of high interest for the development for therapeutic drugs [5]. There are five known S1P receptor types. Expression patterns of the five S1P receptors (S1PRs) vary in tissues and during development and aging. $S1P_1$, $S1P_2$, and $S1P_3$ are ubiquitously expressed, whereas expression of $S1P_4$ and $S1P_5$ is highly restricted to distinct cell types [6]. Since three of the five known S1P receptor types are expressed ubiquitously, specificity of drugs targeting S1P receptors is essential to predict the therapeutic and potential side effects as each S1P receptor displays different physiological effects upon activation (Fig. 12.1).

S1PR1 is one of the most widely studied receptors of S1P. It is ubiquitously expressed, and it has influence in many different pathways. It is of high importance in the regulation of the adaptive and innate immune responses [7]. Its role in autoimmune responses is well established, and several findings support the idea that S1PR1 plays a role in immune responses to infectious diseases by affecting recruitment and

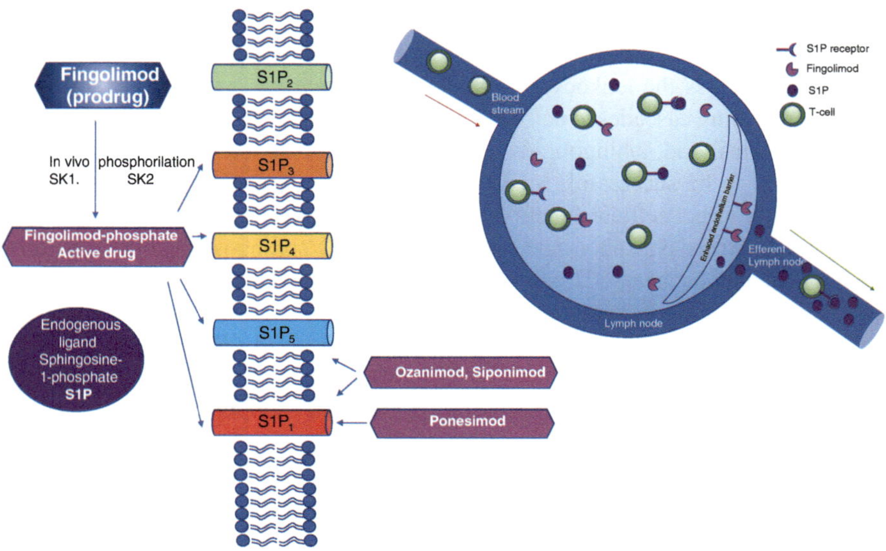

Fig. 12.1 Mechamism of action of fingolimod

trafficking of innate immune cells, macrophage polarization, and plasmacytoid dendritic cell functions.

S1PR2 is present in innate cells, mainly macrophages, monocytes, and granulocytes.

It is known to oppose the activity of S1PR1 by repelling instead of attracting cells in response to S1P. Its main role in innate immune cells is to increase antibody-mediated phagocytosis of fungi and inhibit phagocytosis of bacteria in alveolar macrophages [8].

S1PR3 mediates S1P-induced increase in mature dendritic cell migration and endocytosis. It has several functions in immunity by affecting dendritic cell maturation, macrophage chemotaxis and killing, as well as neutrophil and eosinophil recruitment. It promotes immune cell recruitment by driving leukocyte rolling on endothelial cells [9].

S1PR4 is widely expressed on immune cells and has a role in plasmacytoid dendritic cell differentiation and activation and neutrophil recruitment. S1PR5 is expressed in the spleen and oligodendrocytes and is the less studied receptor, and the way it influences trafficking needs further study [10].

Multiple sclerosis is a chronic inflammatory disease of the central nervous system (CNS) leading to demyelination and neurodegeneration, with the presence of focal lesions in the gray and white matter and diffuse neurodegeneration in the entire brain. The presentation of multiple sclerosis is highly variable in individuals. There are several forms of the disease described: the classic relapsing-remitting (RRMS) form with the appearance of recurring clinical symptoms followed by total or partial recovery. Approximately 50% of patients that don't receive any specific treatment have progressive symptoms with clinical deterioration around 10 years after the onset of the disease, a stage called secondary progressive multiple sclerosis (SPMS). In about 15% of patients with multiple sclerosis however, disease progression is relentless from onset, primary progressive multiple sclerosis (PPMS). All typical pathological features of MS are seen in all stages of the disease [11].

The exact pathogenesis of MS is controversial. Study findings suggest that MS is an immune-mediated disorder involving numerous antigens of the CNS and also an autoimmune disease of the CNS [12]. The large confluent demyelinated lesions in the white and gray matter of the CNS, the main pathologic hallmark of MS, have a prominent immunologic response dominated by CD8+ and CD4+ T cells. Patients with MS also have oligoclonal bands in the cerebrospinal fluid, revealing the presence of immunoglobulin-producing B cells, that also play a role in the pathogenesis of MS. Levels of demyelination are not strictly correlated to disease stage, neurologic deficits, or lesion pathology. Pathology suggests that inflammation drives tissue injury at every stage of the disease. Focal inflammatory infiltrates in the meninges and the perivascular spaces produce soluble factors, which induce demyelination or neurodegeneration by activation of the microglia. The final process by which demyelination and neurodegeneration take place is oxidative injury and mitochondrial damage. Perivascular inflammatory infiltrates consist mainly of lymphocytes and plasma cells, whereas active tissue damage is associated with macrophages and activated microglia. The lymphocyte population is mainly T cells with a smaller contribution of B cells and plasma cells [12].

Mechanism of Action

The most common form of MS is relapsing remitting, where the characteristic pathological hallmark is the appearance of one or more focal demyelinating lesions in the central nervous system usually associated with an acute exacerbation of neurological dysfunction. The trigger is the activation and clonal expansion of pro-inflammatory T lymphocytes in the peripheral circulation by an unidentified myelin-related antigen [13], which then can cross the vascular epithelium by binding to the vascular cell adhesion molecule and enter the CNS. Once activated by epitopes on myelin, chemokines and cytokines are released to attract other T cells and to activate surrounding microglial cells and macrophages, destroying the myelin sheath. Once the episode is over, the lesion may remyelinate; however, there are long-term consequences, as the axon is exposed to neurotoxic factors with irreversible damage. The repeated neuronal loss in the gray matter leads to brain atrophy and progressive disability [13]. Moreover, the acute inflammatory episode activates a persistent inflammatory state, leading to diffuse inflammation in the brain parenchyma, typical of MS with progressive presentations [14].

Therapeutic approaches are therefore focused on inflammation and neurodegeneration both present from early stages of the disease. S1PR modulators seem to target both scenarios.

Several S1PR modulators have been approved by the FDA as they have demonstrated to be able to reduce disease activity or progression in multiple sclerosis. They act as functional antagonists of sphingosine by blockade of the S1PR signaling pathway. Binding of these agents to this receptor subtype on lymphocytes has an anti-inflammatory effect.

The receptor's main role is the migration of lymphocytes through the lymph nodes, with the egression of naïve and memory T and B lymphocytes to the circulation [15]. This process is gated by CCR7 receptor present only on the surface of naïve and memory T and B lymphocytes. When effector memory lymphocytes are stimulated by an antigen, they lose the CCR7 on their surface and therefore can leave the lymph node toward the circulation, and this process is mediated by the activation of S1P (Fig. 12.1).

Treatment with S1PR modulators activates S1PR at the surface of lymphocytes, leading to a GRK2-mediated phosphorylation of C-terminal tail of S1PR, inducing internalization of the receptor. This results in depletion of S1PR at the surface of lymphocytes, as S1PR is exposed to proteasomal degradation. The consequence is the blocked recirculation of lymphocytes from secondary lymphoid organs to blood, since lymphocytes egress by chemotactic response to S1P concentration gradient (high in blood and low in lymph node) through S1PR. This results in naïve and memory T and B lymphocytes being stacked at the lymph node, but still allowing the circulation of effector memory lymphocytes [4].

Both S1P and fingolimod phosphate have been shown to induce lymphopenia via the agonistic activation of S1PR and subsequent internalization of S1PR in the lymphocytes. S1PR modulators have a long-lasting effect; this is due to internalized S1PR undergoing proteasomal degradation, with the absence of S1PR until de novo synthesized [4]. In the case of S1P, the internalized S1PR is recycled back to the cell surface within hours.

Current Indications for the Use

Several of the drugs developed under this mechanism have been evaluated for different conditions; however, the main indication of this group of drugs is for MS (Table 12.1).

Fingolimod was the first S1P1 modulator approved by the FDA back in 2010. Fingolimod's intended action is through binding of the S1P1 receptor on lymphocyte surfaces and has nonselective modulation of S1P3, S1P4, and S1P5.

Table 12.1 Main studies analyzing sphingosine-1-phosphate receptor modulators (fingolimod, siponimod, ozanimod, ponesimod)

Name of trial, author, year of publication	Type of study	Molecule	Study population	Outcomes	Comments
FREEDOMS Kappos et al. 2010	Phase 3 multicenter clinical trial	Oral **fingolimod** vs. placebo	1033 relapsing-remitting MS	Reduced the risk of disability progression, HR = 0.70, $P = 0.02$. The cumulative probability of CDP was 17.7% with fingolimod and 24.1% with placebo and fingolimod resulted in fewer new or enlarged T2 lesions, fewer gadolinium-enhancing lesions, and less brain volume loss ($P < 0.001$)	Oral fingolimod improved the relapse rate, the risk of disability progression, and end points on MRI
FREEDOMS II Calabresi PA et al. 2014	Phase 3 multicenter clinical trial	Oral **fingolimod** vs. placebo	1083 Patients with relapsing-remitting MS	Fingolimod reduced the ARR 0.21, compared with placebo 0.40; $P < 0.0001$)	Oral fingolimod improved the relapse rate with no effect on disability progression
TRANSFORMS Cohen JA et al. 2010	Phase 2 multicenter clinical trial	Oral **fingolimod** vs. intramuscular interferon beta-1a	1153 Patients with relapsing-remitting MS	The AAR was significantly lower in both groups receiving fingolimod 0.20 in the 1.25-mg group and 0.16 in the 0.5-mg group, than in the interferon group 0.33, $P < 0.001$ for both comparisons	Superior efficacy of oral fingolimod with respect to relapse Rates and MRI outcomes

Table 12.1 (continued)

Name of trial, author, year of publication	Type of study	Molecule	Study population	Outcomes	Comments
INFORMS Lublin F et al. 2016	Phase 3 multicenter clinical trial	Oral **fingolimod** vs. placebo	970 patients with secondary progressive MS	CDP had occurred in 77.2% of patients in the fingolimod group vs 80.3% of patients in the placebo group (risk reduction 5.05%, HR 0.95, $p = 0.544$)	The anti-inflammatory effects of fingolimod did not slow disease progression in primary progressive multiple sclerosis
EXPAND Kappos L et al. 2018	Phase 3 multicenter clinical trial	**Siponimod** versus placebo	1651 patients with secondary progressive MS	26% of patients receiving siponimod and 32% of patients receiving placebo had 3-month CDP (hazard ratio 0.79, relative risk reduction 21%; $p = 0.013$)	Siponimod reduced the risk of disability progression
SUNBEAM Corni G et al. 2019	Phase 3 multicenter clinical trial	**Ozanimod** versus interferon beta-1a	1346 patients with relapsing MS	Adjusted ARRs were 0.35 for interferon beta-1a, 0.18 for ozanimod 1.0 mg (rate ratio of 0.52 vs interferon beta-1a; $p < 0.0001$), and 0.24 (0.19–0.31) for ozanimod 0.5 mg (rate ratio 0.69 vs. interferon beta-1a; $p = 0.0013$)	Ozanimod was well Tolerated and demonstrated a significantly lower relapse rate than interferon beta-1a

Table 12.1 (continued)

Name of trial, author, year of publication	Type of study	Molecule	Study population	Outcomes	Comments
RADIANCE Cohen JA et al. 2017	Phase 2/3 multicenter clinical trial	**Ozanimod** versus interferon beta-1a	1320 patients with relapsing MS	Adjusted ARRs were 0.17 with ozanimod 1.0 mg, 0.22 with ozanimod 0.5 mg, and 0.28 with interferon beta-1a, with rate ratios versus interferon beta-1a of 0.62 ($p < 0.0001$) for ozanimod 1.0 mg and 0.79 ($p = 0.0167$) for ozanimod 0.5 mg	Ozanimod was well Tolerated and associated with a significantly lower rate of clinical relapses than intramuscular interferon beta-1a
OPTIMUM Kappos L et al. 2019	Phase 3 multicenter clinical trial	**Ponesimod** vs. teriflunomide	1133 patients with relapsing MS	ARR ponesimod versus teriflunomide were 0.202 and 0.290, corresponding to a RRR with ponesimod of 30.5% ($P = 0.0003$). Respective mean change from baseline in fatigue symptom and impact questionnaire score was 0.01 vs. 3.57 ($P = 0.0019$). Mean number of active lesions per year on MRI was 1.405 vs. 3.164 (RRR 56%, $P < 0.0001$)	**Ponesimod was superior to teriflunomide with regard to ARR, fatigue symptoms, MRI activity, brain atrophy**

AAR annualized relapse rate, *CDP* confirmed disability progression, *HR* hazard ratio, *MRI* magnetic resonance imaging, *MS* multiple sclerosis, *RRR* relative rate reduction
FDA approved for MS
Fingolimod 2010
Siponimod 2019
Ozanimod 2020
Ponesimod 2020

(continued)

Two big studies have evaluated the efficacy of fingolimod. In the FREEDOMS phase 3 trial, fingolimod was shown to decrease annualized relapse rate (ARR) by 54% and 60%, respectively, for 0.5 mg and 1.25 mg doses compared to placebo. Fingolimod also significantly reduced gadolinium-enhancing MRI lesions (approximately 90%) and new/enlarged T2 lesions (approximately 50%) at 24 months [16]. These results were largely confirmed in a second placebo-controlled phase 3 trial, FREEDOMS II, where fingolimod reduced the annualized relapse rate (ARR) (0.21; 95% CI, 0.17–0.25) compared with placebo (0.40; 95% CI, 0.34–0.48; $P < 0.0001$) [17].

In the TRANSFORMS trial, both doses of fingolimod (0.5 mg and 1.25 mg) were demonstrated to be superior to interferon beta-1a in decreasing the ARR by 52% and 38%, respectively. The proportion of relapse-free participants and time to confirmed relapse were greater in both fingolimod groups. On MRI, the numbers of GdE lesions and new/enlarged T2 lesions were significantly lower in the fingolimod groups compared to IFN-β1a. Brain volume reductions were significantly less with both fingolimod doses than with IFNβ-1[a] [18].

When fingolimod was assessed in patients with secondary progressive MS, in the INFORMS trial, fingolimod did not slow disease progression. Confirmed disability progression had occurred in 77.2% (95% CI 71.87–82.51) of patients in the fingolimod group versus 80.3% (73.31–87.25) of patients in the placebo group (risk reduction 5.05%; hazard ratio 0.95, 95% CI 0.80–1.12; $p = 0.544$) [19]. Fingolimod is currently being evaluated in clinical trials for chemotherapy-induced peripheral neuropathy, breast carcinoma, intracerebral hemorrhage, stroke, RETT syndrome, and COVID-19.

Siponimod is a selective S1PR modulator with affinity for S1PR1 and S1PR5 that was FDA approved in 2019 for the treatment of adults with relapsing forms of MS, including clinically isolated syndrome, relapsing-remitting MS, and active secondary progressive MS. In the phase III clinical trial, 26% of the patients receiving siponimod and 32% of the patients receiving placebo had 3-month confirmed disability progression (hazard ratio 0.79, 95% CI 0.65–0.95; relative risk reduction 21%; $p = 0.013$) [20]. Siponimod has also been studied for dermatomyositis; however, the study was terminated prematurely after interim analysis for futility, as it did not provide any evidence for efficacy in this condition. It is also being studied for intracranial hemorrhage; however, recruiting has been stopped temporarily due to COVID-19 pandemic.

Ozanimod is a selective S1PR modulator with affinity for S1PR1 and S1PR5. Ozanimod was one of the latest SP1 modulators to be approved by the FDA in 2020 for the indication of relapsing forms of MS. In the phase II clinical trial, RADIANCE, ozanimod vs. placebo reduced the mean number of gadolinium-enhancing lesions (1.5 ± 3.7 vs. 11.1 ± 29.9; odds ratio 0.16, 95% CI 0.08–0.30; $P < 0.0001$) [21]. In the phase III RADIANCE trial, it was compared to intramuscular interferon β-1a for 24 months showing reduced ARR by 21% ($P = 0.001$) [22]. In another phase III clinical trial, ozanimod vs. intramuscular interferon β-1a reduced ARR by 31% ($P = 0.0013$) [23]. In both trials, ozanimod was compared to interferon β-1a and ozanimod reduced volume loss in the whole brain, cortical gray matter, and the thalamus. Apart from MS, ozanimod is being investigated as a therapy for Crohn's disease and ulcerative colitis, and there are several phase III clinical trials recruiting patients currently. Phase II clinical trial has shown endoscopic, histological, and clinical improvements within 12 weeks of initiating ozanimod therapy in patients with moderately to severely active Crohn's disease [24]. Ozanimod also resulted in a slightly higher rate of clinical remission of ulcerative colitis than placebo in another phase II clinical trial [25].

Ponesimod is highly selective for the S1PR1 subtype and the latest of this group of modulators to be approved by the Food and Drug Administration (FDA). Its indication is for relapsing multiple sclerosis. It was compared to teriflunomide for relapsing MS, showing an ARR by 30.5% over 108 weeks (0.202 vs. 0.290; $P = 0.0003$). Those treated with ponesimod also had significant reductions in fatigue compared to the teriflunomide group, measured by the Fatigue Symptom and Impact Questionnaire-Relapsing Multiple Sclerosis (FSIQ-RMS), (mean FSIQ-RMS score − 3.57; $P = 0.0019$), and reduced combined active lesions by 56% compared with teriflunomide (1.4 vs. 3.16; $P < 0.0001$) [26]. Ponesimod has also been proposed as treatment for psoriasis, showing benefit in phase II clinical trials [27]; however, further studies are granted.

The Described Risk of Infections

Patients with multiple sclerosis have been reported to have an increased risk of infections compared with the general population, regardless of treatment [28]. Although fingolimod is a highly effective disease-modifying therapy for multiple sclerosis, it has been associated with an increased risk of infections comparing with injectable therapies as interferon beta and glatiramer acetate [18, 29–31]. Nevertheless, the magnitude of the potential risk increase was not well established in randomized clinical trials and post-marketing surveillance [18]. Importantly, the Swedish nationwide register-based cohort study found that patients with multiple sclerosis treated with fingolimod had an incidence rate of severe infections per 1000 person-years of 14.3 (95% CI: 10.8–18.5), defined as any infection recorded as the main reason for a hospitalization [32]. Viral infections, especially varicella-zoster (VZV) infection, were common, followed by urinary tract infections and pneumonia of any origin [32] (Table 12.2).

Varicella-zoster (VZV) is the most frequent infectious complication in patients receiving fingolimod, followed by herpes simplex virus (HSV) infection. Varicella-zoster virus antibodies are likely to provide a first line of defense against a new respiratory mucosal inoculation of the virus, whereas VZV-specific T-cell responses are the major host defense against symptomatic reactivation of latent VZV, which results in herpes zoster (HZ). The latter clinical presentation (HZ) is the most common in patients receiving fingolimod, mainly due to the reduced number of circulating VZV-specific T cells during treatment. Although rates of VZV infections in clinical trials were low with fingolimod, there were higher than in placebo recipients [16–18]. Rates reported in the post-marketing setting are comparable, and it

Table 12.2 Type of infections described in patients treated with fingolimod

	Frequency of reported infection
Virus	Common
Varicella-zoster virus	Common
Herpes simplex virus	Uncommon
Molluscum contagiosum	Uncommon
Progressive multifocal leukoencephalopathy (JV virus)	Uncommon
Kaposi sarcoma (herpes 8 virus)	Uncommon
Hepatitis C virus reactivation	
Bacteria	Uncommon
Listeria spp.	
Fungi	Uncommon
Cryptococcus spp.	
Parasites	Uncommon
Leishmania spp.	Uncommon
Toxoplasma spp.	

seems that there is no sign of risk accumulation with longer exposure. Most reported infections are usually mild and limited to the skin or mucosa, and serious or complicated cases of herpes zoster were uncommon. Nevertheless, some severe forms have been also reported [33, 34].

Other infections that have been associated with fingolimod use are cryptococcal infection [35–37], visceral leishmaniasis [38], and extensive molluscum contagiosum infection [39]. Furthermore, isolated case reports have been reported describing cerebral toxoplasmosis, listeriosis, progressive multifocal leukoencephalopathy, hepatitis C virus reactivation, and Kaposi's sarcoma related to fingolimod use [40–45].

Finally, some data of infection due to coronavirus disease 2019 (COVID-19) in patients receiving fingolimod have been recently reported. Although some authors published some indolent cases [46, 47], others disclosed severe courses [48, 49]. Therefore, possible benefits of reducing inflammation when using immunomodulation and immunosuppression therapies in patients with COVID-19 should be carefully weighed up against the risk of inhibiting antiviral immune response, with a consequent perpetuation and worsening of the illness. Thus, more data is needed to know exactly the role of fingolimod in COVID-19 patients.

References

1. Hannun YA, Obeid LM. Principles of bioactive lipid signalling: lessons from sphingolipids. Nat Rev Mol Cell Biol. 2008;9(2):139–50.
2. Samson GPB, Legler DF. Membrane compartmentalization and scaffold proteins in leukocyte migration. Front Cell Dev Biol. 2020;8:285.
3. Spiegel S, Milstien S. The outs and the ins of sphingosine-1-phosphate in immunity. Nat Rev Immunol. 2011;11(6):403–15.
4. Park SJ, Im DS. Sphingosine 1-phosphate receptor modulators and drug discovery. Biomol Ther. 2017;25(1):80–90.

5. Cyster JG, Schwab SR. Sphingosine-1-phosphate and lymphocyte egress from lymphoid organs. Annu Rev Immunol. 2012;30:69–94.
6. Blaho VA, Hla T. An update on the biology of sphingosine 1-phosphate receptors. J Lipid Res. 2014;55(8):1596–608.
7. Pyne S, Pyne NJ. Sphingosine 1-phosphate signalling in mammalian cells. Biochem J. 2000;349(Pt 2):385–402.
8. Adada M, Canals D, Hannun YA, Obeid LM. Sphingosine-1-phosphate receptor 2. FEBS J. 2013;280(24):6354–66.
9. Nussbaum C, Bannenberg S, Keul P, Gräler MH, Gonçalves-De-Albuquerque CF, Korhonen H, et al. Sphingosine-1-phosphate receptor 3 promotes leukocyte rolling by mobilizing endothelial P-selectin. Nat Commun. 2015;6:6416.
10. Bryan AM, Del Poeta M. Sphingosine-1-phosphate receptors and innate immunity. Cell Microbiol. 2018;20(5):e12836.
11. Lublin FD, Reingold SC, Cohen JA, Cutter GR, Sørensen PS, Thompson AJ, et al. Defining the clinical course of multiple sclerosis: the 2013 revisions. Neurology. 2014;83(3):278–86.
12. Lemus HN, Warrington AE, Rodriguez M. Multiple sclerosis: mechanisms of disease and strategies for myelin and axonal repair. Neurol Clin. 2018;36(1):1–11.
13. Sospedra M, Martin R. Immunology of multiple sclerosis. Annu Rev Immunol. 2005;23:683–747.
14. Bordet R, Camu W, De Seze J, Laplaud DA, Ouallet JC, Thouvenot E. Mechanism of action of s1p receptor modulators in multiple sclerosis: the double requirement. Rev Neurol (Paris). 2020;176(1-2):100–12.
15. Chun J, Hartung HP. Mechanism of action of oral fingolimod (FTY720) in multiple sclerosis. Clin Neuropharmacol. 2010;33(2):91–101.
16. Kappos L, Radue E-W, O'Connor P, Polman C, Hohlfeld R, Calabresi P, et al. A placebo-controlled trial of Oral fingolimod in relapsing multiple sclerosis. N Engl J Med. 2010;362(5):387–401.
17. Calabresi PA, Radue EW, Goodin D, Jeffery D, Rammohan KW, Reder AT, et al. Safety and efficacy of fingolimod in patients with relapsing-remitting multiple sclerosis (FREEDOMS II): a double-blind, randomised, placebo-controlled, phase 3 trial. Lancet Neurol. 2014;13(6):545–56.
18. Cohen JA, Barkhof F, Comi G, Hartung H-P, Khatri BO, Montalban X, et al. Oral fingolimod or intramuscular interferon for relapsing multiple sclerosis. N Engl J Med. 2010;362(5):402–15.
19. Lublin F, Miller DH, Freedman MS, Cree BAC, Wolinsky JS, Weiner H, et al. Oral fingolimod in primary progressive multiple sclerosis (INFORMS): a phase 3, randomised, double-blind, placebo-controlled trial. Lancet. 2016;387(10023):1075–84.
20. Kappos L, Bar-Or A, Cree BAC, Fox RJ, Giovannoni G, Gold R, et al. Siponimod versus placebo in secondary progressive multiple sclerosis (EXPAND): a double-blind, randomised, phase 3 study. Lancet. 2018;391(10127):1263–73.
21. Cohen JA, Arnold DL, Comi G, Bar-Or A, Gujrathi S, Hartung JP, et al. Safety and efficacy of the selective sphingosine 1-phosphate receptor modulator ozanimod in relapsing multiple sclerosis (RADIANCE): a randomised, placebo-controlled, phase 2 trial. Lancet Neurol. 2016;15(4):373–81.
22. Cohen JA, Comi G, Selmaj KW, Bar-Or A, Arnold DL, Steinman L, et al. Ozanimod vs. interferon β-1a: clinical and MRI results of RADIANCE part B - a 2-year phase 3 trial in relapsing multiple sclerosis. Mult Scler. 2017;25(9):1255–62.
23. Comi G, Kappos L, Selmaj KW, Bar-Or A, Arnold DL, Steinman L, et al. Safety and efficacy of ozanimod versus interferon beta-1a in relapsing multiple sclerosis (SUNBEAM): a multicentre, randomised, minimum 12-month, phase 3 trial. Lancet Neurol. 2019;18(11):1009–20.
24. Feagan BG, Sandborn WJ, Danese S, Wolf DC, Liu WJ, Hua SY, et al. Ozanimod induction therapy for patients with moderate to severe Crohn's disease: a single-arm, phase 2, prospective observer-blinded endpoint study. Lancet Gastroenterol Hepatol. 2020;5(9):819–28.

25. Sandborn WJ, Feagan BG, Wolf DC, D'Haens G, Vermeire S, Hanauer SB, et al. Ozanimod induction and maintenance treatment for ulcerative colitis. N Engl J Med. 2016;374(18):1754–62.
26. Kappos L, Burcklen M, Freedman MS, Fox R, Havrdova EK, Hennessy B, et al. Efficacy and safety of ponesimod compared to teriflunomide in patients with relapsing multiple sclerosis: results of the randomized, active-controlled, double-blind, parallel-group phase 3 OPTIMUM study. Mult Scler J. 2019;
27. Vaclavkova A, Chimenti S, Arenberger P, Holló P, Sator PG, Burcklen M, et al. Oral ponesimod in patients with chronic plaque psoriasis: a randomised, double-blind, placebo-controlled phase 2 trial. Lancet. 2014;384(9959):2036–45.
28. Montgomery S, Hillert J, Bahmanyar S. Hospital admission due to infections in multiple sclerosis patients. Eur J Neurol. 2013;20(8):1153–60.
29. Grebenciucova E, Pruitt A. Infections in patients receiving multiple sclerosis disease-modifying therapies. Curr Neurol Neurosci Rep. 2017;17(11):88.
30. Winkelmann A, Loebermann M, Reisinger EC, Hartung HP, Zettl UK. Disease-modifying therapies and infectious risks in multiple sclerosis. Nature reviews. Neurology. 2016;12(4):217–33.
31. Soelberg SP. Safety concerns and risk management of multiple sclerosis therapies. Acta Neurol Scand. 2017;136(3):168–86.
32. Luna G, Alping P, Burman J, Fink K, Fogdell-Hahn A, Gunnarsson M, et al. Infection risks among patients with multiple sclerosis treated with fingolimod, Natalizumab, Rituximab, and Injectable Therapies. JAMA Neurol. 2020;77(2):184–91.
33. Pfender N, Jelcic I, Linnebank M, Schwarz U, Martin R. Reactivation of herpesvirus under fingolimod: a case of severe herpes simplex encephalitis. Neurology. 2015;84(23):2377–8.
34. Hagiya H, Yoshida H, Shimizu M, Motooka D, Nakamura S, Iida T, et al. Herpes zoster laryngitis in a patient treated with fingolimod. J Infect Chemother. 2016;22(12):830–2.
35. Forrestel AK, Modi BG, Longworth S, Wilck MB, Micheletti RG. Primary cutaneous cryptococcus in a patient with multiple sclerosis treated with fingolimod. JAMA Neurology. 2016;73(3):355–6.
36. Seto H, Nishimura M, Minamiji K, Miyoshi S, Mori H, Kanazawa K, et al. Disseminated cryptococcosis in a 63-year-old patient with multiple sclerosis treated with fingolimod. Intern Med. 2016;55(22):3383–6.
37. Ward MD, Jones DE, Goldman MD. Cryptococcal meningitis after fingolimod discontinuation in a patient with multiple sclerosis. Mult Scler Relat Disord. 2016;9:47–9.
38. Artemiadis AK, Nikolaou G, Kolokythopoulos D, Tegos N, Terentiou A, Triantafyllou N, et al. Visceral leishmaniasis infection in a fingolimod-treated multiple sclerosis patient. Mult Scler. 2015;21(6):795–6.
39. Behle V, Wobser M, Goebeler M, Stoevesandt J. Extensive molluscum contagiosum virus infection in a young adult receiving fingolimod. Mult Scler. 2016;22(7):969–71.
40. Faulkner M. Risk of progressive multifocal leukoencephalopathy in patients with multiple sclerosis. Expert Opin Drug Saf. 2015;14(11):1737–48.
41. Gyang TV, Hamel J, Goodman AD, Gross RA, Samkoff L. Fingolimod-associated PML in a patient with prior immunosuppression. Neurology. 2016;86(19):1843–5.
42. Enriquez-Marulanda A, Valderrama-Chaparro J, Parrado L, Diego Vélez J, Maria Granados A, Luis Orozco J, et al. Cerebral toxoplasmosis in an MS patient receiving fingolimod. Mult Scler Relat Disord. 2017;18:106–8.
43. Tecellioglu M, Kamisli O, Kamisli S, Erdogmus UA, Özcan C. Listeria monocytogenes rhombencephalitis in a patient with multiple sclerosis during fingolimod therapy. Mult Scler Relat Disord 2019; \:409-411
44. Walker S, Brew B. Kaposi sarcoma in a fingolimod-treated patient with multiple sclerosis. J Clin Neurosci. 2016;31:217–8.

45. Tagawa A, Ogawa T, Tetsuka S, Otsuka M, Hashimoto R, Kato H, et al. Hepatitis C virus (HCV) reactivation during fingolimod treatment for relapsing and remitting multiple sclerosis. Mult Scler Relat Disord. 2016;9:155–7.
46. Luca B, Tommaso G, Bavaro DF, Laura M, Annalisa S, Gioacchino A, et al. Seroconversion and indolent course of COVID-19 in patients with multiple sclerosis treated with fingolimod and teriflunomide. J Neurol Sci. 2020;416:117011.
47. Barzegar M, Mirmosayyeb O, Nehzat N, Sarrafi R, Khorvash F, Maghzi AH, et al. COVID-19 infection in a patient with multiple sclerosis treated with fingolimod. Neurol Neuroimmunol Neuroinflamm. 2020;7(4):e753.
48. Valencia-Sanchez C, Wingerchuk DM. A Fine balance: immunosuppression and immunotherapy in a patient with multiple sclerosis and COVID-19, vol. 42. Mult Scler Relat Disord; 2020. p. 102182.
49. Foerch C, Friedauer L, Bauer B, Wolf T, Adam EH. Severe COVID-19 infection in a patient with multiple sclerosis treated with fingolimod. Mult Scler Relat Disord. 2020;42:102180.

Immune Checkpoint Inhibitors 13

Keith C. K. Lau, Benson Weyant, and Carlos Cervera

Introduction to Immune Checkpoint Blockade

Appropriate and effective functioning of the immune system requires a delicate balance between activation against foreign antigens and tolerance to self-molecules. The disruption of this balance is evident in immunosuppressed or immunocompromised individuals who have significantly increased susceptibility to infectious agents or reactivation of immunologically suppressed pathogens. A prime example of this phenomenon is observed in human immunodeficiency virus (HIV)-acquired immunodeficiency syndrome (AIDS) patients who are prone to opportunistic fungal infections such as cryptococcal meningitis. On the other hand, the lack of an appropriate self-antigen tolerance can manifest into severe autoimmune diseases such as type I diabetes mellitus.

The defining characteristics of foreign antigen specificity and self-tolerance are mediated by the adaptive immunity and their main cellular effectors – lymphocytes. An essential component in the maintenance of the immunological balance of specificity and tolerance is the immune costimulatory checkpoints that are crucial in regulating lymphocyte activation and function. Cytotoxic T-lymphocyte antigen (CTLA)-4 and the programmed cell death (PD)-1/PD-L1 axes are two

Keith C. K. Lau and Benson Weyant contributed equally with all other contributors.

K. C. K. Lau
Faculty of Medicine and Dentistry, University of Alberta, Edmonton, CA, Canada
e-mail: klau@ualberta.ca

B. Weyant
Department of Medicine, University of Alberta Hospital, Edmonton, CA, Canada
e-mail: weyant@ualberta.ca

C. Cervera (✉)
Division of Infectious Diseases, Department of Medicine, University of Alberta Hospital, Edmonton, CA, Canada
e-mail: cerveraa@ualberta.ca

C. Cervera, J. M. Aguado (eds.), *Infectious Complications in Biologic and Targeted Therapies*, https://doi.org/10.1007/978-3-031-11363-5_13

well-characterized immune checkpoints which are foundational as immunotherapeutic targets and will be discussed in further detail.

CTLA-4 Immune Checkpoint

Activation and subsequent regulation of T-lymphocytes are determined through a combination of stimulatory and/or inhibitory signals. One such regulatory checkpoint is dependent on the CD28 receptor, which is important in the antigen priming and activation of naïve T cells. These immune cells utilize T-cell receptors (TCR) for recognition of a specific antigen presented on the appropriate major histocompatibility complex (MHC) molecule, which provides an initial activating signal (i.e., signal 1). However, signal 1 alone is insufficient for T-lymphocyte activation, and additional costimulatory interactions between the lymphocyte and antigen presentation cells (APC) are required. More specifically, the CD28 molecule present on the cell surface of naïve T cells can interact with B7-1 (CD80) and/or B7-2 (CD86) located on the APCs (Fig. 13.1a). These interactions serve as additional activation

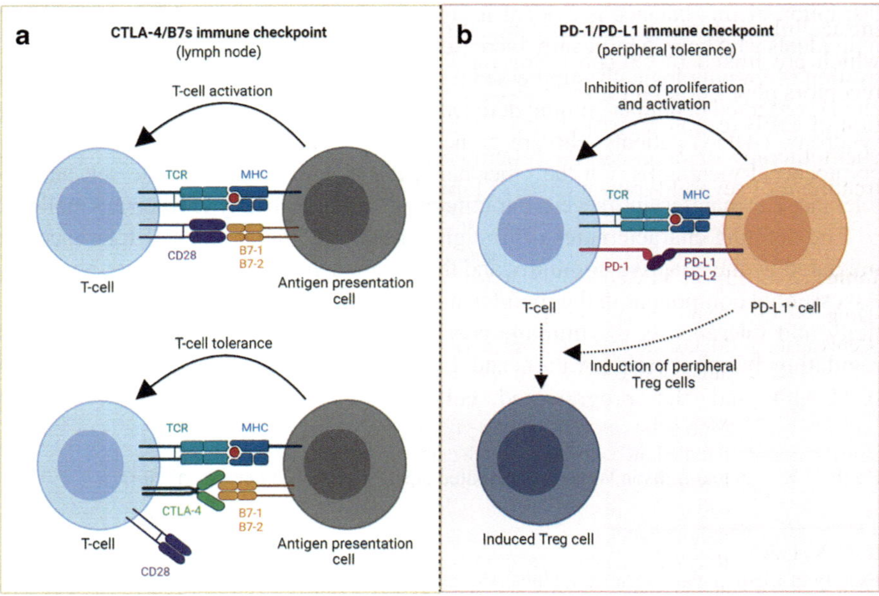

Fig. 13.1 Immune checkpoints fundamental for immunotherapeutic targeting using checkpoint inhibitors. (**a**) CTLA-4/B7s axis is characterized by the interaction of CTLA-4 with B7-1 and/or B7-2. Activation of T cells arises with signal 1 (TCR + MHC) in combination with costimulatory signal 2 (CD28 + B7-1/B7-2) present on antigen-presenting cells. However, CTLA-4 serves to outcompete CD28 for interactions with B7s thereby inducing T-cell tolerance and inactivity. (**b**) PD-1/PD-L1 checkpoint is primarily associated with peripheral tolerance (e.g., tumor tissues). PD-1 on activated T cells interacts with PD-L1 expressed by a variety of cells including tumor cells and immunosuppressive cells. This association results in inhibition of T-cell activity, proliferation, and function thereby inducing T-cell exhaustion or anergy. In addition, peripheral Treg cells are induced which further suppress peripheral T-cell responses. (Figure prepared using Biorender.com)

signals (i.e., signal 2) that subsequently induce naïve T-cell activation and differentiation against the presenting antigen.

Shortly after T cell activation via TCR binding to MHC, CTLA-4 expression is induced. CTLA-4 serves as an inhibitory signal receptor that can bind selectively to the B7-1 and B7-2 ligands (Fig. 13.1a). Through interactions with these ligands, CTLA-4 utilizes a combination of cell-intrinsic and cell-extrinsic mechanisms for immune regulation. CTLA-4 expression on cells can directly outcompete the costimulatory receptor CD28, thereby blocking activation signals to subsequently dampen T lymphocytes. Furthermore, CTLA-4 ligation to B7-1 and B7-2 also modulates intracellular signaling pathways which prevent appropriate activation via TCR signal transduction [1].

CTLA-4 also possesses cell-extrinsic immune modulatory mechanisms. A particular feature of CTLA-4 is the capability of inducing trans-endocytosis of the B7–1 and B7–2 ligands. In brief, CTLA-4 can essentially remove the B7 ligands from APCs thereby effectively reducing the presence and levels of the B7 ligands required for T-cell activation [2]. An important subset of cellular immune mediators is the regulatory T (Treg) cells that may utilize B7 trans-endocytosis as an aspect of their immunosuppressive activities [1, 3]. Indeed, CTLA-4 function and expression have been shown to contribute toward Treg cell-mediated suppression of host immune responses and the induction of immune tolerance.

However, it is important to highlight the essential physiological role of CTLA-4 in immunological balance. Indeed, the appropriate function of CTLA-4 is best demonstrated by murine models lacking functional copies of this gene (CTLA-$4^{-/-}$). These CTLA-4 double knockout mice would succumb to extensive lymphoproliferation that invades multiple organ systems shortly after birth [4]. Similarly, autoimmune diseases in humans such as type I diabetes mellitus have been associated with dysfunctional or mutated CTLA-4 [1, 5].

PD-1/PD-L1 Immune Checkpoint

The second prototypical immune checkpoint is the interaction of PD-1 with endogenous ligands, mainly PD-L1 and to a lesser extent PD-L2. The PD-1/PD-L1 axis serves as a potent negative feedback loop in which pro-inflammatory cytokines can induce the expression of PD-L1 in both immune cells and nonimmune tissues/cells. Although PD-1 is constitutively expressed in naïve T lymphocytes, both PD-1 and PD-L1 expression can be upregulated upon their activation [6]. The ligation of PD-1 with PD-L1 inhibits T-lymphocyte activation and function through disruption of TCR signaling pathways, metabolic activity, cytokine production, as well as cellular proliferation and survival (Fig. 13.1b) [6, 7].

With the variety of different tissue expression patterns in both immune and nonimmune cells, the PD-1/PD-L1 immune checkpoint is primarily focused upon the peripheral tissues and tolerance. Indeed, PD-1/PD-L1 interaction can also induce the differentiation of naïve T cells into a particular subset of Treg cells that are induced peripherally (Fig. 13.1b) [6]. Another feature contributing to peripheral tolerance is the presence of exhausted or anergic T cells. Extensive expression of PD-1 is characteristic of this unique subset of cells with reduced immune activity and function [6, 7]. Similar to CTLA-4, it is important to note the significance of PD-1 toward appropriate immunological balance as demonstrated by murine models that develop autoimmune conditions when PD-1 is dysfunction or deficient [7].

Brief History of Immune Checkpoint Inhibitors

Unfortunately, a variety of infectious agents and neoplastic diseases have developed mechanisms that exploit these immune checkpoints to evade the immune system, thereby advancing their replication, proliferation, and growth. Chronic infections from viral pathogens including HIV and hepatitis B virus often induce immune tolerance and anergy to facilitate their persistence. Long-term exposure to viral antigens such as HBV surface protein is associated with the sustained expression of PD-1 and creation of exhausted or anergic T cells [6]. Similarly, a variety of malignant cancers frequently recruit and foster immune cells in their tumor microenvironment that expresses high levels of PD-1 or PD-L1 [6]. Often, the tumor cells themselves overexpress or amplify PD-L1 to attenuate antitumor T-cell responses in order to evade immune-mediated destruction [6, 7].

To counteract the ineffective antitumor effects observed within malignant diseases, immune checkpoint inhibitors (ICI) were developed and have made significant progress within the field of cancer therapeutics. Indeed, this progress resulted in the 2018 Nobel Prize in Medicine which recognized the immense clinical potential and impact of these anticancer immunotherapies. The conceptualization of using inhibitors specifically targeting of CTLA-4 and PD-1 originated in the 1990s.

Shortly after the discovery of CTLA-4 as an inhibitor of T-cell activation, Allsion and his colleagues hypothesized that CTLA-4 might be hindering effective endogenous antitumor immunity [8]. Indeed, the seminal publications from their group demonstrated the powerful antitumor effects and potential of antibodies targeting CTLA-4 [8]. Successful studies in preclinical models of anti-CTLA-4 in a variety of cancers eventually led to human clinical trials, the first of which began in 2003 with ipilimumab (Bristol-Myers Squibb's Yervoy®). In 2011, ipilimumab was the first ICI approved by the FDA for use in unresectable or metastatic melanoma (Table 13.1) [9]. Subsequent clinical trials with ipilimumab have been completed which now has expanded uses beyond advanced melanoma, as well as combination therapies with anti-PD-1 therapy (i.e., nivolumab) [9]. Building off the success in melanoma, ipilimumab (and other anti-CTLA-4 agents) are being explored in other malignancies either as monotherapy or in a combination therapy with other immunotherapies or chemotherapies (www.clinicaltrials.gov). Aside from ipilimumab, the other notable anti-CTLA-4 agent thus far with some clinical success is tremelimumab (by AstraZeneca) which is undergoing continual research in a variety of trials as a monotherapy or combination therapy. A more comprehensive description of clinical indications of anti-CTLA-4 agents will be discussed in Sect. 3.1 and 3.2.

Table 13.1 Immune checkpoint inhibitors approved for clinical use in the USA (FDA) and Canada (Health Canada) at the time of writing (November 2020). Data obtained from FDA medication guides (https://www.accessdata.fda.gov/scripts/cder/daf/index.cfm?event=medguide.page) and Health Canada drug product database (https://www.canada.ca/en/health-canada/services/drugs-health-products/drug-products/drug-product-database.html)

Target	Agents (brand name)	Indications[a]	Year of initial FDA approval
CTLA-4	Ipilimumab (Yervoy®)	Melanoma	2011
PD-1	Nivolumab (Opdivo®)	Melanoma, NSCLC, *SCLC*[b], RCC, *cHL*, HNSCC, *UC*[b], *CRC*[b], *HCC*, ESCC[b]	2014
	Pembrolizumab (Keytruda®)	Melanoma, NSCLC, *SCLC*[b], HNSC, cHL, PMBCL, UC, *MSI-H*, *GC*[b], ESCC[b], *CC*[b], *HCC*[b], *MCC*[b], RCC, *ENC*, *TMB-H*[b], cSCC[b]	2014
	Cemiplimab(Libtayo®)	cSCC	2018
CTLA-4 + PD-1	Ipilimumab + nivolumab	RCC, *CRC*[b], *HCC*[b], *NSCLC*[b], mesothelioma[b]	2015
PD-L1	Atezolizumab(Tecentriq®)	*UC*, NSCLC, *BC*, SCLC, HCC, melanoma[b]	2016
	Avelumab (Bavencio®)	*MCC*, UC, RCC[b]	2017
	Durvalumab (Imfinzi®)	*UC*, NSCLC, SCLC	2017

[a]*BC* breast cancer, *CC* cervical cancer, *cHL* classical Hodgkin's lymphoma, *CRC* colorectal cancer, *cSCC* cutaneous squamous cell carcinoma, *ENC* endometrial carcinoma, *ESCC* esophageal squamous cell carcinoma, *GC* gastric cancer, *HCC* hepatocellular carcinoma, *HNSC* head and neck squamous cell carcinoma, *MSI-H* microsatellite instability high, *NSCLC* non-small cell lung cancer, *PMBCL* primary mediastinal B-cell lymphoma, *RCC* renal cell carcinoma, *SCLC* small cell lung cancer, *TMB-H* tumor mutational burden-high cancer, *UC* urothelial carcinoma

[b]Currently only approved for use in the USA, but not Canada

Italics indicates FDA approval is contingent on verification and confirmatory trials (accelerated approval). Typically, Health Canada approval follows the FDA although medications may not be immediately approved by Health Canada or they may remain NOC/c (notice of compliance with conditions) for a period of time after FDA approval

Discovery of PD-1 itself and its immune modulatory function was spearheaded by the work of Honjo and his colleagues in the 1990s. Subsequent identification of PD-L1 and PD-L2 as ligands of PD-1 was achieved in 2000 and 2001, respectively. These important findings led to the creation of anti-PD-1 and anti-PD-L1 antibodies which were tested in murine models of cancer. The remarkable preclinical results quickly led to human clinical trials which began in 2006 with nivolumab (marketed as Opdivo® by Bristol-Myers Squibb), an anti-PD-1-based immunotherapy. Nivolumab was eventually approved in 2014 by the FDA for use as therapy for advanced melanoma (Table 13.1, Sect. 3.4) [9]. Due to a combination of improved therapeutic efficiency, range of activity, and reduced drug-related adverse effects, anti-PD-1 and anti-PD-L1 therapeutic candidates have surpassed that of anti-CTLA-4 [9]. Indeed, nivolumab was approved shortly after pembrolizumab (Keytruda® by Merck) which received recognition as the first ICI targeting PD-1 for clinical use (see Sect. 3.3). Since 2018, a third anti-PD-1 monoclonal antibody cemiplimab (Libtayo® by Regeneron) is now clinically available (Table 13.1, Sect. 3.5). Furthermore, atezolizumab (Roche's Tecentriq®), avelumab (Bavenio® by EMD Serono/Pfizer), and durvalumab (Imfinzi® by AstraZeneca) were FDA approved as human therapeutics in 2016, 2017, and 2017, respectively. These three anti-PD-L1-based immunotherapies are recognized for their utility against a growing list of malignant diseases (Table 13.1, Sect. 3.6–3.8).

Considering the different immune pathways targeted by anti-CTLA-4 and anti-PD-1 agents, combination therapy of the two was explored beginning with ipilimumab and nivolumab. The simultaneous targeting of these separate pathways has been successful in terms of enhancing the antitumor efficacy observed with monotherapy use [3, 9]. Indeed, ipilimumab and nivolumab are now clinically indicated for use in a variety of non-melanoma malignancies (Table 13.1, Sect. 3). The success of ipilimumab and nivolumab opened the doorway for additional research into combinatory therapies with other immunotherapy agents. For example, pembrolizumab and ipilimumab are currently within a phase III clinical trial as first-line therapy for non-small cell lung cancer (NCT03302234). These developments in combination therapies allow for further expansion of the clinical uses of ICIs to improve cancer immunotherapies.

Although the clinical advancements of ICIs thus far have primarily been focused upon malignant neoplastic diseases, it is important to highlight that ICIs are also being explored for use in chronic viral infections (see Sect. 5). With the immunosuppressive similarities between persistent viral infections and cancer, a number of studies in chronic diseases such as HIV or HBV have been initiated (www.clinicaltrials.gov; example search terms: HIV or HBV with PD-1, CTLA-4, PD-L1, ipilimumab, nivolumab, etc.).

The field of ICIs is exceptionally promising with an explosion of therapeutic options with an increasing range of activity against malignant diseases. Since the discoveries of CTLA-4 and PD-1/PD-L1 immune checkpoints, additional inhibitory regulators of T-cell function and markers of exhausted T-cells have been identified. Some of the more prominent contenders include but are not limited to LAG-3, TIGIT, and B7-H3 [10]. Moving forward, additional research into these molecules and checkpoints will likely produce an increasing variety of different therapeutic possibilities for the next generation of immunotherapies and the prospect of combination therapies. Indeed, a variety of clinical trials including phase II and III trials are currently underway for antibodies targeting LAG3, TIGIT, and B7-H3 as either monotherapies or combination therapies [10]. Appropriately understanding the clinical outcomes and risks of ICI use will be of utmost importance as this field of immune-modulating therapies rapidly expands.

Mechanism of Action of Immune Checkpoint Inhibitors

All ICIs currently approved for clinical use are biologic agents, namely, monoclonal antibodies, that specifically interfere with CTLA-4, PD-1, or PD-L1 signaling. Overall, the blockade of these checkpoints aims to reinvigorate the immune system by removing the brakes to the antitumor responses. Recognizing the mechanism of action of these monoclonal antibody therapies is essential to understand the potential adverse effects as well as inform the development of improved ICIs.

Ipilimumab, the anti-CTLA-4 biologic, functions through a combination of two main mechanisms. The binding of the monoclonal antibody to CTLA-4 introduces a direct block that prevents interactions of this receptor to the endogenous ligands B7-1 and B7-2 [1, 3]. As a result, CTLA-4 can no longer serve as a competitive inhibitor for the costimulatory CD28 nor induce intracellular signaling changes that prevent T-cell activation. Through this interaction, ipilimumab functions to allow activation and priming of T cells toward tumor antigens (Fig. 13.2a). In addition, a secondary effect of anti-CTLA-4 is Treg cell depletion. The specific binding of ipilimumab can induce antibody-dependent cellular cytotoxicity (ADCC) of Tregs, which generally express CTLA-4, thereby reducing their immunosuppressive effects on antitumor immunity (Fig. 13.2a) [3]. This secondary mechanism of action is important to note as the lack of ADCC activity might be responsible for the reduced efficacy of tremelimumab, an additional anti-CTLA-4 agent that has yet to receive approval for clinical use [1, 3].

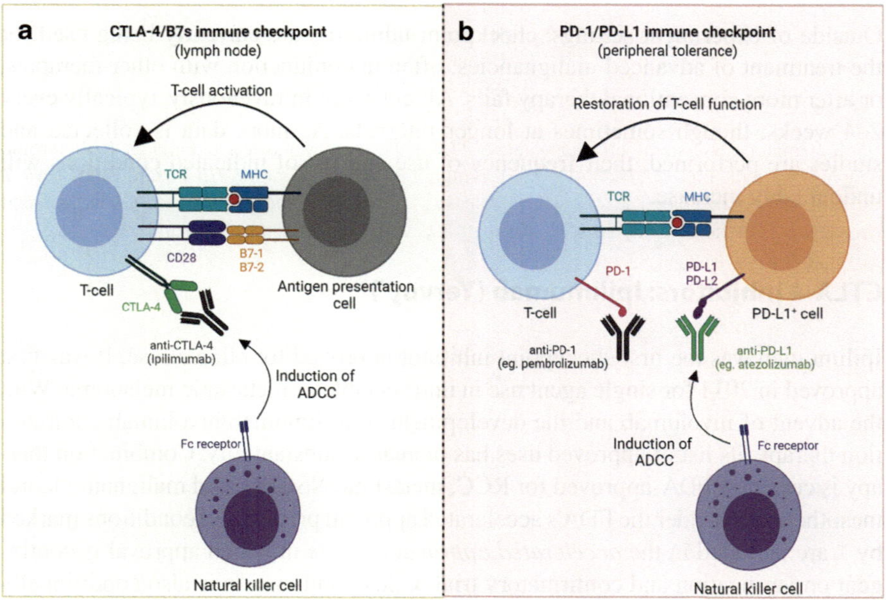

Fig. 13.2 Mechanism of action of immune checkpoint inhibitors targeting the CTLA-4/B7s and PD-1/PD-L1 axes. (**a**) Monoclonal antibodies targeting CTLA-4 (e.g., ipilimumab) serve to sterically hinder interaction with B7s thus eliminating the competition with the costimulatory CD28. In addition, ipilimumab serves to identify CTLA-4⁺ T cells which are targeted by antibody-dependent cellular cytotoxicity (ADCC) mediated by binding of the anti-CTLA-4 Fc. (**b**) PD-1/PD-L1 checkpoint is inhibited with the use of either anti-PD-1 (e.g., pembrolizumab) or anti-PD-L1 (e.g., atezolizumab). Attenuating PD-1/PD-L1 interactions allows for restoration of T-cell function and activity. Anti-PD-L1 agents are also associated with the induction of ADCC thereby directly removing PD-L1-expressing malignant cells. (Figure prepared using Biorender.com)

The basis of anti-PD-1 immunotherapy is to disrupt the PD-1/PD-L1 immune checkpoint axis. By preventing the interaction of these two cell surface molecules, their inhibitory effects on T cells can be attenuated. An important aspect of anti-PD-1 therapy is the targeting of exhausted T cells which are characterized, at least in part, with sustained elevated expression of PD-1 [3]. By inhibiting the signals transduced through PD-1 and PD-L1, exhausted T cells can regain their function and proliferative capabilities (Fig. 13.2b). Thus, T cells previously exposed to tumor antigens that were subsequently rendered anergic or tolerant can be restored into antitumor effectors. It is noteworthy to mention that the three currently approved anti-PD-1 therapies (nivolumab, pembrolizumab, and cemiplimab) are IgG4 antibodies which lack effective cytotoxic capabilities (i.e., ADCC and complement dependent cytotoxicity) [1]. As the endogenous ligand for PD-1, biologic therapies targeting PD-L1 have similar mechanisms of action. However, an additional feature of anti-PD-L1 biologic agents is the benefit of ADCC which also directly induces cell death in tumor cells that express PD-L1 (Fig. 13.2b).

Indications

Outside of experiment settings, checkpoint inhibitors are currently being used for the treatment of advanced malignancies, often in conjunction with other therapies, or after more conventional therapy fails. All are given intravenously, typically every 2–4 weeks, though sometimes at longer intervals. As more data is collected and studies are performed, their frequency of use and list of indicated conditions will undoubtably increase.

CTLA-4 Inhibitors: Ipilimumab (Yervoy®)

Ipilimumab was the first checkpoint inhibitor approved for clinical use. It was first approved in 2011 for single agent use in unresectable or metastatic melanoma. With the advent of nivolumab and the development of ipilimumab/nivolumab combination therapy, its list of approved uses has increased substantially. Combination therapy is currently FDA-approved for RCC, metastatic NSCLC, and malignant pleural mesothelioma. Under the FDA's accelerated approval process (all conditions marked by * are included in the *accelerated approval process* in which approval is contingent on verification and confirmatory trials), this combination is also conditionally approved for several other cancers including HCC and MSI-H or mismatch repair deficient metastatic CRC.

Tremelimumab

Tremelimumab has been tested as mono- or part of combination therapy for several cancers such as NSCLC, SCLC, and UC. Unfortunately, none of these trials have found success and lead to FDA approval. Despite this, research continues, and promising results for a phase II trial in advanced HCC have been reported recently (NCT02519348).

PD-1 Inhibitors: Pembrolizumab (Keytruda®)

When pembrolizumab was approved for use in 2014, it was the first of the PD-1 inhibitor class. Like ipilimumab, it was first indicated for the treatment of unresectable melanoma. In 2017, it would make history when studies showed it could treat microsatellite instability-high (MSI-H) or mismatch repair-deficient malignancies. Microsatellite instability is the measure of the number of genetic mutations in a tumor cell's microsatellite DNA sequences, used a marker of prognosis. Pembrolizumab's approval for MSI-H malignancies marked the first time a medication could be used for a cancer based on a biomarker, rather than the origin location in the body. Later in 2020, pembrolizumab would receive its second biomarker-based approval from the FDA. This time, it was for unresectable or metastatic tumors with a high tumor mutational burden (TMB-H), defined as >10 mutations/megabase. While some indications for Pembrolizumab are based on biomarkers, others are based on location of the cancer or the location in addition to a biomarker such as tumor proportion score (TPS), the percentage of tumor cells that express PD-L1. Typically, the medication is indicated if either conventional treatment has failed or biomarker requirements are met. Pembrolizumab is also currently approved for NSCLC, SCLC, HNSCC, HL, PMLBCL, UC, GC*, ESCC, CC* HCC*, MCC*, RCC, ENC*, and cSCC.

Nivolumab (Opdivo®)

Nivolumab was approved shortly after Pembrolizumab. Like the earlier ICIs, it was originally approved for use in advanced melanoma. It would later have its approval expanded to NSCLC and then SCLC. As monotherapy, it can also be used for HNSCC and ESCC. Together with ipilimumab, it is approved for use in malignant pleural mesothelioma, metastatic NSCLC, and RCC. Accelerated approval has been granted by the FDA for use in UC, cHL, MSI-H, or mismatch repair-deficient CRC and HCC.

Cemiplimab (Libtayo®)

Cemiplimab, the latest PD-1 inhibitor, was approved for use in 2018. Being a newer medication, it has fewer indicated uses than other ICIs. Currently, it is only approved for metastatic cSCC or locally advanced cutaneous SCC in patients who are not candidates for surgery or radiation.

PD-L1 Inhibitors: Atezolizumab (Tecentriq®)

Atezolizumab was approved for use in 2016, the first of the PD-L1 inhibitor class. Its initial indication was for use in UC*, and it has since been approved for NSCLC, triple-negative BC*, SCLC, HCC, and melanoma. Atezolizumab is often used as part of a cancer regimen alongside chemotherapy agents carboplatin and etoposide, in addition to newer agents such as bevacizumab, cobimetinib, and vemurafenib.

Avelumab (Bavencio®)

Avelumab's first indicated use was in metastatic MCC in 2017*. This made it the first ICI not originally approved for use in advanced skin cancer (either melanoma or cSCC). Other approved indications include UC and advanced RCC.

Durvalumab (Imfinzi®)

Like atezolizumab, durvalumab is currently approved for use in UC*. NSCLC and SCLC were later added to its list of indications.

Checkpoint Inhibitors and Infections

Mechanisms Predisposing to Infection

There are several possible mechanisms through which immune checkpoint inhibitors can predispose individuals to infection, each with their own level of evidence to support them.

The first, and most common mechanism, is through immune-related adverse events (irAEs). By "boosting" the immune system, ICIs can cause autoimmune inflammatory reactions. Due to the ubiquitous nature of the immune system, any organ system can be involved, though most commonly are the gastrointestinal tract (colitis, diarrhea, pancreatitis, and hepatitis), lungs (pneumonitis and sarcoidosis), endocrine glands (hypo−/hyperthyroidism, thyroiditis, hypophysitis, diabetes mellitus, Addison's disease, and adrenal insufficiency), skin (rash and vitiligo) [11]. The exact mechanism behind these adverse events is unclear, but these autoimmune events make sense from a mechanistic perspective. The healthy immune system is constantly trying to find equilibrium between detecting intruders (microbes, cancer) and not reacting to the host. A balance that most of the time is carefully struck. Checkpoint molecules are part of this crucial balancing act, by "deactivating" immune cells when they are no longer needed. However, when a host develops a malignancy, the scales can be tipped toward inactivation. Studies have shown that tumor cells are able to upregulate checkpoint molecules [6], an adaptation that likely helps avoid an immune-mediated demise. When we use ICIs, we are shifting the balance toward immune-system activation, which can lead to the collateral damage of autoimmune events. These events usually occur several weeks-months after starting an ICI; however, they can occur at any point, even after discontinuation [12]. Treatment for irAEs typically involves the use of corticosteroids, and if corticosteroids are ineffective, then another immunosuppressive therapy may be required. In this mechanism, it is the treatment of the side effects (irAEs) rather than the ICI itself that predisposes to infection. Interestingly, the different classes of ICIs do not seem to have identical side effect profiles. CTLA-4 inhibitors tend to cause more GI symptoms or hypophysitis, whereas the PD-1 inhibitors cause more pneumonitis and arthralgias.

The second way that ICIs can predispose to infection is through immune-mediated cytopenia. Like other irAEs, the exact mechanism is unclear. The frequency of these hematopoietic immune events has been found to be around 0.5% [13], and they can present in a wide spectrum of conditions such as immune thrombocytopenia, autoimmune hemolytic anemia, neutropenia, aplastic anemia, and hemophagocytic syndrome. Not only do these events usually warrant immune suppression on their own, but neutropenia can also predispose patients to opportunistic infections. One review found that of 11 cases of ICI-induced neutropenia, 6 were complicated by severe infection [13]. These immune-mediated cytopenia's were typically reversible and usually treated with some combination of granulocyte-colony stimulating factor, corticosteroids, IVIG, or other immunosuppressants.

Lastly, it has been suggested that ICIs can lead to the development/reactivation of tuberculosis (TB) independent of immune suppression for irAEs. Several cases have been published on patients, not on immunosuppressants, who develop acute pulmonary TB after taking ICIs for metastatic malignancies. There are many confounding factors to consider when looking at TB infection in patients on ICIs. For one, patients are often started on ICIs after first undergoing many cycles of chemotherapy. Second, cancer itself is a risk factor for infection. Diagnosis can also be difficult as TB and lung cancer share many symptoms and pneumonitis is a documented side effect of the PD-1/PD-L1 inhibitors. There are some preclinical trials to support this notion as studies in mice have suggested that PD-1/PD-L1 play a protective role against the reactivation of TB [14]. One theory is that ICIs activate mycobacterium-specific T cells, leading to an immune reconstitution syndrome. Looking beyond case reports, the data suggests that TB reactivation is very rare in patients on ICIs. One retrospective study observed 1144 patients taking ICIs over a 4-year period and found that only three patients developed tuberculosis, and two of them were taking immunosuppressants prior to their diagnosis [15]. Another retrospective study looked at 908 patients on PD-1/PD-L1 inhibitors and found two cases of TB, neither had been on immunosuppressants [16].

Risk of Infection

Assessing the absolute risk of infection with ICIs is difficult for several reasons. Rates of infection are typically secondary outcomes in trials, often lacking detail in the types of infections or how they were diagnosed. The patients on these medications commonly have many comorbidities, are usually seriously ill, and may have completed several cycles of chemotherapy.

Initial studies were done on ipilimumab, as it was the first ICI approved for human use. The phase 2 trials for ipilimumab in melanoma patients did not show an increased risk of infection [17]. A head-to-head trial of ipilimumab plus dacarbazine versus placebo plus dacarbazine also found no increased risk of infections, though there were significantly more adverse events [18].

The largest study, a retrospective study done by Castillo et al. [19], looked at 740 patients receiving ICIs for melanoma and found that 54 (7.3%) developed serious infections (defined as requiring hospital admission or parenteral antibiotics). The risk factors identified for a serious infection were corticosteroid use (OR 7.71), infliximab use (OR 4.74), or the use of ipilimumab and nivolumab together. Pembrolizumab was inversely associated with the risk of serious infections. These different infection rates are likely attributable to the variable risk of irAEs as 69% of patients treated with ipilimumab plus nivolumab received corticosteroids compared to only 6% of the patients who received pembrolizumab alone. Bacterial infections were the most common (pneumonia, bacteremia, *C. difficile*-associated diarrhea and intra-abdominal infections), but there were also cases of fungal (invasive pulmonary aspergillosis, pneumocystis pneumonia, and candidemia), viral (herpes zoster, CMV colitis, and EBV), and parasitic (single case of *Strongyloides*) infections.

Komodo et al. [20] did a retrospective analysis on 111 patients taking either nivolumab, pembrolizumab, or ipilimumab and found that 14% developed a serious infection. Patients who were on steroids had a much higher risk of developing a serious infection. Bacterial infections were the most common cause of serious infections (pneumonia, genitourinary infections, SSTIs, and bacteremia), and there were only a few cases of viral infections (enterovirus and rhinovirus).

Another study, done by Fujita et al. [21], reviewed 167 patients with NSCLC who had been treated with nivolumab. They found that 19.2% of the patients developed an infection that required the use of antimicrobials. Of these infections, most were bacterial, but there were some viral and fungal infections as well. This study found that only type 2 diabetes, and not steroid use, was associated with an increased risk of infection. Several limitations to this study were brought up by the authors themselves. The main limitation is that it was difficult to distinguish pneumonia for pneumonitis, and their definition of infection included patients who were empirically given antibiotics. This could explain the higher incidence of infection and why there was no association found with immunosuppressant use.

Current Guidelines

Due to the minor risk of infection associated with ICIs, society guidelines such as the European Society of Medical Oncology [22] and the American Society of Clinical Oncology [23] do not recommend treating patients with infectious prophylactic mediations (either antiviral or anti-pneumocystis). However, prophylaxis is still recommended in patients who are being treated with prolonged immune suppression for ICI-induced irAEs, that same as for any individual on prolonged immunosuppressants. Along with this, some guidelines suggest testing for latent TB, in addition to hepatitis B and C, in case immune suppression is required in the future.

Using Checkpoint Inhibitors to Treat Infections

Not only do cancer cells upregulate checkpoint molecules, but checkpoint molecule expression is also increased on lymphocytes in many infectious disease states. This phenomenon is often referred to as immune exhaustion, and given that ICIs can be used to boost the immune system to help detect and fight cancer, a reasonable proposition would be that they could also treat infections. The mechanism for this makes sense, but most, if not all, of the pivotal trials used to investigate efficacy and safety had active infections as an exclusion criterion. To date, there have been no large-scale RCTs for this, but there have been some promising preclinical and phase 1 trials.

Sepsis

Sepsis is an active area of investigation for checkpoint inhibitors. Checkpoint molecule expression is known to be increased in septic patients [24]. The idea is that ICIs would boost the immune system's response and enhance clearance of bacterial or even fungal infections. Several animal models have shown that ICIs improve survival when provoked with a bacterial or lipopolysaccharide challenge. A meta-analysis by Busch et al. [25] looked at mouse models of sepsis and found that ICIs significantly increased the OR of survival in 10/19 of the studies (OR = 3.37 [1.55–7.31]). Of note was that ten of the studies were from the same lab group, and all the studies had a high risk of bias. Due to the somewhat promising preclinical data, two phase I trials were conducted in 2019. One with nivolumab [26] and another with BMS-936559 [27], a PD-L1 inhibitor. Both trials showed that the medication was well tolerated, with no evidence of worsening symptoms or cytokine storm. However, being phase I trials, there were no comparison or placebo arms, so definitive conclusions cannot be drawn about their efficacy at this point.

HIV

Research with HIV and ICIs has been done looking into two main categories, the safety and efficacy of ICIs in treating cancers in HIV+ individuals, and whether ICIs can be used to treat HIV itself. In answering the first question, a meta-analysis done in 2019 looked at 73 patients and concluded that there was no association with adverse changes in HIV viral load or CD4 count [28]. It was also found that the checkpoint inhibitors remained effective against their respective malignancies. The answer to the second question is more nuanced and is still an area of active research.

While antiretroviral therapy can effectively suppress HIV and prevent the development of AIDS, it remains an incurable infection. One of the mechanisms through which HIV is able to persist in its host and remain latent is through T-cell exhaustion and checkpoint inhibitor upregulation [29]. In addition to downregulating T-cell proliferation, in vitro studies have shown that PD-1 activation in CD4+ T cells inhibits HIV viral replication. Studies have also shown that overexpression of checkpoint molecules partially regresses with antiretroviral treatment. It is thought that the use of ICIs would not only activate HIV-specific CD8 T cells, but it would also increase the production of the HIV virus from reservoir cells, shifting the disease state away from latency. A meta-analysis by Baptiste et al. [29] evaluated 176 HIV+ individuals taking ICIs and found that in 92%, the viral load remained stable, and it increased in 6% and decreased in 2%. It was found that CD4 counts remained stable in 61%, and they increased in 24% and decreased in 15%. In 2017, a phase I study was conducted on HIV patients, comparing BMS-936559 (a PD-L1 inhibitor) and placebo [30]. They found that there was an increase in HIV-1-specific CD8 T cells in two out of six of the patients, though the results were not significant when the whole treatment arm was analyzed. Overall ICIs have shown some benefit in decreasing the HIV reservoir, though it is unlikely that their use alone will be substantial enough.

JC Virus

Currently the only treatment available for progressive multifocal leukoencephalopathy (PML) is immune reconstitution. This can come with its own risks, depending on the initial reason for immune suppression, and is not always an option for everyone. In 2019, a case report was published about a patient with Hodgkin lymphoma, on nivolumab, who developed PML and then went into remission [31]. This was followed shortly by a small trial in which eight patients with PML were given three doses of pembrolizumab as an experimental treatment [32]. Five of the eight patients had clinical improvement or stabilization of their symptoms. Of these five patients, four of them had a persistently decreased JC viral load in the CSF, with the other being a temporary decrease. A possible confounder was that the studies could not rule out the possibility of pembrolizumab assisting in the treatment of the underlying malignancies. Unfortunately, this study was followed by several case reports of PML developing in patients being treated with nivolumab [33], and more research will be required in this area.

Hepatitis B

Due to hepatitis B virus's (HBV) causative relationship with hepatocellular carcinoma (HCC), the use of ICIs has been studied in patients with chronic HBV. Metanalysis has shown that ICIs, while they can cause reversible hepatic injury, are safe for use in patients with either chronic HBV or HCV [34]. Like in other chronic infections discussed earlier, HBV is associated with increased checkpoint molecule expression on T lymphocytes. Ex vivo studies have shown that checkpoint inhibition increases HBV-specific T-cell proliferation and the production of protective antibodies [35]. Given this relation, it is thought that HBV clearance could be enhanced with the use of ICIs. A phase I study done in 2019 gave patients with chronic HBV low-dose nivolumab and found that it caused a decreased in HBsAg titers in 91% of the subjects, with one patient seroconverting [36].

Invasive Fungal Infections

Mucormycosis is a serious life-threatening fungal infection caused by fungi in the order Mucorales. These infections are typically seen in the immunosuppressed or the critically ill where they can be challenging to treat. In 2017, the first report of mucormycosis being treated with an ICI was published [37]. The case involved a young woman who survived a terrorist bombing, only to develop invasive intra-abdominal mucormycosis that was nonresponsive to standard treatment. Investigations showed lymphopenia, low monocyte HLA-DR (a T-cell ligand) expression, and increased PD-1 expression on T cells. For this, her treating team gave her interferon-γ and a single dose of nivolumab. The patient made a full recovery, and subsequent investigation showed a reversal of the aforementioned abnormalities. Since then, another case has been described in a woman with AML who developed an invasive infection with aspergillus and lichtheimia [38]. She was treated similarly with interferon-γ and nivolumab. There were signs of recovery, but eventually the patient declined medical treatment due to AML progression. These cases show that under the right circumstances, invasive fungal diseases can be treated with ICIs, though large-scale investigation is still required.

COVID-19

With the COVID-19 pandemic changing almost every aspect of people's lives, it is no wonder that that researchers are investigating the use of ICIs in this viral illness. One large difference between the SARS-CoV-2 virus and other viral infections discussed in this chapter is that rather than remaining latent in its host, COVID-19 causes mortality through a cytokine storm. This is caused by an exaggerated response of the immune system, leading to systemic inflammation which can cause acute respiratory distress syndrome (ARDS) among other complications. Like the other infections in the chapter, COVID has been associated with T-cell exhaustion [39]. Lymphopenia, another complication associated with COVID, is thought due to T-cell exhaustion and abnormal cytokine production. Like all aspects of COVID-19, this is an area of active research. Retrospective analyses on COVID patients who were previously taking ICIs are mixed, and some have shown no difference in severity [40, 41] while others found the opposite [42]. As of writing, there are several registered trials that are assessing the effectiveness of treating COVID-19 with ICIs such as nivolumab (NCT04343144) and pembrolizumab (NCT04335305), though none have been published. Some researchers have suggested that the best benefit from ICIs in COVID-19 might be when paired with an immunosuppressant like tocilizumab (IL-6 inhibitor). This would allow the ICI to prevent T-cell exhaustion, and an IL-6 inhibitor could manage the cytokine storm. A phase II trial has recently been registered to test this hypothesis (NCT04335305). With the incredible resources and speed of COVID research, it is inevitable that we will soon have more answers.

Mouse Models of Infection

In addition to the potential applications of ICIs in human infections, there are several promising uses that have been demonstrated in mice. In a mouse model of infection with *Histoplasma capsulatum*, Lázár-Molnár et al. found that PD-1-deficient mice all survived while wild-type mice died from disseminated infection [43]. Their study also found that most of the wild-type mice survived when given a PD-1 inhibitor. Similarly, for mice with persistent *Cryptococcus neoformans* infections, using a PD-1 inhibitor significantly improved fungal clearance [44]. In mice infected with *Echinococcus multilocularis* (the causative organism of alveolar echinococcosis, which causes cyst formation in the liver, among other organs), PD-1 blockade was associated with a decreased parasite load and fewer liver lesions [45]. These models all showed impressive response to treatment and, given that the side effect profile of ICIs is well known, look for human case reports in the future.

Summary

Checkpoint molecules are cell ligands or receptors that are expressed on lymphocytes, the main cellular component of the adaptive immune system. Activation of checkpoint molecules (PD-1/PD-L1 and CTLA-4) shifts the immune system away from activation and toward tolerance or dormancy. Various cancers and infections have adapted to take advantage of this by causing the upregulation of checkpoint molecules, thereby decreasing lymphocyte function. The medication class of checkpoint inhibitors (ICIs) consists of monoclonal antibodies against checkpoint molecules or their receptors. The use of these antibodies has been shown to prolong survival in many cancers, with much more tolerable side effects compared to traditional chemotherapies. The main complications of ICIs are immune-related adverse events (irAEs). These autoimmune side effects are caused by the shift of the immune system away from self-tolerance, and they can affect almost any organ system. While ICIs by themselves rarely increase infection risk, the treatment of these irAEs (typically with immunosuppressants) is a significant risk factor for various types of infection. In addition to their ever-increasing role in cancer treatment, ICIs have recently shown promise in treating various types of infection, including but not limited to sepsis, HIV, JC virus, and mucormycosis. With the list of potential uses in oncology and infectious diseases growing exponentially, it is important for researchers and clinicians to know and understand this interesting class of medications.

References

1. Lee HT, Lee SH, Heo YS. Molecular interactions of antibody drugs targeting PD-1, PD-L1, and CTLA-4 in immuno-oncology. Molecules. 2019;24(6):1190. https://doi.org/10.3390/molecules24061190.
2. Qureshi OS, Zheng Y, Nakamura K, et al. Trans-endocytosis of CD80 and CD86: a molecular basis for the cell-extrinsic function of CTLA-4. Science. 2011;332(6029):600–3. https://doi.org/10.1126/science.1202947.
3. Wei SC, Duffy CR, Allison JP. Fundamental mechanisms of immune checkpoint blockade therapy. Cancer Discov. 2018;8(9):1069–86. https://doi.org/10.1158/2159-8290.CD-18-0367.
4. Waterhouse P, Penninger JM, Timms E, et al. Lymphoproliferative disorders with early lethality in mice deficient in Ctla-4. Science. 1995;270(5238):985–8. https://doi.org/10.1126/science.270.5238.985.
5. Chen Z, Fei M, Fu D, et al. Association between cytotoxic T lymphocyte antigen-4 polymorphism and type 1 diabetes: a meta-analysis. Gene. 2013;516(2):263–70. https://doi.org/10.1016/j.gene.2012.12.030.
6. Bardhan K, Anagnostou T, Boussiotis VA. The PD1: PD-L1/2 pathway from discovery to clinical implementation. Front Immunol. 2016;7:550. https://doi.org/10.3389/fimmu.2016.00550.
7. Sun C, Mezzadra R, Schumacher TN. Regulation and function of the PD-L1 checkpoint. Immunity. 2018;48(3):434–52. https://doi.org/10.1016/j.immuni.2018.03.014.
8. Leach DR, Krummel MF, Allison JP. Enhancement of antitumor immunity by CTLA-4 blockade. Science. 1996;271(5256):1734–6. https://doi.org/10.1126/science.271.5256.1734.
9. Hargadon KM, Johnson CE, Williams CJ. Immune checkpoint blockade therapy for cancer: an overview of FDA-approved immune checkpoint inhibitors. Int Immunopharmacol. 2018;62:29–39. https://doi.org/10.1016/j.intimp.2018.06.001.
10. Pant A, Medikonda R, Lim M. Alternative checkpoints as targets for immunotherapy. Curr Oncol Rep. 2020;22(12) https://doi.org/10.1007/s11912-020-00983-y.
11. Man J, Ritchie G, Links M, Lord S, Lee CK. Treatment-related toxicities of immune checkpoint inhibitors in advanced cancers: a meta-analysis. Asia Pac J Clin Oncol. 2018;14(3):141–52. https://doi.org/10.1111/ajco.12838.
12. Postow MA, Sidlow R, Hellmann MD. Immune-related adverse events associated with immune checkpoint blockade. N Engl J Med. 2018;378(2):158–68. https://doi.org/10.1056/nejmra1703481.
13. Michot JM, Lazarovici J, Tieu A, et al. Haematological immune-related adverse events with immune checkpoint inhibitors, how to manage? Eur J Cancer. 2019;122:72–90. https://doi.org/10.1016/j.ejca.2019.07.014.
14. Barber DL, Mayer-Barber KD, Feng CG, Sharpe AH, Sher A. CD4 T cells promote rather than control tuberculosis in the absence of PD-1–mediated inhibition. J Immunol. 2011;186(3):1598–607. https://doi.org/10.4049/jimmunol.1003304.

15. Im Y, Lee J, Kim SJ, Koh WJ, Jhun BW, Lee SH. Development of tuberculosis in cancer patients receiving immune checkpoint inhibitors. Respir Med. 2020;161:105853. https://doi.org/10.1016/j.rmed.2019.105853.
16. Picchi H, Mateus C, Chouaid C, et al. Infectious complications associated with the use of immune checkpoint inhibitors in oncology: reactivation of tuberculosis after anti PD-1 treatment. Clin Microbiol Infect. 2018;24(3):216–8. https://doi.org/10.1016/j.cmi.2017.12.003.
17. Redelman-Sidi G, Michielin O, Cervera C, et al. ESCMID study Group for Infections in compromised hosts (ESGICH) consensus document on the safety of targeted and biological therapies: an infectious diseases perspective (immune checkpoint inhibitors, cell adhesion inhibitors, sphingosine-1-phosphate receptor modulators and proteasome inhibitors). Clin Microbiol Infect. 2018;24:S95–S107. https://doi.org/10.1016/j.cmi.2018.01.030.
18. Robert C, Thomas L, Bondarenko I, et al. Ipilimumab plus dacarbazine for previously untreated metastatic melanoma. N Engl J Med. 2011;364(26):2517–26. https://doi.org/10.1056/nejmoa1104621.
19. Del Castillo M, Romero FA, Argüello E, Kyi C, Postow MA, Redelman-Sidi G. The spectrum of serious infections among patients receiving immune checkpoint blockade for the treatment of melanoma. Clin Infect Dis. 2016;63(11):1490–3. https://doi.org/10.1093/cid/ciw539.
20. Komoda K, Ross JA, Margolin K, et al. 1556 Infectious disease complications with use of checkpoint inhibitors in solid organ malignancies. *Open forum*. Infect Dis. 2018;5(suppl_1):S484. https://doi.org/10.1093/ofid/ofy210.1384.
21. Fujita K, Kim YH, Kanai O, Yoshida H, Mio T, Hirai T. Emerging concerns of infectious diseases in lung cancer patients receiving immune checkpoint inhibitor therapy. Respir Med. 2019;146:66–70. https://doi.org/10.1016/j.rmed.2018.11.021.
22. Haanen JBAG, Carbonnel F, Robert C, et al. Management of toxicities from immunotherapy: ESMO clinical practice guidelines for diagnosis, treatment and follow-up. Ann Oncol. 2017;28:iv119–42. https://doi.org/10.1093/annonc/mdx225.
23. Brahmer JR, Lacchetti C, Schneider BJ, et al. Management of immune-related adverse events in patients treated with immune checkpoint inhibitor therapy: American society of clinical oncology clinical practice guideline. J Clin Oncol. 2018;36(17):1714–68. https://doi.org/10.1200/JCO.2017.77.6385.
24. Patil NK, Guo Y, Luan L, Sherwood ER. Targeting immune cell checkpoints during sepsis. Int J Mol Sci. 2017;18(11):2413. https://doi.org/10.3390/ijms18112413.
25. Busch LM, Sun J, Cui X, Eichacker PQ, Torabi-Parizi P. Checkpoint inhibitor therapy in preclinical sepsis models: a systematic review and meta-analysis. Intensive Care Med Exp. 2020;8(1):1–19. https://doi.org/10.1186/s40635-019-0290-x.
26. Hotchkiss RS, Colston E, Yende S, et al. Immune checkpoint inhibition in sepsis: a phase 1b randomized study to evaluate the safety, tolerability, pharmacokinetics, and pharmacodynamics of nivolumab. Intensive Care Med. 2019;45(10):1360–71. https://doi.org/10.1007/s00134-019-05704-z.
27. Hotchkiss RS, Colston E, Yende S, et al. Immune checkpoint inhibition in sepsis: a phase 1b randomized, placebo-controlled, single ascending dose study of Antiprogrammed cell death-ligand 1 antibody (BMS-936559). Crit Care Med. 2019;47(5):632–42. https://doi.org/10.1097/CCM.0000000000003685.
28. Kim C, Cook MR. Safety and efficacy of immune checkpoint inhibitor therapy in patients with HIV infection and advanced-stage cancer: a systematic review. JAMA Oncol. 2019;5(7):1049–53. https://doi.org/10.1001/jamaoncol.2018.6737.
29. Abbar B, Baron M, Katlama C, et al. Immune checkpoint inhibitors in people living with HIV: what about anti-HIV effects? AIDS. 2020;34(2):167–75. https://doi.org/10.1097/QAD.0000000000002397.
30. Gay CL, Bosch RJ, Ritz J, et al. Clinical trial of the anti-PD-L1 antibody BMS-936559 in HIV-1 infected participants on suppressive antiretroviral therapy. J Infect Dis. 2017;215(11):1725–33. https://doi.org/10.1093/infdis/jix191.

31. Hoang E, Bartlett NL, Goyal MS, Schmidt RE, Clifford DB. Progressive multifocal leukoencephalopathy treated with nivolumab. J Neurovirol. 2019;25(2):284–7. https://doi.org/10.1007/s13365-019-00738-x.
32. Cortese I, Muranski P, Enose-Akahata Y, et al. Pembrolizumab treatment for progressive multifocal leukoencephalopathy. N Engl J Med. 2019;380(17):1597–605. https://doi.org/10.1056/nejmoa1815039.
33. Martinot M, Ahle G, Petrosyan I, et al. Progressive multifocal leukoencephalopathy after treatment with nivolumab. Emerg Infect Dis. 2018;24(8):1594–6. https://doi.org/10.3201/eid2408.180460.
34. Pu D, Yin L, Zhou Y, et al. Safety and efficacy of immune checkpoint inhibitors in patients with HBV/HCV infection and advanced-stage cancer: a systematic review. Medicine (Baltimore). 2020;99(5):e19013. https://doi.org/10.1097/MD.0000000000019013.
35. Salimzadeh L, Le Bert N, Dutertre CA, et al. PD-1 blockade partially recovers dysfunctional virus-specific B cells in chronic hepatitis B infection. J Clin Invest. 2018;128(10):4573–87. https://doi.org/10.1172/JCI121957.
36. Gane E, Verdon DJ, Brooks AE, et al. Anti-PD-1 blockade with nivolumab with and without therapeutic vaccination for virally suppressed chronic hepatitis B: a pilot study. J Hepatol. 2019;71(5):900–7. https://doi.org/10.1016/j.jhep.2019.06.028.
37. Grimaldi D, Pradier O, Hotchkiss RS, Vincent JL. Nivolumab plus interferon-γ in the treatment of intractable mucormycosis. Lancet Infect Dis. 2017;17(1):18. https://doi.org/10.1016/S1473-3099(16)30541-2.
38. Mueller N, Banck J, Mellinghoff S, et al. P09.09 PD-1 checkpoint blockade for treatment of mucormycosis and invasive aspergillosis in a stem cell transplant recipient. J Immunother Cancer. 2020;8(Suppl 2):A56–7. https://doi.org/10.1136/jitc-2020-itoc7.109.
39. Diao B, Wang C, Tan Y, et al. Reduction and functional exhaustion of T cells in patients with coronavirus disease 2019 (COVID-19). Front Immunol. 2020;11:827. https://doi.org/10.3389/fimmu.2020.00827.
40. Luo J, Rizvi H, Egger JV, Preeshagul IR, Wolchok JD, Hellmann MD. Impact of PD-1 blockade on severity of COVID-19 in patients with lung cancers. Cancer Discov. 2020;10(8):1121–8. https://doi.org/10.1158/2159-8290.CD-20-0596.
41. Rogiers A, Tondini C, Grimes JM, et al. Abstract S02-01: clinical characteristics and outcomes of coronavirus 2019 disease (COVID-19) in cancer patients treated with immune checkpoint inhibitors (ICI). Clin Cancer Res. 2020;26(18 Supplement):S02-01. https://doi.org/10.1158/1557-3265.COVID-19-S02-01.
42. Robilotti EV, Babady NE, Mead PA, et al. Determinants of COVID-19 disease severity in patients with cancer. Nat Med. 2020;26(8):1218–23. https://doi.org/10.1038/s41591-020-0979-0.
43. Lázár-Molnár E, Gácser A, Freeman GJ, Almo SC, Nathenson SG, Nosanchuk JD. The PD-1/PD-L costimulatory pathway critically affects host resistance to the pathogenic fungus histoplasma capsulatum. Proc Natl Acad Sci U S A. 2008;105(7):2658–63. https://doi.org/10.1073/pnas.0711918105.
44. Roussey JA, Viglianti SP, Teitz-Tennenbaum S, Olszewski MA, Osterholzer JJ. Anti–PD-1 antibody treatment promotes clearance of persistent cryptococcal lung infection in mice. J Immunol. 2017;199(10):3535–46. https://doi.org/10.4049/jimmunol.1700840.
45. Wang J, Jebbawi F, Bellanger A-P, Beldi G, Millon L, Gottstein B. Immunotherapy of alveolar echinococcosis via PD-1/PD-L1 immune checkpoint blockade in mice. Parasite Immunol. 2018;40(12):e12596. https://doi.org/10.1111/pim.12596.

α4-Integrin (and Other Leukocyte Integrin)-Targeting Agents

14

Eleftheria E. Kampouri, Jonathan Tschopp, and Oriol Manuel

Abbreviations

CD	Crohn's disease
CDI	*Clostridioides difficile* infection
CMV	Cytomegalovirus
CNS	Central nervous system
CSF	Cerebrospinal fluid
ELISA	Enzyme-linked immunosorbent assay
HAV	Hepatitis A virus
HBV	Hepatitis B virus
HSV	Herpes-simplex virus
IBD	Inflammatory bowel disease
ICAM-1	Intercellular adhesion molecule 1
JCV	JC virus
LAD	Leukocyte adhesion deficiency
LFA-1	Lymphocyte function-associated antigen-1

Eleftheria E. Kampouri and Jonathan Tschopp contributed equally with all other contributors.

E. E. Kampouri · J. Tschopp
Infectious Diseases Service, Lausanne University Hospital (CHUV) and University of Lausanne, Lausanne, Switzerland
e-mail: Eleftheria-Evdokia.Kampouri@chuv.ch; jonathan.tschopp@chuv.ch

O. Manuel (✉)
Infectious Diseases Service, Lausanne University Hospital (CHUV) and University of Lausanne, Lausanne, Switzerland

Transplantation Center, Lausanne University Hospital (CHUV) and University of Lausanne, Lausanne, Switzerland
e-mail: oriol.manuel@chuv.ch

C. Cervera, J. M. Aguado (eds.), *Infectious Complications in Biologic and Targeted Therapies*, https://doi.org/10.1007/978-3-031-11363-5_14

MAdCAM1	Mucosal address cell adhesion molecule
MRI	Magnetic resonance imaging
MS	Multiple sclerosis
PLEX	Plasma exchange
PML	Progressive multifocal leukoencephalopathy
TB	Tuberculosis
TNF-α	Tumor necrosis factor α
UC	Ulcerous colitis
VCAM-1	Vascular cell adhesion molecule 1
VLA-4	Very late antigen-4
VZV	Varicella-zoster virus

Introduction

Integrins are transmembrane receptors that play a key role in cell adhesion and intracellular signaling. Integrins located on the leukocyte surface are essential for the recruitment of leukocytes from the vasculature to the tissues and are successfully used as therapeutic targets to modulate inflammation [1, 2]. The first drugs targeting the integrin molecules were the α4-integrin subunit inhibitor natalizumab and the lymphocyte function-associated antigen-1 (LFA-1) β2-integrin inhibitor efalizumab [1]. Their main mechanism of action is based on blocking the migration of lymphocytes and therefore decreasing the inflammatory reaction in the brain and the intestinal mucosa. These drugs were initially developed for treating autoimmune disorders, such as multiple sclerosis (MS) and inflammatory bowel disease (IBD) for natalizumab, and psoriasis for efalizumab [1]. Early in the introduction process of the drug, several cases of PML were reported with the use of natalizumab and efalizumab, which led to the withdrawal of both drugs. After a review process taking into consideration the efficacy of the drug for progressive MS and the stratification of the individual risk for developing PML, natalizumab was reintroduced for therapy of severe forms of MS, in particular in patients with low risk for the development of PML [2]. However, natalizumab is only rarely used in patients with IBD due to the availability of equally effective and safer drugs [3]. Vedolizumab, a novel α4-integrin-targeted agent, specifically blocking α4β7 integrin only present in the intestinal mucosa, has not been associated with PML and is approved for IBD [4, 5]. In this chapter, we will review the mechanism of action and potential infection risk of natalizumab and vedolizumab, and we will describe the proposed preventive and therapeutic measures for decreasing the risk of infection in patients receiving these drugs.

Integrins Overview

Integrins: A Complex Structure with Unique Biology

Integrins represent an important family of transmembrane receptors that mediate cell–cell and cell–extracellular matrix interactions and play a key role in cell adhesion. These complex receptors are type I αβ-heterodimers comprising two subunits, and each integrin is named for the one α-chain and one β-chain that compose it. To date, 24 different heterodimers have been identified in humans, derived from the combination of 18 α and 8 β subunits. The complex structure contributes to the distinct functions of each integrin as well as their distribution and tissue specificity. All integrins carry out two main functions: cell adhesion and intracellular signaling [1].

In contrast to most receptors, transmitting information from the cell's exterior to the interior, integrins propagate signals in a bidirectional way. The heterodimeric receptors undergo large conformational changes in the extracellular domains in response to signaling events inside the cell, initiated by various intracellular adaptor molecules. This process, known as "inside-out signaling," leads to integrin activation and an increased affinity for their ligands and is therefore essential for ligand binding and cell adhesion. In the absence of activating signals, integrins have an inactive, bent conformation, and the ligand-binding site is not exposed, thus not readily accessible to ligands. In the opposite direction, ligand binding induces integrin clustering (a process which brings the signaling domains of integrin-proximal proteins close together), which in turn leads to the initiation of intracellular signal transduction, implicating various intracellular enzymes and involved in multiple cellular functions in a process commonly known as "outside-in signaling" [1, 6] (Fig. 14.1).

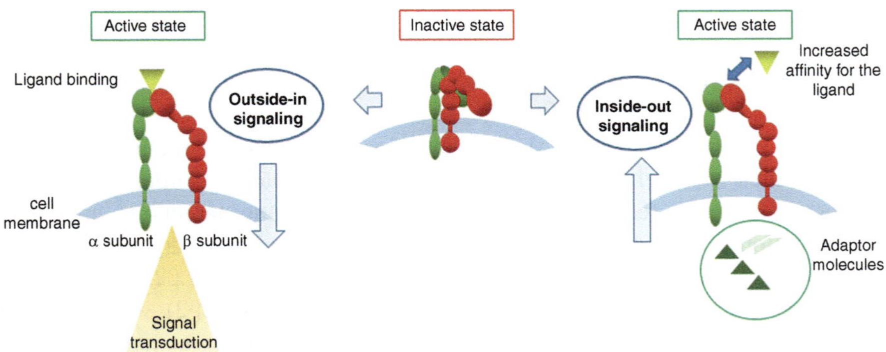

Fig. 14.1 Mechanism of action of integrins. Integrins propagate signals in a bidirectional way: large conformational changes in the extracellular domains occur as a response to signaling events inside the cell ("inside-out signaling"), leading to integrin activation which is required for ligand binding and cell adhesion. In the absence of activating signals, integrins have an inactive, bent conformation, and the ligand-binding site is not readily accessible. In the opposite direction, ligand binding induces integrin clustering, leading to integrin-mediated intracellular signal transduction ("outside-in signaling")

Leukocyte Integrins

Six integrins are exclusively expressed on the surface of leukocytes αLβ2, αMβ2, αxβ2, αDβ2, α4β7, and αEβ7, while the seventh one, α4β1, is also expressed in several other cells [1, 7]. These molecules serve distinct functions and purposes in the immune system and are involved in multiple steps of the leukocyte adhesion cascade [7]. αLβ2, also known as LFA-1, is required for the formation of the immunological synapse, facilitating the interaction between T cells and antigen-presenting cells, but is also involved in many other facets of the immune response, including adhesion, activation, and trafficking of leukocyte populations [8]. αMβ2 integrin is essential for neutrophil function as well as for complement-mediated phagocytosis and is involved in the defense against bacterial and fungal infections [9]. The role of αxβ2 is central in the regulation of the inflammatory function of recruited tissue macrophages [9]. αDβ2 is expressed on monocytes/macrophages and particularly those found in atherosclerotic lesions (foam cells) [10]. α4β7 and αEβ7 integrins direct lymphocyte trafficking from vessels to the intestinal mucosa [11]. Finally, α4β1integrin also known as very late antigen-4 (VLA-4) [12] binds to ligands present on endothelial cells and mediates adhesion of leukocytes to all inflamed tissues and organs, including the central nervous system. The central role of integrins in inflammation is further highlighted by the severe immune dysregulation observed in patients with leukocyte adhesion deficiency (LAD) syndromes. Patients with LAD-I due to mutations in the β2 subunit present impaired immunity and recurrent infections [13].

Integrins as Therapeutic Targets

In light of the prominent role of leukocyte integrins in leukocyte recruitment in tissues and their role in the pathogenesis of many inflammatory disorders, these molecules were early recognized as promising therapeutic targets to modulate inflammation. Four leukocyte integrins have been therapeutically targeted by monoclonal antibodies in clinical trials: α4β7, α4β1, αEβ7, and αLβ2. Natalizumab (anti-α4), vedolizumab (anti-α4β7), and efalizumab (anti-αLβ2) were the first developed therapeutic agents [1]. New molecules with different targets or new applications of molecules directed to the same targets are continuously emerging in parallel with a deeper understanding of the function of integrins [1, 6]. For instance, new monoclonal antibodies and small molecules targeting β7-containing integrins and their ligands are in development for the treatment of inflammatory bowel disease (IBD).

Leukocyte integrins are not the only ones therapeutically targeted. The platelet integrin αIIbβ3 was the first one to be targeted in the 1990s by abciximab, an antigen-binding fragment (Fab) of a chimeric mouse human monoclonal antibody, used for the prevention of thrombotic complications before or after percutaneous coronary intervention in selected patients [14]. Two additional antagonists, eptifibatide [15] and tirofiban [16], followed. Even though these drugs are not largely used due to the availability of more effective and safe treatments, they laid the foundation for further integrin antagonist development. Finally, the use of integrins as therapeutic targets in oncological treatments and as probes in imaging to evaluate prognosis and treatment response is emerging ($\alpha v\beta 3$, $\alpha v\beta 5$, $\alpha v\beta 6$, $\alpha 5\beta 1$), renewing interest in this family of adhesive molecules [1]. Monoclonal antibodies inhibiting leukocyte integrins remain the most successful examples of therapeutic targeting of integrins in clinical practice and the most interesting ones from an infectious complications point of view and will be the focus of this chapter.

Leukocyte-Integrin-Targeting Agents

Monoclonal Antibodies: Mechanism of Action

Natalizumab (Tysabri; Biogen Idec and Elan Corporation), the first successful drug targeting leucocyte integrins, is a humanized IgG4 monoclonal antibody, which binds with the $\alpha 4$ subunit present in $\alpha 4\beta 7$ and $\alpha 4\beta 1$ integrins, thus inhibiting the binding of their physiological ligands. $\alpha 4\beta 1$ (or VLA-4) is expressed on practically all leukocytes, except for mature granulocytes. Via its complex interactions with the vascular cell adhesion molecule 1 (VCAM-1) and fibronectin, $\alpha 4\beta 1$ participates in leukocyte slow rolling, adhesion, and transmigration via the endothelium to all inflamed tissues and organs, as well as in pro-inflammatory signaling in the endothelial cells. The second target of natalizumab, $\alpha 4\beta 7$ integrin, binds to mucosal address cell adhesion molecule (MAdCAM1) which is predominantly expressed on the endothelial cells of the intestinal vasculature thus mediating lymphocyte homing to the gut mucosa [1].

Vedolizumab (Entyvio; Millennium Pharmaceuticals), a humanized IgG1 monoclonal antibody, targets an epitope formed by both $\alpha 4$ and $\beta 7$ subunits and is therefore a specific antagonist of $\alpha 4\beta 7$ integrin, inhibiting the homing of T lymphocytes to the intestinal mucosa [17]. The clinical indication of natalizumab and vedolizumab will be discussed in the next section.

Abrilumab, a second human monoclonal IgG2 antibody directed against a combinatorial epitope only present in $\alpha 4\beta 7$, has been shown in a phase 2b randomized controlled trial to induce remission in patients with ulcerative colitis (UC) [18].

Etrolizumab is a humanized IgG1 monoclonal antibody directed against the $\beta 7$ unit, present in both $\alpha 4\beta 7$ and $\alpha E\beta 7$ integrins. $\alpha 4\beta 7$ integrin interacts with MAdCAM1 and is the most significant determinant of lymphocyte recruitment in the intestine, while $\alpha E\beta 7$ via its binding to E-cadherin mediates the adhesion of intraepithelial lymphocytes to the epithelial cells. $\alpha E\beta 7$ is also present on dendritic cells producing anti-inflammatory cytokines involved in the development of regulatory T cells [19]. Blocking both pathways effectively inhibits the trafficking of lymphocytes into the gut and provides a promising therapeutic strategy for UC (phase II study) and Crohn's disease (CD) (ongoing phase III trials) [20, 21].

Efalizumab (Raptiva; Genentech), a recombinant humanized monoclonal antibody, binds to the αL unit of the $\alpha L\beta 2$ (LFA-1), preventing the binding of T cells to

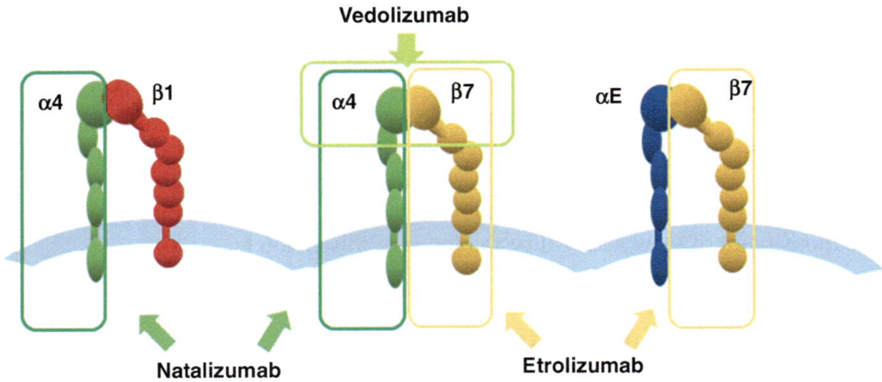

Fig. 14.2 The three integrins, α4β7, α4β1, and αEβ7 that are targeted by monoclonal antibodies. Natalizumab targets the α4 subunit (green) present in α4β1 and α4β7 integrins. Etrolizumab targets the β7 subunit (yellow) present in α4β7 and αEβ7. Vedolizumab targets an epitope formed by both the α4 and β7 subunits (light green) and inhibits specifically the α4β7 integrin (adapted from [1])

the intercellular adhesion molecule 1 (ICAM-1), which is found on antigen-presenting cells, endothelial cells, and keratinocytes [1]. Figure 14.2 illustrates the targets of monoclonal antibodies targeting leukocyte integrins currently used or in late-stage clinical trials.

Other Therapeutic Agents

Besides monoclonal antibodies, efforts have been devoted to the development of peptide or small-molecule antagonists, including allosteric inhibitors designed to inhibit the activation of integrins by blocking the large conformational changes of their extracellular domains. These allosteric inhibitors failed to enter clinical trials due to limited specificity and unexpected systemic toxicity [1]. Non-allosteric, small-molecule inhibitors are actively investigated. AJM300 is a small molecule inhibiting the α4 subunit and has been proven successful in inducing remission in UC [22]. Finally, another small molecule, lifitegrast, binds to αLβ2, blocking the binding of ICAM1 which is overexpressed in corneal and conjunctival tissues in patients with dry eye disease and is used locally as ophthalmic solution to reduce inflammation in those patients [23].

Approved Indications of Integrin-Targeting Agents

Two leukocyte integrin antagonists are currently available on the market, namely, natalizumab and vedolizumab. A third one, efalizumab, was initially approved for the treatment of chronic plaque psoriasis but was withdrawn from the market in 2009 due to major risk of adverse events [24].

Natalizumab

The prominent role of α4β1 for the entry of T lymphocytes in the CNS provides the theoretical background for its use as a target for CNS diseases [2]. In 1992, Yednock and al. first described the use of antibodies against the α4β1 integrin to inhibit the migration of leukocytes into the CNS in a murine experimental model of autoimmune encephalitis [25]. Natalizumab was developed subsequently for the treatment of multiple sclerosis (MS), an idiopathic inflammatory disease of the CNS characterized by demyelinating lesions affecting mostly the white matter of the brain and spinal cord. For decades, MS was treated with nonspecific anti-inflammatory and immunomodulatory drugs such as corticosteroids, interferon β1b, and glatiramer acetate. In more recent years, progress was made in the understanding of the pathophysiology of MS, notably the key role played by activated T lymphocytes recruited from the blood to the CNS and the ensuing inflammatory reaction due to the release of pro-inflammatory cytokines. In this context, natalizumab was studied in randomized controlled trials and proved to be effective in reducing CNS inflammatory lesions and relapses in patients with severe relapsing-remitting MS, either as monotherapy [26] or as part of a combination therapy [27]. Natalizumab was approved in 2004 in the USA and in Europe for the treatment of severe relapsing-remitting MS with no response on first-line therapies, and in severe primary relapsing MS [28].

Due to its dual action also targeting the α4β7 integrin, natalizumab was investigated as a therapeutic agent in CD, a type of IBD characterized by mucosal ulceration and inflammation that can involve any portion of the gastrointestinal tract. Natalizumab was shown to be more effective than placebo in inducing and maintaining remission in moderate to severe CD in multiple clinical studies [29–31] and was approved for this indication in patients who had an inadequate response to or were unable to tolerate conventional CD therapies and tumor necrosis factor α (TNF-α) inhibitors. Nevertheless, the use of natalizumab for CD is now limited because of safer therapeutic options [3].

Vedolizumab

The successful use of natalizumab in CD provided the incentive for the development of other molecules targeting more specifically the α4β7 integrin without the collateral targeting of α4β1, which mediates the most serious adverse events. Vedolizumab was therefore developed to be used specifically in IBD. The pathogenesis of IBD is complex and incompletely understood but involves genetic susceptibility, environmental triggers, and aberrant interactions between the immune system and gut microorganisms, leading to an augmented permeability of the mucosal barrier and homing of activated lymphocytes, creating a vicious circle of local inflammation [32]. Nonspecific anti-inflammatory therapies such as corticosteroids, aminosalicylates, and oral immunomodulators were the cornerstone of the treatment of IBD. In the recent years, more potent and specific agents showed encouraging results in moderate to severe disease, such as Janus kinase inhibitors, TNF-α inhibitors, and integrin antagonists.

Vedolizumab demonstrated promising results for the treatment of IBD in early studies [33] that were confirmed in two randomized controlled trials demonstrating its superiority compared to placebo in achieving maintenance in UC (GEMINI 1 study) and CD (GEMINI 2 study) [4, 5]. Based on these data, vedolizumab was approved in 2014 for both moderate to severe UC and moderate to severe CD. Since then, its efficacy has been confirmed in subsequent randomized (GEMINI 3 study) [34] and multiple cohort studies.

Infectious Complications of Integrin-Targeting Agents

Natalizumab

The clinical impact of integrin inhibition on infection risk is largely derived from the experience with natalizumab, the first-in-class drug available on the market. Initial data from pivotal clinical trials were surprisingly reassuring regarding the global infectious risk of natalizumab, as no major increase in infections was noted. In 2006, post-marketing data revealed two of cases of progressive multifocal encephalopathy (PML) in patients receiving natalizumab [35]. This rare but life-threatening complication led to its transient withdrawal from the market in 2005 to perform safety analyses, before it was reintroduced in 2006 together with a global risk management plan (TOUCH prescribing program). More than 800 cases of natalizumab-induced PML have been described since then, with an estimate incidence of approximately 0.4% of patients treated with natalizumab (https://medinfo.biogen.com/s/).

PML is a rare disease caused by the reactivation of the JC virus (JCV) in brain cells [36]. This small DNA virus from the polyomaviridae family seems to be acquired during youth and usually leads to asymptomatic infection or a nonspecific influenza-like illness. The reported seroprevalence varies between 39% in the United States [37] and 48–69% in European countries [38]. After the primary infection, it establishes a persistent asymptomatic infection in urothelial cells as well as in oligodendrocytes and astrocytes. JCV causes no disease in immunocompetent individuals as JCV replication is controlled by specific cytotoxic T cells. Intermittent asymptomatic JCV viruria can be detected in healthy persons [39].

PML was first described in 1958 as a very rare disease affecting highly immunocompromised patients with hematological malignancies [40], but its relationship with JCV was only described in 1971 [36]. PML became better recognized during the AIDS pandemic, as it affected up to 5% of persons with AIDS, and it was associated with high mortality [41].

PML is mostly a white matter inflammatory disease, but it can sometimes involve the gray matter as well, when JCV replication involves granule cell neurons. The symptoms vary widely depending on the affected area of the brain but most frequently consist in altered mental status, motor deficits, ataxia, or visual symptoms, further complicating the diagnosis when these symptoms occur in a patient with MS. Brain MRI in patients with PML typically shows subcortical T2-enhancing lesions not corresponding to cerebrovascular territories, and without mass effect or contrast enhancement. Some degree of contrast enhancement has been seen in PML associated with natalizumab use that can be difficult to differentiate from active MS lesions [42]. The diagnosis of PML can be confirmed by a positive JCV PCR in the cerebrospinal fluid (CSF). Although the sensitivity and specificity of JCV PCR are excellent, a negative test cannot rule out PML [43]. In cases of high clinical and radiological suspicion, but negative JCV PCR in the CSF, a definitive diagnosis may require a brain biopsy, which characteristically shows a histopathological triad of demyelination, bizarre astrocytes, and enlarged oligodendroglial nuclei [44].

There is no specific therapy against PML, and the management primarily relies on restoring immunity. In the case of PML induced by natalizumab, early removing the drug with plasma exchange (PLEX) or immunoadsorption is the most important therapeutic strategy. Nevertheless, the quick restoration of immunity by drug removal can be complicated by an immune reconstitution inflammatory syndrome (IRIS) that can lead to cerebral edema and death if left untreated [45]. This entity has been mostly described in patients managed with PLEX and is usually treated aggressively with the administration of high-dose corticosteroids. The reported mortality of natalizumab-associated PML is lower than in AIDS-related PML, ranging from 18 to 23% [46]. However, most survivors have residual moderate to severe disabilities [47]. Of note, a small case series published in 2019 showed potential benefit of immunotherapy with the checkpoint inhibitor pembrolizumab in eight patients with confirmed PML, but none of these cases were related to the use of natalizumab [48].

Natalizumab has been also associated with an increased risk of herpes viruses reactivation, in particular herpes-simplex virus (HSV) and varicella-zoster virus (VZV). Most cases are mild mucocutaneous diseases, but some cases of life-threatening HSV or VZV encephalitis have also been reported [49–51]. A high index of suspicion for HSV and VZV reactivation is therefore needed in patients receiving natalizumab, and acyclovir should be initiated promptly if necessary. Given the relatively low incidence of HSV and VZV reactivation, routine antiviral prophylaxis with acyclovir/valaciclovir in patients receiving natalizumab is not recommended. Other infections such as tuberculosis (TB) have exceptionally been described in patients receiving natalizumab [52]. No increase in the incidence of gastrointestinal infections has been reported in patients treated with natalizumab.

Vedolizumab

The larger source of data regarding vedolizumab safety comes from the GEMINI long-term safety study, which consists in the continued follow-up of patients included in the three GEMINI studies, as well as the enrollment of vedolizumab-naive patients. The final analysis was published in 2020 and included more than 2000 patients with up to 9 years of follow-up, and a total of 7999 person-years (PYs) [53]. In this study, the rate of serious infections was 18/1000 PYs in patients with UC and 33/1000 PYs with CD, as compared to the higher rate of serious infections of 38/1000 PYs in patients with IBD receiving no treatment [54]. Infectious complications in patients receiving vedolizumab consisted mostly in anal abscesses, pneumonia, gastroenteritis, and appendicitis.

The only reported opportunistic infection associated with the use of vedolizumab was an increased number of *Clostridioides difficile* infections (CDI) ranging from 3.6/1000 PYs (CD) to 4.9/1000 PYs (UC), with most cases being mild to moderate. There was no case of intestinal TB and only a few cases of primary TB in patients living in high-endemic countries. Overall, the rate of infection following vedolizumab exposure was significantly lower than with TNF-α inhibitors [55]. Only one case of PML has been described in over 470,000 PYs of vedolizumab exposure and occurred in a patient with multiple other risk factors (HIV infection, CD4 count <300 cell/mm^3, prior immunosuppression) [56]. No increase in risk of herpesvirus was observed in patients with IBD treated with vedolizumab, including HSV, VZV, and cytomegalovirus (CMV). Thus, neither antiviral prophylaxis nor preemptive strategies against CMV are recommended in this population.

Efalizumab

As with natalizumab, early data on efalizumab safety profile were reassuring, with no major risk of infection reported [57]. Only a marginal increase in minor infections was reported in some studies, mostly viral upper respiratory tract infections, streptococcal pharyngitis, and mild mucocutaneous infections [58]. In 2008, the FDA issued a warning after three confirmed cases of PML were diagnosed in patients who had been receiving efalizumab for more than 3 years. Efalizumab was eventually withdrawn from the market in 2009 due to this concern and the availability of less toxic alternatives for the treatment of psoriasis.

Figure 14.3 summarizes the infectious complications reported for each molecule.

	Infectious risk	Infection
Natalizumab	High	PML (JCV)
	Intermediate	HSV infection VZV infection
	No increase	Bacterial infections Mycobacterial infections Fungal infections Parasitic infections Other viral infections
Vedolizumab	High	None
	Intermediate	*Clostridioides difficile* infection
	No increase	Other bacterial infections Mycobacterial infections Fungal infections Parasitic infections Other viral infections
Efalizumab	High	JCV (PML)
	Intermediate	*Streptococcus pyogenes* pharyngitis Viral upper respiratory tract infections Impetigo Cellulitis
	No increase	Other bacterial infections Mycobacterial infections Fungal infections Parasitic infections Other viral infections

Fig. 14.3 Infection risk and complications by therapeutic molecule. *JCV* JC virus; *PML* progressive multifocal encephalopathy; *HSV* herpes simplex virus; *VZV* varicella zoster virus

Prevention Strategies in MS Patients Receiving Natalizumab

PML Risk Stratification

The prevention of PML in patients receiving natalizumab relies on a stringent risk stratification system and serial MRI monitoring [59]. Risk stratification is based on three components identified by the intensive global risk management program and later validated in large cohorts [60], namely (1) JCV positive serostatus, (2) cumulate use of immunosuppressive drugs, and (3) natalizumab treatment duration, especially beyond 2 years [59–61]. Patients with all of the above factors present the highest risk for PML [60] and require the most intensive monitoring strategy. Monitoring is recommended during treatment and for 6 months after discontinuation of natalizumab, as some cases of PML have been reported up to 6 months after cessation of treatment [59, 62].

JCV Serostatus and MRI

JCV serostatus before the initiation of natalizumab represents the single most important risk factor for subsequent PML development. Determining JCV serostatus is the cornerstone of risk stratification algorithms to define the intensity of PML monitoring needed (Fig. 14.4). The presence of anti-JCV specific IgG is a prerequisite for PML development, and the risk of PML is negligible in their absence. In a study using data from post-marketing sources, clinical studies and an independent Swedish registry, the incidence of PML was 0.09 cases or less per 1000 patients (95% CI, 0 to 0.48) in the absence of anti-JCV antibodies. At the other extreme, patients with positive antibodies, a history of immunosuppression and more than 2 years of natalizumab treatment, presented the highest incidence of 11.1 cases per 1000 patients (96% CI, 8.3 to 14.5) [60].

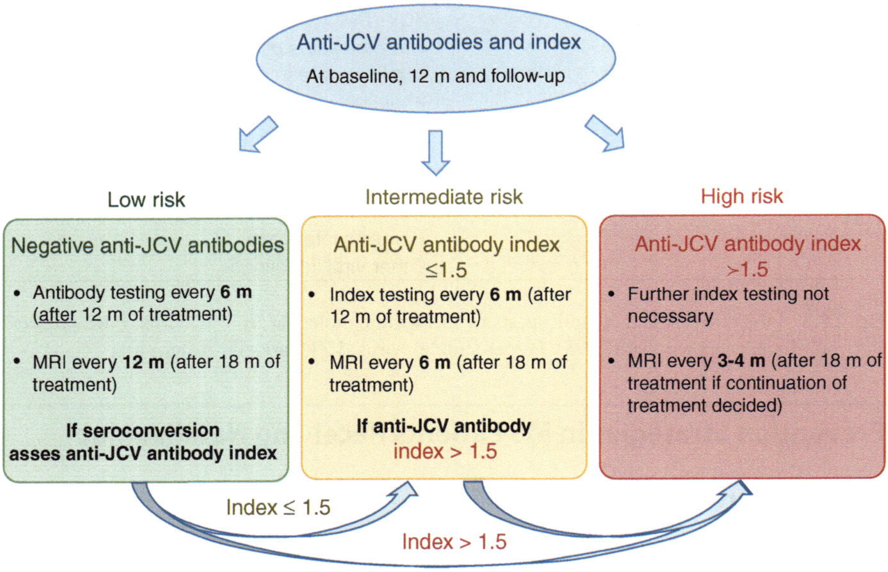

Fig. 14.4 Algorithm for PML prevention and monitoring according to anti-JCV antibody stratification in patients with no history of immunosuppressive treatment, adapted from [59]. All patients should undergo anti-JCV antibody or index testing and brain MRI at baseline and at 12 months. No additional testing is routinely recommended in the first year of treatment. Thereafter antibody or index testing should be performed every 6 months for seronegative and patients with index ≤1.5, respectively. After 18 months of treatment, the frequency of MRI testing is determined by risk category. A dynamic evaluation of PML risk based on index testing is recommended, with a modification of monitoring strategy when patients change "risk category" from a lower to a higher one (curved arrows). Anti-JCV antibody status is only one component of PML risk stratification. Previous immunosuppressive treatment and natalizumab therapy beyond 2 years are the other two, and the presence of these additional risk factors should prompt evaluation of more frequent MRI testing (every 3–4 months as "high-risk patients"). Monitoring is recommended for the whole duration of treatment plus another 6 months. More frequent monitoring and additional workup are indicated in case of new or worsening symptoms

The quantitative anti-JCV serum antibody index allows a more accurate differentiation between negative and positive samples and more reliable results than assays providing only absolute cutoff values [63]. This index refers to the normalized ratio between the signal derived from IgG antibodies in the serum of the patient and the signal from an anti-JCV positive cutoff calibrator sample. An index value of <0.20 is regarded as negative, a value >0.40 positive, and values between 0.20 and 0.40 are considered indeterminate. A longitudinal study including data from 2522 non-PML and 71 PML patients showed that the anti-JCV antibody index value was significantly higher in non-immunosuppressed patients who developed PML compared with non-PML patients ($p < 0.0001$) [63]. An index of ≤1.5 is associated with a lower incidence of PML, and this cutoff could be used to determine monitoring intensity [59, 61, 63]. An anti-JCV antibody index of >1.5 is not a contraindication for treatment continuation, as many patients with a high index will not develop PML. Therefore, the antibody index has a high sensitivity and a low specificity in predicting PML [64].

The risk of anti-JCV antibodies seroconversion was evaluated in a large Dutch cohort of MS patients on natalizumab treatment. Out of 179 patients with available longitudinal blood samples, 86 (48%) tested negative initially and 23 patients among them (26.7%) subsequently seroconverted, contributing to an estimated annual rate of seroconversion of 7.1% and cumulatively leading to more than 25% of seronegative patients becoming seropositive in 4 years [65]. Based on these data, testing for anti-JCV antibodies and anti-JCV index is recommended every 6 months beyond the first year of treatment in seronegative patients (low risk) and patients with a baseline index of ≤1.5, respectively (intermediate). In the risk of developing PML being very low during the first year of treatment (1 in 10,000 to 1 in 1000), no anti-JCV antibody monitoring is routinely recommended during this interval [63].

JCV antibodies are traditionally qualitatively assessed using a two-step enzyme-linked immunosorbent assay (ELISA) method [66]. A second-generation ELISA is commercially available (STRATIFY JCV Dx Select; Focus Diagnostics), though mostly in reference centers, presenting an improved performance, especially in low antibody concentrations where its enhanced resolution allows to significantly decrease "indeterminate" results [67].

The second essential element of monitoring is brain MRI, which is highly performant for the early detection of PML, even months before symptom development [59]. Current recommendation regarding MRI frequency is based on expert opinion. A baseline MRI is recommended for all patients and at least annually during treatment. After the first year, the frequency of MRI depends on the risk category but is generally recommended every 6 months in low- and intermediate-risk patients and every 3–4 months in high-risk patients [59, 61].

Previous Immunosuppression

Previous immunosuppression is associated with a considerably higher incidence of PML which is estimated at 0.88/1000 patients in the presence of previous immunosuppression versus 0.31/1000 patients in the absence of immunosuppression [60]. The exact mechanism via which previous immunosuppression increases the risk of PML is not fully understood. A possible explanation is that a prolonged impairment of cell-mediated immunity permits viral reactivation and the accumulation of genetic rearrangements leading to the emergence of neuropathogenic JCV prototypes (as opposed to the non-pathogenic archetype ones), which are more frequently present in patients having received immunosuppression before natalizumab [68].

Duration of Natalizumab Treatment

The risk of PML increases with longer duration of treatment, reaching a peak in incidence of 2 cases per 1000 patients in patients receiving natalizumab for more than 48 months [60]. The greatest increase appears after 24 months (and until 48 months) with an incidence of 5.2/1000 patients versus 0.6/1000 patients in the first 24 months of treatment [63]. However, patients having received a single or only a few infusions of natalizumab are usually analyzed in the group of duration inferior to 24 months, contributing to an artificially lower estimation of risk of PML in this group. Long-term data beyond 4 years of treatment are scarce, so that the risk of PML is not clearly delineated in patients with longer exposures [64].

Additional Biomarkers for Risk Stratification

Despite the advances in prevention strategies, PML continues to be a limiting factor for the use of natalizumab, underlining the need for more accurate prediction models. In this setting, many immunological biomarkers have been proposed [64, 69]. CD62L/L-selectin, a cell-adhesion molecule expressed on T lymphocytes, has been identified as a potential tool for PML prediction, with low CD62L in blood mononuclear cells being associated with a 55-fold increase in the relative risk of PML [70]. The presence of lipid-specific immunoglobulin M bands in the CSF, a recognized marker in highly inflammatory MS, was independently associated with decreased PML risk (OR 45.9, 95% CI 5.9–339.3, $p < 0.0001$) [71]. This marker is independent of JCV serostatus as opposed to CD62L and could be a promising in risk stratification.

Additional Preventive Strategies

Given the low effect of natalizumab and vedolizumab in the net state of immunosuppression, additional preventive measures such as the use of antimicrobial and antiviral prophylaxis with co-trimoxazole or valaciclovir, respectively, are not routinely recommended [61].

The risk of hepatitis B virus (HBV) reactivation has not been accurately determined with the use of natalizumab and vedolizumab. No cases of HBV infection are reported in the major clinical trials with both molecules [72, 73], and only one case of fatal acute liver failure due to HBV is reported with natalizumab in the post-marketing setting (though serologic markers do not allow to distinguish between primary infection and reactivation in this case) [74]. Although preventive strategies for HBV are not well established, screening for the presence of HBV infection with HBsAg and anti-HBc before initiation of treatment is appropriate in order to assess the risk of HBV reactivation (based on the presence of HBsAg and the agent used) and decide whether a preventive strategy needs to be introduced [72].

Finally, natalizumab and vedolizumab do not seem to modify vaccine response [75, 76], though a reduction in immunogenicity of the oral cholera vaccine has been observed with vedolizumab in one study [76]. Of note, live vaccines are not contraindicated. As additional immunosuppressive agents can be required in the setting of MS and IBD, an update of the vaccine schedule including HBV/HAV and measles-mumps-rubella-varicella (MMR-V) vaccines in seronegative patients, as well as pneumococcal conjugate vaccine and diphtheria-tetanus-pertussis vaccine (dTP), is recommended.

Conclusions

Leukocyte integrins are privileged therapeutic targets for inflammatory modulation in MS and IBD and are currently targeted by two monoclonal antibodies, natalizumab and vedolizumab. The advent of these molecules has substantially improved the prognosis of patients living with MS and IBD but also highlights the challenge of the use of biologicals in modern medicine. On the one hand, integrins-targeting agents specifically inhibit leukocyte integrins resulting in an excellent efficacy for decreasing MS activity without increasing the net state of immunosuppression. On the other hand, the very same aimed therapeutic effect mediated by the blockade of leukocyte recruitment to the brain is also the principal determinant of the risk for developing PML, a life-threatening disease. Assessment of risk/benefit ratio and the absence of other therapeutic options for severe forms of MS have resulted in the reintroduction of the drug in the clinical practice. While the use of an accurate risk stratification and universal prevention strategies has led to improved management of patients receiving natalizumab, the use of novel specific biomarkers may help to further characterize the risk for PML in these patients. The evaluation of novel therapeutic approaches for natalizumab-associated PML, including immunomodulatory drugs such as checkpoint inhibitors, adoptive T-cell transfer, and anti-JCV specific antivirals, is highly needed to decrease the burden of disease.

References

1. Ley K, Rivera-Nieves J, Sandborn WJ, Shattil S. Integrin-based therapeutics: biological basis, clinical use and new drugs. Nat Rev Drug Discov. 2016;15(3):173–83. https://doi.org/10.1038/nrd.2015.10.
2. Ransohoff RM. Natalizumab for multiple sclerosis. N Engl J Med. 2007;356(25):2622–9. https://doi.org/10.1056/NEJMct071462.
3. Nelson SM, Nguyen TM, McDonald JW, MacDonald JK. Natalizumab for induction of remission in Crohn's disease. Cochrane Database Syst Rev. 2018;8:CD006097. https://doi.org/10.1002/14651858.CD006097.pub3.
4. Feagan BG, Rutgeerts P, Sands BE, Hanauer S, Colombel JF, Sandborn WJ, et al. Vedolizumab as induction and maintenance therapy for ulcerative colitis. N Engl J Med. 2013;369(8):699–710. https://doi.org/10.1056/NEJMoa1215734.
5. Sandborn WJ, Feagan BG, Rutgeerts P, Hanauer S, Colombel JF, Sands BE, et al. Vedolizumab as induction and maintenance therapy for Crohn's disease. N Engl J Med. 2013;369(8):711–21. https://doi.org/10.1056/NEJMoa1215739.
6. Baiula M, Spampinato S, Gentilucci L, Tolomelli A. Novel ligands targeting alpha4beta1 integrin: therapeutic applications and perspectives. Front Chem. 2019;7:489. https://doi.org/10.3389/fchem.2019.00489.
7. Mitroulis I, Alexaki VI, Kourtzelis I, Ziogas A, Hajishengallis G, Chavakis T. Leukocyte integrins: role in leukocyte recruitment and as therapeutic targets in inflammatory disease. Pharmacol Ther. 2015;147:123–35. https://doi.org/10.1016/j.pharmthera.2014.11.008.
8. Nicolls MR, Gill RG. LFA-1 (CD11a) as a therapeutic target. Am J Transplant. 2006;6(1):27–36. https://doi.org/10.1111/j.1600-6143.2005.01158.x.
9. Jawhara S, Pluskota E, Cao W, Plow EF, Soloviev DA. Distinct effects of integrins alphaX-beta2 and alphaMbeta2 on leukocyte subpopulations during inflammation and antimicrobial responses. Infect Immun. 2017;85(1) https://doi.org/10.1128/IAI.00644-16.
10. Van der Vieren M, Le Trong H, Wood CL, Moore PF, St John T, Staunton DE, et al. A novel leukointegrin, alpha d beta 2, binds preferentially to ICAM-3. Immunity. 1995;3(6):683–90. https://doi.org/10.1016/1074-7613(95)90058-6.
11. Berlin C, Berg EL, Briskin MJ, Andrew DP, Kilshaw PJ, Holzmann B, et al. Alpha 4 beta 7 integrin mediates lymphocyte binding to the mucosal vascular addressin MAdCAM-1. Cell. 1993;74(1):185–95. https://doi.org/10.1016/0092-8674(93)90305-a.
12. Hemler ME, Huang C, Schwarz L. The VLA protein family. Characterization of five distinct cell surface heterodimers each with a common 130,000 molecular weight beta subunit. J Biol Chem. 1987;262(7):3300–9.
13. Abram CL, Lowell CA. Leukocyte adhesion deficiency syndrome: a controversy solved. Immunol Cell Biol. 2009;87(6):440–2. https://doi.org/10.1038/icb.2009.32.
14. Coller BS. Platelet GPIIb/IIIa antagonists: the first anti-integrin receptor therapeutics. J Clin Invest. 1997;100(11 Suppl):S57–60.
15. Phillips DR, Scarborough RM. Clinical pharmacology of eptifibatide. Am J Cardiol. 1997;80(4A):11B–20B. https://doi.org/10.1016/s0002-9149(97)00572-9.
16. Cook JJ, Gardell SJ, Holahan MA, Sitko GR, Stump GL, Wallace AA, et al. Antithrombotic efficacy of thrombin inhibitor L-374,087: intravenous activity in a primate model of venous thrombus extension and oral activity in a canine model of primary venous and coronary artery thrombosis. J Pharmacol Exp Ther. 1999;289(1):503–10.
17. Wyant T, Fedyk E, Abhyankar B. An overview of the mechanism of action of the monoclonal antibody vedolizumab. J Crohns Colitis. 2016;10(12):1437–44. https://doi.org/10.1093/ecco-jcc/jjw092.
18. Sandborn WJ, Cyrille M, Hansen MB, Feagan BG, Loftus EV Jr, Rogler G, et al. Efficacy and safety of Abrilumab in a randomized, placebo-controlled trial for moderate-to-severe ulcerative colitis. Gastroenterology. 2019;156(4):946–57 e18. https://doi.org/10.1053/j.gastro.2018.11.035.

19. Hadley GA, Higgins JM. Integrin alphaEbeta7: molecular features and functional significance in the immune system. Adv Exp Med Biol. 2014;819:97–110. https://doi.org/10.1007/978-94-017-9153-3_7.
20. Sandborn WJ, Vermeire S, Tyrrell H, Hassanali A, Lacey S, Tole S, et al. Etrolizumab for the treatment of ulcerative colitis and Crohn's disease: an overview of the phase 3 clinical program. Adv Ther. 2020;37(7):3417–31. https://doi.org/10.1007/s12325-020-01366-2.
21. Vermeire S, O'Byrne S, Keir M, Williams M, Lu TT, Mansfield JC, et al. Etrolizumab as induction therapy for ulcerative colitis: a randomised, controlled, phase 2 trial. Lancet. 2014;384(9940):309–18. https://doi.org/10.1016/S0140-6736(14)60661-9.
22. Yoshimura N, Watanabe M, Motoya S, Tominaga K, Matsuoka K, Iwakiri R, et al. Safety and efficacy of AJM300, an Oral antagonist of alpha4 integrin, in induction therapy for patients with active ulcerative colitis. Gastroenterology. 2015;149(7):1775–83 e2. https://doi.org/10.1053/j.gastro.2015.08.044.
23. Donnenfeld ED, Karpecki PM, Majmudar PA, Nichols KK, Raychaudhuri A, Roy M, et al. Safety of Lifitegrast ophthalmic solution 5.0% in patients with dry eye disease: a 1-year, multicenter, randomized, placebo-controlled study. Cornea. 2016;35(6):741–8. https://doi.org/10.1097/ICO.0000000000000803.
24. Carson KR, Focosi D, Major EO, Petrini M, Richey EA, West DP, et al. Monoclonal antibody-associated progressive multifocal leucoencephalopathy in patients treated with rituximab, natalizumab, and efalizumab: a review from the research on adverse drug events and reports (RADAR) project. Lancet Oncol. 2009;10(8):816–24. https://doi.org/10.1016/S1470-2045(09)70161-5.
25. Yednock TA, Cannon C, Fritz LC, Sanchez-Madrid F, Steinman L, Karin N. Prevention of experimental autoimmune encephalomyelitis by antibodies against alpha 4 beta 1 integrin. Nature. 1992;356(6364):63–6. https://doi.org/10.1038/356063a0.
26. Polman CH, O'Connor PW, Havrdova E, Hutchinson M, Kappos L, Miller DH, et al. A randomized, placebo-controlled trial of natalizumab for relapsing multiple sclerosis. N Engl J Med. 2006;354(9):899–910. https://doi.org/10.1056/NEJMoa044397.
27. Rudick RA, Panzara MA. Natalizumab for the treatment of relapsing multiple sclerosis. Biologics. 2008;2(2):189–99. https://doi.org/10.2147/btt.s1956.
28. Clerico M, Artusi CA, Liberto AD, Rolla S, Bardina V, Barbero P, et al. Natalizumab in multiple sclerosis: long-term management. Int J Mol Sci. 2017;18(5) https://doi.org/10.3390/ijms18050940.
29. Targan SR, Feagan BG, Fedorak RN, Lashner BA, Panaccione R, Present DH, et al. Natalizumab for the treatment of active Crohn's disease: results of the ENCORE trial. Gastroenterology. 2007;132(5):1672–83. https://doi.org/10.1053/j.gastro.2007.03.024.
30. Sandborn WJ, Colombel JF, Enns R, Feagan BG, Hanauer SB, Lawrance IC, et al. Natalizumab induction and maintenance therapy for Crohn's disease. N Engl J Med. 2005;353(18):1912–25. https://doi.org/10.1056/NEJMoa043335.
31. Ghosh S, Goldin E, Gordon FH, Malchow HA, Rask-Madsen J, Rutgeerts P, et al. Natalizumab for active Crohn's disease. N Engl J Med. 2003;348(1):24–32. https://doi.org/10.1056/NEJMoa020732.
32. Zhang YZ, Li YY. Inflammatory bowel disease: pathogenesis. World J Gastroenterol. 2014;20(1):91–9. https://doi.org/10.3748/wjg.v20.i1.91.
33. Parikh A, Fox I, Leach T, Xu J, Scholz C, Patella M, et al. Long-term clinical experience with vedolizumab in patients with inflammatory bowel disease. Inflamm Bowel Dis. 2013;19(8):1691–9. https://doi.org/10.1097/MIB.0b013e318281f538.
34. Sands BE, Feagan BG, Rutgeerts P, Colombel JF, Sandborn WJ, Sy R, et al. Effects of vedolizumab induction therapy for patients with Crohn's disease in whom tumor necrosis factor antagonist treatment failed. Gastroenterology. 2014;147(3):618–27 e3. https://doi.org/10.1053/j.gastro.2014.05.008.
35. Yousry TA, Major EO, Ryschkewitsch C, Fahle G, Fischer S, Hou J, et al. Evaluation of patients treated with natalizumab for progressive multifocal leukoencephalopathy. N Engl J Med. 2006;354(9):924–33. https://doi.org/10.1056/NEJMoa054693.

36. Padgett BL, Walker DL, ZuRhein GM, Eckroade RJ, Dessel BH. Cultivation of papova-like virus from human brain with progressive multifocal leucoencephalopathy. Lancet. 1971;1(7712):1257–60. https://doi.org/10.1016/s0140-6736(71)91777-6.
37. Kean JM, Rao S, Wang M, Garcea RL. Seroepidemiology of human polyomaviruses. PLoS Pathog. 2009;5(3):e1000363. https://doi.org/10.1371/journal.ppat.1000363.
38. Bozic C, Subramanyam M, Richman S, Plavina T, Zhang A, Ticho B. Anti-JC virus (JCV) antibody prevalence in the JCV epidemiology in MS (JEMS) trial. Eur J Neurol. 2014;21(2):299–304. https://doi.org/10.1111/ene.12304.
39. Egli A, Infanti L, Dumoulin A, Buser A, Samaridis J, Stebler C, et al. Prevalence of polyomavirus BK and JC infection and replication in 400 healthy blood donors. J Infect Dis. 2009;199(6):837–46. https://doi.org/10.1086/597126.
40. Astrom KE, Mancall EL, Richardson EP Jr. Progressive multifocal leuko-encephalopathy; a hitherto unrecognized complication of chronic lymphatic leukaemia and Hodgkin's disease. Brain. 1958;81(1):93–111. https://doi.org/10.1093/brain/81.1.93.
41. Power C, Gladden JG, Halliday W, Del Bigio MR, Nath A, Ni W, et al. AIDS- and non-AIDS-related PML association with distinct p53 polymorphism. Neurology. 2000;54(3):743–6. https://doi.org/10.1212/wnl.54.3.743.
42. Sahraian MA, Radue EW, Eshaghi A, Besliu S, Minagar A. Progressive multifocal leukoencephalopathy: a review of the neuroimaging features and differential diagnosis. Eur J Neurol. 2012;19(8):1060–9. https://doi.org/10.1111/j.1468-1331.2011.03597.x.
43. Swinnen B, Saegeman V, Beuselinck K, Wouters A, Cypers G, Meyfroidt G, et al. Predictive value of JC virus PCR in cerebrospinal fluid in the diagnosis of PML. Diagn Microbiol Infect Dis. 2019;95(3):114859. https://doi.org/10.1016/j.diagmicrobio.2019.06.011.
44. Berger JR, Aksamit AJ, Clifford DB, Davis L, Koralnik IJ, Sejvar JJ, et al. PML diagnostic criteria: consensus statement from the AAN neuroinfectious disease section. Neurology. 2013;80(15):1430–8. https://doi.org/10.1212/WNL.0b013e31828c2fa1.
45. Kappos L, Bates D, Edan G, Eraksoy M, Garcia-Merino A, Grigoriadis N, et al. Natalizumab treatment for multiple sclerosis: updated recommendations for patient selection and monitoring. Lancet Neurol. 2011;10(8):745–58. https://doi.org/10.1016/S1474-4422(11)70149-1.
46. Clerico M, Artusi CA, Di Liberto A, Rolla S, Bardina V, Barbero P, et al. Long-term safety evaluation of natalizumab for the treatment of multiple sclerosis. Expert Opin Drug Saf. 2017;16(8):963–72. https://doi.org/10.1080/14740338.2017.1346082.
47. Dahlhaus S, Hoepner R, Chan A, Kleiter I, Adams O, Lukas C, et al. Disease course and outcome of 15 monocentrically treated natalizumab-associated progressive multifocal leukoencephalopathy patients. J Neurol Neurosurg Psychiatry. 2013;84(10):1068–74. https://doi.org/10.1136/jnnp-2013-304897.
48. Cortese I, Muranski P, Enose-Akahata Y, Ha SK, Smith B, Monaco M, et al. Pembrolizumab treatment for progressive multifocal leukoencephalopathy. N Engl J Med. 2019;380(17):1597–605. https://doi.org/10.1056/NEJMoa1815039.
49. Fine AJ, Sorbello A, Kortepeter C, Scarazzini L. Central nervous system herpes simplex and varicella zoster virus infections in natalizumab-treated patients. Clin Infect Dis. 2013;57(6):849–52. https://doi.org/10.1093/cid/cit376.
50. Fragoso YD, Brooks JB, Gomes S, de Oliveira FT, da Gama PD. Report of three cases of herpes zoster during treatment with natalizumab. CNS Neurosci Ther. 2013;19(4):280–1. https://doi.org/10.1111/cns.12067.
51. Kwiatkowski A, Gallois J, Bilbault N, Calais G, Mackowiak A, Hautecoeur P. Herpes encephalitis during natalizumab treatment in multiple sclerosis. Mult Scler. 2012;18(6):909–11. https://doi.org/10.1177/1352458511428082.
52. Dahdaleh D, Altmann DM, Malik O, Nicholas RS. Breathlessness, night sweats, and weight loss on natalizumab. Lancet. 2012;380(9843):726–7. https://doi.org/10.1016/S0140-6736(12)61401-9.
53. Loftus EV Jr, Feagan BG, Panaccione R, Colombel JF, Sandborn WJ, Sands BE, et al. Long-term safety of vedolizumab for inflammatory bowel disease. Aliment Pharmacol Ther. 2020;52(8):1353–65. https://doi.org/10.1111/apt.16060.

54. Colombel JF, Sands BE, Rutgeerts P, Sandborn W, Danese S, D'Haens G, et al. The safety of vedolizumab for ulcerative colitis and Crohn's disease. Gut. 2017;66(5):839–51. https://doi.org/10.1136/gutjnl-2015-311079.
55. McAuliffe ME, Lanes S, Leach T, Parikh A, Faich G, Porter J, et al. Occurrence of adverse events among patients with inflammatory bowel disease in the HealthCore integrated research database. Curr Med Res Opin. 2015;31(9):1655–64. https://doi.org/10.1185/03007995.2015.1065242.
56. Card T, Xu J, Liang H, Bhayat F. What is the risk of progressive multifocal leukoencephalopathy in patients with ulcerative colitis or Crohn's disease treated with vedolizumab? Inflamm Bowel Dis. 2018;24(5):953–9. https://doi.org/10.1093/ibd/izx097.
57. Langley RG, Carey WP, Rafal ES, Tyring SK, Caro I, Wang X, et al. Incidence of infection during efalizumab therapy for psoriasis: analysis of the clinical trial experience. Clin Ther. 2005;27(9):1317–28. https://doi.org/10.1016/j.clinthera.2005.09.007.
58. Scheinfeld N. Efalizumab: a review of events reported during clinical trials and side effects. Expert Opin Drug Saf. 2006;5(2):197–209. https://doi.org/10.1517/14740338.5.2.197.
59. McGuigan C, Craner M, Guadagno J, Kapoor R, Mazibrada G, Molyneux P, et al. Stratification and monitoring of natalizumab-associated progressive multifocal leukoencephalopathy risk: recommendations from an expert group. J Neurol Neurosurg Psychiatry. 2016;87(2):117–25. https://doi.org/10.1136/jnnp-2015-311100.
60. Bloomgren G, Richman S, Hotermans C, Subramanyam M, Goelz S, Natarajan A, et al. Risk of natalizumab-associated progressive multifocal leukoencephalopathy. N Engl J Med. 2012;366(20):1870–80. https://doi.org/10.1056/NEJMoa1107829.
61. Redelman-Sidi G, Michielin O, Cervera C, Ribi C, Aguado JM, Fernandez-Ruiz M, et al. ESCMID study Group for Infections in compromised hosts (ESGICH) consensus document on the safety of targeted and biological therapies: an infectious diseases perspective (immune checkpoint inhibitors, cell adhesion inhibitors, sphingosine-1-phosphate receptor modulators and proteasome inhibitors). Clin Microbiol Infect. 2018;24(Suppl 2):S95–S107. https://doi.org/10.1016/j.cmi.2018.01.030.
62. Wattjes MP, Killestein J. Progressive multifocal leukoencephalopathy after natalizumab discontinuation: few and true? Ann Neurol. 2014;75(3):462. https://doi.org/10.1002/ana.24110.
63. Plavina T, Subramanyam M, Bloomgren G, Richman S, Pace A, Lee S, et al. Anti-JC virus antibody levels in serum or plasma further define risk of natalizumab-associated progressive multifocal leukoencephalopathy. Ann Neurol. 2014;76(6):802–12. https://doi.org/10.1002/ana.24286.
64. Schwab N, Schneider-Hohendorf T, Melzer N, Cutter G, Wiendl H. Natalizumab-associated PML: challenges with incidence, resulting risk, and risk stratification. Neurology. 2017;88(12):1197–205. https://doi.org/10.1212/WNL.0000000000003739.
65. Vennegoor A, van Rossum JA, Leurs C, Wattjes MP, Rispens T, Murk JL, et al. High cumulative JC virus seroconversion rate during long-term use of natalizumab. Eur J Neurol. 2016;23(6):1079–85. https://doi.org/10.1111/ene.12988.
66. Gorelik L, Lerner M, Bixler S, Crossman M, Schlain B, Simon K, et al. Anti-JC virus antibodies: implications for PML risk stratification. Ann Neurol. 2010;68(3):295–303. https://doi.org/10.1002/ana.22128.
67. Lee P, Plavina T, Castro A, Berman M, Jaiswal D, Rivas S, et al. A second-generation ELISA (STRATIFY JCV DxSelect) for detection of JC virus antibodies in human serum and plasma to support progressive multifocal leukoencephalopathy risk stratification. J Clin Virol. 2013;57(2):141–6. https://doi.org/10.1016/j.jcv.2013.02.002.
68. Cortese I, Reich DS, Nath A. Progressive multifocal leukoencephalopathy and the spectrum of JC virus-related disease. Nat Rev Neurol. 2021;17(1):37–51. https://doi.org/10.1038/s41582-020-00427-y.
69. Antoniol C, Stankoff B. Immunological markers for PML prediction in MS patients treated with natalizumab. Front Immunol. 2014;5:668. https://doi.org/10.3389/fimmu.2014.00668.

70. Schwab N, Schneider-Hohendorf T, Pignolet B, Spadaro M, Gorlich D, Meinl I, et al. PML risk stratification using anti-JCV antibody index and L-selectin. Mult Scler. 2016;22(8):1048–60. https://doi.org/10.1177/1352458515607651.
71. Villar LM, Costa-Frossard L, Masterman T, Fernandez O, Montalban X, Casanova B, et al. Lipid-specific immunoglobulin M bands in cerebrospinal fluid are associated with a reduced risk of developing progressive multifocal leukoencephalopathy during treatment with natalizumab. Ann Neurol. 2015;77(3):447–57. https://doi.org/10.1002/ana.24345.
72. Epstein DJ, Dunn J, Deresinski S. Infectious complications of multiple sclerosis therapies: implications for screening, prophylaxis, and management. Open forum. Infect Dis. 2018;5(8):ofy174. https://doi.org/10.1093/ofid/ofy174.
73. Ng SC, Hilmi IN, Blake A, Bhayat F, Adsul S, Khan QR, et al. Low frequency of opportunistic infections in patients receiving vedolizumab in clinical trials and post-marketing setting. Inflamm Bowel Dis. 2018;24(11):2431–41. https://doi.org/10.1093/ibd/izy153.
74. Hillen ME, Cook SD, Samanta A, Grant E, Quinless JR, Rajasingham JK. Fatal acute liver failure with hepatitis B virus infection during natalizumab treatment in multiple sclerosis. Neurol Neuroimmunol Neuroinflamm. 2015;2(2):e72. https://doi.org/10.1212/NXI.0000000000000072.
75. Kaufman M, Pardo G, Rossman H, Sweetser MT, Forrestal F, Duda P. Natalizumab treatment shows no clinically meaningful effects on immunization responses in patients with relapsing-remitting multiple sclerosis. J Neurol Sci. 2014;341(1–2):22–7. https://doi.org/10.1016/j.jns.2014.03.035.
76. Wyant T, Leach T, Sankoh S, Wang Y, Paolino J, Pasetti MF, et al. Vedolizumab affects antibody responses to immunisation selectively in the gastrointestinal tract: randomised controlled trial results. Gut. 2015;64(1):77–83. https://doi.org/10.1136/gutjnl-2014-307127.

Tyrosine-Kinase Inhibitors

15

Cybele Lara R. Abad and Raymund R. Razonable

Introduction

Tyrosine kinases are a family of membrane-bound or intracellular molecules that regulate a variety of important cellular functions. They are involved in transferring phosphate groups to tyrosine residues in substrate proteins transducing intracellular signals engaged in many cellular functions, including the modulation of growth factors related to carcinogenesis. Many tyrosine kinase inhibitors (TKIs) play a key role in cell cycle regulation and carry significant potential for oncogenesis if mutated [1]. As such, protein kinases have become one of the most intensively investigated target classes for therapeutic intervention with consensus guidelines for clinicians who care for immune compromised hosts [2]. So far, more than ten classes of small molecular weight protein kinase inhibitors have been approved for cancer treatment, and over 100 kinase inhibitors are currently in clinical development [3].

The first TKI, imatinib, was approved in 2001 as an inhibitor of breakpoint cluster region (BCR)-v-abl Abelson murine leukemia viral oncogene homolog (ABL) tyrosine kinase fusion protein (BCR-ABL). It represents the first-in-class agent targeting this specific mutation and subsequently spawned a new class of targeted therapies [1]. There are now many other approved TKIs for patients with hematologic or other malignancies. In this chapter, we review this family of small molecules with special attention to BCR-ABL TKI inhibitors. We also highlight the unique features of TKIs and focus on their specific indications, the risks of infection and recommendations for prophylaxis.

C. L. R. Abad
Division of Infectious Diseases, Department of Medicine, University of the Philippines-Manila, Philippine General Hospital, Manila, Philippines

R. R. Razonable (✉)
Department of Health Sciences Research and The William J. Von Liebig Center for Transplantation and Clinical Regeneration, Mayo Clinic, Rochester, MN, USA
e-mail: razonable.raymund@mayo.edu

C. Cervera, J. M. Aguado (eds.), *Infectious Complications in Biologic and Targeted Therapies*, https://doi.org/10.1007/978-3-031-11363-5_15

The Tyrosine Kinase Inhibitor Family

Tyrosine kinases are involved in intracellular signaling cascades and play a crucial role in initiating or perpetuating a signaling cascade within the cell, leading to cell growth, transformation, activation, or apoptosis. Inhibitors of these enzymes, known as TKIs, are small molecules that have been considered as "targeted therapies" because of their specific mechanisms of action [4] as seen in (Fig. 15.1). The tyrosine kinases are often selectively overexpressed in malignancies due to point mutations or chromosomal rearrangements. Hence, TKIs have mostly been developed for the treatment of malignancies. TKIs have good oral bioavailability and may be prone to cytochrome P450 drug-drug interactions [5, 6]. TKIs, because of their unique mechanism of action, have the potential to increase the risk of several infectious complications, which are detailed in Table 15.1.

BCR-ABL Inhibitors

There are currently five agents in this class—imatinib, dasatinib, nilotinib, bosutinib, and ponatinib—which are all used to treat primary hematologic malignancies that arise as a result of the BCR-ABL gene and fusion protein. BCR-ABL inhibitors also target other receptor tyrosine kinases and a wide range of non-receptor kinases [7]. They all share a common mechanism of binding to the ATP-binding site of the mutant BCR-ABL fusion protein with high affinity.

Receptor targets	Biological agents
Janus kinase	Tofacitinib Baricitinib Ruxolitinib
Bruton's tyrosine kinase	Ibrutinib Acalabrutinib
BCR-ABL	Imatinib Dasatinib Nilotinib Ponatinib Bosutinib
Anaplastic lymphoma kinase	Crizotinib Ceritinib Alectinib Brigatinib
Phosphoinositide 3-kinase	Idelalisib Copanlisib
Spleen tyrosine kinase	Fostamatinib

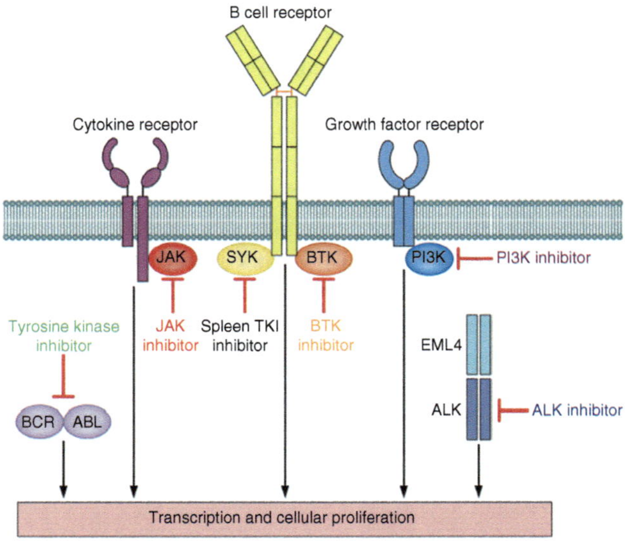

Fig. 15.1 Action points of specific TKI [with permission from Davis et al.]

Mechanism of Action (MOA) and Indications

Imatinib was the first TKI approved for chronic myelogenous leukemia (CML). It competitively inhibits the ATP-binding site of the BCR-ABL tyrosine kinase, inhibiting the phosphorylation of tyrosine proteins involved in BCR-ABL signal transduction. It also specifically acts on the receptor for platelet-derived-growth factor (PDGFR) and c-KIT tyrosine kinases. As a result, it is also clinically useful for certain diseases such as gastrointestinal stromal tumors (GIST) and systemic mastocytosis, as well as diseases such as hypereosinophilic syndromes (HES) and chronic myelomonocytic leukemia (CMML) [1].

Dasatinib is a second-generation inhibitor of BCR-ABL kinases approved for the treatment of Ph + CML or acute lymphocytic leukemia (ALL) [8–10]. It was

Table 15.1 Summary of tyrosine kinase inhibitors

Tyrosine kinase inhibitor	Mechanism of action	Indication	Pathophysiology of infection	Infection risk
BCR-ABL inhibitor				
Imatinib	Competitive inhibitor of Bcr-Abl, PDGFr, c-kit	CML, GIST, MDS, Eos leukemia HES, mastocytosis	Induces neutropenia, Inhibits T-cell proliferation And activation Reduces specific CD8+ responses and cause Dysfunction of dendritic Cells	Higher neutropenia risk Mild upper respiratory infections Usually in first year Increased risk of VZV, HBV Rare cases of fungal and TB infection
Dasatinib	Dual SRC/ABL inhibitor, TEC family kinases, and BTK	Ph + CML, Ph + CLL		**Higher risk of infection than imatinib** CMV reactivation with HSCT
Nilotinib	Selective, competitive inhibitor of Bcr-Abl **More potent than imatinib**	Ph + CML		Less risk of infection
Bosutinib	Competitive inhibitor of Bcr-Abl	Ph + CML		Higher neutropenia risk **Pleural effusion** Pneumonia
Ponatinib	Competitive inhibitor of Bcr-Abl	Ph + CML or **T315I mutant** CML or ALL		Higher neutropenia risk Limited data

(continued)

Table 15.1 (continued)

Tyrosine kinase inhibitor	Mechanism of action	Indication	Pathophysiology of infection	Infection risk
JAK inhibitor				
Tofacitinib	Competitive inhibitor of JAK1, 2,3	RA, PsA, UC	Reduce T-cell number and function, inhibit T-cell proliferation, and impair NK cell maturation	Increased risk of mild infection, usually pneumonia, SSTI, HZ Serious infection was 3.1 events/100 patient-years
Baricitinib	Selective and reversible JAK1 and 2 inhibitor	RA		**Highest risk for HZ**
Ruxolitinib	Inhibitor of JAK1 and 2	MF, PCV		HZ, tuberculosis
Upadacitinib	Selective JAK1 inhibitor	Moderate to severe RA refractory to MTX		Limited data
BTK inhibitor				
Ibrutinib	Selective, reversible inhibitor of BTK protein	CLL, SLL, MCL, WM, MZL, cGVHD	Primary B cell dysfunction	Neutropenia **Pneumonia**, **URTI**, SSTI IFI
Acalabrutinib	Irreversible BTK inhibitor	MCL		Grade 3 or 4 infections
PI3K inhibitor				
Idelalisib	Reversible inhibitor of PI3K-δ	CLL, SLL, FL	B- and T-cell dysfunction	**Fatal pneumonia or sepsis** PJP, IFI
Copanlisib	Second generation, PI3K-α and δ isoforms	FL		Pneumonia PJP IFI

Table 15.1 (continued)

Tyrosine kinase inhibitor	Mechanism of action	Indication	Pathophysiology of infection	Infection risk
ALK inhibitor				
Crizotinib	ALK or ROS1	NSCLC	Not specified	No significant increase in risk of infection **Interstitial pneumonitis Increased risk for infected complex renal cysts**
Ceritinib	ALK	Locally advanced or metastatic NSCLC		None reported
Alectinib	ALK	Advanced or previously treated NSCLC		**Nasopharyngitis**
Brigatinib	ALK	Advanced NSCLC		None reported
SyK inhibitor				
Fostamatinib	Intracellular SyK inhibitor	ITP, RA	Regulates both T-cell and B-cell expansion and proliferation; diminished proliferation of antigen-specific CD4+ T cells and reduced production of inflammatory cytokines such as IFN λ and IL-17	Neutropenia. No significant increase in infection risk

ALK anaplastic lymphoma kinase, *BCR-ABL* breakpoint cluster region (BCR)-v-abl Abelson murine leukemia, *BTK* Bruton tyrosine kinases, *JAK* Janus-associated kinase, *PI3K* phosphatidylinositol 3-kinase inhibitors, *SYK* spleen tyrosine kinase
In bold—unique features of the drug/class

developed as a dual SRC/ABL inhibitor, but it also affects a wider array of kinases, including TEC family kinases and Bruton tyrosine kinase (BTK) [11]. This increase in off-target activity may be responsible for in vitro data that hint at a strongest immunosuppressive effect for this TKI [12].

Nilotinib is a second-generation BCR-ABL inhibitor that is also approved for use in the treatment of Ph + CML [13, 14]. It is an analogue of imatinib with more potent BCR-ABL kinase inhibition.

Bosutinib is a small, orally bioavailable molecule, inhibiting both SRC and BCR-ABL with activity against imatinib-resistant CML cell lines [15]. It is approved for use in various phases of CML [16, 17]. Bosutinib has demonstrated activity and manageable tolerability in a phase I/II study of patients with chronic phase CML following resistance/intolerance to imatinib only, or imatinib plus dasatinib and/or nilotinib [15, 18–20].

Ponatinib is a TKI active against disease resistant to other BCR-ABL TKIs [21]. It is approved for use in patients with CML or PH+ ALL resistant to other therapies, or with the T315I mutation.

Risk of Infection

Imatinib is known to induce neutropenia, inhibit T-cell proliferation and activation, reduce specific CD8+ responses to CMV and EBV, and cause dysfunction of dendritic cells [22–24]. The phase 3 IRIS study in 2003 [25] using imatinib as initial treatment of newly diagnosed chronic phase CML among 553 patients showed 60.8% all-grade neutropenia with imatinib, of which only 14.3% were grades 3 (i.e., neutrophil count between 500–1000/mm^3 and 4 (neutrophil count <500/mm^3), based on the Common Toxicity Criteria of the National Cancer Institute. Mild respiratory infections were commonly low grade and viral in origin. Long-term data showed that nearly all infection complications occurred within the first year. Only 1 patient each was reported as having treatment-related neutropenia, febrile neutropenia, and an anorectal infection in the first year of treatment, whereas only 1 patient each developed appendicitis and cellulitis in years 6 and 11, respectively [26].

Patients receiving imatinib for GIST did not have significant infection risk, although grade 3 or higher neutropenia occurred in 7% [27, 28]. There were also no significant infectious complications in a phase II study investigating its use in other malignancies [29].

However, long-term experience with imatinib has demonstrated increased risk of HBV or VZV reactivation, occurring in 2% of patients in a single retrospective study [30]. In another, 13–16% of patients developed a variety of infections, most commonly VZV and pneumonia [31]. Sporadic cases of tuberculosis [9, 32, 33], leishmaniasis [34], *cryptococcosis*, and other fungal infections have also been reported [35, 36].

Dasatinib appears to be associated with a greater risk of infection compared to other BCR-ABL inhibitors. In a clinical trial [37], infections of any grade occurred in 27 (11%) of dasatinib-treated patients compared to 18 (7%) imatinib-treated patients. Five patients versus 1 patient died due to infection, in the dasatinib and imatinib arm, respectively; however, the investigators deemed these infections unrelated to the drug. Interestingly, the majority of infections did not occur during the period of neutropenia.

In a safety analysis of two major clinical trials [38] inclusive of 1150 patients, serious infections were rare and only one grade 3–4 opportunistic infection was observed for dasatinib. However, a comparative analysis of dasatinib with nilotinib demonstrated that there was a higher proportion of infection-related healthcare resource utilization costs among those receiving dasatinib than in those receiving nilotinib, largely attributable to a larger proportion of infection-related inpatient-days [39].

The risk of CMV reactivation appears to be increased following hematopoietic stem cell transplantation (HSCT); in one study of 109 patients, dasatinib was associated with an increased incidence of CMV reactivation in the first year after transplantation (adjusted hazard ratio = 7.65, 95% CI, 1.84–31.7) [40].

Nilotinib was not associated with a greater risk of infection and caused less neutropenia compared to imatinib among patients with newly diagnosed CML. This was corroborated by subsequent cohorts [41–43]. Phase II studies examining its use in treated patients with chronic phase CML also failed to demonstrate evidence of significant infections, although neutropenia more commonly occurred [44, 45].

In a review of 169 patients with CML receiving first-line nilotinib therapy or therapy after imatinib failure, 9 (10%) patients among the frontline therapy group developed any infection, whereas 29 of 79 (37%) patients treated with nilotinib after imatinib failure developed any infection [46].

Phase I/II studies of *bosutinib* monotherapy in patients with imatinib-resistant chronic phase CML found no evidence of infectious complications but reported grade 3 or higher neutropenia in 18% of patients [15]. On long-term follow-up of this cohort [47], serious adverse events (SAEs) occurred in 59% (99/167) of patients with the most frequently occurring individual SAEs (>5% of patients overall) being pneumonia (10%), pyrexia (7%), febrile neutropenia (6%), thrombocytopenia (6%), disease progression (5%), headache (5%), and pleural effusion (5%). The only newly occurring individual SAE reported in more than two patients within year 2, 3, or 4 was pneumonia (three patients with events in year 2).

Ponatinib is relatively new, and post-marketing surveillance is limited. However, in phase II studies investigating its use in previously treated patients with CML or ALL did not demonstrate increased risk for infectious complications, although grade 3 or 4 neutropenia occurred in 12–26% [48], or in 14% of patients, respectively [49].

Prevention of Infection

Given the potentially increased risk of HBV reactivation infection among patients treated with TKIs, all patients should be screened for HBV prior to starting treatment [7] (Table 15.2). Those with evidence of HBV infection should initiate antiviral therapy or prophylaxis with entecavir or tenofovir, which should continue up to 6–12 months after cessation of immune suppressive therapy [50]. Susceptible patients should be vaccinated according to society guidelines [51], although the response may be impaired because of the underlying condition or because of the TKI.

Janus-Associated Kinases (JAK) Inhibitors

JAKs are a family of four non-receptor protein tyrosine kinases—JAK1, JAK2, JAK3, and tyrosine-kinase 2—which mediate signaling of cytokine receptors [52]. The pathways are involved in the growth, development, and differentiation of various cells but are crucial to the function of immune and hematopoietic cells [53]. There are three currently available JAK inhibitors—tofacitinib, baricitinib, and ruxolitinib. Their mechanisms of action, indications, and infection risk are summarized in Table 15.1.

Table 15.2 Recommendations for screening and prophylaxis

TKI class	Screening/monitoring	Prophylaxis	Vaccination
TKI	Hepatitis B	Consider treatment of chronic hepatitis B (HbsAg+) up to 6–12 months after cessation of therapy	Routine, age-appropriate vaccination
JAK	LTBI Hepatitis B	No specific recommendations	VZV vaccine
BTK	Hepatitis B	Consider PCP or other fungal prophylaxis if heavily treated or with prior exposure Chronic hep B (HbsAg+)	Influenza, pneumococcal vaccines
PI3K	Hepatitis B LTBI *Monitoring* CMV (monthly) ANC (q2 weeks)	Universal prophylaxis for PJP During treatment and for 2–6 months after cessation of therapy	Influenza, pneumococcal vaccines
ALK	No specific recommendations		
SyK	No specific screening recommendations Monitor ANC monthly	No specific recommendations	

ALK anaplastic lymphoma kinase, *BCR-ABL* breakpoint cluster region (BCR)-v-abl Abelson murine leukemia, *BTK* Bruton tyrosine kinases, *JAK* Janus-associated kinase, *PI3K* phosphatidylinositol 3-kinase inhibitors; SyK, spleen tyrosine kinase [10, 11]

MOA and Indication

Tofacitinib is a reversible competitive inhibitor of JAK1, JAK2, and JAK3 that inhibits lymphocyte proliferation and cytokine production, affecting the maturation of monocyte-derived dendritic cells and capacity to stimulate T cells [54, 55]. It was approved by the US Food and Drug Administration (FDA) for the treatment of rheumatoid arthritis (RA) and psoriatic arthritis (PsA) [56, 57].

Baricitinib, the second JAK inhibitor approved by the FDA for use in the treatment of RA [58, 59], is a selective and reversible JAK1 and 2 inhibitor. It suppresses the differentiation of plasmablasts, Th1, and Th17 cells [60]. *Ruxolitinib* is an inhibitor of JAK 1 and 2, approved for treatment of myelofibrosis and polycythemia vera (PCV) [61, 62]. *Upadacitinib*, a selective JAK-1 inhibitor, was recently approved in 2019 for the treatment of moderate to severe RA nonresponsive to methotrexate.

Risk of Infection

All JAK inhibitors may reduce T-cell number and function, inhibit T-cell proliferation, and impair NK cell maturation, which may be responsible for the increased risk of infectious complications [63]. In general, JAK inhibitors are associated with an increased risk of mild infections, such as respiratory tract infections, a small but increased risk of serious infections (3 per 100 patient years), and a consistent signal for a heightened risk for herpes zoster and tuberculosis [64].

In a review of pooled data from phase 2, phase 3 (P2P3), and long-term extension (LTE) studies of tofacitinib, among 4789 patients with RA, the overall rate of serious infection was 3.1 events/100 patient-years [65]. Age, corticosteroid dose, diabetes, and tofacitinib dose were independently linked to the risk of serious infection. Lymphocyte counts of $<0.5 \times 10^3/mm^3$ were rare but were associated with an increased risk of treated and/or serious infection. The most frequent infection was pneumonia, but skin and soft tissue infections were also commonly reported. Nonserious or serious herpes zoster virus infections were reported in 346 patients in the P2P3LTE population (incidence rate 4.27 events per 100 patient-years [95% CI 3.85–4.75]), while only 25 patients experienced an opportunistic infection (0.30 events per 100 patient-years [95% CI 0.20–0.44]). TB was reported in 16 patients (6 cases in the pooled P3 population [all receiving higher-dose tofacitinib at 10 mg twice daily], and 10 in the LTE group [5 receiving tofacitinib at a dosage of 5 mg twice daily and 5 receiving tofacitinib at a dosage of 10 mg twice daily]). The risk of serious infection did not increase over time with an incidence rate of 3.09 events/100 patient-years at 8.5 years follow-up.

Twenty-one studies were included in a recent meta-analysis [66] specifically evaluating the risk of serious infection and herpes zoster among RA patients receiving JAK inhibitors—11 tofacitinib (5888 patients), 6 baricitinib (3520 patients), and 4 upadacitinib studies (1736 patients). For serious infections, the incidence rates were relatively low at 1.97 (95% CI: 1.41, 2.68), 3.16 (95% CI: 2.07, 4.63), and 3.02 (95% CI: 0.98, 7.04), respectively. For herpes zoster, the incidence rates were 2.51 (95% CI: 1.87, 3.30), 3.16 (95% CI: 2.07, 4.63), and 2.41 (95% CI: 0.66, 6.18), respectively. The risk of herpes zoster appears to be higher overall than the general population, and it was numerically greatest with baricitinib.

Prevention of Infection

Screening for and treatment of latent tuberculosis infection and hepatitis B infection are advised in all patients before commencing treatment (Table 15.2). Given the higher risk of varicella zoster virus (VZV), vaccination against VZV with recombinant vaccine should also be considered for patients with positive serology or prior history of illness 2–3 weeks prior to starting therapy [67] (Table 15.2).

Bruton's Tyrosine Kinase (BTK) Inhibitors

BTK is a non-receptor protein kinase expressed in B cells, myeloid cells, mast cells, and platelets. B-cell receptor (BCR) signaling via BTK is imperative for B-cell activation, proliferation, and survival (945). There are two currently approved agents in this class – ibrutinib and acalabrutinib (Table 15.1).

MOA and Indication

Ibrutinib is a selective and reversible inhibitor of the BTK protein, approved for the treatment of CLL, small lymphocytic lymphoma (SLL), and mantle cell lymphoma (MCL), Waldenstrom's macroglobulinemia (WM), marginal zone lymphoma (MZL), and chronic graft versus host disease (cGVHD) [68, 69].

Acalabrutinib is an irreversible BTK inhibitor for the treatment of MCL. The highly selective and potent BTK inhibition provided by acalabrutinib is thought to translate into an improved safety profile compared with other targeted therapies [70, 71].

Risk of Infection

Infections in patients treated with ibrutinib relate primarily to B-cell dysfunction [72]. However, invasive fungal infection has also frequently been reported in association with BTK inhibitors, possibly as a result of its off-target effect on other kinases [72, 73].

In one study [74], 70% of 195 patients with relapsed or refractory CLL/SLL treated with ibrutinib developed an infection. Neutropenia occurred in 42 patients (22%), and pneumonia and urinary tract infections occurred in 14–17%.

The use of ibrutinib as first-line therapy for CLL/SLL was not clearly associated with an increased risk of infection in clinical trials, although severe pneumonia did occur [75]. In another study of 64 patients given ibrutinib for relapse or refractory MZL, 19% of patients experienced grade 3 or higher infections, most commonly pneumonia (8%) and cellulitis (5%) [76].

In a meta-analysis of prospective studies evaluating the use of ibrutinib among patients with a lymphoid malignancy [77], infectious complications were reported in almost all (44/48, 92%) trials. Infectious adverse events of any grade occurred in 56% of patients (approximately $N = 900$) treated with single-agent ibrutinib and in 52% of patients (approximately $N = 250$) receiving combination therapy. Grade 3–4 infectious adverse events occurred in 26% of patients on a single agent, and 20% of patients receiving combination therapy. The rate of grade 5 infectious adverse events was 2% in both cohorts. Eighteen of 22 single-agent trials and 15 of 28 combination therapy trials noted grade 3–4 pneumonia. The patient-affected rates for grade 3–4 pneumonia were 13% in single-agent studies and 8% in the combination setting. Grade 5 pneumonia occurred in 2% of all patients. These fatal infectious events included opportunistic pathogens such as *Pneumocystis jirovecii*, *Histoplasma capsulatum*, *Cryptococcus neoformans*, *Nocardia* species, and *Aspergillus* species.

In a more recent systematic review of phase III randomized controlled trials only [78], (7 studies, $n = 2167$ patients), ibrutinib was associated with a significantly increased risk of infection (any grade and grade 3–5) in patients with B-cell malignancies [pooled risk ratio (RR) = 1.34, 95% confidence interval [CI], 1.06–1.69, $P = 0.015$; and RR = 1.35, 95% CI, 1.05–1.74, $P = 0.018$, respectively]. In patients with CLL, a significantly increased risk of grade 3–5 infection was noted in the ibrutinib group [pooled RR = 1.24, 95% CI, 1.02–1.50, $P = 0.028$]. Pneumonia and URTI were the two most commonly reported infections in the studies included in this analysis.

A recent study looked at 124 patients treated with acalabrutinib in the phase II ACE-LY-004 trial [70], who were adjusted to match average baseline characteristics of populations from studies using alternative targeted treatment regimens for relapsed/refractory MCL for either monotherapy or combination therapies. The overall safety profile of acalabrutinib was similar to or better than that of the monotherapies; however, there was an increased risk of grade 3/4 infections versus the combination bendamustine + rituximab, and an increased risk of anemia compared with lenalidomide + rituximab and ibrutinib + rituximab.

Prevention of Infection

Recommendations for antifungal prophylaxis are currently not well defined. Further systemic and large-scale evaluation of the risk for pneumocystis pneumonia and other fungal infections are required before formal guidance can be issued. In general, pneumocystis prophylaxis may be given to those who have received prior chemoimmunotherapy, have refractory disease, or other risk factors such as concomitant high-dose steroid use [79, 80]. All patients should be screened for serological evidence of hepatitis B virus prior to commencement of ibrutinib, with prophylaxis provided to those who are hepatitis B surface antigen positive [81]. Vaccination against influenza and pneumococcus is recommended prior to initiation of therapy, but immune response is typically poor because of the underlying condition [82–84] (Table 15.2).

Phosphatidylinositol 3-Kinase (PI3K) Inhibitors

Phosphatidylinositol 3-kinase (PI3K) is a signaling pathway activated downstream of BCR. Along with protein kinase B (AKT) and mammalian target of rapamycin (mTOR), it is responsible for B-cell proliferation, cell survival, and angiogenesis [85]. There are two currently available agents in this class—idelalisib and copanlisib.

MOA and Indication

Idelalisib is a reversible inhibitor of PI3K-δ and is approved for use in the treatment of CLL, SLL, and follicular lymphoma (FL) [86–88]. Inhibition of PI3K-δ impairs both B- and T-cell-mediated function [81, 89, 90].

Copanlisib is a second-generation, intravenous PI3K inhibitor with predominant activity in PI3K-α and δ isoforms [91] approved for relapsed FL.

Risk of Infection

Pneumonia is one of the most common infectious complications associated with idelalisib use, with an incidence of about 20%; majority are grade 3 or higher [92]. Atypical infections, such as pneumocystis pneumonia, invasive fungal infection, and noninfectious (autoimmune) pneumonitis also occur [93].

In a retrospective analysis among 2198 patients receiving idelalisib [94], the overall incidence of pneumocystis pneumonia infection was 2.5% in patients receiving idelalisib, with or without rituximab, with or without bendamustine, compared to only 0.2% in patients receiving only rituximab with or without bendamustine. In this cohort, pneumocystis pneumonia prophylaxis reduced the incidence from 3.4% to 1.3%.

Fatal and serious infections have been reported in 21–48% of patients receiving idelalisib [86], and a warning was issued related to this risk. The increased risk of infection related death from either sepsis or pneumonia frequently occurred within the first 180 days of starting treatment [95]. Given this substantial risk, the FDA recommended that it is not indicated for first-line treatment of malignancy or in combination with bendamustine and/or rituximab for patients with FL [86].

Two phase II studies have evaluated the infection profile of copanlisib; in the smaller study [96] ($n = 33$), neutropenia occurred in 34.5% with grade 3 or higher neutropenia in majority (29.8%); infections were reported in 64.3% of patients, with grade 3 or higher infections including pneumonia in 14.3%, febrile neutropenia in 3.6%, and urinary tract and skin and soft tissue infections in 2.4%. In the larger study ($n = 142$) [97], pneumonia occurred in 21% of patients overall, and 15% experience grade 3 or higher pneumonia. In both cohorts, infection from unusual organisms such as *P. jirovecii*, *C. neoformans*, and *Aspergillus* species also occurred.

Prevention of Infection

Universal prophylaxis against *P. jirovecii* is recommended for all patients during treatment and for 2–6 months after cessation of idelalisib therapy [81] (Table 15.2). Monthly preemptive monitoring for CMV among those with positive IgG serology is also recommended upon initiation of idelalisib treatment [86–88]. Monitoring of absolute neutrophil count should be monitored at least every 2 weeks for the first 6 months of treatment, and the drug should not be started in patients with an ongoing or active infection [86–88]. Screening for latent TB infection and HBV are also recommended although there is insufficient data regarding the risk of reactivation infection. Both pneumococcal and influenza vaccination are also recommended [98]. Until further data are available, the recommendations for idelalisib should also be applied to copanlisib (Table 15.2).

Anaplastic Lymphoma Kinase (ALK) Inhibitors

The ALK gene codes for the ALK receptor tyrosine kinase whose exact function is unknown but may be related to neuronal cell proliferation [64]. Activation of this gene usually occurs via chromosomal rearrangement, and ALK rearrangements are seen in 3–5% of non-small cell lung cancers (NSCLC), most commonly in adenocarcinomas.

MOA and Indication

Crizotinib was the first ALK inhibitor approved for the treatment of advanced non-small cell lung carcinoma (NSCLC) with an ALK or ROS1 gene rearrangement [99–101]. The other ALK inhibitors currently approved for use are summarized in Table 15.1.

Risk of Infection

Data from two randomized controlled trials [102, 103] did not show evidence of increased risk of infection with crizotinib, although neutropenia occurred in 11–13%

of patients. Upper respiratory tract infections also occurred at a higher rate but were not associated with significant morbidity or mortality [102]. A unique feature of crizotinib is the propensity to develop complex renal cysts, which may be secondarily infected [104]. Interstitial pneumonitis has also been reported with all ALK inhibitors [103, 105–108].

Prevention of Infection

At this time, there are no specific recommendations regarding prevention of infectious complications from the use of ALK inhibitors.

Spleen (Syk) TKI

Spleen tyrosine kinase (Syk) is an intracellular cytoplasmic tyrosine kinase that is widely expressed in hematopoietic stem cells, particularly B cells [109]. It also plays a pivotal role in signaling and activating Fc receptors [110], regulating both T-cell and B-cell expansion and proliferation, and mediating signaling in inflammatory cells [111]. In vitro, Syk inhibition leads to diminished proliferation of antigen-specific CD4+ T cells and reduced production of inflammatory cytokines such as IFN λ and IL-17 [112].

MOA and Indication

Fostamatinib is the only currently approved agent in this class for use in patients with chronic immune thrombocytopenia (ITP) [113]; it is used off label for RA [111]. Its active metabolite, R406, inhibits signal transduction by Fcγ receptors involved in the antibody-mediated destruction of platelets by immune cells in chronic ITP [110], which results in increased platelet counts in this population.

Risk of Infection

Given the role of Syk in the immune response, one would expect its inhibition to have the potential to make the patient critically ill, but this has not been the case thus far [64]. Early phase II studies in patients receiving fostamatinib reported dose-related neutropenia in 6 [109] to 15% [114] of patients, higher than those receiving placebo.

In a small phase II study of 16 patients with chronic, refractory ITP [115], the use of various doses of fostamatinib led to a small but statistically significant decrease in total WBC, without increasing the infection risk. Two paired phase III studies compared fostamatinib with placebo using different doses [116], and rates of moderate to severe infections were similar compared to placebo at 8% vs. 6%. The risk of mild respiratory infections was slightly higher for patients on fostamatinib at 11% compared to 6% of those on placebo.

Prevention of Infection

There are currently no specific recommendations about preventive measures for patients taking fostamatinib. However, monthly monitoring of the absolute neutrophil count is recommended, with dose reduction or temporary cessation of the drug if it falls to <1 × 10^9/liter [113].

Conclusion

Several TKI are now available for use as primary therapy for hematologic malignancies and autoimmune diseases and has made the treatment of these diseases easier and more successful. However despite this targeted approach, the risk of infection remains, and is higher for those with refractory disease and those with history of prior immune suppression. The types of infection differ depending on the TKI class, although infection risk with TKIs appears to be related to the degree of neutropenia, and include viral or fungal pneumonia and other respiratory tract infections. Reactivation infections, such as tuberculosis and hepatitis B, can also occur, and a thorough evaluation and screening of these patients prior to initiation therapy must be performed.

References

1. Kin A, Schiffer CA. Infectious complications of tyrosine kinase inhibitors in hematological malignancies. Infect Dis Clin N Am. 2020;34(2):245–56.
2. Reinwald M, Silva JT, Mueller NJ, Fortún J, Garzoni C, de Fijter JW, et al. ESCMID study Group for Infections in compromised hosts (ESGICH) consensus document on the safety of targeted and biological therapies: an infectious diseases perspective (intracellular signaling pathways: tyrosine kinase and mTOR inhibitors). Clin Microbiol Infect. 2018;24(Suppl 2):S53–s70.
3. Zsila F, Fitos I, Bencze G, Kéri G, Orfi L. Determination of human serum alpha1-acid glycoprotein and albumin binding of various marketed and preclinical kinase inhibitors. Curr Med Chem. 2009;16(16):1964–77.
4. Hartmann JT, Haap M, Kopp HG, Lipp HP. Tyrosine kinase inhibitors—a review on pharmacology, metabolism and side effects. Curr Drug Metab. 2009;10(5):470–81.
5. Pajares B, Torres E, Trigo JM, Sáez MI, Ribelles N, Jiménez B, et al. Tyrosine kinase inhibitors and drug interactions: a review with practical recommendations. Clin Transl Oncol. 2012;14(2):94–101.
6. Drenberg CD, Baker SD, Sparreboom A. Integrating clinical pharmacology concepts in individualized therapy with tyrosine kinase inhibitors. Clin Pharmacol Ther. 2013;93(3):215–9.
7. Knoll BM, Seiter K. Infections in patients on BCR-ABL tyrosine kinase inhibitor therapy: cases and review of the literature. Infection. 2018;46(3):409–18.
8. Sprycel (dasatinib) 2018. Prescribing information. Reference ID 4179887. Food and Drug Administration, Silver Spring, MD. https://www.accessdata.fda.gov/drugsatfda_docs/label/2017/021986s020lbl.pdf. Accessed October 2020.
9. Therapeutic Goods Administration. Australian product information—Sprycel (dasatinib) 2018. Therapeutic Goods Administration, Woden, Australia. https://www.ebs.tga.gov.au/ebs/picmi/picmirepository.nsf/pdf?OpenAgent&id%03CP-2010-PI-02657-3. Accessed October 2020.
10. European Medicines Agency. Sprycel, INN—dasatinib. Product information. European Medicines Agency, Amsterdam, The Netherlands. https://www.ema.europa.eu/documents/product-information/sprycel-epar-product-information_en.pdf. Accessed October 2020 [Internet]. 2018 [cited October 2020].

11. Hantschel O, Rix U, Superti-Furga G. Target spectrum of the BCR-ABL inhibitors imatinib, nilotinib and dasatinib. Leuk Lymphoma. 2008;49(4):615–9.
12. Hayashi Y, Nakamae H, Katayama T, Nakane T, Koh H, Nakamae M, et al. Different immunoprofiles in patients with chronic myeloid leukemia treated with imatinib, nilotinib or dasatinib. Leuk Lymphoma. 2012;53(6):1084–9.
13. Therapeutic Goods Administration. 2018. Australian product information— Tasigna (nilotinib). Therapeutic goods Administration, Woden, Australia. https://www.ebs.tga.gov.au/ebs/picmi/picmirepository.nsf/pdf?OpenAgent&id%03CP-2009-PI-00292-3. Accessed October 2020.
14. Anonymous. 2018. Tasigna (nilotinib). Prescribing information. Reference ID 4309495. Food and Drug Administration, Silver Spring, MD.https://www.accessdata.fda.gov/drugsatfda_docs/label/2018/022068s029lbl.pdf. Accessed October 2020.
15. Cortes JE, Kantarjian HM, Brümmendorf TH, Kim DW, Turkina AG, Shen ZX, et al. Safety and efficacy of bosutinib (SKI-606) in chronic phase Philadelphia chromosome-positive chronic myeloid leukemia patients with resistance or intolerance to imatinib. Blood. 2011;118(17):4567–76.
16. European Medicines Agency. 2018. Bosulif, INN—bosutinib. Product information. European Medicines Agency, Amsterdam, The Netherlands. http://www.ema.europa.eu/docs/en_GB/document_library/EPAR_Product_Information/human/002373/WC500141721.pdf. Accessed October 2020.
17. Anonymous 2018. Bosulif (bosutinib). Prescribing information. Reference ID 4197387. Food and Drug Administration, Silver Spring, MD. https://www.accessdata.fda.gov/drugsatfda_docs/label/2017/ 203341s009lbl.pdf. Accessed October 2020.
18. Gambacorti-Passerini C, Brümmendorf TH, Kim DW, Turkina AG, Masszi T, Assouline S, et al. Bosutinib efficacy and safety in chronic phase chronic myeloid leukemia after imatinib resistance or intolerance: minimum 24-month follow-up. Am J Hematol. 2014;89(7):732–42.
19. Kantarjian HM, Cortes JE, Kim DW, Khoury HJ, Brümmendorf TH, Porkka K, et al. Bosutinib safety and management of toxicity in leukemia patients with resistance or intolerance to imatinib and other tyrosine kinase inhibitors. Blood. 2014;123(9):1309–18.
20. Khoury HJ, Cortes JE, Kantarjian HM, Gambacorti-Passerini C, Baccarani M, Kim DW, et al. Bosutinib is active in chronic phase chronic myeloid leukemia after imatinib and dasatinib and/or nilotinib therapy failure. Blood. 2012;119(15):3403–12.
21. Cortes JE, Kantarjian H, Shah NP, Bixby D, Mauro MJ, Flinn I, et al. Ponatinib in refractory Philadelphia chromosome-positive leukemias. N Engl J Med. 2012;367(22):2075–88.
22. Appel S, Boehmler AM, Grünebach F, Müller MR, Rupf A, Weck MM, et al. Imatinib mesylate affects the development and function of dendritic cells generated from CD34+ peripheral blood progenitor cells. Blood. 2004;103(2):538–44.
23. Dietz AB, Souan L, Knutson GJ, Bulur PA, Litzow MR, Vuk-Pavlovic S. Imatinib mesylate inhibits T-cell proliferation in vitro and delayed-type hypersensitivity in vivo. Blood. 2004;104(4):1094–9.
24. Seggewiss R, Loré K, Greiner E, Magnusson MK, Price DA, Douek DC, et al. Imatinib inhibits T-cell receptor-mediated T-cell proliferation and activation in a dose-dependent manner. Blood. 2005;105(6):2473–9.
25. O'Brien SG, Guilhot F, Larson RA, Gathmann I, Baccarani M, Cervantes F, et al. Imatinib compared with interferon and low-dose cytarabine for newly diagnosed chronic-phase chronic myeloid leukemia. N Engl J Med. 2003;348(11):994–1004.
26. Hochhaus A, Larson RA, Guilhot F, Radich JP, Branford S, Hughes TP, et al. Long-term outcomes of imatinib treatment for chronic myeloid leukemia. N Engl J Med. 2017;376(10):917–27.
27. Blanke CD, Rankin C, Demetri GD, Ryan CW, von Mehren M, Benjamin RS, et al. Phase III randomized, intergroup trial assessing imatinib mesylate at two dose levels in patients with unresectable or metastatic gastrointestinal stromal tumors expressing the kit receptor tyrosine kinase: S0033. J Clin Oncol. 2008;26(4):626–32.

28. Demetri GD, von Mehren M, Blanke CD, Van den Abbeele AD, Eisenberg B, Roberts PJ, et al. Efficacy and safety of imatinib mesylate in advanced gastrointestinal stromal tumors. N Engl J Med. 2002;347(7):472–80.
29. Heinrich MC, Joensuu H, Demetri GD, Corless CL, Apperley J, Fletcher JA, et al. Phase II, open-label study evaluating the activity of imatinib in treating life-threatening malignancies known to be associated with imatinib-sensitive tyrosine kinases. Clin Cancer Res. 2008;14(9):2717–25.
30. Mattiuzzi GN, Cortes JE, Talpaz M, Reuben J, Rios MB, Shan J, et al. Development of varicella-zoster virus infection in patients with chronic myelogenous leukemia treated with imatinib mesylate. Clin Cancer Res. 2003;9(3):976–80.
31. Breccia M, Girmenia C, Latagliata R, Loglisci G, Santopietro M, Federico V, et al. Low incidence rate of opportunistic and viral infections during imatinib treatment in chronic myeloid leukemia patients in early and late chronic phase. Mediterr J Hematol Infect Dis. 2011;3(1):e2011021.
32. Daniels JM, Vonk-Noordegraaf A, Janssen JJ, Postmus PE, van Altena R. Tuberculosis complicating imatinib treatment for chronic myeloid leukaemia. Eur Respir J. 2009;33(3):670–2.
33. Senn L, Kovacsovics T, Tarr PE, Meylan P. Peritoneal tuberculosis after imatinib therapy. Arch Intern Med. 2009;169(3):312–3.
34. Quixada A, Filho PA, Filho TP, Duarte FB, Moreira-Nunes CA, Lemes RP. Pancytopenia during tyrosine kinase inhibitor treatment—coexistence of chronic myeloid leukemia and visceral leishmaniasis: a case report. J Med Case Rep. 2016;10:207.
35. Crisan AM, Ghiaur A, Stancioaca MC, Bardas A, Ghita C, Manea CM, et al. Mucormycosis during imatinib treatment: case report. J Med Life. 2015;8(3):365–70.
36. Speletas M, Vyzantiadis TA, Kalala F, Plastiras D, Kokoviadou K, Antoniadis A, et al. Pneumonia caused by Candida krusei and Candida glabrata in a patient with chronic myeloid leukemia receiving imatinib mesylate treatment. Med Mycol. 2008;46(3):259–63.
37. Kantarjian HM, Shah NP, Cortes JE, Baccarani M, Agarwal MB, Undurraga MS, et al. Dasatinib or imatinib in newly diagnosed chronic-phase chronic myeloid leukemia: 2-year follow-up from a randomized phase 3 trial (DASISION). Blood. 2012;119(5):1123–9.
38. Al-Ameri A, Kantarijan H., Burton E. Low risk of infectious events in patients (pts) with chronic myeloid leukemia (CML) in chronic phase (CP) treated with dasatinib. Abstract 3291 ASH Annual Meeting 2009.
39. Seiter K, Latremouille-Viau D, Guerin A, Ndife B, Habucky K, Tang DH, et al. Burden of infections among chronic myeloid leukemia patients receiving Dasatinib or nilotinib: a real-world retrospective healthcare claims study in the United States. Adv Ther. 2018;35(10):1671–85.
40. Prestes DP, Arbona E, Nevett-Fernandez A, Woolley AE, Ho VT, Koo S, et al. Dasatinib use and risk of cytomegalovirus reactivation after allogeneic hematopoietic-cell transplantation. Clin Infect Dis. 2017;65(3):510–3.
41. Hochhaus A, Rosti G, Cross NC, Steegmann JL, le Coutre P, Ossenkoppele G, et al. Frontline nilotinib in patients with chronic myeloid leukemia in chronic phase: results from the European ENEST1st study. Leukemia. 2016;30(1):57–64.
42. Hochhaus A, Saglio G, Hughes TP, Larson RA, Kim DW, Issaragrisil S, et al. Long-term benefits and risks of frontline nilotinib vs imatinib for chronic myeloid leukemia in chronic phase: 5-year update of the randomized ENESTnd trial. Leukemia. 2016;30(5):1044–54.
43. Larson RA, Hochhaus A, Hughes TP, Clark RE, Etienne G, Kim DW, et al. Nilotinib vs imatinib in patients with newly diagnosed Philadelphia chromosome-positive chronic myeloid leukemia in chronic phase: ENESTnd 3-year follow-up. Leukemia. 2012;26(10):2197–203.
44. le Coutre PD, Giles FJ, Hochhaus A, Apperley JF, Ossenkoppele GJ, Blakesley R, et al. Nilotinib in patients with Ph+ chronic myeloid leukemia in accelerated phase following imatinib resistance or intolerance: 24-month follow-up results. Leukemia. 2012;26(6):1189–94.
45. Nicolini FE, Turkina A, Shen ZX, Gallagher N, Jootar S, Powell BL, et al. Expanding nilotinib access in clinical trials (ENACT): an open-label, multicenter study of oral nilotinib

in adult patients with imatinib-resistant or imatinib-intolerant Philadelphia chromosome-positive chronic myeloid leukemia in the chronic phase. Cancer. 2012;118(1):118–26.
46. Al-Ameri AM, Cortes JE, Kantarjian H, Burton E, Quintas-Cardama A, Jabbour E, et al. Infectious events in patients with chronic myeloid leukemia treated with nilotinib as a front line therapy and after imatinib failure. Blood. 2010;116:1233.
47. Gambacorti-Passerini C, Kantarjian HM, Kim DW, Khoury HJ, Turkina AG, Brümmendorf TH, et al. Long-term efficacy and safety of bosutinib in patients with advanced leukemia following resistance/intolerance to imatinib and other tyrosine kinase inhibitors. Am J Hematol. 2015;90(9):755–68.
48. Cortes JE, Kim DW, Pinilla-Ibarz J, le Coutre P, Paquette R, Chuah C, et al. A phase 2 trial of ponatinib in Philadelphia chromosome-positive leukemias. N Engl J Med. 2013;369(19):1783–96.
49. Jain P, Kantarjian H, Jabbour E, Gonzalez GN, Borthakur G, Pemmaraju N, et al. Ponatinib as first-line treatment for patients with chronic myeloid leukaemia in chronic phase: a phase 2 study. Lancet Haematol. 2015;2(9):e376–83.
50. Reddy KR, Beavers KL, Hammond SP, Lim JK, Falck-Ytter YT. American Gastroenterological Association Institute guideline on the prevention and treatment of hepatitis B virus reactivation during immunosuppressive drug therapy. Gastroenterology. 2015;148(1):215–9; quiz e16–7
51. Rubin LG, Levin MJ, Ljungman P, Davies EG, Avery R, Tomblyn M, et al. 2013 IDSA clinical practice guideline for vaccination of the immunocompromised host. Clin Infect Dis. 2014;58(3):309–18.
52. Cai B, Cai JP, Luo YL, Chen C, Zhang S. The specific roles of JAK/STAT signaling pathway in sepsis. Inflammation. 2015;38(4):1599–608.
53. Hodge JA, Kawabata TT, Krishnaswami S, Clark JD, Telliez JB, Dowty ME, et al. The mechanism of action of tofacitinib - an oral Janus kinase inhibitor for the treatment of rheumatoid arthritis. Clin Exp Rheumatol. 2016;34(2):318–28.
54. Kubo S, Yamaoka K, Kondo M, Yamagata K, Zhao J, Iwata S, et al. The JAK inhibitor, tofacitinib, reduces the T cell stimulatory capacity of human monocyte-derived dendritic cells. Ann Rheum Dis. 2014;73(12):2192–8.
55. Maeshima K, Yamaoka K, Kubo S, Nakano K, Iwata S, Saito K, et al. The JAK inhibitor tofacitinib regulates synovitis through inhibition of interferon-γ and interleukin-17 production by human CD4+ T cells. Arthritis Rheum. 2012;64(6):1790–8.
56. Anonymous. 2018. Xeljanz (tofacitinib). Prescribing information. Reference ID 4308396. Food and Drug Administration, Silver Spring, MD. https://www.accessdata.fda.gov/drugsatfda_docs/label/2018/203214s021,208246s007lbl.pdf. Accessed October 2020.
57. European Medicines Agency. 2018. Xeljanz, INN—tofacitinib citrate. Product information. European Medicines Agency, Amsterdam, The Netherlands. http://www.ema.europa.eu/docs/en_GB/document_library/EPAR_-_Product_Information/human/004214/WC500224911.pdf. Accessed October 2020.
58. European Medicines Agency. 2018. Olumiant, INN—baricitinib. Product information. European Medicines Agency, Amsterdam, The Netherlands. http://www.ema.europa.eu/docs/en_GB/document_library/EPAR_-_Product_Information/human/004085/WC500223723.pdf. Accessed October 2020.
59. Anonymous. 2018. Olumiant (baricitinib). Prescribing information. Reference ID 4271150. Food and Drug Administration, Silver Spring, MD. https://www.accessdata.fda.gov/drugsatfda_docs/label/2018/207924Orig1s000lbl.pdf. Accessed October 2020.
60. Kubo S, Nakayamada S, Sakata K, Kitanaga Y, Ma X, Lee S, et al. Janus kinase inhibitor Baricitinib modulates human innate and adaptive immune system. Front Immunol. 2018;9:1510.
61. Therapeutic Goods Administration. 2018. Australian product information—Jakavi (ruxolitinib). Therapeutic Goods Administration, Woden, Australia. https://www.ebs.tga.gov.au/ebs/picmi/picmirepository.nsf/ pdf?OpenAgent&id_CP-2013-PI-01918-1&d_201809111016933. October 2020.

62. Anonymous. 2018. Jakafi (ruxolitinib). Prescribing information. Reference ID 4191667. Food and Drug Administration, Silver Spring, MD. https://www.accessdata.fda.gov/drugsatfda_docs/label/2017/202192s015lbl.pdf. Accessed October 2020.
63. McLornan DP, Khan AA, Harrison CN. Immunological consequences of JAK inhibition: friend or foe? Curr Hematol Malig Rep. 2015;10(4):370–9.
64. Davis JS, Ferreira D, Paige E, Gedye C, Boyle M. Infectious complications of biological and small molecule targeted immunomodulatory therapies. Clin Microbiol Rev. 2020;33(3)
65. Cohen S, Radominski SC, Gomez-Reino JJ, Wang L, Krishnaswami S, Wood SP, et al. Analysis of infections and all-cause mortality in phase II, phase III, and long-term extension studies of tofacitinib in patients with rheumatoid arthritis. Arthritis Rheumatol. 2014;66(11):2924–37.
66. Bechman K, Subesinghe S, Norton S, Atzeni F, Galli M, Cope AP, et al. A systematic review and meta-analysis of infection risk with small molecule JAK inhibitors in rheumatoid arthritis. Rheumatology (Oxford). 2019;58(10):1755–66.
67. Winthrop KL, Park SH, Gul A, Cardiel MH, Gomez-Reino JJ, Tanaka Y, et al. Tuberculosis and other opportunistic infections in tofacitinib-treated patients with rheumatoid arthritis. Ann Rheum Dis. 2016;75(6):1133–8.
68. Anonymous. 2018. Imbruvica (ibrutinib). Prescribing information. Reference ID 4222705. Food and Drug Administration, Silver Spring, MD. https://www.accessdata.fda.gov/drugsatfda_docs/label/2018/210563s000lbl.pdf. Accessed October 2020.
69. Therapeutic Goods Administration. 2018. Australian product information—Imbruvica (ibrutinib). Therapeutic goods Administration, Woden, Australia. https://www.ebs.tga.gov.au/ebs/picmi/picmirepository.nsf/pdf?OpenAgent&id%03CP-2015-PI-01676-1&d%0320180825l016933. Accessed October 2020.
70. Telford C, Kabadi SM, Abhyankar S, Song J, Signorovitch J, Zhao J, et al. Matching-adjusted indirect comparisons of the efficacy and safety of acalabrutinib versus other targeted therapies in relapsed/refractory mantle cell lymphoma. Clin Ther. 2019;41(11):2357–79.e1.
71. Wu J, Zhang M, Liu D. Acalabrutinib (ACP-196): a selective second-generation BTK inhibitor. J Hematol Oncol. 2016;9:21.
72. Hilal T, Gea-Banacloche JC, Leis JF. Chronic lymphocytic leukemia and infection risk in the era of targeted therapies: linking mechanisms with infections. Blood Rev. 2018;32(5):387–99.
73. Varughese T, Taur Y, Cohen N, Palomba ML, Seo SK, Hohl TM, et al. Serious infections in patients receiving ibrutinib for treatment of lymphoid cancer. Clin Infect Dis. 2018;67(5):687–92.
74. Byrd JC, Brown JR, O'Brien S, Barrientos JC, Kay NE, Reddy NM, et al. Ibrutinib versus ofatumumab in previously treated chronic lymphoid leukemia. N Engl J Med. 2014;371(3):213–23.
75. Burger JA, Tedeschi A, Barr PM, Robak T, Owen C, Ghia P, et al. Ibrutinib as initial therapy for patients with chronic lymphocytic leukemia. N Engl J Med. 2015;373(25):2425–37.
76. Noy A, de Vos S, Thieblemont C, Martin P, Flowers CR, Morschhauser F, et al. Targeting Bruton tyrosine kinase with ibrutinib in relapsed/refractory marginal zone lymphoma. Blood. 2017;129(16):2224–32.
77. Tillman BF, Pauff JM, Satyanarayana G, Talbott M, Warner JL. Systematic review of infectious events with the Bruton tyrosine kinase inhibitor ibrutinib in the treatment of hematologic malignancies. Eur J Haematol. 2018;100(4):325–34.
78. Ball S, Das A, Vutthikraivit W, Edwards PJ, Hardwicke F, Short NJ, et al. Risk of infection associated with ibrutinib in patients with B-cell malignancies: a systematic review and meta-analysis of randomized controlled trials. Clin Lymphoma Myeloma Leuk. 2020;20(2):87–97.e5.
79. Gribben JG, Bosch F, Cymbalista F, Geisler CH, Ghia P, Hillmen P, et al. Optimising outcomes for patients with chronic lymphocytic leukaemia on ibrutinib therapy: European recommendations for clinical practice. Br J Haematol. 2018;180(5):666–79.
80. Reinwald M, Boch T, Hofmann WK, Buchheidt D. Risk of infectious complications in Hemato-oncological patients treated with kinase inhibitors. Biomark Insights. 2015; 10(Suppl 3):55–68.

81. Teh BW, Tam CS, Handunnetti S, Worth LJ, Slavin MA. Infections in patients with chronic lymphocytic leukaemia: mitigating risk in the era of targeted therapies. Blood Rev. 2018;32(6):499–507.
82. Andrick B, Alwhaibi A, DeRemer DL, Quershi S, Khan R, Bryan LJ, et al. Lack of adequate pneumococcal vaccination response in chronic lymphocytic leukaemia patients receiving ibrutinib. Br J Haematol. 2018;182(5):712–4.
83. Douglas AP, Trubiano JA, Barr I, Leung V, Slavin MA, Tam CS. Ibrutinib may impair serological responses to influenza vaccination. Haematologica. 2017;102(10):e397–e9.
84. Sun C, Gao J, Couzens L, Tian X, Farooqui MZ, Eichelberger MC, et al. Seasonal influenza vaccination in patients with chronic lymphocytic leukemia treated with ibrutinib. JAMA Oncol. 2016;2(12):1656–7.
85. Greenwell IB, Ip A, Cohen JB. PI3K inhibitors: understanding toxicity mechanisms and management. Oncology (Williston Park). 2017;31(11):821–8.
86. Anonymous. 2018. Zydelig (idelalisib). Prescribing information. Reference ID 4213201. Food and Drug Administration, Silver Spring, MD. https://www.accessdata.fda.gov/drugsatfda_docs/label/2018/205858s009lbl.pdf. Accessed October 2020.
87. European Medicines Agency. 2018. Zydelig, INN—idelalisib. Product information. European Medicines Agency, Amsterdam, The Netherlands. http://www.ema.europa.eu/docs/en_GB/document_library/EPAR_-_Product_Information/human/003843/WC500175377.pdf. Accessed October 2020.
88. Therapeutic Goods Administration. 2018. Product information—Zydelig (idelalisib). Therapeutic goods Administration, Woden, Australia https://www.ebs.tga.gov.au/ebs/picmi/picmirepository.nsf/pdf?OpenAgent&id%03CP-2015-PI-01225-1&d%03201809151016933. Accessed October 2020.
89. Martinelli S, Maffei R, Fiorcari S, Quadrelli C, Zucchini P, Benatti S, et al. Idelalisib impairs T-cell-mediated immunity in chronic lymphocytic leukemia. Haematologica. 2018;103(12):e598–601.
90. Mensah FA, Blaize JP, Bryan LJ. Spotlight on copanlisib and its potential in the treatment of relapsed/refractory follicular lymphoma: evidence to date. Onco Targets Ther. 2018;11:4817–27.
91. Liu N, Rowley BR, Bull CO, Schneider C, Haegebarth A, Schatz CA, et al. BAY 80-6946 is a highly selective intravenous PI3K inhibitor with potent p110α and p110δ activities in tumor cell lines and xenograft models. Mol Cancer Ther. 2013;12(11):2319–30.
92. de Weerdt I, Koopmans SM, Kater AP, van Gelder M. Incidence and management of toxicity associated with ibrutinib and idelalisib: a practical approach. Haematologica. 2017;102(10):1629–39.
93. Coutré SE, Barrientos JC, Brown JR, de Vos S, Furman RR, Keating MJ, et al. Management of adverse events associated with idelalisib treatment: expert panel opinion. Leuk Lymphoma. 2015;56(10):2779–86.
94. Sehn LH, Hallek M, Jurczak W, Brown JR, Barr PM, Catalano J, et al. A retrospective analysis of Pneumocystis jirovecii pneumonia infection in patients receiving idelalisib in clinical trials. Blood. 2016;128:3705.
95. Australian Government Department of Health. 2017. Idelalisib (zydelig): safety advisory—change to indications and addition of warnings. https://www.tga.gov.au/alert/idelalisib-zydelig. Accessed October 2020.
96. Dreyling M, Morschhauser F, Bouabdallah K, Bron D, Cunningham D, Assouline SE, et al. Phase II study of copanlisib, a PI3K inhibitor, in relapsed or refractory, indolent or aggressive lymphoma. Ann Oncol. 2017;28(9):2169–78.
97. Dreyling M, Santoro A, Mollica L, Leppä S, Follows GA, Lenz G, et al. Phosphatidylinositol 3-kinase inhibition by Copanlisib in relapsed or refractory indolent lymphoma. J Clin Oncol. 2017;35(35):3898–905.
98. Cuneo A, Barosi G, Danesi R, Fagiuoli S, Ghia P, Marzano A, et al. Management of adverse events associated with idelalisib treatment in chronic lymphocytic leukemia and follicular lymphoma: a multidisciplinary position paper. Hematol Oncol. 2019;37(1):3–14.

99. European Medicines Agency. 2018. Xalkori, INN—crizotinib. Product Information. European Medicines Agency, Amsterdam, The Netherlands. http://www.ema.europa.eu/docs/en_GB/document_library/EPAR_-_Product_Information/human/002489/WC500134759.pdf. Accessed October 2020.
100. Anonymous. 2018. Xalkori (crizotinib). Prescribing information. Reference ID 4216933. Food and Drug Administration, Silver Spring, MD. https://www.accessdata.fda.gov/drugsatfda_docs/label/2018/202570s023lbl.pdf. Accessed October 2020.
101. Therapeutic Goods Administration. 2018. Australian product information—Xalkori (crizotinib). Therapeutic goods Administration, Woden, Australia. https://www.ebs.tga.gov.au/ebs/picmi/picmirepository.nsf/pdf?OpenAgent&id%03CP-2013-PI-02261-1. Accessed October 2020.
102. Shaw AT, Kim DW, Nakagawa K, Seto T, Crinó L, Ahn MJ, et al. Crizotinib versus chemotherapy in advanced ALK-positive lung cancer. N Engl J Med. 2013;368(25):2385–94.
103. Solomon BJ, Mok T, Kim DW, Wu YL, Nakagawa K, Mekhail T, et al. First-line crizotinib versus chemotherapy in ALK-positive lung cancer. N Engl J Med. 2014;371(23):2167–77.
104. Yoneshima Y, Okamoto I, Arimura-Omori M, Kimura S, Hidaka-Fujimoto N, Iwama E, et al. Infected complex renal cysts during crizotinib therapy in a patient with non-small cell lung cancer positive for ALK rearrangement. Investig New Drugs. 2015;33(2):510–2.
105. Faderl S, Talpaz M, Estrov Z, O'Brien S, Kurzrock R, Kantarjian HM. The biology of chronic myeloid leukemia. N Engl J Med. 1999;341(3):164–72.
106. Ikeda S, Yoshioka H, Arita M, Sakai T, Sone N, Nishiyama A, et al. Interstitial lung disease induced by alectinib (CH5424802/RO5424802). Jpn J Clin Oncol. 2015;45(2):221–4.
107. Kim DW, Mehra R, Tan DSW, Felip E, Chow LQM, Camidge DR, et al. Activity and safety of ceritinib in patients with ALK-rearranged non-small-cell lung cancer (ASCEND-1): updated results from the multicentre, open-label, phase 1 trial. Lancet Oncol. 2016;17(4):452–63.
108. Yamamoto Y, Okamoto I, Otsubo K, Iwama E, Hamada N, Harada T, et al. Severe acute interstitial lung disease in a patient with anaplastic lymphoma kinase rearrangement-positive non-small cell lung cancer treated with alectinib. Investig New Drugs. 2015;33(5):1148–50.
109. Weinblatt ME, Kavanaugh A, Genovese MC, Musser TK, Grossbard EB, Magilavy DB. An oral spleen tyrosine kinase (Syk) inhibitor for rheumatoid arthritis. N Engl J Med. 2010;363(14):1303–12.
110. Braselmann S, Taylor V, Zhao H, Wang S, Sylvain C, Baluom M, et al. R406, an orally available spleen tyrosine kinase inhibitor blocks fc receptor signaling and reduces immune complex-mediated inflammation. J Pharmacol Exp Ther. 2006;319(3):998–1008.
111. Kunwar S, Devkota AR, Ghimire DK. Fostamatinib, an oral spleen tyrosine kinase inhibitor, in the treatment of rheumatoid arthritis: a meta-analysis of randomized controlled trials. Rheumatol Int. 2016;36(8):1077–87.
112. Platt AM, Benson RA, McQueenie R, Butcher JP, Braddock M, Brewer JM, et al. The active metabolite of spleen tyrosine kinase inhibitor fostamatinib abrogates the $CD4^+$ T cell-priming capacity of dendritic cells. Rheumatology (Oxford). 2015;54(1):169–77.
113. Anonymous. 2018. Tavalisse (fostamatinib disodium hexahydrate).Reference ID 4249943. Prescribing information. Food and Drug Administration, Silver Spring, MD. https://www.accessdata.fda.gov/drugsatfda_docs/label/2018/209299lbl.pdf. Accessed October 2020.
114. Weinblatt ME, Kavanaugh A, Burgos-Vargas R, Dikranian AH, Medrano-Ramirez G, Morales-Torres JL, et al. Treatment of rheumatoid arthritis with a Syk kinase inhibitor: a twelve-week, randomized, placebo-controlled trial. Arthritis Rheum. 2008;58(11):3309–18.
115. Podolanczuk A, Lazarus AH, Crow AR, Grossbard E, Bussel JB. Of mice and men: an open-label pilot study for treatment of immune thrombocytopenic purpura by an inhibitor of Syk. Blood. 2009;113(14):3154–60.
116. Bussel J, Arnold DM, Grossbard E, Mayer J, Treliński J, Homenda W, et al. Fostamatinib for the treatment of adult persistent and chronic immune thrombocytopenia: results of two phase 3, randomized, placebo-controlled trials. Am J Hematol. 2018;93(7):921–30.

Bcl-2, JAK and mTOR Inhibitors

16

Nicolas J. Mueller and Sara H. Burkhard

mTOR Inhibitors

The mammalian target of rapamycin (mTOR) was discovered through the study of its inhibitor rapamycin, a substance with antitumor and immunosuppressive activity [1] (Fig. 16.1). mTOR associates with a set of proteins to form the mTOR complexes (mTORC) 1 and 2 and acts as the catalytic core. Whereas mTORC1 is efficiently inhibited by rapamycin, mTORC2 is relatively resistant [1]. mTORC1 initiates anabolic processes required for energy storage and cell growth through the promotion of protein, lipid, and nucleotide synthesis. Simultaneously, mTORC1 suppresses catabolism by inhibiting autophagy and degradation of ubiquitinated proteins [2]. mTORC1 activity increases upon nutrient intake and stimulation of growth factor signaling pathways. The latter converge on inhibiting the tuberous sclerosis complex (TSC) 1 and 2, a negative regulator of mTORC1 activity. TSC is exemplary suppressed downstream of insulin growth factor IGF involving PI3K and Akt activation. In addition, signaling pathways such as the Ras/ERK/MAP kinase cascade, involved in cell proliferation, inhibit TSC and thereby stimulate mTORC1 activity. In contrast, DNA damage and the lack of energy and oxygen will prevent mTORC1 activation [2]. Less is known about the role of mTORC2. This complex stimulates proliferation and cell migration and ensures cell survival, most prominently by activating the PI3K/Akt pathway, but also phosphorylates protein kinases involved in cytoskeleton remodeling and ion transport. Just as with mTORC1, mTORC2 activity is stimulated by insulin/PI3K signaling, implying a positive feedback loop. Via Akt signaling, the mTORC1 and 2 pathways are intertwined as mTORC1 inhibits insulin/PI3K mediated mTORC2 activation [2].

N. J. Mueller (✉) · S. H. Burkhard
Department of Infectious Diseases and Hospital Epidemiology, University Hospital Zurich, Zurich, Switzerland
e-mail: nicolas.mueller@usz.ch; Sarahelene.Burkhard@usz.ch

C. Cervera, J. M. Aguado (eds.), *Infectious Complications in Biologic and Targeted Therapies*, https://doi.org/10.1007/978-3-031-11363-5_16

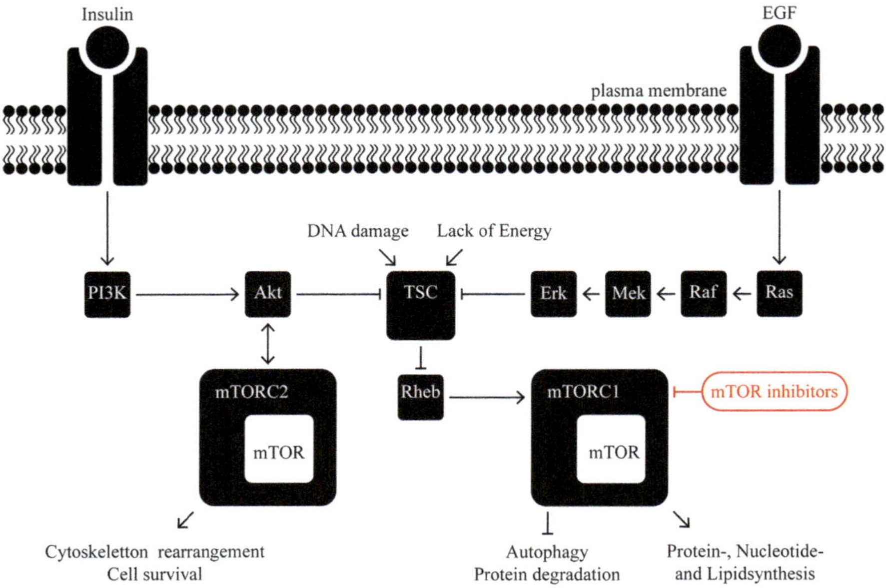

Fig. 16.1 mTOR is the catalytic center of the protein complexes mTORC1 and 2. mTORC1 is activated by the Ras homolog enriched in brain (Rheb) that is in turn inhibited by TSC 1 and 2. TSC is integral to upstream signaling pathways of which cascades responding to DNA damage and energy stress activate TSC. Growth signals, such as the Ras/ERK/MAPK pathway, exemplary stimulated by the epidermal growth factor EGF and the PI3K/Akt pathway initiated by insulin binding to its receptor, inhibit TSC. This results in the activation of mTORC 1 and consequently an anabolic state of the cell by protein, nucleotide, and lipid synthesis, by regulating protein degradation and inhibiting autophagy. mTORC2 is involved in a positive feedback loop involving Akt and has implications on cell survival and cytoskeleton rearrangement. mTOR inhibitors mainly inhibit mTORC1, while mTORC2 is relatively resistant to their effect

The complex effects of mTORC1 and 2 signaling have implications on immune function, the aging process, and the pathogenesis of Alzheimer's disease, diabetes, obesity, and cancer [3]. Whereas the metabolic effects of mTOR-mediated signaling concern all eukaryotic cells, mTOR activity has specific consequences for innate and adaptive immune cells [4]. In T cells, mTORC1 and 2 are activated upon antigen recognition by the T-cell receptor (TCR). mTOR also acts downstream of co-stimulatory molecules and cytokines, signal 2 and 3, that are essential for T-cell activation and proliferation [4]. Inhibition of mTOR activity during antigen presentation was shown to result in T-cell anergy [5] and supports the differentiation of regulatory T cells [6]. In contrast, mTOR inhibition promotes the formation of CD8$^+$ T-cell memory [4]. Due to the largely immunosuppressive effects, the mTOR inhibitor rapamycin, clinically known as sirolimus, was initially approved as an immunosuppressive substance to prevent graft rejection in kidney transplant recipients in 1999. The drug showed negative effects on the growth of vascular smooth muscle cells and was consequently approved for the coating of coronary artery stents, where it inhibits occlusion. mTOR also plays a critical role in tumorigenesis and in a multitude of cancers mTOR activity is increased [7]. As depicted above, various oncogenic signaling pathways are intertwined with mTORC1 and 2. Exemplary, increased mTOR activity can result from mutations enhancing the Ras/ERK MAPK or PI3K/Akt pathways. Metabolic adaption in cancer cells via mTOR signaling facilitates proliferation and migration and promotes vessel growth in tumors [3]. Hoping to develop a potent anticancer treatment, rapamycin analogues were developed. Compared to sirolimus, everolimus shows increased oral bioavailability, while the prodrug temsirolimus is administered intravenously [8]. Despite the great expectations, these substances showed limited effect in only a few cancer subsets, such as renal cell carcinoma, mantle cell lymphoma, tuberous sclerosis complex patients, and pancreatic neuroendocrine tumors [1]. This is likely explained by the abrogation of the negative feedback loop of mTORC1 on the PI3K/Akt pathway, incomplete inhibition of the phosphorylation of mTORC1 effectors, and relative resistance of mTORC2 to mTOR inhibitors [1]. Scientists are hoping to overcome these limitations by combination of therapies and the development of pan-mTOR inhibitors blocking activity of both mTORC1 and 2 [1]. Temsirolimus is currently approved for the treatment of renal cell carcinoma, and everolimus is used both in posttransplant immunosuppressive regimens and treatment of breast, renal, and neuroendocrine cancers, while another analogue to sirolimus, ridaforolimus, has not reached approval.

Early studies of sirolimus compared to placebo or azathioprine in addition to cyclosporine and corticosteroids in kidney allograft recipients showed no significant difference in the rate of infections, although more mucosal ulcers were observed. On a clinical basis, these mucosal lesions were linked to the herpes simplex virus [9, 10]. Later, impaired wound healing was described in conjunction with sirolimus treatment, leading to a significant increase in perigraft tissue collection and wound infection [11], although the study population was limited in number. Larger randomized trials confirmed the delay in wound healing upon sirolimus administration compared to cyclosporine [12, 13] and tacrolimus [13]. In addition, they revealed a decrease in cytomegalovirus (CMV) infections in the sirolimus group, while high-risk patients (CMV seronegative patients receiving a transplant from a seropositive donor) were equally distributed or even overrepresented in the sirolimus group [12, 13]. Similar results were also reported for everolimus used to prevent kidney graft rejection. A study powered to compare CMV incidence found a 75–90% reduction in patients treated with everolimus versus mycophenolate-based regimens. These patients did not receive antiviral CMV prophylaxis [14]. Both direct antiviral effects of mTOR inhibitors and changes in CMV immune control have since been suggested to be causative [15]. In a large randomized open-label trial, kidney transplant recipients were stratified regarding the risk of CMV infection (donor and recipient serology) and prophylactic antiviral therapy. Even after adjusting for CMV risk, the rate of infection was significantly lower in the group receiving everolimus versus mycophenolic acid. Interestingly, a reduced rate of BK viruria or viremia was also observed in the everolimus group. Together, this resulted in a lower frequency of all viral infections, while no differences were observed for fungal or bacterial infections [16].

In a meta-analysis of 28 randomized controlled trials, Mallat and colleagues confirmed the lower incidence of CMV infection in mTOR versus calcineurin inhibitor-treated renal transplant patients. The risk ratio was calculated at 0.54, thus almost half the risk of CMV infection [15]. A meta-analysis comparing mTOR inhibitors to mycophenolate or azathioprine came to similar conclusions regarding CMV infections [17]. Due to this anti-CMV effect, switching the immunosuppressive regimen from calcineurin inhibitors to mTOR inhibitors is one strategy suggested to control CMV infections in solid organ-transplanted patients [18]. For BKV infections, however, the meta-analysis mentioned above found no significant difference between mTOR and calcineurin inhibitor-treated patients, likely due to underreporting of the disease in the studies analyzed [15]. While Montero et al. did not report on BKV infections, they compared the discontinuation rates, which were consistently higher in the mTOR inhibitor than the mycophenolate or azathioprine arm. As this highlights tolerability issues connected to mTOR inhibitors, many studies found discontinuation rates to correlate with the dose of mTOR inhibitor administered [17]. While Mallat and colleagues reported no difference in frequency of infections other than BKV and CMV [15], Montero and colleagues saw significant risk reduction for all infections in the first year of mTOR inhibition. The risk in the compared groups, however, equalized after long-term treatment, albeit fewer studies could be included in this analysis [17]. In contrast, an open-label trial, converting immunosuppressive regimens of kidney-transplanted patients form a calcineurin inhibitor to a sirolimus-based treatment, showed more overall infectious adverse events after the switch. Significant differences were observed for pneumonia, stomatitis, presumptive herpes simplex infection, and fever. Such adverse events were particularly frequent in the first 6 months after therapy conversion, while rates equalized between the groups after this time period [19]. The risk of *Pneumocystis jirovecii* pneumonia linked to mTOR inhibition has also been debated in the literature. A meta-analysis of 15 case-control, cohort studies and randomized controlled studies concluded that mTOR inhibition was associated with an elevated PCP risk. A significant increase of cases was observed after the first year posttransplantation [20], whereas this difference reflects on the net state of immunosuppression or is substance specific remains elusive.

Due to the combination of drugs required to avoid allograft rejection, the study of mTOR inhibitors in this setting involves subjects with a potent therapeutic immunosuppression. In contrast, in patients with neoplastic disorders, the effect of a monotherapy with mTOR inhibitors could be compared to placebo. In addition, tumor patients are generally treated with higher-dose mTOR inhibitors compared to transplant recipients. In randomized phase 3 studies, patients receiving everolimus to treat metastatic renal cell cancer or pancreatic neuroendocrine tumors showed higher rates of infections, stomatitis, and noninfectious pneumonitis [21, 22], of which the latter conditions predispose to infections due to a breakdown of barrier function and can be mistaken for an infection. Three patients with renal cell cancer died due to candida sepsis, presumed bacterial sepsis, or bronchopulmonary aspergillosis [23]. In the population with pancreatic neuroendocrine tumors, a case of tuberculosis, bronchopulmonary aspergillosis, and hepatitis B reactivation was described upon everolimus treatment [22]. A meta-analysis of eight phase 2 and 3 trials treating cancer with either everolimus or temsirolimus yielded an incidence of 33.1% for all-grade infections and 5.6% for serious infections under mTOR inhibition. Comparing mTOR inhibition to the placebo control, a significantly elevated relative risk of 2 and 2.6 was calculated for all-grade infections and high-grade infections, respectively. The relative risks did not significantly differ between the everolimus and the temsirolimus group. Frequently reported infections were localized in the respiratory, genitourinary, and gastrointestinal tract, the skin, and soft tissue or were described as sepsis [24]. A rare genetic disease, called tuberous sclerosis complex, is caused by a mutation in the TSC gene, yields an overactive mTORC1, and results in the formation of benign tumors in multiple organs. In such patients, stomatitis, mouth ulcerations, and pneumonitis were detected more frequently in the everolimus compared to the placebo group [25] consistent with the studies in cancer patients. Rates of respiratory tract infections were particularly high in everolimus-treated patients [25–27]. The frequency of these adverse events decreased during long-term treatment [26]. Table 16.1 lists the trials highlighted above, while relevant infections and action points are summarized in Table 16.2.

Table 16.1 Clinical trials and pooled analyses referenced in Chap. 2

	Year of publication	Author	Trial characteristics	Trial Registration Number	Number of patients	Condition	Substances compared
mTOR inhibitors	2000	Kahan et al.	Randomized, double-blind		719	Renal TPL	Sirolimus vs. azathioprin
	2001	MacDonald et al.	Randomized, double-blind, phase 3		576	Renal TPL	Sirolimus vs. placebo + CNI + corticosteroids
	2004	Dean et al.	Randomized		123	Renal TPL	Sirolimus vs. tacrolimus
	2007	Büchler et al.	Randomized		150	Renal TPL	Sirolimus vs. cyclosporin
	2007	Ekberg et al.	Randomized, open-label	NCT00231764	1645	Renal TPL	Sirolimus vs. cyclosporine vs. tacrolimus
	2009	Schena et al.	Randomized, open-label		830	Renal TPL	Conversion from cyclosporine to sirolimus
	2015	Tedesco-Silva et al.	Randomized, open label	NCT01354301	288	Renal TPL	Everolimus regimen vs. standard treatment
	2019	Tedesco-Silva et al.	Randomized, open-label, 2-arm study	NCT01950819	2026	Renal TPL	Everolimus + CNI + MMF vs. CNI + MMF
	2017	Mallat et al.	Pooled analysis		6211	Renal TPL	Sirolimus/everolimus
	2019	Montero et al.	Pooled analysis		7356	Renal TPL	Sirolimus/everolimus vs. tacrolimus/cyclosporin
	2019	Ghadimi et al.	Pooled analysis		37,597	Solid organ TPL	Sirolimus/everolimus
	2008	Motzer et al.	Randomized, double-blind, phase 3	NCT00410124	410	RCC	Everolimus vs. placebo
	2010	Motzer et al.	Randomized, double-blind, phase 3	NCT00410124	416	RCC	Everolimus vs. placebo
	2011	Yao et al.	Randomized, double-blind, phase 3	NCT00510068	410	Pancreatic neuroendocrine tumours	Everolimus vs. placebo
	2013	Kaymakcalan et.al	Pooled analysis		3180	Varoius cancers	Everolimus/temsirolimus
	2013	Franz et al.	Randomized, double-blind, phase 3	NCT00789828	117	Tuberous sclerosis complex	Everolimus vs. placebo
	2016	Franz et al.	Open-label, single arm	NCT00789828	117	Tuberous sclerosis complex	Everolimus
	2016	French et al.	Randomized, double-blind, phase 3	NCT01713946	366	Tuberous sclerosis complex	Everolimus vs. placebo

JAK inhibitors	2012	Verstovsek et al.	Randomized, double-blind, phase 3	NCT00952289	309	Myelofibrosis	Ruxolitinib vs. placebo
	2012	Harrison et al.	Randomized, open-label, phase 3	NCT00934544	219	Myelofibrosis	Ruxolitinib vs. best available therapy
	2016	Harrison et al.	Randomized, open-label, phase 3	NCT00934544	219	Myelofibrosis	Ruxolitinib vs. best available therapy
	2017	Verstovsek et al.	Randomized, double-blind, phase 3	NCT00952289	299	Myelofibrosis	Ruxolitinib vs. placebo
	2020	Al Ali et al.	Open-label, single arm, phase 3b	NCT01493414	1144	Myelofibrosis	Ruxolitinib
	2020	Zeiser et al.	Randomized, open-label, phase 3	NCT02913261	309	Acute graft-versus-host disease	Ruxolitinib vs. investigators choice
	2015	Vannucchi et al.	Randomized, open-label, phase 3	NCT01243944	222	Polycythemia vera	Ruxolitinib vs. standard treatment
	2020	Kiladjian et al.	Randomized, open-label, phase 3	NCT01243944	222	Polycythemia vera	Ruxolitinib vs. standard treatment
	2012	Fleischmann et al.	Randomized, double-blind, phase 3	NCT00814307	611	Rheumatoid arthritis	Tofacitinib vs. placebo
	2014	Lee et al.	Randomized, double-blind, phase 3	NCT01039688	958	Rheumatoid arthritis	Tofacitinib vs. methotrexate
	2014	Cohen et al.	Pooled analysis		4789	Rheumatoid arthritis	Tofacitinib vs. tofacitinib + MTX or other csDMARDs
	2016	Winthrop et al.	Pooled analysis		5671	Rheumatoid arthritis	Tofacitinib vs. placebo vs. adalimumab vs. MTX
	2017	Winthrop et al.	Pooled analysis		6192	Rheumatoid arthritis	Tofacitinib ± csDMARDs
	2015	Bachelez et al.	Randomized, double-blind, phase 3	NCT01241591	1106	Plaque psoriasis	Tofacitinib vs. etanercept vs. placebo
	2017	Mease et al.	Randomized, double-blind, phase 3	NCT01877668	422	Psoriatic arthritis	Tofacitinib vs. placebo vs. adalimumab
	2017	Sandborn et al.	3 randomized, double-blind, phase 3		1732	Ulcerative colitis	Tofacitinib vs. placebo
	2018	Winthrop et al.	Pooled analysis		1157	Ulcerative colitis	Tofacitinib
	2012	Vincenti et al.	Randomized, phase 2	NCT00483756	331	Renal TPL	Tofacitinib vs. cyclosporine
	2016	Genovese et al.	Randomized, double-blind, phase 3	NCT01721044	527	Rheumatoid arthritis	Baricitinib vs. placebo
	2017	Dougados et al.	Randomized, double-blind, phase 3	NCT01721057	684	Rheumatoid arthritis	Baricitinib vs. placebo
	2017	Taylor et al.	Randomized, double-blind, phase 3	NCT01710358	1307	Rheumatoid arthritis	Baracitinib vs. placebo vs. adalimumab
	2019	Smolen et al.	Pooled analysis		3492	Rheumatoid arthritis	Baricitinib vs. placebo
	2019	Genovese et al.	Randomized, double-blind, phase 3	NCT02873936	448	Rheumatoid arthritis	Filgotinib vs. placebo
	2018	Burmester et al.	Randomized, double-blind, phase 3	NCT02675426	661	Rheumatoid arthritis	Upadacitinib vs. placebo
	2019	Fleischmann et al.	Randomized, double-blind, phase 3	NCT02629159	1629	Rheumatoid arthritis	Upadacitinib vs. placebo vs. adalimumab + MTX
	2019	Tanaka et al.	Randomized, double-blind, phase 3	NCT02308163	507	Rheumatoid arthritis	Peficitinib vs. placebo vs. etanercept

(continued)

Table 16.1 (continued)

	Year of publication	Author	Trial characteristics	Trial Registration Number	Number of patients	Condition	Substances compared
BCL-2 inhibitors	2016	Roberts et al.	Open-label, phase 1	NCT01328626	116	Relapsed or refractory CLL or SLL	Venetoclax
	2018	Seymour et al.	Randomized, open-label, phase 3	NCT02005471	389	Relapsed/refractory CLL	Venetoclax + rituximab vs. bendamustine + rituximab
	2018	Stilgenbauer et al.	Open-label, phase 2	NCT01889187	158	Relapsed/refractory CLL with 17p deletion	Venetoclax
	2019	Fisher et al.	Randomized, open-label, phase 3	NCT02242942	432	Previously untreated CLL	Venetoclax + obinutuzumab vs. chlorambucil + obinutuzumab
	2020	DiNardo et al.	Randomized, double-blind, phase 3	NCT02993523	431	Previously untreated AML	Venetoclax + azacitidine vs. + placebo + azacitidine

MTX methotrexate, *csDMARDs* conventional synthetic disease-modifying anti-rheumatic drugs, *TPL* transplantation, *CNI* calcineurin inhibitor, *MMF* mycophenolate, *RCC* renal cell carcinoma, *CLL* chronic lymphatic leukaemia, *SLL* small lymphocytic lymphoma, *AML* acute myeloid leukaemia

Table 16.2 Infectious risk connected with mTOR, JAK, and BCL-2 inhibiting substances

Substance	Infection/condition	Risk	Suggested management
mTOR inhibitors	Overall viral infections	Elevated	Yearly influenza vaccination
	Herpes simplex/zoster	Elevated	Prophylaxis in subjects with additional risk (e.g. after transplantation)
	CMV	Decreased	
	BKV	Possibly decreased	
	HBV	Elevated	Screening for HBV
			Treatment in patients with detectable HBV DNA and/ or HBs-ag
			HBV DNA monitoring in patients with undetectable HBV DNA and/or HBs-ag but positive HBc-antibody
	Overall bacterial infections	Elevated	Consider prophylaxis in subjects with additional risk (e.g. neutropenic patients)
	Tuberculosis	Elevated	Screening for latent tuberculosis in patients from non-endemic regions
			Treatment of latent tuberculosis upon positive screening or in patients form endemic regions
	Fungal infections	Rare cases	Consider prophylaxis in subjects with additional risk (e.g. neutropenic patients)
	Pneumocystis jirovecii pneumonia	Possibly elevated	Prophylaxis in subjects with additional risk (e.g. upon corticosteroid use, after transplantation)
	Impaired wound healing, mucositis, pneumonitis	Elevated	Risk of superinfection

(continued)

Table 16.2 (continued)

Substance	Infection/condition	Risk	Suggested management
JAK inhibitors	Overall viral infections	Elevated	Yearly influenza vaccination
	Herpes zoster	Elevated	Screening for VZV IgG
			VZV or HZ vaccination before treatment
			Prophylaxis in subjects with additional risk (e.g. after transplantation)
	CMV	Elevated in presence of potent immunosuppression	Prophylaxis in subjects with additional risk (e.g. after transplantation)
	BKV, EBV	Possibly elevated in presence of potent immunosuppression	Monitoring
	HBV	Elevated	Screening for HBV
			Treatment in patients with detectable HBV DNA and/or HBs-ag
			HBV DNA monitoring in patients with undetectable HBV DNA and/or HBs-ag but positive HBc-antibody
	Overall bacterial infections	Elevated	Consider prophylaxis in subjects with additional risk (e.g. neutropenic patients)
	Tuberculosis	Elevated	Screening for latent tuberculosis in patients from non-endemic regions
			Treatment of latent tuberculosis upon positive screening or in patients form endemic regions
	Fungal infections	Rare cases	Consider prophylaxis in subjects with additional risk (e.g. neutropenic patients)
	Pneumocystis jirovecii pneumonia	Elevated	Prophylaxis in subjects with additional risk (e.g. upon corticosteroid use, after transplantation)
BCL-2 inhibitors	Neutropenia	Elevated	Risk for neutropenic fever

VZV varicella zoster virus, *HZ* herpes zoster, *CMV* cytomegalovirus, *BKV* BK virus, *EBV* Epstein-Barr-virus, *HBV* hepatitis B virus

JAK Inhibitors

Janus kinases (JAKs) are involved in the intracellular signal transduction downstream of cytokine, colony-stimulating factor, growth factor, and hormone receptors (Fig. 16.2). Such receptors are essential for hematopoiesis, metabolism, and immunity [28]. Upon interaction with the respective ligand, the receptors oligomerize, bringing JAKs, non-covalently bound to the cytoplasmic domain of the receptor, into close proximity. This leads to the phosphorylation of JAKs, the cytokine receptors, and target molecules such as signal transducers and activators of transcription (STAT). STAT, upon activation, dimerize and translocate into the nucleus where they regulate transcription of a variety of genes [29]. The JAK-STAT pathway was first discovered in conjunction with interferon signaling [30], highlighting its importance in the pathogenesis of autoimmunity, infection, and cancer. There are four mammalian members of the JAK family—JAK 1, JAK 2, JAK 3, and TYK2—involved in the signaling of many more receptors [28]. JAK 3 exemplary binds to the common γ chain (γc) of cytokine receptors and hereby is essential for signaling downstream of interleukin (IL) -2, −4, −7, −9, −15, and −21 [28]. Defective signal

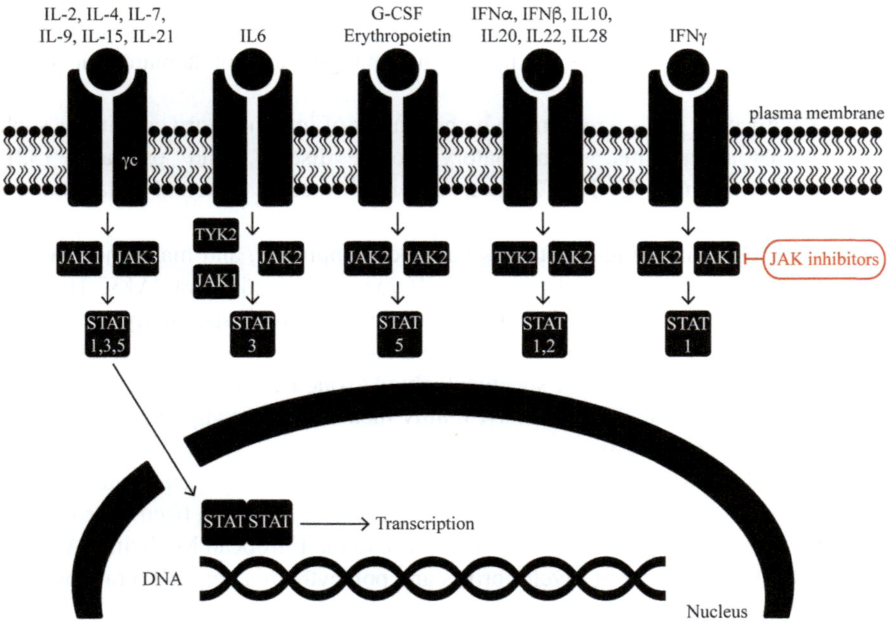

Fig. 16.2 The four members of the JAK family (JAK1, 2, 3, and Tyk2) are activated downstream of growth factors (e.g., G-CSF and erythropoietin) and cytokines (various interleukins (IL) and interferons (IFN) binding to their corresponding receptor. Among other proteins, STATs are phosphorylated by JAKs, dimerize, and induce transcription in the nucleus. Different receptors will engage a distinct set of JAKs, which will further determine the STAT protein activated and the genes targeted. JAK inhibitors inhibit one or multiple JAK family members. JAK inhibitors applied for hematological malignancies aim for JAK2 downstream of growth receptor signaling, while in autoimmune disease, JAK1 and 3, involved in cytokine signaling, are targeted

transduction, caused by JAK 3 loss of function mutations, leads to severe combined immunodeficiency (SCID) in mice and humans, illustrating the nonredundant role of JAK 3 for immune function [28]. Human SCID is commonly the result of the X chromosome-linked mutation of the γc gene [31]. JAK 3 mutations result in the same phenotype due to the deficient development, homeostasis, and activation of T and NK cells [28]. TYK 2 dysfunction due to germ line mutations has rarely been described in humans and seems to vary regarding the phenotypic presentation of immunodeficiency syndromes [28]. JAK 1 and 2 associate with a larger variety of receptors involved in immune signaling, hematopoiesis, growth, and organ development. Just as for JAK 3, JAK 1 activity is required for the signal transduction downstream of γc cytokine receptors but additionally associated with receptors of the IL-6 family cytokines, IL-10, IL-13, and IL-22, type 1 and 2 interferons (IFN) and GCSF. JAK 2 is essential for signaling via the IL-6 and IL-3 family receptors, IL-12, IL-23, IL-13, and INFγ and receptors involved in hematopoiesis (e.g., erythropoietin, GCSF) [28]. Genetic knockout of both JAK 1 and 2 in mice results in a lethal phenotype [28, 29], which is why there is no human correlate for disease. In contrast, a gain of function mutation in JAK genes, particularly for JAK 2, can result in neoplastic growth, primarily of hematopoietic origin [28]. JAK 2 has been implicated in the pathogenesis of leukemia, lymphoma, thrombocytemia, and particularly in polycythemia vera and myelofibrosis. Increased JAK 1 and 3 activity is reported in the development of monoclonal malignancies of hematological origin [28].

JAK activation plays a role in the pathogenesis of inflammatory conditions such as rheumatoid arthritis, inflammatory bowel disease, and psoriasis [32]. Polymorphisms in JAK2-STAT3 have been implicated in different inflammatory conditions [28].

Several JAK inhibiting substances have been approved, and many more are in clinical trials, each compound targeting different combinations of JAKs. The first generation of JAK inhibitors (JAKinibs) are broader in their specificity and inhibit the activation of multiple JAKs [33]. In the attempt to avoid side effects later, substances were developed to more specifically bind to one JAK. Despite these improvements, all JAKinibs inhibit other JAK family members when applied at high dose, thus displaying similar adverse effects [32].

The JAK1-JAK2 inhibitor ruxolitinib was the first substance being evaluated for the treatment of myelofibrosis in clinical trials [28]. It has since been approved by the US Food and Drug Administration (FDA) and the European Medicines Agency (EMA) for the treatment of myelofibrosis and polycythemia vera. Two randomized clinical trials comparing ruxolitinib to placebo [34] or the best available treatment [35] did not suggest an added risk for infection under ruxolitinib. The long-term study of the patient population, however, revealed a link between ruxolitinib treatment and herpes zoster [36, 37]. Similar results were obtained in a phase 3 open-label study, in which polycythemia vera patients resistant or intolerant to hydroxyurea treatment were observed. Herpes zoster, mostly grade 1 or 2, was reported in 6% versus 0% in patients given ruxolitinib or standard care, respectively [38]. The 5-year follow-up study confirmed the link of ruxolitinib with herpes zoster, as the patients who crossed over from best available treatment to the study drug approached herpes zoster rates of the ruxolitinib group (3.9% vs. 4.7%). With the exception of herpes zoster, the study showed a reduction in all infections in ruxolitinib-treated patients compared to control [39]. A large single-arm, open-label, phase 3b study, in patients with myelofibrosis under ruxolitinib treatment, showed low rates of infections [40]. These mostly low-grade infections involved pneumonia, urinary tract infections, herpes zoster, and nasopharyngitis. They observed five cases of tuberculosis, one hepatitis B reactivation, but no patient developed progressive multifocal leukencephalopathy [40]. In patients with acute corticosteroid refractory graft versus host disease (GVHD), ruxolitinib was compared to the investigator's choice of salvage therapy, and more CMV infections were observed in the ruxolitinib group compared to control (26% vs. 21%). This difference was not demonstrated for grade 3 and 4 infections [41].

The majority of data concerning the safety of JAKinibs are derived from studies of tofacitinib, a JAK 1/3 inhibitor. It is now approved for the treatment of rheumatoid arthritis, psoriasis arthritis, and ulcerative colitis. A phase 3 trial in rheumatoid arthritis described an increased rate of serious infections under the tofacitinib compared to placebo. The infections involved skin (including one case of herpes zoster), respiratory tract, urinary tract, and liver [42]. Higher rates of all-grade infections and serious infections were also reported in tofacitinib groups compared to placebo in ulcerative colitis patients [43]. In rheumatoid arthritis patients, herpes zoster infections developed in 4% of the tofacitinib versus 1.1% of the methotrexate-treated subjects. A dose-dependent effect was suggested as the group receiving 5 mg tofacitinib developed herpes zoster in 3.5%, compared to 4.5% in the 10 mg group. Bronchitis and influenza were also observed more frequently in tofacitinib- versus methotrexate-treated patients [44]. In psoriasis patients, two phase 3 trials comparing tofacitinib, etanercept, and placebo [45] or tofacitinib, adalimumab, and placebo [46], the treated groups showed similar rates of adverse events [45, 46]. Over the study period, only a few patients experienced serious infections including diverticulitis, an extradural abscess, pneumonia, and paronychia [45], and influenza, appendicitis, and pneumonia [46] in the tofacitinib groups. Whereas Bachelez et al. did not see a difference in herpes zoster rates between the treated groups, Mease et al. only observed herpes zoster infection upon tofacitinib treatment. A pooled analysis investigated rates of infections in phase 2/3 and long-term extension studies treating rheumatoid arthritis patients with tofacitinib [47]. With 3.09 events per 100 patient-years upon treatment, tofacitinib was comparable to other biologic agents regarding serious infections. The most common serious infections were pneumonia and infections of skin or soft tissue. The majority of infections were, however, moderate in severity, and exposure-adjusted event rates in the phase 3 studies were comparable between tofacitinib- and placebo-treated groups. Consistent with previous results, tofacitinib treatment was linked to herpes zoster infections. While most cases were mild, four cases of zoster ophthalmicus and two cases of multi-dermatomal disease were described. There were three cases of HBV infection with one accounting for a possible reactivation. 41 opportunistic infections were reported including patients suffering from tuberculosis, esophageal candidiasis,

CMV infection, cryptococcal infection, *Pneumocystis jirovecii* pneumonia, nontuberculous mycobacteria infections, multi-dermatomal herpes zoster, and BKV encephalitis [47]. Winthrop et al. aimed at characterizing severity, geographical distribution, and the role of concomitant therapy of herpes zoster infections in patients treated with tofacitinib for rheumatoid arthritis from phase 1 to 3 and long-term studies. In 6192 patients (16,839 patient-years), 636 cases of herpes zoster were identified of which 94% were involving one dermatome, and disease was generally manageable with antiviral treatment. Concomitant corticosteroid administration, baseline age, and dose of daily tofacitinib were independent risk factors [48]. Similar results were observed in ulcerative colitis patients, although lower patient numbers only allowed identifying age and prior failure of TNF inhibitors as independent risk factors [49]. Herpes zoster was observed more frequently in east-Asian countries, implying underlying genetic differences to be causative, and gene polymorphisms have been suggested [48]. Both studies showed no evidence for a herpes zoster-related risk accumulation over exposure time [48, 49]. In a phase 2 clinical trial of de novo kidney-transplanted patients, tofacitinib was compared to cyclosporine in addition to basiliximab induction mycophenolic acid and corticosteroids [50]. Overall, serious infections were observed more frequently in the tofacitinib group. While there was no difference between the groups for upper airway and urinary tract infections, there was significantly more CMV disease under tofacitinib. Although low in numbers, BKV nephropathy and PTLD developed more often in tofacitinib-treated patients, reflecting on the potential over-immunosuppression [50]. In a pooled analysis of phase 2, 3, and long-term extension clinical trials of tofacitinib-treated rheumatoid arthritis cases, such infections related to immunosuppression were investigated [51]. In a population of 5671 patients, 60 opportunistic infections were described, all within the tofacitinib-treated group. These encompassed cases of tuberculosis, esophageal candidiasis, disseminated herpes zoster manifestations, CMV infections, *Pneumocystis jirovecii* pneumonias, nontuberculous mycobacteria infections, cryptococcal diseases, BK encephalitis, and toxoplasmosis. Among 286 patients with a positive screening for latent tuberculosis, and consequent 9-month isoniazid treatment, no case of active tuberculosis was observed. Out of the 26 subjects developing tuberculosis, 24 had negative screenings at inclusion. Of the tuberculosis cases, 81% emerged in endemic regions [51], although no subjects lived in countries with the highest incidence according to the WHO.

Another reversible JAK1/3 inhibitor, baricitinib, showed very low frequencies of serious infections and herpes zoster in placebo-controlled studies of patients with rheumatoid arthritis [52, 53]. Similar to other JAKinibs, respiratory infections [52, 53] and urinary tract infections [53] were among the most frequent adverse events. A comparison of baricitinib and adalimumab showed similar rates of serious infections and herpes zoster [54]. A pooled analysis of phase 1–3 and long-term studies showed an increase in infections only in patients treated with high-dose baricitinib (4 mg) compared to placebo. Higher-exposure-adjusted incidence rates were shown for upper respiratory tract infections, herpes zoster, and herpes simplex. Serious infections, such as pneumonia herpes zoster, urinary tract infections, and cellulitis were the most common in the baricitinib group, but incidence rates were similar in patients receiving placebo. Under baricitinib, ten patients developed tuberculosis [55]. With a lack of head-to-head analysis, it remains unclear whether incidences of specific infections differ between tofacitinib and baricitinib.

Similar to others, the pan-JAKinibs peficitinib treatment was connected to an increased incidence of serious infections compared to placebo in rheumatoid arthritis, but comparable to patients under etanercept treatment. It is only for herpes zoster infections that peficitinib showed a higher incidence than both the placebo and etanercept group [56]. Peficitinib is approved in Japan for the treatment of rheumatoid arthritis.

A higher incidence of infections was reported in rheumatoid arthritis patients treated with the specific JAK 1 inhibitor upadacitinib compared to placebo, although no difference was observed for serious infections opportunistic infections or herpes zoster [57]. The serious infections in the upadacitinib groups involved one case for each enterocolitis, upper respiratory tract infection, wound infection, and a primary varicella zoster infection leading to VZV pneumonia. The high-dose upadacitinib group included three patients with oral candidiasis [57]. A phase 3 trial comparing upadacitinib with placebo and adalimumab on a methotrexate background treatment saw similar frequencies of infections and serious infections for both treatment groups. Herpes zoster was the only infection with higher rates in the upadacitinib compared to the placebo and adalimumab group [58]. Similar results were shown for filgotinib, another JAK 1 inhibitor, as more infections were observed in the treatment versus the placebo group in rheumatoid arthritis patients. Herpes zoster, although only few cases, was only observed in the filgotinib groups [59]. Table 16.1 lists the trials highlighted above, while relevant infections and action points are summarized in Table 16.2.

BCL-2 Inhibitors

B-cell lymphoma 2 (BCL-2) family proteins are involved in the regulation of the mitochondrial pathway of apoptosis (Fig. 16.3). They share a combination of one to four conserved BCL-2 homology (BH) domains, which determine their anti- or proapoptotic function [60]. The interplay of the BCL-2 family members creates a balance between cell survival and death, which can be shifted by physiological signals and pathological dysregulation of the proteins involved. Within the family, the antiapoptotic BCL-2 was discovered first in follicular lymphomas and diffuse large B-cell lymphomas. In such tumors, a chromosomal translocation results in cancer cell survival through a BCL-2 gain of function. Since this discovery, other antiapoptotic BCL-2 family members, such as B-cell lymphoma extra large (BCL-X_L), BCL-W, and myeloid cell leukemia 1 (MCL1), have been characterized. Such antiapoptotic BCL-2 proteins counteract the proapoptotic function of BCL-2 antagonist killer 1 (BAK) and BCL-2-associated X protein (BAX). This, in turn, prevents an increased permeability of the mitochondrial membrane, the release of cytochrome C into the cytoplasm, and subsequent activation of the caspase cascade resulting in

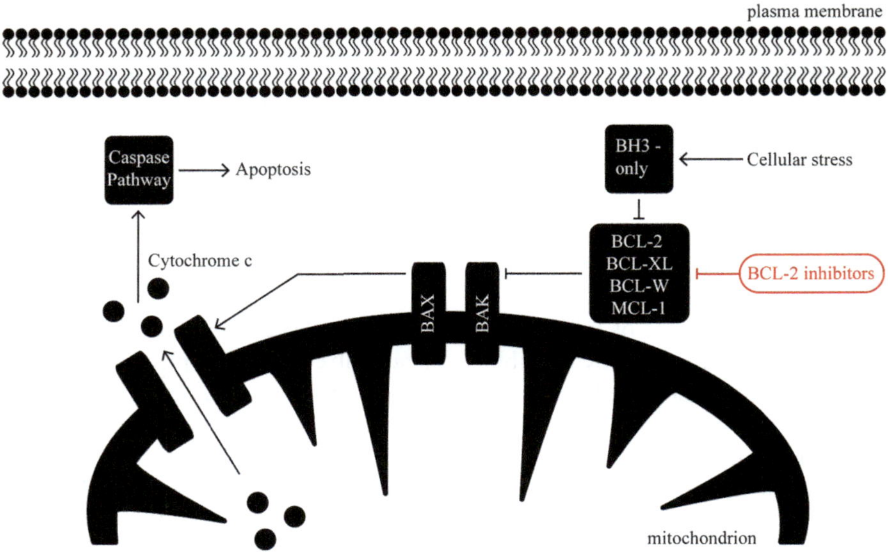

Fig. 16.3 Pro-survival BCL-2 family members, such as BCL-2, BCL-XL, BCL-W, and MCL-1, inhibit their proapoptotic counterparts BAK and BAX. This in turn inhibits the permeabilization of the mitochondrial membrane, the release of cytochrome c into the cytoplasm, and subsequently prevents apoptosis by the activation of the caspase cascade. Pro-survival BCL-2 proteins are inhibited by BH3-only proteins, which are activated by cellular stress. BCL-2 inhibitors mimic the function of BH3-only proteins, promoting apoptosis and thereby counteracting deregulated survival signals in cancer cells. While early BCL-2 inhibitors affected multiple pro-survival BCL-2 proteins leading to adverse thrombocytopenia, venetoclax specifically inhibits BCL-2, avoiding this adverse event

apoptosis [60]. Upstream, pro-survival BCL-2 proteins are inhibited by BCL-2 family members only containing the BH3 domain, therefore referred to as BH3-only proteins. Apart from this indirect induction of apoptosis, some BH3-only proteins can directly interact with BAK and BAX [61]. BH3-only proteins are activated by intracellular stress signals, such as DNA damage, oxidative stress, or the lack of growth factor signaling. Exemplary, in response to DNA damage, the tumor suppressor p53 induces transcription of certain BH3-only proteins. A mutation resulting in p53 loss of function is observed in as many as 50% of cancers [62]. Due to this frequent dysregulation of BCL-2 activity in malignancies, pharmacological substances aiming to inhibit BCL-2 function were developed. Such small molecules were termed BH3 mimetics, as they reproduce the mechanism by which BH3-only proteins inhibit pro-survival BCL-2 signaling [63]. The first promising BH3-mimetic was termed ABT-737 and was followed by navitoclax, a substance with improved oral bioavailability compared to its predecessor. Both drugs mainly inhibit BCL-2, BCL-X_L, and BCL-W. Despite antitumor efficacy in phase 1 trials, navitoclax never reached approval due to its negative impact on thrombocyte survival, an on-target effect involving inhibition of BCL-X_L function [63]. To avoid this undesirable effect, more recent BH3-mimetics were designed to show higher specificity.

The BCL-2-selective inhibitor venetoclax provoked a solid antitumor response, while thrombocytopenia was less severe [64]. Venetoclax is the first BH3-mimetic approved by the FDA and the EMA for patients with chronic lymphatic leukemia [63]. More recently, the combination therapy with several anticancer substances has reached approval. Moreover, venetoclax is being studied in various other cancer types. While no other drugs interfering with BCL-2 protein-associated apoptosis are in clinical use, the development MCL-1 inhibitors is of great interest, and several drugs are in clinical trials.

Due to the recent approval for venetoclax, up to now, there is a limited amount of articles studying safety. In a dose-escalation phase 1 trial of CLL and small lymphocytic lymphoma, patients that relapsed after or proved refractory to initial treatment were administered with venetoclax. Neutropenia was a frequent adverse event, in some cases progressing to episodes of febrile neutropenia. Upper respiratory tract infections and pneumonia were other infections reported [65]. Similar observations were made in a phase 2 study in CLL patients with a genetic 17p deletion, a finding related to poor prognosis [66]. In addition to the febrile neutropenia and respiratory infections, this trial reported cutaneous herpes zoster and *Pneumocystis jirovecii* pneumonia, although the latter was only observed in patients previously treated with the chemotherapeutic fludarabine. Four patients succumb to a RSV infection, *Klebsiella* sepsis, septic shock, and pneumonia [66]. In a randomized, double-blind phase 3 trial in AML patients, venetoclax was compared to placebo, while all patients received azacitidine, a hypomethylating agent. Neutropenia, febrile neutropenia, and all-grade infections were observed more frequently in the venetoclax group, while there was no difference in rates of pneumonia and sepsis compared to control [67]. In most studies, venetoclax was investigated in comparison to other antitumor therapeutics frequently used to treat CLL patients. Receiving a combination of rituximab (an anti-CD20 antibody) with either venetoclax or the alkylating agent bendamustine, grade 3/4 neutropenia was more common in the venetoclax group, while grade 3/4 febrile neutropenia and infections were more frequent under bendamustine treatment [68]. Comparing venetoclax with the alkylating agent chlorambucil, both in combination with the anti-CD20 antibody obinutuzumab accounted for similar rates of neutropenia, febrile neutropenia, and infections [69]. Table 16.1 lists the trials highlighted above, while relevant infections and action points are summarized in Table 16.2.

References

1. Benjamin D, Colombi M, Moroni C, Hall MN. Rapamycin passes the torch: a new generation of mTOR inhibitors. Nat Rev Drug Discov. 2011;10(11):868–80. https://doi.org/10.1038/nrd3531.
2. Saxton RA, Sabatini DM. mTOR signaling in growth, metabolism, and disease. Cell. 2017;168:960–76. https://doi.org/10.1016/j.cell.2017.02.004.
3. Hua H, Kong Q, Zhang H, Wang J, Luo T, Jiang Y. Targeting mTOR for cancer therapy. J Hematol Oncol. 2020;12(1):71. https://doi.org/10.1186/s13045-019-0754-1.

4. Chi H. Regulation and function of mTOR signalling in T cell fate decisions. Nat Rev Immunol. 2012;12:325–38. https://doi.org/10.4049/jimmunol.177.9.5890.
5. Zheng Y, Collins SL, Lutz MA, Allen AN, Kole TP, Zarek PE, et al. A role for mammalian target of rapamycin in regulating t cell activation versus anergy. J Immunol. 2007;178:2163–70. https://doi.org/10.1097/01.tp.0000185299.72295.90.
6. Haxhinasto S, Mathis D, Benoist C. The AKT–mTOR axis regulates de novo differentiation of CD4+Foxp3+ cells. J Exp Med. 2008;205:565–74. https://doi.org/10.1128/JVI.70.8.5701-5705.1996.
7. Mossmann D, Park S, Hall MN. mTOR signalling and cellular metabolism are mutual determinants in cancer. Nat Rev Cancer. 2020;18:744–57. https://doi.org/10.1038/s41568-018-0074-8.
8. MacKeigan JP, Krueger DA. Differentiating the mTOR inhibitors everolimus and sirolimus in the treatment of tuberous sclerosis complex. Neuro-Oncology. 2015;17:1550–9. https://doi.org/10.1093/annonc/mds602.
9. Kahan BD. Efficacy of sirolimus compared with azathioprine for reduction of acute renal allograft rejection: a randomised multicentre study. Lancet. 2000;356:194–202. https://doi.org/10.1016/S0140-6736(00)02480-6.
10. MacDonald AS. RAPAMUNE global study group. A worldwide, phase III, randomized, controlled, safety and efficacy study of a sirolimus/cyclosporine regimen for prevention of acute rejection in recipients of primary mismatched renal allografts. Transplantation. 2001;71:271–80. https://doi.org/10.1097/00007890-200101270-00019.
11. Dean PG, Lund WJ, Larson TS, Prieto M, Nyberg SL, Ishitani MB, et al. Wound-healing complications after kidney transplantation: a prospective, randomized comparison of sirolimus and tacrolimus. Transplantation. 2004;77:1555–61. https://doi.org/10.1097/01.TP.0000123082.31092.53.
12. Büchler M, Caillard S, Barbier S, Thervet E, Toupance O, Mazouz H, et al. Sirolimus versus cyclosporine in kidney recipients receiving thymoglobulin ®, mycophenolate mofetil and a 6-month course of steroids. Am J Transplant. 2007;7:2522–31. https://doi.org/10.1128/JVI.75.13.6022-6032.2001.
13. Ekberg H, Tedesco-Silva H, Demirbas A, Vítko Š, Nashan B, Gürkan A, et al. Reduced exposure to calcineurin inhibitors in renal transplantation. N Engl J Med. 2007;357:2562–75. https://doi.org/10.1056/NEJMoa067411.
14. Tedesco- Silva H, Felipe C, Ferreira A, Cristelli M, Oliveira N, Sandes-Freitas T, et al. Reduced incidence of cytomegalovirus infection in kidney transplant recipients receiving everolimus and reduced tacrolimus doses. Am J Transplant. 2015;15:2655–64. https://doi.org/10.1097/00007890-201407151-01810.
15. Mallat SG, Tanios BY, Itani HS, Lotfi T, McMullan C, Gabardi S, et al. CMV and BKPyV infections in renal transplant recipients receiving an mTOR inhibitor–based regimen versus a CNI-based regimen: a systematic review and meta-analysis of randomized, controlled trials. Clin J Am Soc Nephrol. 2017;12:1321–36. https://doi.org/10.1111/ajt.13710.
16. Tedesco-Silva H, Pascual J, Viklicky O, Basic-Jukic N, Cassuto E, Kim DY, et al. Safety of everolimus with reduced calcineurin inhibitor exposure in de novo kidney transplants: an analysis from the randomized TRANSFORM study. Transplantation. 2019;103:1953–63. https://doi.org/10.1097/TP.0000000000002626.
17. Montero N, Quero M, Melilli E, Pérez-Sáez MJ, Redondo-Pachón D, Bestard O, et al. Mammalian target of rapamycin inhibitors combined with calcineurin inhibitors as initial immunosuppression in renal transplantation. Transplantation. 2019;103:2031–56. https://doi.org/10.1097/TP.0000000000002769.
18. Kotton CN, Kumar D, Caliendo AM, Huprikar S, Chou S, Danziger-Isakov L, et al. The third international consensus guidelines on the management of cytomegalovirus in solid-organ transplantation. Transplantation. 2018;102:900–31. https://doi.org/10.1097/TP.0000000000002191.
19. Schena FP, Pascoe MD, Alberu J, del Carmen Rial M, Oberbauer R, Brennan DC, et al. Conversion from calcineurin inhibitors to sirolimus maintenance therapy in renal allograft

recipients: 24-month efficacy and safety results from the CONVERT trial. Transplantation. 2009;87:233–42. https://doi.org/10.1097/TP.0b013e3181927a41.
20. Ghadimi M, Mohammadpour Z, Dashti-Khavidaki S, Milajerdi A. M-TOR inhibitors and risk of pneumocystis pneumonia after solid organ transplantation: a systematic review and meta-analysis. Eur J Clin Pharmacol. 2020;75(11):1471–80. https://doi.org/10.1007/s00228-019-02730-0.
21. Motzer RJ, Escudier B, Oudard S, Hutson TE, Porta C, Bracarda S, et al. Efficacy of everolimus in advanced renal cell carcinoma: a double-blind, randomised, placebo-controlled phase III trial. Lancet. 2008;372:449–56. https://doi.org/10.1016/S0140-6736(08)61039-9.
22. Yao JC, Shah MH, Ito T, Bohas CL, Wolin EM, Van Cutsem E, et al. Everolimus for advanced pancreatic neuroendocrine tumors. N Engl J Med. 2011;364:514–23. https://doi.org/10.1056/NEJMoa1009290.
23. Motzer RJ, Escudier B, Oudard S, Hutson TE, Porta C, Bracarda S, et al. Phase 3 trial of everolimus for metastatic renal cell carcinoma. Cancer. 2010;116:4256–65. https://doi.org/10.1056/NEJMoa065044.
24. Kaymakcalan MD, Je Y, Sonpavde G, Galsky M, Nguyen PL, Heng DYC, et al. Risk of infections in renal cell carcinoma (RCC) and non-RCC patients treated with mammalian target of rapamycin inhibitors. Br J Cancer. 2013;108(12):2478–84. https://doi.org/10.1038/bjc.2013.278.
25. Franz DN, Belousova E, Sparagana S, Bebin EM, Frost M, Kuperman R, et al. Efficacy and safety of everolimus for subependymal giant cell astrocytomas associated with tuberous sclerosis complex (EXIST-1): a multicentre, randomised, placebo-controlled phase 3 trial. Lancet. 2013;381:125–32. https://doi.org/10.1016/S0140-6736(12)61134-9.
26. Franz DN, Belousova E, Sparagana S, Bebin EM, Frost MD, Kuperman R, et al. Long-term use of everolimus in patients with tuberous sclerosis complex: final results from the EXIST-1 study. PLoS One. 2016;11:e0158476. https://doi.org/10.1371/journal.pone.0158476.
27. French JA, Lawson JA, Yapici Z, Ikeda H, Polster T, Nabbout R, et al. Adjunctive everolimus therapy for treatment-resistant focal-onset seizures associated with tuberous sclerosis (EXIST-3): a phase 3, randomised, double-blind, placebo-controlled study. Lancet. 2016;388:2153–63. https://doi.org/10.1016/S0140-6736(16)31419-2.
28. O'Shea JJ, Holland SM, Staudt LM. JAKs and STATs in immunity, immunodeficiency, and cancer. N Engl J Med. 2013;368:161–70. https://doi.org/10.1056/NEJMra1202117.
29. Levy DE, Darnell JE Jr. STATs: transcriptional control and biological impact. Nat Rev Mol Cell Biol. 2002;3:651–62. https://doi.org/10.1016/S0092-8674(00)81443-9.
30. Stark GR, Darnell JE. The JAK-STAT pathway at twenty. Immunity. 2012;36:503–14. https://doi.org/10.1016/j.immuni.2012.03.013.
31. Cossu F. Genetics of SCID. Ital J Pediatr. 2010;36:76. https://doi.org/10.1186/1824-7288-36-76.
32. Winthrop KL. The emerging safety profile of JAK inhibitors in rheumatic disease. Nat Rev Rheumatol. 2017;13:234–43. https://doi.org/10.1038/nrrheum.2017.23.
33. Fragoulis GE, McInnes IB, Siebert S, JAK-inhibitors. New players in the field of immune-mediated diseases, beyond rheumatoid arthritis. Rheumatology. 2019;58:i43–54. https://doi.org/10.1016/j.hemonc.2017.07.002.
34. Verstovsek S, Mesa RA, Gotlib J, Levy RS, Gupta V, DiPersio JF, et al. A double-blind, placebo-controlled trial of ruxolitinib for myelofibrosis. N Engl J Med. 2012;366:799–807. https://doi.org/10.1056/NEJMoa1110557.
35. Harrison C, Kiladjian JJ, Ali Al HK, Gisslinger H, Waltzman R, Stalbovskaya V, et al. JAK inhibition with ruxolitinib versus best available therapy for myelofibrosis. N Engl J Med. 2012;366:787–98. https://doi.org/10.1056/NEJMoa1110556.
36. Harrison CN, Vannucchi AM, Kiladjian J-J, Al-Ali HK, Gisslinger H, Knoops L, et al. Long-term findings from COMFORT-II, a phase 3 study of ruxolitinib vs best available therapy for myelofibrosis. Leukemia. 2016;30:1701–7. https://doi.org/10.1038/leu.2016.148.
37. Verstovsek S, Mesa RA, Gotlib J, Gupta V, DiPersio JF, Catalano JV, et al. Long-term treatment with ruxolitinib for patients with myelofibrosis: 5-year update from the randomized,

double-blind, placebo-controlled, phase 3 COMFORT-I trial. J Hematol Oncol. 2017;10:55. https://doi.org/10.1186/s13045-017-0417-z.
38. Vannucchi AM, Kiladjian JJ, Griesshammer M, Masszi T, Durrant S, Passamonti F, et al. Ruxolitinib versus standard therapy for the treatment of polycythemia vera. N Engl J Med. 2015;372:426–35. https://doi.org/10.1056/NEJMoa1409002.
39. Kiladjian JJ, Zachee P, Hino M, Pane F, Masszi T, Harrison CN, et al. Long-term efficacy and safety of ruxolitinib versus best available therapy in polycythaemia vera (RESPONSE): 5-year follow up of a phase 3 study. Lancet Haematol. 2020;7:e226–37. https://doi.org/10.1016/S2352-3026(19)30207-8.
40. Ali Al HK, Griesshammer M, Foltz L, Palumbo GA, Martino B, Palandri F, et al. Primary analysis of JUMP, a phase 3b, expanded-access study evaluating the safety and efficacy of ruxolitinib in patients with myelofibrosis, including those with low platelet counts. Br J Haematol. 2020;189:888–903. https://doi.org/10.1111/bjh.16462.
41. Zeiser R, Bubnoff von N, Butler J, Mohty M, Niederwieser D, Or R, et al. Ruxolitinib for glucocorticoid-refractory acute graft-versus-host disease. N Engl J Med. 2020;382:1800–10. https://doi.org/10.1056/NEJMoa1917635.
42. Fleischmann R, Kremer J, Cush J, Schulze-Koops H, Connell CA, Bradley JD, et al. Placebo-controlled trial of tofacitinib monotherapy in rheumatoid arthritis. N Engl J Med. 2012;367:495–507. https://doi.org/10.1056/NEJMoa1109071.
43. Sandborn WJ, Su C, Sands BE, D'Haens GR, Vermeire S, Schreiber S, et al. Tofacitinib as induction and maintenance therapy for ulcerative colitis. N Engl J Med. 2017;376:1723–36. https://doi.org/10.1056/NEJMoa1606910.
44. Lee EB, Fleischmann R, Hall S, Wilkinson B, Bradley JD, Gruben D, et al. Tofacitinib versus methotrexate in rheumatoid arthritis. N Engl J Med. 2014;370:2377–86. https://doi.org/10.1056/NEJMoa1310476.
45. Bachelez H, van de Kerkhof PCM, Strohal R, Kubanov A, Valenzuela F, Lee J-H, et al. Articles tofacitinib versus etanercept or placebo in moderate-to- severe chronic plaque psoriasis: a phase 3 randomised non-inferiority trial. Lancet. 2015;386:552–61. https://doi.org/10.1016/S0140-6736(14)62113-9.
46. Mease P, Hall S, FitzGerald O, van der Heijde D, Merola JF, Avila-Zapata F, et al. Tofacitinib or adalimumab versus placebo for psoriatic arthritis. N Engl J Med. 2017;377:1537–50. https://doi.org/10.1056/NEJMoa1615975.
47. Cohen S, Radominski SC, Gomez Reino JJ, Wang L, Krishnaswami S, Wood SP, et al. Analysis of infections and all-cause mortality in phase II, phase III, and long-term extension studies of tofacitinib in patients with rheumatoid arthritis. Arthrit Rheumatol. 2014;66:2924–37. https://doi.org/10.1002/art.34582.
48. Winthrop KL, Curtis JR, Lindsey S, Tanaka Y, Yamaoka K, Valdez H, et al. Herpes zoster and tofacitinib: clinical outcomes and the risk of concomitant therapy. Arthrit Rheumatol. 2017;69:1960–8. https://doi.org/10.1097/ICO.0000000000000362.
49. Winthrop KL, Melmed GY, Vermeire S, Long MD, Chan G, Pedersen RD, et al. Herpes zoster infection in patients with ulcerative colitis receiving tofacitinib. Inflamm Bowel Dis. 2018;24:2258–65. https://doi.org/10.1093/ibd/izy131.
50. Vincenti F, Tedesco- Silva H, Busque S, O'Connell P, Friedewald J, Cibrik D, et al. Randomized phase 2b trial of tofacitinib (CP-690,550) in de novo kidney transplant patients: efficacy, renal function and safety at 1 year. Am J Transplant. 2012;12:2446–56. https://doi.org/10.1111/j.1600-6143.2007.01749.x.
51. Winthrop KL, Park S-H, Gul A, Cardiel MH, Gomez-Reino JJ, Tanaka Y, et al. Tuberculosis and other opportunistic infections in tofacitinib-treated patients with rheumatoid arthritis. Ann Rheum Dis. 2016;75:1133–8. https://doi.org/10.1136/annrheumdis-2015-207319.
52. Dougados M, van der Heijde D, Chen Y-C, Greenwald M, Drescher E, Liu J, et al. Baricitinib in patients with inadequate response or intolerance to conventional synthetic DMARDs: results from the RA-BUILD study. Ann Rheum Dis. 2017;76:88–95. https://doi.org/10.1136/annrheumdis-2016-210094.

53. Genovese MC, Kremer J, Zamani O, Ludivico C, Krogulec M, Xie L, et al. Baricitinib in patients with refractory rheumatoid arthritis. N Engl J Med. 2016;374:1243–52. https://doi.org/10.1056/NEJMoa1507247.
54. Taylor PC, Keystone EC, van der Heijde D, Weinblatt ME, del Carmen Morales L, Reyes Gonzaga J, et al. Baricitinib versus placebo or adalimumab in rheumatoid arthritis. N Engl J Med. 2017;376:652–62. https://doi.org/10.1056/NEJMoa1608345.
55. Smolen JS, Genovese MC, Takeuchi T, Hyslop DL, Macias WL, Rooney T, et al. Safety profile of baricitinib in patients with active rheumatoid arthritis with over 2 years median time in treatment. J Rheumatol. 2019;46:7–18. https://doi.org/10.3899/jrheum.171361.
56. Tanaka Y, Takeuchi T, Tanaka S, Kawakami A, Iwasaki M, Song YW, et al. Efficacy and safety of peficitinib (ASP015K) in patients with rheumatoid arthritis and an inadequate response to conventional DMARDs: a randomised, double-blind, placebo-controlled phase III trial (RAJ3). Ann Rheum Dis. 2019;78:1320–32. https://doi.org/10.1136/annrheumdis-2019-215163.
57. Burmester GR, Kremer JM, Van den Bosch F, Kivitz A, Bessette L, Li Y, et al. Safety and efficacy of upadacitinib in patients with rheumatoid arthritis and inadequate response to conventional synthetic disease-modifying anti-rheumatic drugs (SELECT-NEXT): a randomised, double-blind, placebo-controlled phase 3 trial. Lancet. 2018;391:2503–12. https://doi.org/10.1016/S0140-6736(18)31115-2.
58. Fleischmann R, Pangan AL, Song I-H, Mysler E, Bessette L, Peterfy C, et al. Upadacitinib versus placebo or adalimumab in patients with rheumatoid arthritis and an inadequate response to methotrexate: results of a phase III, double-blind, randomized controlled trial. Arthrit Rheumatol. 2019;71:1788–800. https://doi.org/10.1002/art.41032.
59. Genovese MC, Kalunian K, Gottenberg J-E, Mozaffarian N, Bartok B, Matzkies F, et al. Effect of filgotinib vs placebo on clinical response in patients with moderate to severe rheumatoid arthritis refractory to disease-modifying antirheumatic drug therapy. JAMA. 2019;322:315. https://doi.org/10.1001/jama.2019.9055.
60. Ashkenazi A, Fairbrother WJ, Leverson JD, Souers AJ. From basic apoptosis discoveries to advanced selective BCL-2family inhibitors. Nat Rev Drug Discov. 2017;16:273–84. https://doi.org/10.1038/nrd.2016.253.
61. Delbridge ARD, Strasser A. The BCL-2 protein family, BH3-mimetics and cancer therapy. Cell Death Differ. 2015;22(7):1071–80. https://doi.org/10.1038/cdd.2015.50.
62. Strasser A, Vaux DL. Cell death in the origin and treatment of cancer. Mol Cell. 2020;78(6):1045–54. https://doi.org/10.1016/j.molcel.2020.05.014.
63. Merino D, Kelly GL, Lessene G, Wei AH, Roberts AW, Strasser A. BH3-mimetic drugs: blazing the trail for new cancer medicines. Cancer Cell. 2018;34:879–91. https://doi.org/10.1016/j.ccell.2018.11.004.
64. Leverson JD, Boghaert ER, Ackler SL, Catron ND, Chen J, Dayton BD, et al. ABT-199, a potent and selective BCL-2 inhibitor, achieves antitumor activity while sparing platelets. Nat Med. 2013;19(2):202–8. https://doi.org/10.1038/nm.3048.
65. Roberts AW, Davids MS, Pagel JM, Kahl BS, Puvvada SD, Gerecitano JF, et al. Targeting BCL2 with venetoclax in relapsed chronic lymphocytic leukemia. N Engl J Med. 2016;374:311–22. https://doi.org/10.1056/NEJMoa1513257.
66. Stilgenbauer S, Eichhorst B, Schetelig J, Hillmen P, Seymour JF, Coutre S, et al. Venetoclax for patients with chronic lymphocytic leukemia with 17p deletion: results from the full population of a phase II pivotal trial. J Clin Oncol. 2018;36:1973–80. https://doi.org/10.1200/JCO.2017.76.6840.
67. DiNardo CD, Jonas BA, Pullarkat V, Thirman MJ, Garcia JS, Wei AH, et al. Azacitidine and venetoclax in previously untreated acute myeloid leukemia. N Engl J Med. 2020;383:617–29. https://doi.org/10.1056/NEJMoa2012971.
68. Seymour JF, Kipps TJ, Eichhorst B, Hillmen P, D'Rozario J, Assouline S, et al. Venetoclax–rituximab in relapsed or refractory chronic lymphocytic leukemia. N Engl J Med. 2018;378:1107–20. https://doi.org/10.1056/NEJMoa1713976.
69. Fischer K, Al-Sawaf O, Bahlo J, Fink A-M, Tandon M, Dixon M, et al. Venetoclax and obinutuzumab in patients with CLL and coexisting conditions. N Engl J Med. 2019;380:2225–36. https://doi.org/10.1056/NEJMoa1815281.

Infection Associated with the Use of CAR T Cells

17

Pedro Puerta-Alcalde, Nicole Garcia-Pouton, and Carolina Garcia-Vidal

Introduction

Adoptive immunotherapy using targeted chimeric antigen receptor (CAR)-modified cells is a novel therapeutic approach with the potential to revolutionize the treatment of patients with several different medical conditions. CAR-modified T cells targeting the B-cell-specific antigen CD19 have been studied in several clinical trials and have demonstrated high rates of complete remission in patients with relapsed or refractory B-cell malignancies, including acute lymphoblastic leukemia (ALL), chronic lymphocytic leukemia (CLL), and non-Hodgkin lymphoma (NHL).

As CAR T cells are not a first-line therapy, most patients receiving them have a baseline immunosuppressed status due to previous therapies and baseline malignancy. Additionally, lymphodepletion chemotherapy is administered prior to CAR T-cell therapy, causing profound cytopenias and mucosal barrier dysfunction. Cytokine release syndrome (CRS) and immune effector cell-associated neurotoxicity syndrome (ICANS) are frequent complications mediated by the elevation of proinflammatory cytokines which take place within the first weeks after CAR T-cell infusion. These life-threatening conditions are often indistinguishable from infections and sepsis, presenting with fever, tachycardia, tachypnea, and hypotension, as well as elevated inflammatory reactants. Intensive care unit admission (ICU) is frequent in this context. Moreover, the treatment of such complications is quite different from that of infections, requiring immunosuppressant therapy mainly with tocilizumab (humanized interleukin-6 receptor monoclonal antibody) and corticosteroids. Finally, CD19 CAR T cells can also deplete nonmalignant B-cells, resulting in varying degrees of B-cell aplasia and hypogammaglobulinemia.

P. Puerta-Alcalde (✉) · N. Garcia-Pouton · C. Garcia-Vidal
Department of Infectious Diseases, Hospital Clínic-IDIBAPS, Barcelona, Spain
e-mail: puerta@clinic.cat; ngpouton@clinic.cat; cgarciav@clinic.cat

C. Cervera, J. M. Aguado (eds.), *Infectious Complications in Biologic and Targeted Therapies*, https://doi.org/10.1007/978-3-031-11363-5_17

In this complex scenario, CAR T-cell recipients are at high risk of infectious complications, and their management regarding screening strategies, prophylaxis, empirical treatments, and de-escalation strategies is challenging. Due to the novelty of this treatment, knowledge on this topic is scarce and most recommendations are based on expert opinion. In this chapter we will briefly review the mechanism of action of CAR T-cell therapy and its main complications, as well as the different infectious complications and possible management strategies within this complex setting. Table 17.1 describes the main studies analyzed in the chapter.

Table 17.1 Main studies evaluating infectious complications in patients receiving CAR T-cell therapy

Study type and hematological malignancy	n	Prior HSCT	Median prior lines of treatment	Main results	Infection severity	Reference and year of publication[a]
Phase I/II study 47 B-ALL, 24 CLL, 62 NHL	133	38%	4	Days 0–28: 23% infections; infection density: 1.19 per 100 days at risk Days 29–90: 14% infections; infection density: 0.67 per 100 days at risk RF for infection: ALL (HR 2.68), ≥4 prior antitumor treatment regimens (HR 3.53), receipt of 2×10^7 CAR T cells per kg (HR 7.25), and severity of CRS (HR 3.83)	50% mild or moderate, 41% severe, 6% life-threatening, 3% fatal	Hill et al. [11] 2018
Phase I study B-ALL	53	36%	3	Days 0–30: 42% infections, mostly bacterial Days 31–180: 31% infection, mostly viral RF for infection: CRS (grade ≥ 3)	NS 5.6% fatal infections	Park et al. [3] 2018
Case series LBCL	3	33%	2	Three patients with concomitant HBV or HCV infection receiving CAR T-cell therapy HBV prophylaxis with entecavir and tenofovir No fulminant hepatitis observed	–	Strati et al. [24] 2019

(continued)

Table 17.1 (continued)

Study type and hematological malignancy	n	Prior HSCT	Median prior lines of treatment	Main results	Infection severity	Reference and year of publication[a]
Retrospective 25 B-ALL, 68 LBCL, 16 MM	109	23%	NS	17% infections in the first 30 days Grade 4–5 infection and grade 3–5 CRS had higher levels of IL-6, but only CRS had also important elevations of ferritin Patients with infection had a second IL-6 peak (>1000 pg/mL) Infection predictive model based in three cytokines: IL-8, IL-1β, and IFN-γ	16% mild or moderate, 26% severe, 58% life-threatening or fatal	Luo et al. [6] 2019
Retrospective LBCL	15	NS	NS	Three patients (20%) had HBV reactivation HBeAg as a marker of infectivity No hepatitis flare	–	Yang et al. [25] 2020
Case series NS hematological malignancy	59	NS	NS	3% (2/59) invasive mold diseases: 1 *Fusarium solani* and 1 probable mucormycosis Both the patients had CRS and neutropenia	Both life-threatening	Haidar et al. [26] 2020
Retrospective 82 B-ALL, 1 LBCL	83	55%	NS	90 days before infusion: 54% infections; infection density: 1.23 per 100 days at risk Days 0–28: 40% infections; infection density: 2.23 per 100 days at risk Days 29–90: 17% infections; infection density: 0.55 per 100 days at risk RF for infection in the first 28 days: Prior HSCT (HR 2.15) and post-infusion hypogammaglobulinemia (HR 2.41)	43% mild-moderate, 45% severe, 13% life-threatening	Vora et al. [16] 2020

(continued)

Table 17.1 (continued)

Study type and hematological malignancy	n	Prior HSCT	Median prior lines of treatment	Main results	Infection severity	Reference and year of publication[a]
Retrospective LBCL	60	27%	4	101 infections (60 bacterial, 38 viral, 2 fungal, and 1 protozoal). Thirty-two during initial CAR T admission and 69 after hospital discharge (70% managed as outpatients) 1-year cumulative incidence of all infections, bacterial, viral, and fungal infections were 63.3, 57.2, 44.7%, and 4.0%, respectively RF for infection: Systemic corticosteroid (HR 2.22) RF for severe bacterial infection: Impaired performance status (HR 2.84) and infection before CAR T infusion (HR 3.98) RF for viral infection: Hypogammaglobulinemia prior to CAR T infusion (HR 5.7)	17% mild, 58% moderate, 24% severe, 1% fatal	Wudhikarn et al. [2] 2020
Retrospective 43 NHL, 17 CLL, 26 B-ALL	86	17%	4	Late events (<90 days to 1 year): 54 patients (61%) had at least 1 infection, for a total of 153 infection events Infection density: 0.55 per 100 days at risk Upper respiratory tract: 48%, lower respiratory tract: 23%	NS, but 80% outpatient, 20% admission, 5% ICU	Cordeiro et al. [10] 2020

HSCT hematopoietic stem-cell transplant, *B-ALL* acute lymphoblastic leukemia B, *CLL* chronic lymphocytic leukemia, *NHL* non-Hodgkin lymphoma, *RF* risk factors, *HR* hazard ratio, *CAR T* chimeric antigen receptor T, *CRS* cytokine release syndrome, *NS* non-specified, *LBCL* large B-cell lymphoma, *HBV* hepatitis B virus, *HCV* hepatitis C virus, *ICU* intensive care unit

[a]Arranged chronologically

Mechanism of Action of CAR T-Cell Therapy

Adoptive T-cell therapy involves the harvesting of T-lymphocytes from a patient's or donor's blood and then stimulating the cells to grow and expand in an in vitro system. These cells are subsequently reinfused back into the patient, primed for action (Fig. 17.1). Typically, T cells act by targeting specific peptides following major histocompatibility complex restrictions. In engineered CARs the binding regions are modified, and thus, the major histocompatibility complex can be avoided, allowing the cell surface antigens to be targeted independently. As a result, the patient's own T-lymphocytes can be activated against any specific target. A lentiviral vector is commonly used to deliver the genetic material into the T-lymphocyte. CAR T constructs include an antibody-based variable region, a transmembrane domain, a CD3ζ signaling domain, and co-stimulatory domains to improve proliferation, cytokine secretion, and in vivo persistence.

The current approach in hematological malignancies uses lymphodepletion chemotherapy, followed by infusion of autologous T cells modified to express a second-generation CD19-CAR incorporating a single-chain variable fragment derived from the murine IgG1 anti-CD19 monoclonal antibody (Fig. 17.1). These infused T cells are a living therapy with the ability to persist in the host for years, potentially preventing future relapses of baseline B-cell malignancy [1].

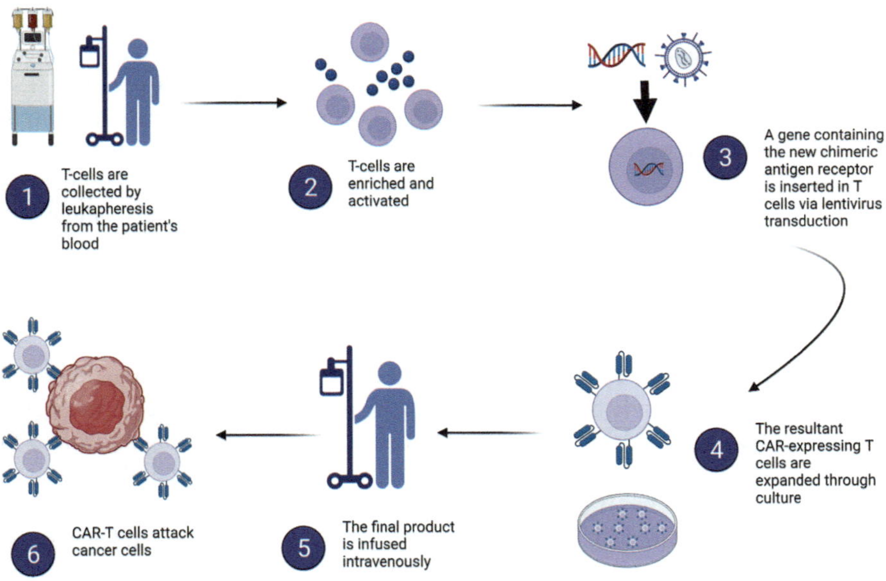

Fig. 17.1 Manufacturing CAR T cells requires several steps. T-lymphocytes are harvested from the patient by leukapheresis. After enriching and activating harvested T cells, the gene codifying the chimeric antigen receptor is inserted via transduction through a lentivirus. Genetically modified T cells are then cultured and expanded, and the final product is infused to the patient. CAR T cells react against cancer cells and can persist in the host for years

Main Toxicities Following CAR T-Cell Therapy

CRS and ICANS

CRS is a potentially life-threatening reaction mediated by the elevation of proinflammatory cytokines, including but not limited to interleukin-6 (IL-6). CRS typically coincides with CAR T-cell expansion, taking place during the first 21 days of CAR T infusion and being generally related to the tumor burden. CRS is very common with incidences ranging from 60% to 80% [2] and severe CRS (≥grade 3) presenting in 12–26% of cases [2, 3]. ICANS is the second most common adverse event related to CAR T-cell therapy and can occur separately from CRS. ICANS incidence is related to the burden of tumoral disease and the patient's age.

CRS and ICANS are commonly managed with tocilizumab (anti-interleukin-6-receptor antibody) and corticosteroids. Besides this additional immunosuppression, CRS causes endothelial damage further increasing the risk of infection [4].

CRS/ICANS can be difficult to distinguish from severe sepsis or infection. In severe sepsis, interferon (IFN)-γ is not commonly significantly elevated, although IL-6 is remarkably high [5]. This may be significantly different from the inflammatory responses of CAR T-cell-induced CRS, although strict interpretations of dynamic markers such as cytokines are challenging. Luo et al. evaluated the inflammatory characteristic signatures in CRS and infection in an attempt to differentiate them [6]. It was found that both grade 4–5 infection and grade 3–5 CRS presented with high levels of IL-6, but only CRS had significant ferritin elevation. Moreover, most patients with life-threatening or fatal infections developed a second IL-6 peak (>1000 pg/mL) immediately after the suppression of the first CRS-related IL-6 peak, with a ferritin increase of less than 50%. Other differences in cytokines were also observed such as IL8, IL-1β, and IFN-γ. After these findings, the authors propose a prediction model based on these three cytokines to help identify infections after CAR T-cell therapy. However, this work needs to be prospectively validated.

Cytopenia

The incidence of severe neutropenia following CAR T-cell infusion ranges from 20 to 80% [7, 8]. In the study by Fried et al. [9], 97% of patients developed neutropenia (72% <500 neutrophils/μL) with a median duration of 19 days, ranging from 0 to 63 days. In several patients, neutropenia was biphasic and linked to SDF-1 levels: a chemokine essential for B-cell development and for trafficking of neutrophils, as well as hematopoietic stem cells. Prolonged cytopenia during several weeks or months after CAR T infusion has been described [10].

Hypogammaglobulinemia

Due to its mechanism of action, CD19 CAR T cells also deplete normal CD19 B-cells in most patients, causing hypogammaglobulinemia. In fact, persistent B-cell aplasia is a marker of persistence of CAR T cells [8]. Additionally, most patients undergo CAR T-cell therapy due to B-cell malignancies, and a significant percentage of them have hypogammaglobulinemia prior to lymphodepletion chemotherapy. Prior IgG deficiency could be associated with an increased risk of developing hypogammaglobulinemia [10].

Different studies have shown that B-cell depletion occurs in 98% of patients within 28 days of CAR T-cell infusion, with 90-day recovery in only 20% [11]. Secondarily, around half of the patients continue to have hypogammaglobulinemia at day 30, with this percentage increasing to over 60% at later follow-up time points [2, 10]. For example, in a trial conducted in children and young adults, 83% of patients had B-cell aplasia at 6 months post-infusion [8]. Hypogammaglobulinemia seems to be more frequent and severe in patients with ALL than NHL.

Long-lived plasma cells that produce most antibodies to previously exposed pathogens may not be impacted by CD19-targeted CAR T-cell therapy due to low surface expression of CD19 [12]. Replacement therapies in patients with hypogammaglobulinemia have varied in the different studies. Immunoglobulin replacement should be considered in those patients with serum IgG levels below 400 mg/dL as well as in those with serum IgG levels between 400 and 600 mg/dL and serious or recurrent infections.

Incidence of Infection

Patients receiving CAR T-cell therapy are at high risk for infection due to underlying malignancy, prior exposure to multiple treatments (sometimes including rituximab), conditioning regimens, prolonged cytopenia, and the use of immunosuppressants to treat CRS. However, data regarding incidence of infections in these patients is scarce and may vary depending on the underlying disease and the CAR T construct.

Pivotal trials reported infections in up to 55% of patients within the first 1 to 2 years and infections of at least grade 3 severity in up to 33% of patients [8, 13–15]. Although most infections occur in the first 28 days, a heightened risk can persist for several months after CAR T infusion following cytopenia and cellular immunity dysfunction.

Hill et al. [11] divided post-CAR T infections into two different periods: early (≤28 days) and late (days 29–90). By day 28, 23% of patients had developed infections, with an infection density of 1.19 per 100 days at risk. Eighty percent of infections occurred within the first 10 days, and bacterial infections were the most common (17%), followed by viral (8%) and fungal (3%) infections. Between days 29 and 90, 14% of patients developed infections, mainly viral (9%), followed by bacterial (6%) and fungal (2%). Infection density in this later period was 0.67 infections for every 100 days at risk. Similarly, Park et al. [3] reported 42% and 31% of patients developed infections until day 30 and from day 31 to 180, respectively. Bacterial infections predominated in the first period, while viral infections were most frequent in the later period. Vora et al. [16] reported infections in children, adolescents, and young adults receiving CAR T-cell therapy. In this study, 40% of patients acquired an infection in the first 28 days (somehow higher than in adults), mainly bacterial (most were bloodstream infections) and viral (most were respiratory viruses). Between days 29 and 90, incidence of infection was around 15%, being mostly caused by respiratory viruses. Wudhikarn et al. [2] documented all the infections in the first year following CAR T-cell therapy and found that the 1-year cumulative incidence of all infections was 63.3%, with 57.2% bacterial, 44.7% viral, and 4% fungal infections. In the first 30 days, bacterial infections were again the most frequent (68%). After the first 30 days, bacterial infections continued to be the most frequent (with similar incidence as viral infections) with most events occurring before post-infusion day 100. Finally, in the study by Cordeiro et al. [10], 61% of patients had at least one infection beyond 90 days after CAR T.

Risk Factors for Infections

Different baseline characteristics and post-CAR T-cell infusion variables have been associated with an increased risk of infection. In the study by Hill et al. [11], ALL (HR 2.68), receipt of ≥4 prior antitumor treatment regimens (HR 3.53), receipt of 2×10^7 CAR T cells per kg (HR 7.25), and more severe CRS (HR 3.83) were independent risk factors for infection. In fact, 73% of those patients experiencing CRS grade ≥ 4 also had an infection. In the study by Park et al. [3], CRS (grade ≥ 3) was the only independent risk factor for infection, being particularly associated with an increased risk of bloodstream infection (BSI—HR 2.67 for infection, HR 19.97 for BSI). In pediatric and young adult patients [16], prior hematopoietic stem cell transplant (HSCT—HR 2.15) and post-CAR T-hypogammaglobulinemia (HR 2.41) were associated with an increased infection risk in the first 28 days. In this study, severe CRS was associated with an increased risk for infection but did not reach statistical significance. Finally, from the study of Wudhikarn et al. who assessed infections until 1-year post-CAR T-cell infusion, the authors evaluated the risk factors for all infections and for severe bacterial infections, as well as viral infections [2]. They found that systemic corticosteroid use was the only independent predictor of overall infections (HR 2.22), while impaired performance status (HR 2.84) and infection before CAR T infusion (HR 3.98) were associated with severe bacterial infection. Patients with low IgG before lymphodepletion chemotherapy had almost sixfold increased risk of viral infection after CAR T cells.

The role of anti-inflammatory monoclonal antibodies (mainly tocilizumab) in the risk for infections is not clear, especially considering the relatively limited dosing of treatment required in the CRS or ICANS setting. The experience regarding patients with autoimmune diseases requiring recurrent doses has shown these antibodies to be quite safe, although a wide range of secondary infections have been described [17]. Despite the fact that older patients and those with comorbidities seem to have a higher risk of CRS and ICANS [18], no studies have shown a clear relation with an increased risk of infection.

In summary, risk factors for infection in patients receiving CAR T-cell therapy are mainly related to the host (baseline disease and prior therapies) and procedure factors (construct and dose of CAR T cells), secondary cytopenia (mainly neutropenia), B-cell aplasia (hypogammaglobulinemia), as well as secondary inflammatory cascade (CRS and ICANS) and its immunosuppressive treatment (corticosteroids and anti-inflammatory monoclonal antibodies).

Main Types of Infection

Most studies reporting infection after CAR T-cell therapy have classified the infection severity as mild, moderate, severe, life-threatening, or fatal, following prior definitions [19]. Briefly, mild infections required no treatment. Moderate infections required only oral treatment. Severe infections required IV antimicrobial therapy or were associated with other clinical circumstances that were considered severe. Life-threatening infections were complicated by symptoms considered life-threatening and fatal infections contributed significantly to death.

Similarly to HSCT, early infections (within 28 days post-HSCT) tend to be bacterial, while late infections are typically caused by viruses and fungi [6]. For example, in the study by Park et al. [3], bacterial infections occurred at a median of 18 days (IQR, 9–29) after CAR T-cell infusion, followed by fungal infections (median 23 days; IQR, 20–29 days) and viral infections (median 48 days; IQR, 20–80 days).

It is challenging to differentiate the risk truly associated with CAR T therapy process from that related to hematological malignancy and prior treatments. For example, in the study by Vora et al. [16], 54% of patients had at least one infection 90 days prior to CAR T infusion. In fact, infection density was higher in this period pre-CAR T than in the 29–90 days period (1.23 vs 0.55 per 100 days at risk). Independently of the incidence, most infections reported after CAR T are classified as moderate or severe, with life-threatening or fatal infections ranging from 1% to 13% in the different studies [2, 6, 11, 16]. Most life-threatening infections were bacterial and mainly bloodstream infections occurring in neutropenic patients.

Two studies to date have reported the incidence and characteristics of late infections after CAR T infusion [2, 10]. Infections occurring later after CAR T-cell therapy (>90 days) are mainly mild or moderate respiratory tract infections, most commonly not requiring the admission of the patients for specific treatment. Of note, Cordeiro et al. [10] found no significant differences in late events between patients with or without ongoing complete response at the time of evaluation.

Table 17.2 displays the main type of infections described.

Table 17.2 Main types of infections described

Bacterial infections
• Most reported infections
• Most episodes occurring during periods of neutropenia
• Bloodstream infections are the most frequent
• Most common life-threatening and fatal infections in the different studies
• *Clostridioides difficile* colitis importance in patients receiving multiple antibiotics
• Differentiating bacterial sepsis from CRS is challenging
• CRS is an important risk factor
• ICU is an additional risk factor in patients with severe CRS
• Persistent hypogammaglobulinemia is a risk factor for encapsulated bacteria
• High-risk for MDR bacteria in the context of prolonged and recurrent admissions, and several prior antibiotic treatments
• Antibiotic prophylaxis is controversial
• Anti-pneumococcal vaccination is recommended
Viral infections
• Most common infections presenting late (>90 days) after infusion
• Upper and lower respiratory tract infections
• Co-infection with bacteria, fungi, and other viruses is frequent
• HSV and VZV reactivation can happen
• SARS-CoV-2 should be ruled out at pertinent time points
• Patients with chronic HBV can undergo CAR T-cell therapy under proper prophylaxis and viremia and liver function monitoring
• Main risk factors for viral infections are severe CRS, prior HSCT, and hypogammaglobulinemia
• Prophylaxis with acyclovir or valacyclovir is recommended in patients seropositive for HSV and VZV
• Seasonal influenza vaccination and HBV in high-risk patients
Fungal infections
• Less reported, but incidence ranging from 2% to 10%
• Fungemia and disseminated disease in patients with other common risk factors (prolonged hospital stay, presence of foreign bodies and instrumentalization, antibiotic selection pressure, etc.)
• Invasive mold disease has been described
• Risk factors for invasive mold disease in the CAR T-cell setting: Prolonged and profound neutropenia, high-dose corticosteroids, prior HSCT, several prior lines of treatment, and CRS
• Antifungal prophylaxis with fluconazole is recommended in severe neutropenic patients
• Anti-mold azole prophylaxis is controversial and should be considered in high-risk patients
• Prophylaxis against *Pneumocystis jirovecii* with trimetroprim-sulfamethoxazole or inhaled pentamidine is recommended until CD4 count is >200/μL

CRS cytokine release syndrome, *ICU* intensive care unit, *MDR* multidrug-resistant, *HSV herpes simplex* virus, *VZV varicella zoster* virus, *SARS-CoV-2* severe acute respiratory syndrome coronavirus 2, *HBV* hepatitis B virus, *CAR T* chimeric antigen receptor T, *HSCT* hematopoietic stem cell transplant

Bacterial Infection

Bacterial infections are the most common infections reported in patients receiving CAR T-cell therapy, with incidences ranging from 10% to 43% and most episodes occurring during periods of neutropenia [3, 8, 11]. As these patients are heavily pretreated and have undergone several prior admissions, and likely received different antibiotic regimens, infections caused by multidrug-resistant microorganisms can arise. For example, in the study by Park et al. [3], multidrug-resistant Gram-negative bacilli, vancomycin-resistant *Enterococcus* (7/13) and *Clostridioides difficile* colitis (five cases), were common. The importance of *C. difficile* colitis in the different studies of patients receiving CAR T-cell therapy is striking, with it being the most commonly isolated agent in some studies [2]. In this setting, stewardship strategies to de-escalate and halt antibiotics, especially in those patients with CRS who do not need antibiotics, are paramount to avoiding this potentially fatal complication [20].

Neutropenic patients presenting with CRS can be indistinguishable from those presenting infection. In this setting, empirical broad-spectrum antibiotics following international neutropenic guidelines are recommended. Thorough knowledge of local epidemiology and rates of multidrug resistance are paramount. However, efforts to differentiate both complications are mandatory. IL-6 and ferritin levels together with other cytokines may be helpful, although prolonged time until having the results may be a limitation. Following the knowledge acquired from other groups of neutropenic patients, de-escalation strategies in 24–72 h can be considered [20, 21].

Viral Infections

Viral infections are the most common infection occurring late after CAR T-cell infusion. Most viral infections are upper and lower respiratory tract infections caused by respiratory viruses. Incidence varies from 6% to 28%, with a median time to presentation of 48 days post-infusion [3, 11]. Clinically, these viruses are almost indistinguishable from each other and commonly present as co-infection with bacteria, fungi, and other viruses. Patients with respiratory symptoms should undergo a chest X-ray and a multiplex PCR workup for respiratory viruses. Studies mainly conducted in allogenic HSCT patients have shown that hypogammaglobulinemia may have an impact in the prognosis of these infections. Apart from oseltamivir treatment in patients with *influenza,* many of these respiratory viruses have no optimal treatment available. Ribavirin can be considered in patients with respiratory syncytial virus, and cidofovir could be helpful in those with adenovirus, although these treatments are associated with significant toxicities.

Herpes simplex virus (HSV) and varicella-zoster virus (VZV) reactivation can happen, although the incidence in the different studies was relatively low, given that most patients received acyclovir or valacyclovir prophylaxis. There are no data on cytomegalovirus (CMV) viremia monitoring, although the risk of end-organ disease seems relatively low. Other herpesviruses and double-stranded DNA viruses such as adenovirus and BK polyomavirus are very infrequent.

The coronavirus disease 2019 (COVID-19) pandemic caused by the severe acute respiratory syndrome coronavirus 2 (SARS-CoV-2) has become a great health challenge, with tremendous impact on our social, economic, and health lives. Experience regarding SARS-CoV-2 infection in patients undergoing CAR T-cell therapy is scarce [22], but data from hematological patients suggest that these patients could have a worsened prognosis. In the current epidemiological context, symptoms of COVID-19 infection should be systematically evaluated. Additionally, PCR screening of SARS-CoV-2 (even in asymptomatic patients) is recommended at pertinent time points: before apheresis, lymphodepleting chemotherapy, and CAR T-cell infusion [23].

Patients with active hepatitis B virus (HBV) or hepatitis C virus (HCV) infection have been excluded from clinical trials of CAR T-cell therapy, due to the potential risk for viral reactivation and fulminant hepatitis. Strati et al. [24] reported on three patients with relapsed/refractory diffuse large B-cell lymphoma and concomitant HBV or HCV infection receiving CAR T. No fulminant hepatitis was observed, although no patient in this study had concomitant liver cirrhosis. Later, Yang et al. [25] reported 15 patients with chronic HBV receiving CAR T cells under antiviral prophylaxis. Three patients (20%) had HBV reactivation. Two of them had HBeAg positive associated with high viral loads, but no hepatitis flare (defined as ALT level more than 100 IU/L) was observed. Following these reports, chronic hepatitis does not seem a clear contraindication for CAR T therapy in otherwise well-controlled patients. As no data exist on T-cell immune reconstitution after CAR T-cell therapy, close monitoring of HBV-DNA load and liver function, together with antiviral prophylaxis, is essential.

Fungal Infections

Rates of invasive fungal disease (IFD) after CAR T-cell therapy range from 2% to 10% in the first 100 days [3, 6, 11]. Later IFD can also occur, for example, Cordeiro et al. [10] reported four IFD in 54 patients (7%) 90 days after CAR T-cell infusion. However, these data are highly influenced by the fact that most studies performed antifungal prophylaxis with fluconazole or an echinocandin.

Impact of CAR T-cell therapy on the risk of invasive mold disease (IMD) is in discussion. In the study conducted in the Fred Hutchinson Cancer Research Center in Seattle [11], IMDs developed in 2% (3/133) of the patients: all had severe CRS and one was neutropenic with a previous HSCT. In the study from Memorial Sloan Kettering in New York [3], 7% (4/53) of patients developed IMD: all were neutropenic and three had CRS. In the study of late complications by Cordeiro et al. [10], two of the four fungal infections recorded were caused by *Aspergillus* spp. Finally, Haidar et al. [26] reported an IMD rate of 3% (2/59), with CRS and neutropenia present in both. Like prophylactic antifungal use, underlying B-cell malignancy remains a major confounder when assessing the risk for fungal infection in these patients.

Latent Infections and Screening Strategies

Patients undergoing CAR T-cell therapy should be screened for latent infections. Human immunodeficiency virus (HIV), HBV, HCV, HSV, CMV, VZV, and *Toxoplasma gondii* serologies should be obtained in all patients. Patients with history of travel to endemic countries for specific infectious diseases should be screened accordingly [27]. Screening for latent tuberculosis remains controversial, and the yield of both interferon-gamma release assays (IGRAs) and enzyme-linked immune absorbent spot (ELISpot) is diminished in these frequently lymphopenic patients. However, we recommend screening for latent tuberculosis in patients living or coming from a country with a high incidence of tuberculosis.

Prophylactic Regimens in Patients Receiving CAR T-Cell Therapy

The role of antibacterial prophylaxis in neutropenic patients is controversial as it diminishes the risk of bacterial infection but may be associated with significant selection pressure for multidrug-resistant microorganisms. Although the role of antibacterial prophylaxis in patients receiving CAR T-cell therapy is not well defined, some centers are performing prophylaxis (mainly with a fluoroquinolone) during the neutropenic phase.

In those patients with positive serologies for HSV 1/2 or VZV, prophylaxis with acyclovir or valacyclovir is endorsed for at least 6 months after CAR T-cell infusion. In patients with HBV infection, prophylaxis with entecavir, lamivudine, or tenofovir is recommended and should be maintained for at least 6 months. Additionally, serum markers of hepatitis should be closely monitored. In patients with HCV infection, specific treatment should be considered prior to CAR T therapy. CMV monitoring should be considered in patients receiving tocilizumab, high-dose corticosteroids, and those with prolonged lymphopenia.

Antifungal prophylaxis with fluconazole is recommended in patients with severe neutropenia. Anti-mold prophylaxis is controversial in this setting since the incidence seems low, and it is associated with increased costs, adverse events, and potential emergence of resistance. Some experts recommend performing a baseline workup for occult IMD prior to CAR T-cell infusion [28]. Mold-active azole prophylaxis (mainly with posaconazole) should be considered in patients with prolonged grade 4 neutropenia (>3 weeks), prior HSCT, prior IMD, several prior lines of treatment, and/or receiving high-dose corticosteroids. Similar to HSCT recipients, patients receiving CAR T-cell therapy with prior invasive fungal disease are probably at an increased risk of recurrent or new fungal infection and should be managed in a highly individualized manner [29].

Prophylaxis against *Pneumocystis jirovecii* with either trimethoprim/sulfamethoxazole or inhaled pentamidine should be considered.

Suggested prophylaxis approach is summarized in Table 17.3.

Table 17.3 Suggested prophylaxis in CAR T-cell therapy recipients

	Suggested strategy	Duration	Comments
Bacterial prophylaxis	• Consider levofloxacin	During grade IV neutropenia (<500/μL)	Bacterial prophylaxis is controversial and should follow local policies for severe neutropenic patients
Viral prophylaxis	• Acyclovir or valacyclovir in patients seropositive for HSV 1/2 and VZV • Entecavir, lamivudine or tenofovir in patients with HBV infection	At least 6 months after CAR T infusion	In patients with HBV, serum markers of hepatitis and viremia should be closely monitored CMV monitoring should be considered in patients receiving tocilizumab, high-dose corticosteroids, and prolonged lymphopenia. However, letermovir prophylaxis is not recommended
Antifungal prophylaxis	• Fluconazole • Trimethoprim-sulfamethoxazole or inhaled pentamidine for PCP • Consider anti-mold prophylaxis: – Posaconazole or isavuconazole – Echinocandin ± nebulized amphotericin B – Intravenous amphotericin B	During grade IV neutropenia (<500/μL) PCP prophylaxis: Until CD4 count is greater than 200/μL	Anti-mold prophylaxis should be considered in patients with grade IV neutropenia for >3 weeks, prior HSCT, prior IMD, several prior lines of treatment, and/or receiving high-dose corticosteroids. First choice for anti-mold prophylaxis is posaconazole. Isavuconazole can be used in case of drug–drug interactions. The other regimens are less well stablished

IV intravenous, *HSV herpes simplex* virus, *VZV varicella zoster* virus, *HBV* hepatitis B virus, *CAR T* chimeric antigen receptor T, *CMV cytomegalovirus*, *HSCT* hematopoietic stem cell transplant, *IMD* invasive mold disease

Vaccination

There exist no current international guidelines regarding vaccination in patients receiving CAR T-cell therapy. Additionally, patients receiving CD19-targeted CAR T-cell therapy are likely to have lower vaccine responses compared with healthy individuals. However, correct vaccination may still prevent infections, decrease their severity, and avoid hospitalizations. Moreover, prolonged B-cell aplasia may heighten the risk for infections caused by encapsulated bacteria.

With the immunological condition of these patients, all live and attenuated vaccines are contraindicated due to potential risk of reactivation. The main recommended vaccinations are (1) seasonal influenza; (2) anti-pneumococcal sequential vaccination: one dose of conjugated vaccine followed by one dose of polysaccharide vaccine >8 weeks later and a second dose of polysaccharide vaccine >5 years later; and (3) HBV, particularly in high-risk populations. Once B-cell aplasia is resolved, full vaccination program can be initiated. Finally, enhancing the immunization of health-caring professionals and cohabiting relatives is essential.

Conclusions

Chimeric antigen receptor (CAR) T-cell therapy against the B-cell-specific antigen CD19 is a promising treatment for patients with relapsing/refractory B-cell malignancies. Patients receiving this treatment are at increased risk of infections due to deteriorated immune status, lymphodepletion chemotherapy, toxicities in form of CRS and ICANS, B-cell aplasia, prolonged hypogammaglobulinemia, and neutropenia. Moderate and severe infections are frequent in this setting. Bacterial infections are the most frequent, followed by viral and fungal. Risk factors for infection relate to both host and procedure factors such as neutropenia, hypogammaglobulinemia, and secondary CRS/ICANS with their respective immunosuppressive treatments including corticosteroids and anti-inflammatory monoclonal antibodies. Systematic screening, prophylactic strategies, and proper vaccination can help diminish the risk of infection.

References

1. Salter AI, Pont MJ, Riddell SR. Chimeric antigen receptor-modified T cells: CD19 and the road beyond [Internet]. Blood. American Society of Hematology; 2018 [cited 2020 Nov 10];131:2621–9. Available from: https://pubmed.ncbi.nlm.nih.gov/29728402/.
2. Wudhikarn K, Palomba ML, Pennisi M, Garcia-Recio M, Flynn JR, Devlin SM, et al. Infection during the first year in patients treated with CD19 CAR T cells for diffuse large B cell lymphoma. Blood Cancer J [Internet]. 2020 [cited 2020 Oct 27];10(8). Available from: https://pubmed.ncbi.nlm.nih.gov/32759935/.
3. Park JH, Romero FA, Taur Y, Sadelain M, Brentjens RJ, Hohl TM, et al. Cytokine release syndrome grade as a predictive marker for infections in patients with relapsed or refractory b-cell acute lymphoblastic leukemia treated with chimeric antigen receptor T cells. Clin Infect Dis [Internet]. 2018 [cited 2020 Oct 25];67(4):533–40. Available from: https://pubmed.ncbi.nlm.nih.gov/29481659/.
4. Budde LE, Zaia JA. CD19 CAR-T therapy and sepsis: dancing with the devil [Internet]. Blood. American Society of Hematology; 2018 [cited 2020 Nov 9]; 131:7–8. Available from: https://pubmed.ncbi.nlm.nih.gov/29301772/.
5. Slaats J, ten Oever J, van de Veerdonk FL, Netea MG. IL-1β/IL-6/CRP and IL-18/ferritin: distinct inflammatory programs in infections [Internet]. PLoS Pathog. Public Library of Science; 2016 [cited 2020 Nov 4]; 12. Available from: https://pubmed.ncbi.nlm.nih.gov/27977798/.
6. Luo H, Wang N, Huang L, Zhou X, Jin J, Li C, et al. Inflammatory signatures for quick diagnosis of life-threatening infection during the CAR T-cell therapy. J Immunother Cancer [Internet]. 2019 [cited 2020 Oct 26];7(1). Available from: https://pubmed.ncbi.nlm.nih.gov/31640816/.
7. Schuster SJ, Bishop MR, Tam CS, Waller EK, Borchmann P, McGuirk JP, et al. Tisagenlecleucel in adult relapsed or refractory diffuse large B-cell lymphoma. N Engl J Med. 2019;380(1):45–56.

8. Maude SL, Laetsch TW, Buechner J, Rives S, Boyer M, Bittencourt H, et al. Tisagenlecleucel in children and young adults with B-cell lymphoblastic leukemia. N Engl J Med [Internet]. 2018 [cited 2020 Nov 6];378(5):439–48. Available from: https://pubmed.ncbi.nlm.nih.gov/29385370/.
9. Fried S, Avigdor A, Bielorai B, Meir A, Besser MJ, Schachter J, et al. Early and late hematologic toxicity following CD19 CAR-T cells. Bone Marrow Transplant [Internet]. 2019 Oct 1 [cited 2020 Nov 4];54(10):1643–50. Available from: https://pubmed.ncbi.nlm.nih.gov/30809033/.
10. Cordeiro A, Bezerra ED, Hirayama A V., Hill JA, Wu Q V., Voutsinas J, et al. Late events after treatment with CD19-targeted chimeric antigen receptor modified T cells. Biol Blood Marrow Transplant [Internet]. 2020 [cited 2020 Oct 26];26(1):26–33. Available from: https://pubmed.ncbi.nlm.nih.gov/31419568/.
11. Hill JA, Li D, Hay KA, Green ML, Cherian S, Chen X, et al. Infectious complications of CD19-targeted chimeric antigen receptor-modified T-cell immunotherapy. Blood [Internet]. 2018 [cited 2020 Sep 28];131(1):121–30. Available from: https://pubmed.ncbi.nlm.nih.gov/29038338/.
12. Hill JA, Seo SK. How I prevent infections in patients receiving CD19-targeted chimeric antigen receptor T cells for B-cell malignancies. Blood [Internet]. 2020 [cited 2020 Nov 2];136(8):925–35. Available from: https://pubmed.ncbi.nlm.nih.gov/32582924/.
13. Neelapu SS, Locke FL, Bartlett NL, Lekakis LJ, Miklos DB, Jacobson CA, et al. Axicabtagene ciloleucel CAR T-cell therapy in refractory large B-cell lymphoma. N Engl J Med [Internet]. 2017 [cited 2020 Nov 9];377(26):2531–44. Available from: https://pubmed.ncbi.nlm.nih.gov/29226797/.
14. Locke FL, Ghobadi A, Jacobson CA, Miklos DB, Lekakis LJ, Oluwole OO, et al. Long-term safety and activity of axicabtagene ciloleucel in refractory large B-cell lymphoma (ZUMA-1): a single-arm, multicentre, phase 1–2 trial. Lancet Oncol [Internet]. 2019 [cited 2020 Nov 9];20(1):31–42. Available from: https://pubmed.ncbi.nlm.nih.gov/30518502/.
15. Schuster SJ, Svoboda J, Chong EA, Nasta SD, Mato AR, Anak Ö, et al. Chimeric antigen receptor T cells in refractory B-cell lymphomas. N Engl J Med [Internet]. 2017 [cited 2020 Nov 9];377(26):2545–54. Available from: https://pubmed.ncbi.nlm.nih.gov/29226764/.
16. Vora SB, Waghmare A, Englund JA, Qu P, Gardner RA, Hill JA. Infectious complications following CD19 chimeric antigen receptor T-cell therapy for children, adolescents, and young adults. Open Forum Infect Dis [Internet]. 2020 [cited 2020 Oct 27];7(5). Available from: https://pubmed.ncbi.nlm.nih.gov/32432149/.
17. Schiff MH, Kremer JM, Jahreis A, Vernon E, Isaacs JD, van Vollenhoven RF. Integrated safety in tocilizumab clinical trials. Arthritis Res Ther [Internet]. 2011 [cited 2020 Nov 9];13(5). Available from: https://pubmed.ncbi.nlm.nih.gov/21884601/.
18. Pasquini MC, Locke FL, Herrera AF, Siddiqi T, Ghobadi A, Komanduri KV, et al. Post-marketing use outcomes of an anti-CD19 chimeric antigen receptor (CAR) T cell therapy, axicabtagene ciloleucel (Axi-Cel), for the treatment of large B cell lymphoma (LBCL) in the United States (US). Blood. 2019;134:764.
19. Young J-AH, Logan BR, Wu J, Wingard JR, Weisdorf DJ, Mudrick C, et al. Infections after transplantation of bone marrow or peripheral blood stem cells from unrelated donors. Biol Blood Marrow Transplant [Internet]. 2016 [cited 2018 Aug 12];22(2):359–70. Available from: http://www.ncbi.nlm.nih.gov/pubmed/26409243.
20. Puerta-Alcalde P, Cardozo C, Suárez-Lledó M, Rodríguez-Núñez O, Morata L, Fehér C, et al. Current time-to-positivity of blood cultures in febrile neutropenia: a tool to be used in stewardship de-escalation strategies. Clin Microbiol Infect. 2019;25(4):447–53.
21. Aguilar-Guisado M, Espigado I, Martín-Peña A, Gudiol C, Royo-Cebrecos C, Falantes J, et al. Optimisation of empirical antimicrobial therapy in patients with haematological malignancies and febrile neutropenia (How Long study): an open-label, randomised, controlled phase 4 trial. Lancet Haematol. 2017;4(12):e573–83.
22. Malard F, Genthon A, Brissot E, van de Wyngaert Z, Marjanovic Z, Ikhlef S, et al. COVID-19 outcomes in patients with hematologic disease. Bone Marrow Transplant. 2020;55(11):2180–4.

23. Los-Arcos I, Iacoboni G, Aguilar-Guisado M, Alsina-Manrique L, Díaz de Heredia C, Fortuny-Guasch C, et al. Recommendations for screening, monitoring, prevention, and prophylaxis of infections in adult and pediatric patients receiving CAR T-cell therapy: a position paper [Internet]. Infection. Springer Science and Business Media Deutschland GmbH; 2020 [cited 2020 Nov 10]. Available from: https://pubmed.ncbi.nlm.nih.gov/32979154/.
24. Strati P, Nastoupil LJ, Fayad LE, Samaniego F, Adkins S, Neelapu SS. Safety of CAR T-cell therapy in patients with B-cell lymphoma and chronic hepatitis B or C virus infection [Internet]. Blood. American Society of Hematology; 2019 [cited 2020 Oct 26];133:2800–2. Available from: https://pubmed.ncbi.nlm.nih.gov/31101626/.
25. Yang C, Xie M, Zhang K, Liu H, Liang A, Young KH, et al. Risk of HBV reactivation post CD19-CAR-T cell therapy in DLBCL patients with concomitant chronic HBV infection. Leukemia [Internet]. 2020 [cited 2020 Oct 26];34(11). Available from: https://pubmed.ncbi.nlm.nih.gov/32533094/.
26. Haidar G, Dorritie K, Farah R, Bogdanovich T, Nguyen MH, Samanta P. Invasive mold infections after chimeric antigen receptor-modified t-cell therapy: a case series, review of the literature, and implications for prophylaxis. Clin Infect Dis [Internet]. 2020 [cited 2020 Oct 27];71(3):672–6. Available from: https://pubmed.ncbi.nlm.nih.gov/31756246/.
27. Sánchez-Montalvá A, Salvador F, Ruiz-Camps I, Barba P, Valcárcel D, Sulleiro E, et al. Imported disease screening prior to chemotherapy and bone marrow transplantation for oncohematological malignancies. Am J Trop Med Hyg [Internet]. 2016 [cited 2020 Nov 10];95(6):1463–8. Available from: https://pubmed.ncbi.nlm.nih.gov/27928093/.
28. Lewis RE, Kontoyiannis DP. Chimeric antigen receptor T cell immunotherapy and need for prophylaxis for invasive mold infections [published online ahead of print 12 January 2020]. Clin Infect Dis. https://doi.org/10.1093/cid/ciaa031.
29. Puerta-Alcalde P, Champlin R, Kontoyiannis DP. How I transplant a patient with a history of invasive fungal disease. Blood [Internet]. 2020 [cited 2020 Oct 19]; Available from: https://pubmed.ncbi.nlm.nih.gov/32845974/.

Part III

Clinical Conditions Associated with the Use of Biologic and Targeted Therapies

Pulmonary Infiltrates

18

Archana Bhaskaran, Britany Kula, and Dima Kabbani

Introduction

Biologic agents have been in clinical use for a few decades since the 1990s, but the number of approved biologic agents is exponentially increasing with better understanding of human biology. Tumor necrosis factor inhibitors (anti-TNFs) have been around for quite some time; however, there are now close to 100 biologic agents most of which have been released in the market in the past 10 years. Biologics are used in the treatment of a wide spectrum of diseases, such as auto-immunity, cancer, and as part of the immunosuppression for transplantation, rejection, and graft versus host disease. Those that target the immune system pose an increased risk for infections.

We have a reasonable amount of data with respect to the infectious complications of the earlier biologics like anti-tumoral necrosis factor (TNF). Apart from randomized controlled trials (RCT), many years of post-marketing data are available by which more uncommon events could be identified. Therefore, the infectious risk they pose have been well delineated. Very limited post-marketing observational data are available for the newer agents, and hence infection risk has not been clearly identified. Until more comprehensive data from RCT becomes available, based on the mechanism of action and the published case reports and case series, clinicians can predict the different types of infection these newer agents can predispose to. It

A. Bhaskaran
Division of Infectious Diseases, Department of Medicine, University of Minnesota, Minneapolis, MN, USA
e-mail: abhaskar@umn.edu

B. Kula · D. Kabbani (✉)
Division of Infectious Diseases, Department of Medicine, University of Alberta, Edmonton, AB, Canada
e-mail: bekula@ualberta.ca; dkabbani@ualberta.ca

C. Cervera, J. M. Aguado (eds.), *Infectious Complications in Biologic and Targeted Therapies*, https://doi.org/10.1007/978-3-031-11363-5_18

is also important to note that sometimes infection risk cannot be elucidated due to confounding by concurrent use of other immunosuppressive medications, immunosuppressive effects of the underlying disease (e.g., neutropenia), and use of prophylaxis and pre-screening for tuberculosis.

TNF inhibitors increase the risk of serious infections by twofold to fourfold [1–3]. The infection risk is higher for all other anti-TNFs compared to etanercept. Bacterial infections are the most common, of which pneumonia is the main cause of infection followed by gastrointestinal, skin and soft tissue, urinary tract, and surgical site infections. Pneumonia accounts for almost half of the serious infections in patients receiving anti-TNFs. There is an increased incidence of tuberculosis and endemic mycosis like histoplasmosis, coccidioidomycosis, and perhaps blastomycosis with TNF inhibitors that led to a black box warning from the FDA in 2008 [4–7]. There have been numerous reports of other invasive fungal infections like *Pneumocystis jirovecii* pneumonia (PCP), aspergillosis, cryptococcosis, and mucormycosis with anti-TNFs [1, 2].

Anti-TNFs provide a case in point for other immunologic biologics like interleukin (IL)-1 inhibitors; IL-6 inhibitors; mammalian target of rapamycin (mTOR) inhibitors; tyrosine kinase inhibitors (TKIs) especially Bruton (TKI); T-cell co-stimulatory blockers like abatacept; Janus kinase (JAK) inhibitors; and anti-CD52 monoclonal antibody in that bacterial are the most common infections with the use of these agents, with pneumonia topping the list [7, 8]. Anti-complement agents like eculizumab increase risk of infection with encapsulated bacteria like *Streptococcus pneumoniae*, *Haemophilus influenzae*, and *Neisseria meningitidis* [7]. Endemic mycosis risk is increased in patients on Bruton's TKI and JAK inhibitors. There is an increased risk of PCP in patients on anti-CD52, Bruton's TKI, phosphoinositide 3-kinase (PI3K) inhibitor, and JAK inhibitors [8]. There have been several reports of invasive fungal infection (aspergillosis, cryptococcosis, mucormycosis) in patients on anti-CD52, Bruton's TKI, JAK inhibitors, and IL-6 inhibitors [6]. The risk of tuberculosis is increased with IL-6 inhibitors, JAK inhibitors, immune checkpoint inhibitors, anti-CD52, and mTOR inhibitors [5, 7–9].

The development of pulmonary infiltrates in patients on biologic therapy could be secondary to infections (listed above), which is the most common, or due to the underlying disease that necessitated biologic therapy (e.g., rheumatoid arthritis), pulmonary toxicity from biologic therapy, or due to other etiologies that occur in the general population (Table 18.1). We will discuss each in further detail below.

Table 18.1 Causes of pulmonary infiltrates

Causes	Specific cause	Biologic agent
Bacterial	Pneumococcus, *Haemophilus influenzae*, *Mycoplasma* spp., *Legionella* spp., *Staphylococcus aureus*, *Pseudomonas aeruginosa*, enteric Gram-negative bacilli, *Nocardia* spp.	Anti-TNF predisposes to *Legionella spp.* Anti-TNF, proteasome inhibitors and rituximab predispose to *Nocardia spp.*
Mycobacterial	Tuberculosis Non-tuberculous mycobacteria	Anti-TNF, IL-6 inhibitors, JAK inhibitors, immune checkpoint inhibitors, anti-CD52 and mTOR inhibitors, rituximab
Viral	Influenza, RSV, parainfluenza, human metapneumovirus	
Fungal	*Pneumocystis* Endemic mycoses *Aspergillus*	Anti-CD52, Bruton's TKI, PI3K inhibitors, and JAK inhibitors Anti-TNF, Bruton's TKI, and JAK inhibitors Immune checkpoint inhibitors, Bruton's TKI
Drug-induced pulmonary toxicity	ILD Drug-induced pneumonitis Pleural effusion Nodules	Anti-TNF Checkpoint inhibitors, rituximab, PI3K inhibitors Dasatinib Anti-TNF
Miscellaneous	Septic emboli (endocarditis), immune reconstitution inflammatory syndrome, pulmonary hemorrhage, pulmonary embolism with infarct, malignancy, healed lesions, nonspecific	

Infectious Pulmonary Complications

Bacterial Infections

Bacterial pneumonia is the most common infectious complication of biologic therapy, and, therefore, it represents an important contributor to the presentation of pulmonary infiltrates. In patients with rheumatoid arthritis (RA), infections are increased in the 6 months following initiation of anti-TNF, with bacterial pneumonia being the most common type of infection [10]. Similarly to the microbiology in the general population, the most common bacteria implicated in community-acquired bacterial pneumonia in patients receiving biologic agents or immune-targeted therapies include *Streptococcus pneumoniae*, *Haemophilus influenzae*, and *Mycoplasma pneumoniae*. More unique to patients receiving these treatments is the increased risk of *Legionella pneumophila* infection [11]. *Staphylococcus aureus* colonization is common in these patients, and hence staphylococcal pneumonia can occur through aspiration or hematogenous seeding from bacteremia. Some of the biologics such as certolizumab can cause neutropenia and hence predispose to less virulent organisms such as *Pseudomonas aeruginosa* pneumonia [12]. Due to frequent access to medical care among patients on biologics, healthcare-associated pneumonia (HCAP) is commonly associated with antibiotic-resistant bacteria. The common causes of HCAP include enterobacteriaceae, *Staphylococcus aureus*, and *Pseudomonas aeruginosa*. Symptomatology that would suggest bacterial infection includes acute onset of symptoms such as fever, cough, sputum production, and dyspnea. Additionally, constitutional symptoms such as fatigue, malaise, and drenching night sweats are common.

Streptococcus pneumoniae is one of the most common pathogens implicated in community-acquired pneumonia in the immunocompetent as well as those prescribed biologics or immune-targeted therapies. This Gram-positive coccus usually aggregates forming pairs (diplococcus) and there are more than 92 serotypes. An external capsule confers virulence and assists in bacterial evasion of host defense [13]. Pneumococcal pneumonia generally presents acutely with fever, productive cough, dyspnea and possibly chest pain, and lobar consolidation on chest radiography. Invasive disease (including bacteremia) is not uncommon. Sputum Gram stain often demonstrates characteristic Gram-positive diplococci in pairs or chains. Sputum culture and, occasionally, blood cultures may grow *S. pneumoniae* allowing for susceptibility testing and serotyping. Rarely, metastatic infection can occur related to underlying infective endocarditis. The classical Austrian syndrome includes a triad of pneumonia, meningitis, and endocarditis. Recommended empiric therapy includes a respiratory fluoroquinolone in clinically stable outpatients. However, most patients will require an IV third-generation cephalosporin (ceftriaxone), beta-lactam/beta-lactamase inhibitor combination therapy, or vancomycin if there is concern for central nervous system disease in inpatients. The risk of beta-lactam resistance has been increasing over time but remains relatively rare overall [13].

Haemophilus influenzae is a Gram-negative coccobacillus that commonly causes community-acquired pneumonia in both the immunocompetent and immunocompromised, such as those on biologics. Since the widespread use of *H. influenzae* B vaccine, there has been a reduction in invasive disease (such as meningitis) caused by this bacterium. However, non-typeable strains still continue to cause invasive and noninvasive respiratory disease internationally [14]. The typical clinical syndrome caused by *H. influenzae* is similar to that of *S. pneumoniae* and consisting of acute onset of respiratory symptoms and fever. Chest radiography may demonstrate ground glass opacification, bronchial wall thickening, or lobar consolidation. Sputum Gram stain showing Gram-negative coccobacillus suggests *H. influenzae* infection, but there are many non-*Haemophilus influenzae* species that can colonize the airway [15]. Growth of the organism in sputum and/or blood culture is diagnostic. Recommended empiric therapy for stable outpatients usually consists of respiratory fluoroquinolones. For more severe cases or inpatients, a third-generation cephalosporin or beta-lactam/beta-lactamase inhibitors are required.

Mycoplasma pneumoniae also causes an acute to subacute bacterial pneumonia syndrome that is generally more insidious than infections caused by *S. pneumoniae* or *H. influenzae*. Symptoms can be comparatively mild with slower onset, many times referred as "walking pneumonia." Chest radiography usually does not show a lobar consolidation but more so bilateral pulmonary infiltrates [16]. An additional clinical feature that is compatible with *M. pneumoniae* infection is a new-onset cold hemolytic anemia starting up to day 7 of illness and that may persist for months post-infection [16]. Manifestations include rash, Raynaud's phenomenon, renal failure, and rarely gangrene. *M. pneumoniae* lacks a cell wall and therefore does not take up Gram stain. Growth of the organism in sputum and/or blood culture is challenging, requires specific media, and can take many days. More often, it can be identified by nuclear acid testing (NAT). Serum immunoglobulins can also be tested for *M pneumoniae* but are nonspecific, and, therefore, repeat testing with a rise in antibodies is required for diagnosis [16]. Recommended empiric therapy is macrolides, respiratory fluoroquinolones, or doxycycline. Given the lack of a cell wall, beta-lactams are not active against *M. pneumoniae*.

Legionella is an uncommon pathogen that similarly leads to an acute bacterial pneumonia syndrome, often accompanied by respiratory failure and shock. It is not unexpected that individuals infected with this pathogen require invasive supportive care in a critical care setting. While relatively rare in the immunocompetent host, in patients receiving therapy with anti-TNF, the risk of legionellosis has been reported at up to 37-fold higher than the baseline population [1, 11, 17]. *L. pneumophila* is the predominant species causing pneumonia and, notably, serogroup 1 causes the bulk of human infection. Occasionally, non-pneumophila *Legionella* species can cause disease. *Legionella* is an intracellular pathogen and does not take up Gram stain [17, 18]. Radiographically, *Legionella* pneumonia is similar to other causes of typical pneumonia. Diagnosis consists of respiratory or urinary antigen detection. However, non *L. pneumophila* serogroup 1 pathogens may not be detected using these assays [16]. NAT is also readily available for the detection of *Legionella*, especially for non-*L. pneumophila* serogroup 1 organisms, and it is recommended to do NAT from lower tract respiratory specimens. Culture is challenging but can be performed at many reference labs. Empiric therapy for diseases caused by *Legionella* consists of a fluoroquinolone or macrolide. Of note, if *Legionella* is identified, public health should be notified to commence environmental investigation given the natural reservoir is stagnant water, and it is particularly notorious for causing outbreaks in congregate living settings.

HCAP should be considered in those individuals on a biologic with frequent healthcare exposure including infusion appointments or hemodialysis. In general, this does confer increased risk of nosocomial pathogens such as enteric Gram-negative bacilli, *Staphylococcus aureus*, and non-lactose fermenters such as *Pseudomonas aeruginosa* or *Acinetobacter baumannii*, but at a lower rate than those with true hospital-acquired pneumonia (HAP) [19]. The incidence of each pathogen and drug resistance patterns, particularly relevant in non-lactose fermenters, varies geographically, and therefore local antibiograms should be reviewed for empiric management if these organisms are suspected. HCAP will generally present with acute to subacute respiratory symptoms. Chest radiography is most likely to show bilateral pulmonary infiltrates rather than a lobar consolidation. Drug resistance should be suspected in those patients with more prolonged healthcare and antimicrobial exposure, frailty, and poorer functional status [19]. Sputum cultures should be obtained, if possible, to guide therapy. The diagnostic yield of blood cultures is low. Broad-spectrum antimicrobial therapy such as a beta-lactam/beta-lactamase inhibitor with anti-pseudomonal coverage is the most frequently recommended empiric antibiotic regimen. When *Staphylococcus aureus* infection is suspected, adding vancomycin is recommended.

Nocardia, a Gram-positive, weak acid fast, filamentous, and branching bacteria, is found in the soil and water. It is an opportunistic pathogen that commonly occurs in patients with transplant and hematologic cancer. Pulmonary nocardiosis has also been described with the use of anti-TNF and patients treated with rituximab and proteasome inhibitors [20–22]. The majority of cases will have pulmonary involvement in the form of either pulmonary nodules (cavitating when large) or reticulonodular or diffuse pneumonic infiltrates with pleural effusions. Dissemination can occur in up to one-third of cases, with the skin and brain being the most common sites of involvement. Cultures can be obtained from sputum, bronchoalveolar lavage, and tissue biopsies, with repeated testing to increase the yield. Testing should include NAT and/or MALDI-TOF MS when possible, to identify to the genus or species level. Antibiotic therapy should be guided by in vitro antibiotic susceptibility testing. Treatment ranges from monotherapy with trimethoprim-sulfamethoxazole to a combination of two to three antibiotics for 2–6 weeks followed by one antibiotic for maintenance therapy.

Mycobacterial Infections

Tuberculosis (TB) incidence is increased about fourfold with the use of anti-TNF. It is higher with infliximab and adalimumab compared to etanercept [1, 4, 5]. It is also increased with the use of IL-6 inhibitors, JAK inhibitors, immune checkpoint inhibitors, anti-CD52, and mTOR inhibitors [9]. Immune checkpoint inhibitors, specifically PD1 and PD-L1 inhibitors, are different from other biologic agents in that T cell activation is enhanced and yet predisposes to tuberculosis, perhaps related to either hypersensitivity similar to immune reconstitution inflammatory response syndrome or immune exhaustion. There is a theoretical risk of tuberculosis with interleukin (IL)-1 inhibitors although not yet evident from clinical data. In IL-17 and IL-12/23 inhibitor trials, there was no increased TB incidence, but subjects were screened for latent TB and treated or excluded [4]. Hence, it is likely that there is an increased risk of tuberculosis with these agents. Only about one-third of the cases of tuberculosis on TNF inhibitors were pulmonary, one-third were extrapulmonary, and another third were disseminated [4]. Therefore, with diagnosis of pulmonary tuberculosis, evidence of extrapulmonary or disseminated disease will need to be investigated. The symptoms of pulmonary tuberculosis include fever, cough, night sweats, and weight loss. Chest X-ray or CT chest can show consolidation, nodules or cavity. Involvement of apex/subapex or superior segment of lower lobe is common in reactivation tuberculosis. At least two to three morning sputum AFB stain/cultures should be submitted. Otherwise, a bronchoalveolar lavage specimen can be tested for the same. Sputum AFB stain is about 60% sensitive and is usually seen in cavitary pulmonary tuberculosis. Growth of *Mycobacterium tuberculosis* in sputum culture is the gold standard but can take 4–6 weeks. *M. tuberculosis* PCR of the respiratory specimen (on both stain-positive and stain-negative cases) can help identify the organism before the culture results become available and has a sensitivity between that of AFB stain and culture. GeneXpert MTB/RIF, which is also a PCR-based test by Cepheid, has a sensitivity and specificity that approaches culture and it also reports rifampin susceptibility, but it may not be available everywhere. Phenotypic susceptibility testing should be done on all isolates to all the anti-tuberculous drugs. Empiric anti-tuberculous therapy should be started when there is high clinical suspicion for TB before cultures are reported. Most physicians stop anti-TNF therapy at the time of diagnosis of TB, but it appears that it can be safely restarted when the patient is better or on completion of tuberculous therapy. IRIS has been reported in patients with tuberculosis receiving anti-TNF, several weeks after discontinuation of the drug after a phase of initial improvement. This has been treated with steroids or re-initiation of anti-TNFs in steroid refractory cases [3]. The duration of anti-tuberculous therapy is uncertain in these patients and infectious disease consultation is recommended.

Non-tuberculous mycobacterial (NTM) infections are also increased by likely the same biologic agents as tuberculosis. In patients on anti-TNF, NTM infections were more common than TB [6, 23, 24]. Patients with non-tuberculous mycobacterial infections are more likely to have RA and chronic lung disease [6, 23]. Only half of the cases of non-tuberculous mycobacterial infections were pulmonary with the remaining being extrapulmonary (skin and soft tissue or bone and joint) and disseminated (8%) [23]. *Mycobacterium avium-intracellulare* infection (MAI) is the most common pathogen accounting for half of the cases [23]. Chronic cough, night sweats, and weight loss are the common presentation of NTM infections. Imaging changes can be either fibro-cavitary or nodular bronchiectatic. A triad of clinical symptoms, NTM growth in cultures (two sputums or one bronchoalveolar lavage (BAL)), and imaging changes is indicative of pulmonary disease that requires treatment with a combination of antimicrobials.

Respiratory Viruses

Infections caused from community-acquired viral respiratory viruses (CARVs) can vary from mild upper tract infection to severe lower pulmonary disease. CARVs include influenza, respiratory syncytial virus (RSV), human metapneumovirus (hMPV), parainfluenza, adenovirus, and entero-rhinovirus. Their incidence on patients using biologics is not known. Although there is an overlap in the imaging appearance of viral and bacterial pulmonary infections, tree-in-bud opacities, multifocal consolidation, and ground glass opacities are more common with viral infections [25, 26]. Diagnosis relies on identification of the virus in nasopharyngeal swabs or BAL specimens. CARVs can be identified by rapid diagnostic tests based on enzyme immunoassay (EIA), immunofluorescence, or multiplex PCR that can detect multiples viruses.

Fungal

Pneumocystis jirovecii was considered a protozoan and recently reclassified as a fungal yeast. It is an opportunistic pathogen causing disease in immunocompromised hosts. It is classically seen in patients on steroids 20 mg daily or more for more than a month. Lungs are the most commonly involved site, but extrapulmonary manifestations can occur. Among biologic agents, anti-CD52, Bruton's TKI, PI3 inhibitors, and JAK inhibitors predispose to PCP. In a retrospective review of PCP complicating rituximab therapy for autoimmune disease, 90% of cases were also on steroids [27]. Symptoms are usually subacute over 1 week to several weeks and include exertional dyspnea, fever, and dry cough. Hypoxia is common at presentation. The chest radiography can be normal in the initial stages and CT scan may be necessary if PCP is suspected. Bilateral interstitial pneumonia emanating from hilum on chest radiography and diffuse ground glass opacities in CT chest are the common findings. Induced sputum or bronchoscopy for diagnosis is usually necessary. Gomori methenamine silver (GMS) stain or *P. jirovecii* immunofluorescent stain of the BAL confirms the diagnosis. Recently, serum β-D-glucan (BDG) has been found to be a very sensitive marker for the diagnosis of PCP. Serum lactate dehydrogenase (LDH) is also usually elevated although this is nonspecific. PCR for *P. jirovecii* in respiratory specimens appears to be very sensitive but may lack specificity, as it can be positive in colonization and disease. Intravenous trimethoprim-sulfamethoxazole is the drug of choice for moderate to severe PCP. Treatment can be switched to oral trimethoprim-sulfamethoxazole when there is improvement or in mild to moderate infections. Duration of treatment is usually 21 days. Steroids can be administered when PaO_2 is <70 mm Hg.

Endemic mycoses (histoplasmosis, coccidiomycosis, and blastomycosis), acquired through inhalation of spores, vary in incidence and geographic distribution. Endemic mycosis risk is increased in patients on anti-TNF, Bruton's TKI, and JAK inhibitors [28–30]. Cases have also been described with anti-IL-1 [3].

Histoplasmosis, caused by *Histoplasma capsulatum,* is the most reported endemic fungi after anti-TNF. Although more common in North and Central America it is occasionally found in Southern Europe, Africa, Asia and Australia. Histoplasmosis presents as disseminated disease in majority of patients on anti-TNF [29]. Pulmonary involvement is prominent on chest imaging, with localized infiltrate or mediastinal lymph node, non-calcified nodule, cavitary lung disease, and a miliary or diffuse pulmonary infiltrate with disseminated disease [29]. Since clinical symptoms are nonspecific, clinician should have a high suspicion for diagnosis. Diagnostic workup includes fungal blood cultures, histoplasma antigen in blood and urine, and serologic testing. If biopsy or bronchoscopy is performed, specimens should be cultured and observed microscopically looking for fungal pathogens.

Coccidiomycosis, caused by *Coccidioides immitis* or *C. posadasii*, is endemic to the deserts of the Southwestern USA and similar desert areas in Central and South America. Pneumonia is the most common presentation. Early infection can present with unilateral infiltrates with or without effusion, hilar lymphadenopathy, and rarely diffuse pneumonia. Pulmonary nodules and cavities can be present early or later in the disease. Extrapulmonary dissemination has been described with anti-TNF and patients on high-dose steroids (equivalent to long-term prednisone at a dose of 20 mg/day or more). Diagnosis can be made by identifying spherules by direct microscopic examination, recovering *Coccidioides* spp. in cultures of clinical specimens or detecting anticoccidial antibodies in serum and other body fluids.

Blastomycosis, which is endemic to the Midwest, South Central, and Southeastern USA and some Canadian provinces (Quebec, Ontario, Manitoba, and Saskatchewan), has been reported in the same frequency as other endemic fungi. Few case reports related to the use of anti-TNF have been published [28, 31].

Aspergillus spp. are ubiquitous in the environment and can cause pulmonary invasive disease, most commonly in patients with hematologic malignancy, stem cell transplant, and solid organ transplant. Tsidoras et al. described cases of aspergillosis in patients receiving anti-TNF (infliximab, etanercept, adalimumab). The majority of these patients were receiving other immunosuppressive agents or had graft vs host disease after stem cell transplant that predisposes to invasive aspergillosis (IA) [28]. Aspergillosis has also been described with golimumab and certolizumab pegol and in patients receiving Bruton's TKI and immune checkpoint blockade for cancer treatment [32–34]. Clinical presentation includes cough, chest, fever, and shortness of breath. Nodules with or without halo sign (ground glass infiltrates surrounding the nodules), nodules with cavitation, and consolidations are changes that can be seen on chest imaging in patients with IA. Diagnosis can be made with cultures taken from sputum or BAL or biopsy specimens, *Aspergillus* galactomannan testing in BAL, and/or molecular testing in BAL (*Aspergillus* PCR). The drug of choice for treatment is voriconazole. Other alternatives include isavuconazole, posaconazole, liposomal amphotericin, and caspofungin or micafungin.

Noninfectious Pulmonary Complications

While the most common causes of pulmonary infiltrates in patients treated with biologic agents are infections, noninfectious etiologies need to be considered. These may be due to underlying disease (pleural disease, interstitial lung disease, airway disease), drug-related toxicity, or secondary to other etiologies that occur in the general population like malignancy, diffuse alveolar hemorrhage, or nonspecific findings related to inflammatory changes in the lungs.

Interstitial Lung Disease

Interstitial lung disease (ILD) is considered an important manifestation of extra-articular connective tissue disease, including systemic sclerosis, rheumatoid arthritis (RA), systemic lupus erythematosus (SLE), mixed connective tissue disease, polymyositis/dermatomyositis, and Sjogren's syndrome [35–37]. ILD is the major cause of morbidity and mortality in these patients and can present at different stages (can even be the first manifestations of the systemic disease), with diverse radiographic patterns and clinical manifestations. Some typical patterns on high-resolution computed tomography (HRCT) include nonspecific interstitial pneumonia (NSIP), usual interstitial pneumonia (UIP), and organizing pneumonia (OP). NSIP and UIP can evolve to a progressive fibrosing form of ILD [35]. The greater extent of fibrosis is associated with lower survival [35]. Although biologic agents are used in treating ILD, anti-TNF and other biologics can sometimes exacerbate ILD or cause do novo ILD in these patients [38, 39].

Pleural Disease

The underlying disease such as with SLE, and RA [37], but also immune-targeted drug such TKI, more with dasatinib compared to imatinib, can produce pleural disease. This can present with pleuritis, pleural effusions, or pleural thickening.

Pulmonary Nodules

Pulmonary nodules are the most characteristic lung changes in patients with RA [36]. Nodules can be solitary or involve both lungs and can be seen regardless of the severity of the arthritis. In addition, etanercept-related pulmonary nodules have been described in few cases, where these nodules decreased or stabilized after stopping etanercept [40].

Drug-Induced Pulmonary Toxicity

Drug-induced pulmonary toxicity has been described with methotrexate and more lately with anti-TNF by exacerbating ILD. Etanercept and infliximab have been described to cause pulmonary granulomas presenting with grand ground opacities on imaging and biopsy showing granulomatous changes that resolve after stopping or changing to a different agent. Few cases of pneumonitis and fibrosing alveolitis have been described with golimumab. However, as all these patients were also taking methotrexate, so it is unclear if the lung toxicity would appear with golimumab monotherapy. Similarly, several cases of pulmonary toxicity have been described with tocilizumab; however a meta-analysis did not show an increase in noninfectious pulmonary side effects related to this drug [38]. Some of the new biologic agents can also cause interstitial pneumonia or pneumonitis, presenting with diffuse interstitial parenchymal changes. The incidence of pneumonitis varies between different agents and the population being studied. Rituximab can cause different patterns of pneumonitis (organizing, desquamative interstitial, and granulomatous) [41]. PI3K inhibitors, and specifically idelalisib, used for the treatment of lymphoma or chronic lymphocytic leukemia have been shown to be associated with pneumonitis in clinical trials [41]. Checkpoint inhibitors cause pneumonitis as a rare immune-mediated complication. Nivolumab and ipilimumab can cause different patterns of pneumonitis ranging from organizing pneumonia, nonspecific interstitial pneumonia, and acute interstitial pneumonia to peri-tumor pneumonitis [41].

Practical Evaluation of Pulmonary Infiltrates

Clinical History

The development of pulmonary infiltrates in patients on biologic agents requires early diagnosis and treatment. A good investigation of the patient's past medical history is vital and should include history of diabetes, renal failure, liver failure, autoimmune conditions, cancer, and the organs involved in disease, among other data. Many of these conditions affect the immune system and can be immune compromising by themselves. For example, uncontrolled diabetes predisposes to bacterial infections and mucormycosis. Renal and liver failure are risk factors for invasive fungal infections. A patient with lung cancer could have a pulmonary infiltrate related to lung cancer, for example, a post-obstructive pneumonia. Patients with RA could have ILD as the cause of pulmonary infiltrate. Medication review is important, including a history of all the immunosuppressive medications the patient has been on, current biologic agent, its dose/frequency, and concurrent use of other immunosuppressive medications. Social history of exposure to tuberculosis, sick contacts, gardening, outdoor activities, hot tub use, and country of birth and countries they have lived in helps establish risk factors for infections like tuberculosis, non-tuberculous mycobacteria, viral infections, invasive fungal infections, endemic mycoses, and *Pseudomonas*, among others. It is important to know if the patient is allergic to antimicrobials which may limit the choice of treatments if indicated.

The tempo of illness can serve as an indicator of the etiology of illness. For example, pyogenic bacterial infections present acutely (days), whereas PCP, endemic mycoses, mold infections, mycobacterial infections, and noninfectious etiologies present subacutely (weeks to months). Although symptoms are usually nonspecific, consisting of cough, chest pain, shortness of breath, etc., some symptoms gave clinicians clue into a particular cause. For example, hemoptysis is usually seen with mold or advanced mycobacterial infections when the etiology is infectious. Low-grade fever for several weeks with night sweats is common with mycobacterial infection. Dry cough and hypoxia are common with PCP, bacterial pneumonia, and noninfectious pneumonitis.

Investigations

We recommend the following investigations in patients on biologics presenting with respiratory or systemic symptoms suspicious of infection:

Blood Investigations

CBC (complete blood count) and CMP (comprehensive metabolic panel) to find out if they are neutropenic, lymphopenic, or thrombocytopenic or if they have kidney or liver dysfunction. Blood culture (pyogenic bacterial pneumonia with secondary bacteremia, endocarditis with septic emboli to lung), serum cryptococcal antigen, serum β-D-glucan (PCP), serum LDH (PCP, histoplasmosis), serum *Aspergillus* galactomannan, endemic mycosis antibodies by complement fixation, and immunodiffusion.

Urine Investigations

Urine *Histoplasma* antigen, urine *Legionella* antigen.

Respiratory Investigations

Nasopharyngeal swab for respiratory viruses PCR, respiratory cultures (sputum or BAL for bacterial, AFB, fungal, *Nocardia*), respiratory viruses PCR in BAL, immunostaining or PCR for *Pneumocystis jirovecii* in BAL, *Aspergillus* galactomannan in BAL, and *Mycoplasma* PCR in respiratory samples.

If the above investigations are noncontributory and the patient is not responding to empiric treatment, a lung biopsy may be necessary. Sending the tissue specimen for histopathology, bacterial, AFB, fungal, *Nocardia* cultures, and saving a non-formalin fixed sample for PCR testing for the future is advised.

Imaging

Radiologic investigation usually starts with a chest radiography (CXR) that might be sufficient in cases with acute presentation. It is important to note that CXR can be normal in early PCP. Computed tomography (CT) scan is much more sensitive and can detect early changes (see Table 18.2). CT can help localizing changes prior to bronchoscopy, biopsy, aspiration, or surgery.

Table 18.2 Etiology of pulmonary infiltrates according to CT scan pattern

Consolidation	Bacteria, *Aspergillus*, endemic fungi
Nodules	Bacterial, *Nocardia*, IFI (*Aspergillus*, mucormycosis), endemic fungi, tuberculosis RA
Micro-nodules	NTM, bacteria, viruses
Cavitation	Mycobacteria, IFI, *Nocardia*, septic emboli, lung abscess, endemic fungi
Ground glass opacities	Viruses, PCP, atypical bacteria ILD, drug toxicity
Nodular interstitial pattern	Miliary tuberculosis, disseminated histoplasma, ILD
Effusion	Bacteria, tuberculosis, *Nocardia* SLE, RA Drugs

Prevention

Transmission of respiratory infections can be decreased by avoiding close contact with individuals that have respiratory infections, frequent hand hygiene before touching mucous membranes, and avoiding smoking and inhalation of tobacco and marijuana due to increased community-acquired bacteria and viruses with tobacco and presence of fungal spores in marijuana. Certain activities can increase the exposure to fungal spores such as planting, mowing the lawn, caving, excavation, construction, and cleaning pigeon or birds' droppings and chicken coops. Avoiding these activities when possible or wearing a mask can decrease the risk of transmission and infection with molds or endemic fungi. Although immunogenicity with pneumococcal and influenza vaccine can be impaired with certain biologic agents, these vaccines are safe and recommended. Pneumococcal vaccines, starting with conjugated PCV20 or PCV13, PCV15 followed by the polysaccharide PPSV23 vaccines, should be given prior to the start of biologic agent. Pneumococcal vaccines are safe to be given after the initiation of biologic agents and ideally would consider administration when the underlying disease is under control. Yearly influenza vaccine should be offered, with an age-appropriate inactivated or recombinant vaccine, preferred over intranasal live attenuated influenza vaccine given the uncertain but possible risk of infection related to the live virus. In patients receiving eculizumab, pneumococcus, *Haemophilus influenzae* B, and meningococcus vaccines should be administered prior the start of treatment. Despite vaccination, infections rates are still high and patients should be offered antibiotic prophylaxis. Screening for latent tuberculosis should be performed prior to starting biologics.

PCP prophylaxis is recommended if concurrent steroid therapy of 20 mg/day or more for more than 1 month, with anti-CD52 and PI3K inhibitors. With Bruton's TKI, PCP prophylaxis should be considered if patients are also on purine analogues or steroids and similarly with JAK inhibitors if patients are also receiving steroids.

References

1. Baddley JW, Cantini F, Goletti D, Gómez-Reino JJ, Mylonakis E, San-Juan R, et al. ESCMID Study Group for Infections in Compromised Hosts (ESGICH) Consensus Document on the safety of targeted and biological therapies: an infectious diseases perspective (Soluble immune effector molecules [I]: anti-tumor necrosis factor-α agents). Clin Microbiol Infect. 2018;24(Suppl 2):S10–s20.
2. Koo S, Marty FM, Baden LR. Infectious complications associated with immunomodulating biologic agents. Hematol Oncol Clin North Am. 2011;25(1):117–38.
3. Furst DE. The risk of infections with biologic therapies for rheumatoid arthritis. Semin Arthritis Rheum. 2010;39(5):327–46.
4. Calabrese C, Winthrop KL. Mycobacterial infections potentiated by biologics. Infect Dis Clin N Am. 2020;34(2):413–23.
5. Godfrey MS, Friedman LN. Tuberculosis and biologic therapies: anti-tumor necrosis factor-α and beyond. Clin Chest Med. 2019;40(4):721–39.
6. Winthrop KL, Baxter R, Liu L, Varley CD, Curtis JR, Baddley JW, et al. Mycobacterial diseases and antitumour necrosis factor therapy in USA. Ann Rheum Dis. 2013;72(1):37–42.

7. Winthrop KL, Mariette X, Silva JT, Benamu E, Calabrese LH, Dumusc A, et al. ESCMID Study Group for Infections in Compromised Hosts (ESGICH) Consensus Document on the safety of targeted and biological therapies: an infectious diseases perspective (Soluble immune effector molecules [II]: agents targeting interleukins, immunoglobulins and complement factors). Clin Microbiol Infect. 2018;24(Suppl 2):S21–s40.
8. Kin A, Schiffer CA. Infectious complications of tyrosine kinase inhibitors in hematological malignancies. Infect Dis Clin N Am. 2020;34(2):245–56.
9. Reinwald M, Silva JT, Mueller NJ, Fortún J, Garzoni C, de Fijter JW, et al. ESCMID Study Group for Infections in Compromised Hosts (ESGICH) Consensus Document on the safety of targeted and biological therapies: an infectious diseases perspective (Intracellular signaling pathways: tyrosine kinase and mTOR inhibitors). Clin Microbiol Infect. 2018;24(Suppl 2):S53–s70.
10. Curtis JR, Patkar N, Xie A, Martin C, Allison JJ, Saag M, et al. Risk of serious bacterial infections among rheumatoid arthritis patients exposed to tumor necrosis factor alpha antagonists. Arthritis Rheum. 2007;56(4):1125–33.
11. Lanternier F, Tubach F, Ravaud P, Salmon D, Dellamonica P, Bretagne S, et al. Incidence and risk factors of Legionella pneumophila pneumonia during anti-tumor necrosis factor therapy: a prospective French study. Chest. 2013;144(3):990–8.
12. José RJ, Mouyis M. Biological therapies in the treatment of inflammatory disease and cancer: impact on pulmonary infection. Ann Res Hospit. 2017;1(6):40.
13. Janoff EN, Musher DM. Streptococcus pneumoniae. In: Mandell, Douglas, and Bennett's principles and practice of infectious diseases. 9th ed. Philadelphia: Elsevier; 2020. p. 2473–91.
14. Langereis JD, de Jonge MI. Invasive disease caused by nontypeable haemophilus influenzae. Emerg Infect Dis. 2015;21(10):1711–8.
15. Murthy TF. Haemophilus species, including H. influenzae and H. ducreyi (Chancroid). In: Blaser JEBRDMJ, editor. Mandell, Douglas, and Bennett's principles and practice of infectious diseases. Philadelphia: Elsevier; 2019. p. 2743–52.
16. Holzman R, Simberkoff M, Leaf H. Mycoplasma pneumoniae and Atypical pneumonia. In: Mandell, Douglas, and Bennett's principles and practice of infectious diseases. 9th ed. Philadelphia: Elsevier; 2019. p. 2332–9.
17. Tubach F, Ravaud P, Salmon-Céron D, Petitpain N, Brocq O, Grados F, et al. Emergence of Legionella pneumophila pneumonia in patients receiving tumor necrosis factor-alpha antagonists. Clin Infect Dis. 2006;43(10):e95–100.
18. Edelstein P, Roy C. Legionnaires disease and Pontiac fever. In: Mandell, Douglas, and Bennett's principles and practice of infectious diseases. 9th ed. Philadelphia: Elsevier. p. 2807–17.
19. Klompas M. Nosocomial pneumonia. In: Mandell, Douglas, and Bennett's principles and practice of infectious diseases. 9th ed. Philadelphia: Elsevier. p. 3576–84.
20. Abreu C, Rocha-Pereira N, Sarmento A, Magro F. Nocardia infections among immunomodulated inflammatory bowel disease patients: a review. World J Gastroenterol. 2015;21(21):6491–8.
21. Redelman-Sidi G, Michielin O, Cervera C, Ribi C, Aguado JM, Fernández-Ruiz M, et al. ESCMID Study Group for Infections in Compromised Hosts (ESGICH) Consensus Document on the safety of targeted and biological therapies: an infectious diseases perspective (Immune checkpoint inhibitors, cell adhesion inhibitors, sphingosine-1-phosphate receptor modulators and proteasome inhibitors). Clin Microbiol Infect. 2018;24(Suppl 2):S95–s107.
22. Ngiu CS, Said MS, Periyasamy P, Low SF. Nocardiosis in a patient with rheumatoid arthritis treated with rituximab and a summary of reported cases. BMJ Case Rep. 2010;2010:bcr1120092421.
23. Winthrop KL, Chang E, Yamashita S, Iademarco MF, LoBue PA. Nontuberculous mycobacteria infections and anti-tumor necrosis factor-alpha therapy. Emerg Infect Dis. 2009;15(10):1556–61.
24. Winthrop KL, Yamashita S, Beekmann SE, Polgreen PM. Mycobacterial and other serious infections in patients receiving anti-tumor necrosis factor and other newly approved

biologic therapies: case finding through the Emerging Infections Network. Clin Infect Dis. 2008;46(11):1738–40.
25. Koo HJ, Lim S, Choe J, Choi SH, Sung H, Do KH. Radiographic and CT features of viral pneumonia. Radiographics. 2018;38(3):719–39.
26. Miller WT Jr, Mickus TJ, Barbosa E Jr, Mullin C, Van Deerlin VM, Shiley KT. CT of viral lower respiratory tract infections in adults: comparison among viral organisms and between viral and bacterial infections. AJR Am J Roentgenol. 2011;197(5):1088–95.
27. Alexandre K, Ingen-Housz-Oro S, Versini M, Sailler L, Benhamou Y. Pneumocystis jirovecii pneumonia in patients treated with rituximab for systemic diseases: report of 11 cases and review of the literature. Eur J Intern Med. 2018;50:e23–e4.
28. Tsiodras S, Samonis G, Boumpas DT, Kontoyiannis DP. Fungal infections complicating tumor necrosis factor alpha blockade therapy. Mayo Clin Proc. 2008;83(2):181–94.
29. Vergidis P, Avery RK, Wheat LJ, Dotson JL, Assi MA, Antoun SA, et al. Histoplasmosis complicating tumor necrosis factor-α blocker therapy: a retrospective analysis of 98 cases. Clin Infect Dis. 2015;61(3):409–17.
30. Wallis RS, Broder MS, Wong JY, Hanson ME, Beenhouwer DO. Granulomatous infectious diseases associated with tumor necrosis factor antagonists. Clin Infect Dis. 2004;38(9):1261–5.
31. Austin A, Tobin E, Judson MA, Hage CA, Hu K, Epelbaum O, et al. Blastomycosis in the capital district of New York state: a newly identified emerging endemic area. Am J Med. 2021;134(2):e101–e8.
32. Davis MR, Thompson GR 3rd, Patterson TF. Fungal infections potentiated by biologics. Infect Dis Clin N Am. 2020;34(2):389–411.
33. Del Castillo M, Romero FA, Argüello E, Kyi C, Postow MA, Redelman-Sidi G. The spectrum of serious infections among patients receiving immune checkpoint blockade for the treatment of melanoma. Clin Infect Dis. 2016;63(11):1490–3.
34. Kyi C, Hellmann MD, Wolchok JD, Chapman PB, Postow MA. Opportunistic infections in patients treated with immunotherapy for cancer. J Immunother Cancer. 2014;2:19.
35. Fischer A, Distler J. Progressive fibrosing interstitial lung disease associated with systemic autoimmune diseases. Clin Rheumatol. 2019;38(10):2673–81.
36. Papiris SA, Manali ED, Kolilekas L, Kagouridis K, Maniati M, Borie R, et al. Investigation of lung involvement in connective tissue disorders. Respiration. 2015;90(1):2–24.
37. Fischer A, du Bois R. Interstitial lung disease in connective tissue disorders. Lancet. 2012;380(9842):689–98.
38. Hadjinicolaou AV, Nisar MK, Bhagat S, Parfrey H, Chilvers ER, Ostör AJ. Non-infectious pulmonary complications of newer biological agents for rheumatic diseases--a systematic literature review. Rheumatology (Oxford). 2011;50(12):2297–305.
39. Perez-Alvarez R, Perez-de-Lis M, Diaz-Lagares C, Pego-Reigosa JM, Retamozo S, Bove A, et al. Interstitial lung disease induced or exacerbated by TNF-targeted therapies: analysis of 122 cases. Semin Arthritis Rheum. 2011;41(2):256–64.
40. Thavarajah K, Wu P, Rhew EJ, Yeldandi AK, Kamp DW. Pulmonary complications of tumor necrosis factor-targeted therapy. Respir Med. 2009;103(5):661–9.
41. Kroschinsky F, Stölzel F, von Bonin S, Beutel G, Kochanek M, Kiehl M, et al. New drugs, new toxicities: severe side effects of modern targeted and immunotherapy of cancer and their management. Crit Care. 2017;21(1):89.

Tuberculosis

19

Tomás Almorza, Jose Maria Aguado, and José L. Pablos

Introduction

Tuberculosis (TB) still represents one of the leading causes of death due to an infectious disease. Its incidence goes from 10 per 10^5 in high-income countries to 100–500 per 10^5 in developing countries. A 10–20% of exposed individuals can eliminate *Mycobacterium tuberculosis* (MT) after exposure [1], whereas in most individuals, MT has the ability to survive in a dormant or latent state for decades. This persistent, latent tuberculosis infection (LTBI) can be detected by a positive tuberculin skin test (TST) or an IFN-γ release assay (IGRA), and 10% of these individuals will develop TB during their lifetime [2].

The prevalence of LTBI varies from less than 5% to more than 30% in "low" or "high" prevalence countries, and therefore, the country where a person lives is the most important risk factor to develop TB [3]. Host factors represent the second factor to explain the incidence of TB. Aging or debilitating conditions are the most common factors associated to the development of TB. People with HIV still represent a 10% of all TB cases worldwide [4]. Therefore, increased transition from LTBI to clinical TB represents an important concern in individuals with different forms of acquired immunodeficiency including immunosuppressive therapies.

T. Almorza
Servicio de Reumatología, Hospital Universitario 12 de Octubre, Madrid, Spain

J. M. Aguado
Unidad de Enfermedades Infecciosas, Hospital Universitario 12 de Octubre, Madrid, Spain

Departamento de Medicina, Universidad Complutense de Madrid (UCM), Madrid, Spain

J. L. Pablos (✉)
Servicio de Reumatología, Hospital Universitario 12 de Octubre, Madrid, Spain

Departamento de Medicina, Universidad Complutense de Madrid (UCM), Madrid, Spain
e-mail: jlpablos@h12o.es

C. Cervera, J. M. Aguado (eds.), *Infectious Complications in Biologic and Targeted Therapies*, https://doi.org/10.1007/978-3-031-11363-5_19

In the context of rheumatic immunomediated or autoimmune diseases, increased rates of TB have been interpreted as the result of the immune disturbances associated to the disease itself and to traditional or current targeted immunosuppressive therapies [5]. Important differences between different therapies exist and have been informative to confirm the relevance of different elements of the immune system in the progression from LTBI to TB.

MT is an intracellular pathogen difficult to eliminate by the immune system. As many other intracellular pathogens, pathogenic mycobacteria have evolved to avoid killing in the phagolysosomal environment of macrophages [6]. The main contention mechanism is the development a robust T-cell response after infection. T-cell responses serve to limit the extension of the disease by granuloma formation and killing of infected macrophages that accumulate in the form of caseum in their center. This process limits MT proliferation, but viable bacilli may persist for decades. If the cellular response weakens, the center of the granuloma changes to a permissive environment for MT proliferation and expansion.

Animal models and human genetic defects have provided relevant information on the cellular and molecular factors involved in the immune response to MT. An example is Mendelian susceptibility to mycobacterial disease (MSMD), a rare monogenic disease characterized by selective predisposition to clinical disease caused by weakly virulent mycobacteria species [7]. In this and in many other monogenic-related conditions, genetic defects in T-cell function, specifically in Th1 cell activation, involving the polarizing (IL-12) and effector (IFN-γ) cytokines underlie the relevance of this pathway. Deficit of the cytokines, regulatory mechanisms, or their intracellular signaling through Jak/STAT results in increased susceptibility to mycobacteria and often to other intracellular pathogens [7].

IFN-γ is a macrophage-activating factor that seems indispensable in experimental models to clear infections by intracellular microbes [8]. Its cellular effects result in the development and activation of pro-inflammatory, "classical," or M1-type macrophages responsible for IL-1β and TNF-α production. TNF-α expression in TB granuloma is abundant and has a clear protective role in the local contention of MT [9, 10]. TNF-α is directly induced in macrophages upon challenge with mycobacteria, and this innate response is critical to control TB [10]. TNF-α is not required for T-cell responses to MT including tuberculin test nor for tuberculous granuloma formation. Instead, it indirectly maintains granuloma integrity by restricting mycobacterial growth within macrophages and preventing their necrosis [11].

The susceptibility factors for LTBI reactivation in adults are more complex and probably more influenced by polygenic or acquired somatic and epigenetic influences that have been more difficult to dissect [12]. The use of different therapies highly specific in the targeting of different elements of the immune system to treat autoimmune rheumatic diseases has provided an excellent experimental model to identify immune factors critical to the defense from mycobacteria and many other pathogens and has changed the clinical strategies to identify and prevent TB in this setting. Among these therapies, biological therapies and new synthetic molecules such as the inhibitors of Janus kinases (Jak) are widely used for chronic arthritis, inflammatory bowel disease, psoriasis, and other autoimmune diseases, where the incidence and characteristics of infections have been closely monitored in the two last decades.

The overall risks of all serious infections vary with background disease and concomitant therapies (i.e., glucocorticoids), with odd ratios (OR) between 1.0 and 1.5. Preventive strategies including vaccination, screening, and monitoring of different infections have been implemented [13]. Safety protocols are similarly applied for all classes of immunomodulatory drugs in different immune-mediated diseases, but the rational and risks are not equivalent. The risk of TB is mainly associated to the use of anti-TNF drugs, the first and most used biological drugs for these diseases, and the differences with other drugs are important. Therefore, the considerations regarding TB risk must be evaluated separately for each therapeutic group.

TNF-α Inhibitors

Anti-TNF agents began to be used in the late 1990s for the therapy of rheumatoid arthritis (RA) and Crohn's disease. The first drug, infliximab (IFX), was widely used in these patients after its commercialization in 1999. The first warning on the risk of TB in IFX users came in 2001, when the Food and Drugs Administration (FDA) reported 70 cases of TB, identified from its spontaneous reporting system [14]. By comparing the reported rate to background rates of tuberculosis in the United States (6.2 cases per 100,000), a significantly greater risk associated to IFX (24.4 cases per 100,000) was observed, although the relative role of the disease (RA) was unclear. Despite no prior LTBI screening for inclusion, the first pivotal trials with IFX and etanercept (ETN) had not detected a significant TB risk, but it is important to point out that they did not include patients in countries with intermediate or high rates of TB [15]. Confirmation of the initial reports came from national registries worldwide that permitted further analysis of the incidence of TB in patients on different anti-TNF drugs in countries with higher LTBI rates and a better knowledge of the risks in RA. In Spain, a country with intermediate TB prevalence (20 per 10^5 in 2000), data obtained from the Database of Biological Products of the Spanish Society of Rheumatology (BIOBADASER) in 2003 showed a fourfold greater incidence of TB in RA not treated with anti-TNF drugs compared to background rates in Spain and a further 20-fold increase in IFX-treated RA patients compared to those not receiving anti-TNF agents [16].

These findings were supported by further analysis of randomized trials and registries where data on TB risk with the different anti-TNF agents suggested that this was a class effect (Table 19.1) [17–21]. Five different anti-TNF agents and many biosimilar drugs are currently available. Most cases of TB occurred in patients treated with IFX, whereas those on ETN, a soluble p75 TNF receptor-Fc molecule, appear to have a significantly lower incidence of TB [22, 23]. This led to the hypothesis of soluble TNF-α receptor-Fc having a lower impact on TB immunity provided by granuloma. A much lower affinity for TNF-α of the receptor compared to the monoclonal antibodies (mAbs), and the potential of complement or cell-mediated cytotoxicity of mAbs on membrane TNF-α expressing macrophages that might

Table 19.1 Risk of TB in different trials and registries of anti-TNF agents

Author, year of publication	Study design	Drugs	Disease	*N* (control)	Risk estimate of tuberculosis
Clinical trials					
Maini et al. (1999) [15] (ATTRACT Study Group)	Randomized, double blind	IFX	RA	428 (88)	OR 0.78 [0.03, 19.36]
Westhovens et al. (2006) [26]	Randomized, double blind	IFX	RA	1084 (363)	OR 2.02 [0.22, 18.13]
St Clair et al. (2004) [27]	Randomized, double blind	IFX	RA	1049 (298)	OR 3.59 [0.19, 66.96]
Baranauskaite et al. (2012) (RESPOND study) [28]	Randomized, double blind	IFX	PsA	115 (58)	OR 3.11 [0.12, 77.85]
Barker et al. (2011) (RESTORE1) [29]	Randomized, open label	IFX	Ps	868 (215)	OR 0.99 [0.04, 24.41]
Rutgeerts et al. (2005) [30]	Randomized, double blind	IFX	UC	364 (121)	OR 1.5 [0.06, 37.17]
Colombel et al. (2010) [31]	Randomized, double blind	IFX	CD	508 (170)	OR 1.52 [0.06, 37.40]
Combe et al. (2006) [32]	Randomized, double blind	ETN	RA	254 (50)	OR 0.74 [0.02, 18.45]
van der Heijde et al. (2006) (TEMPO study) [33]	Randomized, double blind	ETN	RA	682 (228)	OR 1.51 [0.06, 37.25]
Keystone et al. (2004) [34]	Randomized, double blind	ADA	RA	617 (200)	OR 1.44 [0.06, 35.44]
Kim et al. (2007) [35]	Randomized, double blind	ADA	RA	128 (63)	OR 2.9 [0.11, 72.73]
van Vollenhoven et al. (2011) [36]	Randomized, open label	ADA	RA	155 (76)	OR 2.92 [0.12, 72.88]
Emery et al. (2009) [37]	Randomized, double blind	GOL	RA	637 (160)	OR 1.01 [0.04, 24.88]
Keystone et al. (2008) [38]	Randomized, double blind	CZP	RA	982 (199)	OR 2.82 [0.16, 51.19]
Smolen et al. (2009) [39]	Randomized, double blind	CZP	RA	617 (127)	OR 2.88 [0.16, 71.06]
Registries					
BIOBADASER (Spain) (2003) [16]	Multicenter registry	Anti-TNF	RD	1540	aRR/aHR 4.13 [2.6, 6.8]
ARTIS (Sweden) (2005) [40]	Multicenter registry	Anti-TNF	RA	1565	aRR/aHR 4.0 [1.3, 12.0]
PharMetrics (USA and Canada) (2006) [41]	Pharmaceutical claims database	Anti-TNF	RA	4.558	aRR/aHR 1.5 [1.1, 1.9]
RATIO (France) (2009) [42]	Multicenter registry	Anti-TNF	RD	57,711	SIR 12.2 [9.7, 15.5] IFX or ADA vs ETN
BSRBR (UK) (2010) [43]	Multicenter registry	Anti-TNF	RA	10,712	aRR/aHR 3.1 [1, 9.5] IFX vs ETN aRR/aHR 4.2 [1.4, 12.4] ADA vs ETN
GISEA (Italy) (2012) [44]	Multicenter registry	Anti-TNF	RD	2769	aRR/aHR 4.91 [2.7, 8.9]

ADA adalimumab, *AS* ankylosing spondylitis, *Anti-TNF* anti-TNF therapy, *aRR* adjusted risk ratio, *aHR* adjusted hazard ratio, *CD* Crohn's disease, *CZP* certolizumab pegol, *ETN* etanercept, *GOL* golimumab, *IFX* infliximab, *OR* odds ratio, *Ps* psoriasis, *PsA* psoriatic arthritis, *RA* rheumatoid arthritis, *RD* rheumatic diseases, *SIR* standardized incidence ratio, *UC* ulcerative colitis release mycobacteria, has been hypothesized to explain these differences [24]. These pharmacodynamic and other pharmacologic differences have also been invoked to explain the different efficacies of mAbs versus ETN in Crohn's disease, where only the mAbs are efficacious [20]. However, differences in the initial use of the different agents in different countries, indications (i.e., IFX but not ETN in Crohn's disease), dosing, and pharmacologic differences such as the schedule and route of administration (IV or SC) cannot be dismissed and make difficult to conclude of the relative risk of ETN compared with anti-TNF mAbs [25].

Since TB preventive recommendations for clinical practice and new clinical trials were initiated in the early 2000s, LTBI has to be formally excluded prior to the use of immunotherapies [25]. Therefore, analyses of TB incidence with later anti-TNF agents and new biologics or targeted immunomodulatory therapies must consider that active prevention strategies significantly reduce but do not completely prevent TB cases [45]. Indeed, the excess of TB reported for all anti-TNF agents (Table 19.1) supports a class effect of all anti-TNF drugs. The largest international registries also yield data consistent with a significantly increased risk, showing OR from 1.5 to 4.5 in countries with different background TB incidences and assuming an at least moderate bias [46–49].

Additional factors may increase the risk of TB in patients with different inflammatory diseases that may also be potential confounders in the different reports. Among these factors, active inflammation has been reported to increase the risk in RA and possibly but less clearly in other diseases [50]. Concomitant treatments may also increase the risk of TB in patients treated with anti-TNF agents, specially the use of glucocorticoids in a dose-dependent manner. The combination therapy of anti-TNF with traditional immunosuppressants such as methotrexate or azathioprine seems to result in a further increase in the risk of TB reactivation as compared with anti-TNF used in monotherapy [47].

Screening and Therapy of LTBI

Once the problem of increased risk of TB reactivation in anti-TNF users was identified, preventive recommendations were established in the early 2000s by different rheumatology societies [13, 46–48]. All agree on the need to screen for LTBI in patients prior to the start of any anti-TNF therapy. Besides an anamnesis directed to potential contacts and previous history of TB diagnosis or therapy, screening is based on the Mantoux tuberculin skin test (TST) and chest radiology. It consists of the intradermal administration of five units of purified protein derivative of tuberculin, and it is considered positive if an induration develops at the injection site of more than 10 mm in the general population and more than 5 mm in certain groups such as immunosuppressed, including those on glucocorticoids. If negative, a two-step TST procedure (booster) with an interval of 7–10 days has to be performed to avoid false-negative results due to anergic situations that are common in patients with active RA or other inflammatory diseases and in patients on glucocorticoids or other immunosuppressive therapies. A chest x-ray to detect the presence of radiological signs of TB must also be performed [25].

In the case of the detection of previously untreated LTBI, either by radiology or by a positive TST, patients are recommended to receive isoniazid treatment at a dose of 5 mg/kg (with a maximum dose of 300 mg daily) once a day for 9 months. Once the patient is on isoniazid, anti-TNF therapy can be started [49].

Evidence of the efficacy of these measures has been provided by a study of the Spanish registry BIOBADASER. In 2002, the Spanish Society of Rheumatology (SER) together with the health authorities implemented the recommendations for the management of LTBI in patients being treated with anti-TNF. A clear benefit was observed after the application of LTBI screening, resulting in a significant reduction of the risk of TB [45]. The strategy did not fully protect against developing TB, and the risk reduction was estimated around 70%. An analysis of the cases occurring after the implementation of the recommendations showed that most occurred in patients with an incomplete screening or prophylaxis regimen [51].

It is also important to consider the potential side effects of LTBI therapy, mainly liver injury as the result of isoniazid. In patients with rheumatic diseases, strict monitoring of liver function is essential, also considering that many patients regularly take other drugs with significant liver toxicity (i.e., methotrexate, leflunomide). The use of 4 months of rifampicin therapy is an alternative more recently established based on clinical evidence [52].

Interferon gamma release assays (IGRA) can be performed by the enzyme-linked immunospot assay (ELISpot) or by the enzyme-linked immunosorbent assay (ELISA) (QuantiFERON-TB Gold) and detect IFN-γ release by T-cells in response to antigens present in MT but not Bacillus Calmette-Guérin (BCG) vaccine nor nontuberculous mycobacteria. These tests to detect LTBI have been more recently introduced as alternative to TST and display a lower sensitivity but higher specificity [53]. Therefore, there may be a relatively low concordance of both tests especially in Bacillus Calmette-Guérin vaccinated patients [54]. Substitution of TST by IGRA for the screening of patients prior to anti-TNF therapy leads to a lower number of patients requiring LTBI therapy without apparently reducing the overall efficacy to prevent TB, but this strategy still requires further validation [55].

Non-anti-TNF Biologics and Other Targeted Immunomodulators

IL-1 Inhibitors

Interleukin-1 family includes 11 molecules, among which IL-1β is a major macrophage pro-inflammatory cytokine that represents an important target of anti-inflammatory therapies. It is one of the main innate immunity effectors, sharing regulatory and signaling mechanisms with the Toll-like receptors, which represent the first line of defense by triggering inflammation upon the recognition of microorganism-associated molecular patterns. It also participates in adaptive immunity by modulating T-helper polarization towards Th17, but not Th1 phenotype [56]. Other members can display complex pro-inflammatory or anti-inflammatory effects that may participate in human disease, but current antagonists of IL-1 are mainly directed to IL-1β. The natural IL-1 receptor antagonist, IL-1RA, is used as therapeutic agent (anakinra), and it can also inhibit IL-1α. IL-1β has a relevant role in multiple inflammatory diseases, from rare systemic autoinflammatory syndromes, where it is the main therapeutic target, to common diseases such as different arthritic diseases, gout, and arteriosclerosis.

In experimental models, IL-1 receptor 1 (IL-1R1) genetic deficiency leads to enhanced susceptibility to acute MT infection, but its role in chronic tuberculous granuloma formation or in granuloma integrity is not known [57].

There are three biological drugs currently available to target IL-1: canakinumab, a mAb that is administered subcutaneously every 4 or 8 weeks depending on the indication; anakinra, the soluble IL-1RA-Fc, which is daily administered by subcutaneous injection; and rilonacept, a fusion protein composed of the ligand-binding domains of the extracellular portions of IL-1R1 and IL-1RAcP linked to the Fc portion of human IgG1, which is weekly and subcutaneously administered. All three molecules target IL-1b, and anakinra and rilonacept also target IL-1a.

Anakinra is the most widely used in clinical practice. It was first approved by the FDA in 2002 for RA, where it is rarely used due to the approval of many other more efficacious drugs, but it is now the elective drug in juvenile idiopathic arthritis and autoinflammatory syndromes. Considering its roles in defense, inhibition of IL-1 was expected to increase the risk of infections, and accordingly, a higher risk of serious inflammatory conditions was first notified in the anakinra pivotal trial that led to its approval for the treatment of RA [58].

One of the largest trials of an IL-1 antagonist is the CANTOS trial, in which 6717 patients were treated with different doses of canakinumab and compared with 3344 patients on placebo, to analyze its potential to prevent cardiovascular events. A significantly increased risk of death attributed to infection or sepsis was observed in the canakinumab groups compared to placebo group [59]. The CANTOS trial was conducted worldwide, including areas with high incidence of TB, and six confirmed cases of tuberculosis occurred. However similar rates were observed in canakinumab and placebo groups, and five of the cases occurred in countries with high TB incidence. In this, as in most trials, patients at high risk were excluded, including those with LTBI at screening.

Therefore, although an increased risk of TB in patients treated with IL1 inhibitors has not been observed, LTBI screening and therapy recommendations as for anti-TNF therapy should be followed.

IL-6 Inhibitors

Interleukin-6 is a pro-inflammatory cytokine, involved in many effector inflammatory responses, and more specifically, it is the main mediator of the systemic response to inflammation. It also contributes to adaptive immunity by shaping T-cell responses towards Th17 phenotype and as B-cell differentiation factor. In experimental models of IL-6 deficiency, it has been shown to participate in the defense against a wide variety of microorganisms: virus, parasites, fungi, and bacteria, including intracellular bacteria such as *Listeria*. Regarding to its participation in TB defense, infection with limited inocula of MT is lethal for IL-6-deficient mice supporting a relevant role for IL-6 in the control of acute infection [60–62].

There are three approved drugs that target IL-6: tocilizumab, siltuximab, and sarilumab with indication in different inflammatory diseases. The first approved antagonist in the anti-IL-6 receptor (IL-6R) mAb is tocilizumab. It was first approved for the therapy of RA where the greatest clinical experience has been obtained. Additional indications are giant cell arteritis, juvenile idiopathic arthritis, and cytokine release syndrome. Sarilumab is also an anti-IL-6R, which is only indicated in RA, while siltuximab is anti-IL-6 mAb indicated for the treatment of Castleman disease.

In randomized trials in RA, the rate of serious infections is increased in tocilizumab patients compared to placebo, with an OR of 1.53 (1.26–1.86), being significantly higher for the 8 mg/kg dose, and in a similar range to that observed with anti-TNF agents. In these trials, no increased incidence of TB by tuberculosis reactivation was observed. However, in the long-term safety follow-up of phase III trials, covering 9000 patient-years, opportunistic infections including TB were only reported in tocilizumab groups [63].

Registries and other post-marketing studies suggest that the risk of developing TB is at least similar to that observed for anti-TNF agents. In Japan post-marketing data from 8000 treated patients, an incidence of 0.13 cases of TB per 100 patient-years was observed [61, 64]. However, in Taiwan, a high TB incidence area, a retrospective cohort study of 1000 patients treated with different targeting therapies did not observe TB cases in the tocilizumab group [65]. Recently, despite its extensive use in COVID-19 under conditions where screening and prophylaxis have been difficult, an excess of cases of TB has not been reported [66].

Current recommendations on LTBI screening and therapy for anti-IL-6 agents are the same as for anti-TNF agents.

IL-12/23 Inhibitors

IL-12 and IL-23 are cytokines primarily produced by innate immune cells such as macrophages and dendritic cells in response to microorganisms or other activation signals. They are members of the same family and are heterodimeric cytokines that share one of their two subunits, protein p40, and differ in the other subunit, p19 in IL-23 and p35 in IL-12. They signal through different receptors restricted to lymphoid cells and are critical in the signals of antigen-presenting cells to T-cells to initiate antigen responses, which also include antigen presentation and co-stimulation. Both cytokine receptors signal through the Jak/STAT system, specifically through Jak2/Tyk2 and STAT3/STAT4 elements. These soluble cytokines are responsible for the differentiation of CD4 Th cells towards Th1 IFNγ−producing cells in the case of IL-12 or Th17 IL-17-producing cells in the case of IL-23. They also have parallel roles in the activation of innate lymphoid cells type-1 (IFN-γ producers) and type-3 (IL-17 producers) [67].

As mentioned in the introduction, the IL-12, Jak/STAT, and Th1-IFNγ axis are critical in the defense against MT, and genetic deficiency in any of these elements causes MSMD. Targeting IFN-γ or IL-12 has not been developed to treat immune-mediated diseases [68]. Instead IL-23 inhibitors are a growing pharmacological group, successful in the therapy of psoriasis, psoriatic arthritis, Crohn's disease, and in different phases of development for many other diseases such as systemic lupus erythematosus and other skin inflammatory diseases where the IL-23/IL-17 axis has been shown to play a relevant pathogenetic role. Genetic defects in the IL-23/Il-17 pathway are characterized by increased susceptibility to *Candida* and extracellular bacteria, but not to TB or other intracellular pathogens.

The most compelling data come from the clinical use of ustekinumab, a mAb directed towards the IL-12 and IL-23 shared p40 subunit, and therefore, a dual IL-12 and IL-23 antagonist, that was approved for the therapy of psoriasis and psoriatic arthritis in 2009. Safety data collected from all randomized trials show no increased risk of infections compared to placebo. Despite the interest on the risk of TB with this drug due to its capacity to neutralize IL-12, only four cases have been reported, and none was identified in a systematic review of randomized trials of patients on ustekinumab [69–73].

As for all other targeted immunomodulatory drugs developed after anti-TNF, it must be pointed out that preventive strategies including LTB screening and therapy were systematically required in clinical trials and were also mandatory in clinical practice. Under these conditions, no cases of TB were observed in 3177 psoriasis ustekinumab-treated patients from five phase III trials in North America, Europe, and Asia [74]. Recently, the large multinational PSOLAR registry of patients with psoriasis treated with different targeted therapies including ustekinumab, from different geographical areas, including areas with a high incidence of TB, only detected two TB cases with all agents, suggesting that at least in cutaneous psoriasis, and following current prophylaxis recommendation, the incidence is very low [75].

Therefore, although the risk of TB reactivation on ustekinumab therapy seems very low, it cannot be fully discarded, and thus, screening of LTBI is still recommended. With novel anti-IL-23 agents, such as mAb guselkumab, that only target the IL-23-specific p19 subunit and have recently been approved for the treatment of psoriasis, only limited data from randomized trials are available. Guselkumab in this indication does not show any cases of TB up to 2 years of follow-up [76].

IL-17 Inhibitors

IL-17 is a family of six cytokines (IL-17A to F) with different receptors and functions. IL-17A and IL-17F to a lesser extent are the members with more relevance in immunomediated inflammatory diseases and defense. They are synthesized by innate immune cells and by lymphoid cells CD8, CD4, NK, and type 3 ILCs. In

CD4 cells, it is produced by Th17-polarized lymphocytes, a phenotype that develops in the presence of inflammatory cytokines IL-6, IL-1, and TGF-β, also requiring IL-23 for its functional maintenance. IL-17A shares with TNF-α its pro-inflammatory effector capacities in many cell types, such as stromal, epithelial, endothelial, or myeloid cells, due to the widespread expression of IL-17A receptors. IL-17A also induces TNF-α expression in myeloid cells, and both cytokines synergize in the final effector pro-inflammatory effects [77].

Although IL-17A is widely expressed in most inflammatory conditions, its antagonists have unveiled its critical pathogenetic role only in psoriasis, including PsA, and spondylarthritis, but not in other diseases such as RA or Crohn's disease, where TNF-α antagonists are more effective [78].

IL-17 roles in defense are well known after the description of primary immunodeficiencies caused by molecular defects in different elements of the Il-23/IL-17 pathway. These patients have an increased susceptibility to chronic mucocutaneous infections due to *Candida* spp. and to recurrent bacterial infections [77].

The first IL-17 antagonist in clinical use is the mAb secukinumab, approved by regulatory agencies in 2015 for the treatment of plaque psoriasis and in 2016 for the treatment of PsA and ankylosing spondylitis (AS). This drug selectively blocks IL-17A and IL-17A/F heterodimers, without effects on other members of the IL-17 family. Approved in 2016, ixekizumab is also an Il-17A mAb, with indication in cutaneous PsC and PsA. Finally, in 2017, another drug of this group, brodalumab, was approved for the treatment of psoriasis. Brodalumab is an anti-IL-17RA receptor mAb that also inhibits the activity of other members of the IL-17 family signaling through this common receptor subunit, including IL-17A, IL-17F, IL-17A/F, and IL-25, which gives it a slightly different profile compared to secukinumab and ixekizumab [78, 79].

The current paradigm of T-cell defense points to Th1-type responses being the main protection to intracellular pathogens as MT, Th2 to parasites, and Th17 to extracellular bacteria and fungi. However, while a primary role in the acute defense against MT infection in mice has been discarded [80], Th17 responses to mycobacteria have shown to be either protective or deleterious in different models of chronic infection [81].

As for all other immunomodulatory drugs developed after anti-TNF agents, screening and therapy of LTBI in clinical trials and clinical practice are the rule. Under these circumstances, the incidence of new cases of TB has been comprehensively evaluated in all secukinumab clinical trials in different indications, including more than 12,000 patients from different geographic areas, including high incidence areas. No cases of active TB or LTBI activation have been identified, and therefore, the risk was estimated to be very low [82]. Again, despite the lack of evidence of greater risk of TB under secukinumab and possibly all other anti-IL-17 therapies, prevention measures are recommended.

T-Cell Co-stimulation Inhibitors

Abatacept is the only drug of this class indicated for the therapy of inflammatory autoimmune diseases. It was commercialized in 2005 with indication only for the treatment of RA. Its mechanism of action is blocking one of the APC/T-cell co-stimulation systems required for T-cell antigen responses [83]. Abatacept is the natural inhibitory molecule CTLA4 coupled to a human immunoglobulin Fc domain, which acts blocking the interaction of CD80/86 ligands in APC with the T-cell receptor CD28 that mediates the co-stimulatory signal needed for activation by antigen recognition. Therefore, it is a T-cell immunity antagonist that interferes with both primary and secondary (memory) responses [84]. A similar drug, belatacept, has been developed for solid organ transplantation [83].

In animal models, CTLA4 therapy does not significantly impact on the course of cytomegalovirus nor *Pneumocystis jirovecii* experimental infection, but it worsens acute herpes virus infection. The effect on TB has been explored in a murine model of chronic MTB infection where abatacept had no impact on TB control, whereas anti-TNF therapy led to a lethal disease in a few weeks in all treated mice [85].

Cases of TB in abatacept-treated patients have not been reported. In a systematic analysis of randomized clinical trials and long-term extension phases and in a large analysis of US administrative registries, TB has only been rarely reported [73, 86]. Despite the absence of evidence on increased risk of TB in abatacept-treated patients, LTBI screening and therapy are recommended by national and international clinical guidelines.

B-Lymphocyte Depletion Therapy

Lymphocyte depletion therapies with different mAbs directed to membrane molecules in B-cells have been developed and are available to treat different autoimmune diseases, such as RA or multiple sclerosis. The largest experience has been reported for the anti-CD20 mAb rituximab (RTX), the first marketed B-cell-depleting therapy for lymphoma in 1997, being later approved for RA in 2006 [87].

RTX produces a profound depletion of mature B-cells that persists for months after a single infusion and that is later recovered from bone marrow B-cell precursors that do not express CD20 and are therefore not depleted. Primary immunization and responses to new antigens (i.e., vaccination) requiring antigen presentation by B-cells are clearly deficient in experimental models and in RTX-treated patients. However, since it does not deplete long-lived plasmatic cells, memory antibody responses are not modified by this therapy [88]. Hypogammaglobulinemia may occur after chronic therapy, but it has not been consistently associated to an increased infection risk [88].

The overall serious infections seem increased in patients treated with RTX for hematologic patients or rheumatic disease, with similar rates to that observed in anti-TNF-treated patients [89, 90]. In addition, opportunistic infections attributed to RTX therapy have been reported, including progressive multifocal leukoencephalopathy, *Pneumocystis jirovecii* infection, and reactivation of HCV, VZV or, HBV [91]. These reports support the concept that RTX therapy causes specific defects in defense to different pathogens, but there are no similar reports that indicate an increased risk for LTB activation.

The protecting role of humoral responses to MT is debated. Experimental data from murine models suggest that the effector functions of antibodies to MTB may be protective by limiting TB inflammatory responses, via Fc inhibitory receptor signaling [92]. Therefore, although the role of B-cell depletion in TB course is not well defined, and despite the absence of evidence of increased risk of TB in RTX-treated patients, recommendations for LTBI screening and prophylaxis are the same as for all immunomodulatory therapies.

JAK Kinase Inhibitors

This is a new pharmacological class with intracellular targets, the Janus kinases or Jak family of tyrosine kinases, that mediate intracellular signaling of a large number of cytokines pertaining to different classes. Targeted cytokines include interferons, IL-6 family, IL-12/23, the γ-receptor group of lymphoid cytokines (IL-2, IL-7, IL-15, IL-21, etc.), and GM-CSF and other hematopoietic cytokines. These drugs are synthetic small molecules and not biological drugs unable to cross cell membranes. It is a rapidly growing family of drugs, approved or under development for many different immune-mediated conditions, including chronic arthritis, systemic autoimmune diseases, dermatological or bowel inflammatory diseases, and myelodysplastic syndromes [93].

Jak family comprises four molecules, including JAK1, JAK2, JAK3, and Tyk2, and different cytokine receptors use different homo- or heterodimeric pairs of these four Jaks [93]. Approved drugs include ruxolitinib, baricitinib, tofacitinib, upadacitinib, and filgotinib, and despite variable biochemical selectivity, all target most of the mentioned cytokines at the cellular level to a certain degree [94]. The main difference with biologics is the duration of pharmacologic effect, with half-lives of a few hours after oral administration. However, persistent immunological effects such as lymphopenia can occur after long-term use [95].

Genetic defects in this family have a great impact in the immune response. Deficits in JAK3 or γ-receptor cause severe immunodeficiency. Tyk2 is another relevant element in defense and genetic deficiency is associated with susceptibility to TB as expected, according to its participation in interferons and IL-12/23 signaling [96]. It is however unclear how partial and transient pharmacological inhibition of the different Jaks would impact on susceptibility to TB or other infections.

Information from clinical trials and their long-term extension pharmacovigilance programs of the first approved drug ruxolitinib showed an increase in the frequency of TB in treated compared with control groups, as well as an increased incidence of other serious and opportunistic infections [97]. In a safety review of all patients treated with tofacitinib in clinical trials (8460 patient-years of exposure), an overall increase in opportunistic infections has been observed, being TB the most frequent [98]. A dose effect was proposed, since most TB cases occurred with the highest dose of 10 mg/12 h that is only currently recommended for the treatment of ulcerative colitis but not for RA. A review of patients treated with baricitinib in clinical trials (7860 patient-years) also identified 11 TB cases, all in endemic areas and with the highest dose of 4 mg/24 h [99].

The estimated incidence with these drugs is therefore in the range of that reported for anti-TNF therapies. Although it is difficult to compare the risks due to the differences in the populations included in multinational trials due to the variation in background TB incidences in the different areas, a potentially increased risk of TB in patients with inhibitors of Jak kinase inhibitor must be considered. Therefore, although there is only long-term safety information for tofacitinib and baricitinib, LTBI screening and prevention measures are mandatory for all drugs of this class.

References

1. Abel L, El-Baghdadi J, Bousfiha AA, Casanova JL, Schurr E. Human genetics of tuberculosis: a long and winding road. Philos Trans R Soc Lond Ser B Biol Sci. 2014;369(1645):20130428.
2. Pai M, Behr M. Latent Mycobacterium tuberculosis infection and interferon-gamma release assays. Microbiol Spectr 2016;4(5).
3. Cohen A, Mathiasen VD, Schön T, Wejse C. The global prevalence of latent tuberculosis: a systematic review and meta-analysis. Eur Respir J. 2019;54(3):1900655.
4. Gilpin C, Korobitsyn A, Migliori GB, Raviglione MC, Weyer K. The World Health Organization standards for tuberculosis care and management. Eur Respir J. 2018;51(3):1800098.
5. Carmona L, Hernández-García C, Vadillo C, Pato E, Balsa A, González-Alvaro I, et al. Increased risk of tuberculosis in patients with rheumatoid arthritis. J Rheumatol. 2003;30(7):1436–9.
6. Smith I. Mycobacterium tuberculosis pathogenesis and molecular determinants of virulence. Clin Microbiol Rev. 2003;16(3):463–96.
7. Casanova JL. Severe infectious diseases of childhood as monogenic inborn errors of immunity. Proc Natl Acad Sci U S A. 2015;112(51):E7128–37.
8. Martinez FO, Gordon S. The M1 and M2 paradigm of macrophage activation: time for reassessment. F1000Prime Rep. 2014;6:13.
9. Flynn JL, Goldstein MM, Chan J, et al. Tumor necrosis factor alpha is required in the protective immune response against Mycobacterium tuberculosis in mice. Immunity. 1995;2:561–72.
10. Cooper AM, Khader SA. The role of cytokines in the initiation, expansion, and control of cellular immunity to tuberculosis. Immunol Rev. 2008;226:191–204.
11. Clay H, Volkman HE, Ramakrishnan L. Tumor necrosis factor signaling mediates resistance to mycobacteria by inhibiting bacterial growth and macrophage death. Immunity. 2008;29:283–94.
12. Dallmann-Sauer M, Correa-Macedo W, Schurr E. Human genetics of mycobacterial disease. Mamm Genome. 2018;29(7–8):523–38.
13. Singh JA, Cameron C, Noorbaloochi S, Cullis T, Tucker M, Christensen R, et al. Risk of serious infection in biological treatment of patients with rheumatoid arthritis: a systematic review and meta-analysis. Lancet. 2015;386(9990):258–65.

14. Keane J, Gershon S, Wise RP, Mirabile-Levens E, Kasznica J, Schwieterman WD, et al. Tuberculosis associated with infliximab, a tumor necrosis factor -neutralizing agent. N Engl J Med. 2001;345:1098–104.
15. Maini R, St Clair EW, Breedveld F, Furst D, Kalden J, Weisman M, et al. Infliximab (chimeric anti-tumour necrosis factor alpha monoclonal antibody) versus placebo in rheumatoid arthritis patients receiving concomitant methotrexate: a randomized phase III trial. ATTRACT Study Group. Lancet. 1999;354:1932–9.
16. Gomez-Reino JJ, Carmona L, Valverde VR, Mola EM, Montero MD, On behalf of the BIOBADASER Group. Treatment of rheumatoid arthritis with tumor necrosis factor inhibitors may predispose to significant increase in tuberculosis risk: a multicenter active-surveillance report. Arthritis Rheum. 2003;48:2122–7.
17. Zhang Z, Fan W, Yang G, et al. Risk of tuberculosis in patients treated with TNF-α antagonists: a systematic review and meta-analysis of randomised controlled trials. BMJ Open. 2017;7:e012567.
18. Salgado E, Gómez-Reino JJ. The risk of tuberculosis in patients treated with TNF antagonists. Expert Rev Clin Immunol. 2011;7(3):329–40.
19. Keane J. TNF-blocking agents, and tuberculosis: new drugs illuminate an old topic. Rheumatology. 2005;44(6):714–20.
20. Baddley JW, et al. ESCMID Study Group for Infections in Compromised Hosts (ESGICH) Consensus Document on the safety of targeted and biological therapies: an infectious diseases perspective (Soluble immune effector molecules [I]: anti-tumor necrosis factor-a agents). Clin Microbiol Infect. 2018;24:S10–20.
21. Klareskog L, Gaubitz M, Rodríguez-Valverde V, Malaise M, Dougados M, Wajdula J, Etanercept Study 301 Investigators. Assessment of long-term safety and efficacy of etanercept in a 5-year extension study in patients with rheumatoid arthritis. Clin Exp Rheumatol. 2011;29(2):238–47.
22. Wallis RS, Broder MS, Wong JY, Hanson ME, Beenhouwer DO. Granulomatous infectious diseases associated with tumor necrosis factor antagonists. Clin Infect Dis. 2004;38(9):1261–5.
23. Mohan AK, Coté TR, Block JA, Manadan AM, Siegel JN, Braun MM. Tuberculosis following the use of etanercept, a tumor necrosis factor inhibitor. Clin Infect Dis. 2004;39(3):295–9.
24. Fallahi-Sichani M, Flynn JL, Linderman JJ, Kirschner DE. Differential risk of tuberculosis reactivation among anti-TNF therapies is due to drug binding kinetics and permeability. J Immunol. 2012;188(7):3169–78.
25. Gardam MA, Keystone EC, Menzies R, Manners S, Skamene E, Long R, Vinh DC. Anti-tumour necrosis factor agents and tuberculosis risk: mechanisms of action and clinical management. Lancet Infect Dis. 2003;3(3):148–55.
26. Westhovens R, Yocum D, Han J, et al. The safety of infliximab, combined with background treatments, among patients with rheumatoid arthritis and various comorbidities: a large, randomized, placebo-controlled trial. Arthritis Rheum. 2006;54:1075–86.
27. St Clair EW, van der Heijde DM, Smolen JS, et al. Active-Controlled Study of Patients Receiving Infliximab for the Treatment of Rheumatoid Arthritis of Early Onset Study Group: Combination of infliximab and methotrexate therapy for early rheumatoid arthritis: A randomized, controlled trial. Arthritis Rheum. 2004;50:3432–43.
28. Baranauskaite A, Raffayová H, Kungurov NV, et al. Infliximab plus methotrexate is superior to methotrexate alone in the treatment of psoriatic arthritis in methotrexate-naive patients: the RESPOND study. Ann Rheum Dis. 2012;71:541–8.
29. Barker J, Hoffmann M, Wozel G, et al. Efficacy and safety of infliximab vs. methotrexate in patients with moderate-to-severe plaque psoriasis: results of an open-label, active-controlled, randomized trial (RESTORE1). Br J Dermatol. 2011;165:1109–17.
30. Rutgeerts P, Sandborn WJ, Feagan BG, et al. Infliximab for induction and maintenance therapy for ulcerative colitis. N Engl J Med. 2005;353:2462–76.
31. Colombel JF, Sandborn WJ, Reinisch W, et al. Infliximab, azathioprine, or combination therapy for Crohn's disease. N Engl J Med. 2010;362:1383–95.

32. Combe B, Codreanu C, Fiocco U, et al. Etanercept and sulfasalazine, alone and combined, in patients with active rheumatoid arthritis despite receiving sulfasalazine: a double-blind comparison. Ann Rheum Dis. 2006;65:1357–62. https://doi.org/10.1136/ard.2005.049650. Epub 2006 Apr 10. PMID: 16606651; PMCID: PMC1798315.
33. van der Heijde D, Klareskog L, Rodriguez-Valverde V, et al. Comparison of etanercept and methotrexate, alone and combined, in the treatment of rheumatoid arthritis: two-year clinical and radiographic results from the TEMPO study, a double-blind, randomized trial. Arthritis Rheum. 2006;54:1063–74.
34. Keystone EC, Kavanaugh AF, Sharp JT, et al. Radiographic, clinical, and functional outcomes of treatment with adalimumab (a human anti-tumor necrosis factor monoclonal antibody) in patients with active rheumatoid arthritis receiving concomitant methotrexate therapy: a randomized, placebo-controlled, 52-week trial. Arthritis Rheum. 2004;50:1400–11.
35. Kim HY, Lee SK, Song YW, et al. A Randomized, Double-Blind, Placebo-Controlled, Phase III Study of the Human Anti-Tumor Necrosis Factor Antibody Adalimumab Administered as Subcutaneous Injections in Korean Rheumatoid Arthritis Patients Treated With Methotrexate. APLAR J Rheumatol. 2007;10:9–16.
36. van Vollenhoven RF, Kinnman N, Vincent E, et al. Atacicept in patients with rheumatoid arthritis and an inadequate response to methotrexate: results of a phase II, randomized, placebo-controlled trial. Arthritis Rheum. 2011;63:1782–92.
37. Emery P, Fleischmann RM, Moreland LW. Golimumab, a human anti-tumor necrosis factor alpha monoclonal antibody, injected subcutaneously every four weeks in methotrexate-naive patients with active rheumatoid arthritis: twenty-four-week results of a phase III, multicenter, randomized, double-blind, placebo-controlled study of golimumab before methotrexate as first-line therapy for early-onset rheumatoid arthritis. Arthritis Rheum. 2009;60:2272–83.
38. Keystone E, Heijde Dv, Mason D Jr, et al. Certolizumab pegol plus methotrexate is significantly more effective than placebo plus methotrexate in active rheumatoid arthritis: findings of a fifty-two-week, phase III, multicenter, randomized, double-blind, placebo-controlled, parallel-group study. Arthritis Rheum. 2008;58:3319–29.
39. Smolen J, Landewé RB, Mease P, et al. Efficacy and safety of certolizumab pegol plus methotrexate in active rheumatoid arthritis: the RAPID 2 study. A randomised controlled trial. Ann Rheum Dis. 2009;68:797–804.
40. Askling J, Fored CM, Brandt L, et al. Risk and case characteristics of tuberculosis in rheumatoid arthritis associated with tumor necrosis factor antagonists in Sweden. Arthritis Rheum. 2005;52:1986-92. PharMetrics (2006)
41. Brassard P, Kezouh A, Suissa S. Antirheumatic drugs and the risk of tuberculosis. Clin Infect Dis. 2006;43:717–22.
42. Tubach F, Salmon D, Ravaud P, et al. Risk of tuberculosis is higher with anti-tumor necrosis factor monoclonal antibody therapy than with soluble tumor necrosis factor receptor therapy: The three-year prospective French Research Axed on Tolerance of Biotherapies registry. Arthritis Rheum. 2009;60:1884–94.
43. Dixon WG, Hyrich KL, Watson KD, et al. BSR Biologics Register. Drug-specific risk of tuberculosis in patients with rheumatoid arthritis treated with anti-TNF therapy: results from the British Society for Rheumatology Biologics Register (BSRBR). Ann Rheum Dis. 2010;69:522–8.
44. Atzeni F, Sarzi-Puttini P, Botsios C, et al. Long-term anti-TNF therapy and the risk of serious infections in a cohort of patients with rheumatoid arthritis: comparison of adalimumab, etanercept and infliximab in the GISEA registry. Autoimmun Rev. 2012;12:225–9.
45. Carmona L, Gomez-Reino JJ, Rodriguez-Valverde V, Montero D, Pascual-Gomez E, Mola EM, et al. Effectiveness of recommendations to prevent reactivation of latent tuberculosis infection in patients treated with tumor necrosis factor antagonists. Arthritis Rheum. 2005;52:1766–72.
46. Yonekura CL, Oliveira RDR, Titton DC, Ranza R, Ranzolin A, Hayata AL, et al. Incidence of tuberculosis among patients with rheumatoid arthritis using TNF blockers in Brazil: data from the Brazilian Registry of Biological Therapies in Rheumatic Diseases (Registro Brasileiro

de Monitoração de Terapias Biológicas - BiobadaBrasil). Rev Bras Reumatol Engl Ed. 2017;57(Suppl 2):477–83.
47. Lorenzetti R, Zullo A, Ridola L, Diamanti AP, Laganà B, Gatta L, et al. Higher risk of tuberculosis reactivation when anti-TNF is combined with immunosuppressive agents: a systematic review of randomized controlled trials. Ann Med. 2014;46(7):547–54.
48. Ledingham J, Wilkinson C, Deighton C. British Thoracic Society (BTS) recommendations for assessing risk and managing tuberculosis in patients due to start anti-TNF-α treatments. Rheumatology (Oxford). 2005;44(10):1205–6.
49. Valesini G, Montecucco C, Cutolo M. Recommendations for the use of biologic (TNF-alpha blocking) agents in the treatment of rheumatoid arthritis in Italy. Clin Exp Rheumatol. 2006;24(4):413–23.
50. Kogure T, Fujinaga H, Niizawa A, Shimada Y, Itoh T, Ochiai H, et al. Rheumatoid arthritis complicated by mycobacterium tuberculosis are there characteristics predisposing to this association? J Clin Rheumatol. 1999;5(1):17–21.
51. Gómez-Reino JJ, Carmona L, Angel Descalzo M, BIOBADASER Group. Risk of tuberculosis in patients treated with tumor necrosis factor antagonists due to incomplete prevention of reactivation of latent infection. Arthritis Rheum. 2007;57(5):756–61.
52. Menzies D, Adjobimey M, Ruslami R, Trajman A, Sow O, Kim H, et al. Four months of rifampin or nine months of isoniazid for latent tuberculosis in adults. N Engl J Med. 2018;379(5):440–53.
53. Auguste P, Tsertsvadze A, Pink J, Court R, McCarthy N, Sutcliffe P, Clarke A. Comparing interferon-gamma release assays with tuberculin skin test for identifying latent tuberculosis infection that progresses to active tuberculosis: systematic review and meta-analysis. BMC Infect Dis. 2017;17(1):200.
54. Zhou G, Luo Q, Luo S, Teng Z, Ji Z, Yang J, Wang F, et al. Interferon-γ release assays or tuberculin skin test for detection and management of latent tuberculosis infection: a systematic review and meta-analysis. Lancet Infect Dis. 2020;20(12):1457–69.
55. Jeong DH, Kang J, Jung YJ, Yoo B, Lee CK, Kim YG, et al. Comparison of latent tuberculosis infection screening strategies before tumor necrosis factor inhibitor treatment in inflammatory arthritis: IGRA-alone versus combination of TST and IGRA. PLoS One. 2018;13:e0198756.
56. Hahn M, Frey S, Hueber AJ. The novel interleukin-1 cytokine family members in inflammatory diseases. Curr Opin Rheumatol. 2017;29:208–13.
57. Satoh T, Otsuka A, Contassot E, French LE. The inflammasome and IL-1b: implications for the treatment of inflammatory diseases. Immunotherapy. 2015;7:243–54.
58. Fleischmann RM, Schechtman J, Bennett R, Handel ML, Burmester GR, Tesser J, et al. Anakinra, a recombinant human interleukin-1 receptor antagonist (r-metHuIL-1ra), in patients with rheumatoid arthritis: a large, international, multicenter, placebo-controlled trial. Arthritis Rheum. 2003;48(4):927–34.
59. Ridker PM, Everett BM, Thuren T, MacFadyen JG, Chang WH, Ballantyne C, et al. CANTOS Trial Group. Antiinflammatory therapy with canakinumab for atherosclerotic disease. N Engl J Med. 2017;377(12):1119–31.
60. Tanaka T, Narazaki M, Kishimoto T. IL-6 in inflammation, immunity, and disease. Cold Spring Harb Perspect Biol. 2014;6(10):a016295.
61. Rose-John S, Winthrop K, Calabrese L. The role of IL-6 in host defence against infections: immunobiology and clinical implications. Nat Rev Rheumatol. 2017;13(7):399–409.
62. Kopf M, Baumann H, Freer G, Freudenberg M, Lamers M, Kishimoto T, et al. Impaired immune and acute-phase responses in interleukin-6-deficient mice. Nature. 1994;368(6469):339–42.
63. Campbell L, Chen C, Bhagat SS, Parker RA, Östör AJ. Risk of adverse events including serious infections in rheumatoid arthritis patients treated with tocilizumab: a systematic literature review and meta-analysis of randomized controlled trials. Rheumatology (Oxford). 2011;50(3):552–62.
64. Koike T, et al. Effectiveness and safety of tocilizumab: postmarketing surveillance of 7901 patients with rheumatoid arthritis in Japan. J Rheumatol. 2014;41:15–23.

65. Lim CH, Chen H-H, Chen Y-H, Chen D-Y, Huang W-N, Tsai J-J, et al. The risk of tuberculosis disease in rheumatoid arthritis patients on biologics and targeted therapy: a 15-year real world experience in Taiwan. PLoS One. 2017;12(6):e0178035.
66. Cortegiani A, Ippolito M, Greco M, Granone V, Protti A, Gregoretti C, et al. Rationale and evidence on the use of tocilizumab in COVID-19: a systematic review. Pulmonology. 2021;27(1):52–66.
67. Langrish CL, McKenzie BS, Wilson NJ, de Waal Malefyt R, Kastelein RA, Cua DJ. IL-12 and IL-23: master regulators of innate and adaptive immunity. Immunol Rev. 2004;202:96–105.
68. Sigidin YA, Loukina GV, Skurkovich B, Skurkovich S. Randomized, double-blind trial of anti-interferon-gamma antibodies in rheumatoid arthritis. Scand J Rheumatol. 2001;30(4):203–7.
69. Shim HH, Cai SCS, Chan W, Low JGH, Tan HH, Ling KL. Mycobacterium abscessus infection during ustekinumab treatment in Crohn's disease: a case report and review of the literature. J Crohns Colitis. 2018;12(12):1505–7.
70. Lynch M, Roche L, Horgan M, Ahmad K, Hackett C, Ramsay B. Peritoneal tuberculosis in the setting of ustekinumab treatment for psoriasis. JAAD Case Rep. 2017;3(3):230–2.
71. Sánchez-Moya AI, Daudén E. Peripheral lymph node recurrence of tuberculosis after ustekinumab treatment. Arch Dermatol. 2012;148(11):1332–3.
72. Tsai TF, Chiu HY, Song M, Chan D. A case of latent tuberculosis reactivation in a patient treated with ustekinumab without concomitant isoniazid chemoprophylaxis in the PEARL trial. Br J Dermatol. 2013;168(2):444–6.
73. Souto A, Maneiro JR, Salgado E, Carmona L, Gomez-Reino JJ. Risk of tuberculosis in patients with chronic immune-mediated inflammatory diseases treated with biologics and tofacitinib: a systematic review and meta-analysis of randomized controlled trials and long-term extension studies. Rheumatology (Oxford). 2014;53(10):1872–85.
74. Tsai TF, Ho V, Song M, Szapary P, Kato T, Wasfi Y, et al. The safety of ustekinumab treatment in patients with moderate-to-severe psoriasis and latent tuberculosis infection. Br J Dermatol. 2012;167(5):1145–52.
75. Kalb RE, Fiorentino DF, Lebwohl MG, Toole J, Poulin Y, Cohen AD, et al. Risk of serious infection with biologic and systemic treatment of psoriasis: results from the psoriasis longitudinal assessment and registry (PSOLAR). JAMA Dermatol. 2015;151:961–9.
76. Puig L, Tsai TF, Bhutani T, Uy J, Ramachandran P, Song M, et al. Safety in moderate-to-severe plaque psoriasis patients with latent tuberculosis treated with guselkumab and anti-tuberculosis treatments concomitantly: results from pooled phase 3 VOYAGE 1 & VOYAGE 2 trials. J Eur Acad Dermatol Venereol. 2020;34(8):1744–9.
77. Blauvelt A, Lebwohl MG, Bissonnette R. IL-23/IL-17A dysfunction phenotypes inform possible clinical effects from anti-IL-17A therapies. J Invest Dermatol. 2015;135(8):1946–53.
78. Mease PJ, Genovese MC, Greenwald MW, et al. Brodalumab, an anti-IL17RA monoclonal antibody, in psoriatic arthritis. N Engl J Med. 2014;370(24):2295–306.
79. Papp KA, Bachelez H, Blauvelt A, et al. Infections from seven clinical trials of ixekizumab, an anti-interleukin-17A monoclonal antibody, in patients with moderate-to-severe psoriasis. Br J Dermatol. 2017;177(6):1537–51.
80. Segueni N, Tritto E, Bourigault ML, Rose S, Erard F, Le Bert M, et al. Controlled Mycobacterium tuberculosis infection in mice under treatment with anti-IL-17A or IL-17F antibodies, in contrast to TNFα neutralization. Sci Rep. 2016;6:36923.
81. Li Y, Wei C, Xu H, Jia J, Wei Z, Guo R, et al. The immunoregulation of Th17 in host against intracellular bacterial infection. Mediat Inflamm. 2018;2018:6587296.
82. Elewski BE, Baddley JW, Deodhar AA, Magrey M, Rich PA, Soriano ER, et al. Association of secukinumab treatment with tuberculosis reactivation in patients with psoriasis, psoriatic arthritis, or ankylosing spondylitis. JAMA Dermatol. 2020;157:e203257.
83. Vincenti F, Luggen M. T cell costimulation: a rational target in the therapeutic armamentarium for autoimmune diseases and transplantation. Annu Rev Med. 2007;58:347–58.
84. Judge TA, Tang A, Spain LM, Deans-Gratiot J, Sayegh MH, Turka LA. The in vivo mechanism of action of CTLA4Ig. J Immunol. 1996;156(6):2294–9.

85. Bigbee L, et al. Abatacept treatment does not exacerbate chronic mycobacterium tuberculosis infection in mice. Arthritis Rheum. 2007;56(8):2557–65.
86. Simon TA, Boers M, Hochberg M, Baker N, Skovron ML, Ray N, et al. Comparative risk of malignancies and infections in patients with rheumatoid arthritis initiating abatacept versus other biologics: a multi-database real-world study. Arthritis Res Ther. 2019;21(1):228.
87. Cohen SB, Emery P, Greenwald MW, Dougados M, Furie RA, Genovese MC, et al. Rituximab for rheumatoid arthritis refractory to anti-tumor necrosis factor therapy: results of a multicenter, randomized, double-blind, placebo-controlled, phase III trial evaluating primary efficacy and safety at twenty-four weeks. Arthritis Rheum. 2006;54(9):2793–806.
88. Mikulska M, et al. ESCMID Study Group for Infections in Compromised Hosts (ESGICH) Consensus Document on the safety of targeted and biological therapies: an infectious diseases perspective (Agents targeting lymphoid cells surface antigens [I]: CD19, CD20 and CD52). Clin Microbiol Infect. 2018;24:S71–82.
89. Lanini S, Molloy AC, Prentice AG, Ippolito G, Kibbler CC. Infections in patients taking Rituximab for hematologic malignancies: two-year cohort study. BMC Infect Dis. 2013;13:317.
90. Shi Y, Wu Y, Ren Y, Jiang Y, Chen Y. Infection risks of rituximab versus non-rituximab treatment for rheumatoid arthritis: a systematic review and meta-analysis. Int J Rheum Dis. 2019;22(8):1361–70.
91. Kelesidis T, Daikos G, Boumpas D, Tsiodras S. Does rituximab increase the incidence of infectious complications? A narrative review. Int J Infect Dis. 2011;15(1):e2–16.
92. Maglione PJ, et al. Fc receptors regulate immune activation and susceptibility during Mycobacterium tuberculosis infection. J Immunol. 2008;180:3329–38.
93. O'Shea JJ, Schwartz DM, Villarino AV, Gadina M, McInnes IB, Laurence A. The JAK-STAT pathway: impact on human disease and therapeutic intervention. Annu Rev Med. 2015;66:311–28.
94. McInnes IB, Byers NL, Higgs RE, et al. Comparison of baricitinib, upadacitinib, and tofacitinib mediated regulation of cytokine signaling in human leukocyte subpopulations. Arthritis Res Ther. 2019;21(1):183.
95. Van Vollenhoven R, Lee EB, Strengholt S, et al. Evaluation of the short-, mid-, and long-term effects of tofacitinib on lymphocytes in patients with rheumatoid arthritis. Arthritis Rheumatol. 2019;71(5):685–95.
96. Casanova JL, Holland SM, Notarangelo LD. Inborn errors of human JAKs and STATs. Immunity. 2012;36(4):515–28.
97. Lussana F, Cattaneo M, Rambaldi A, Squizzato A. Ruxolitinib-associated infections: a systematic review and meta-analysis. Am J Hematol. 2018;93(3):339–47.
98. Cohen S, Radominski SC, Gomez-Reino JJ, Wang L, Krishnaswami S, Wood SP, et al. Analysis of infections and all-cause mortality in phase II, phase III, and long-term extension studies of tofacitinib in patients with rheumatoid arthritis. Arthritis Rheumatol. 2014;66(11):2924–37.
99. Winthrop KL, Harigai M, Genovese MC, Lindsey S, Takeuchi T, Fleischmann R, et al. Infections in baricitinib clinical trials for patients with active rheumatoid arthritis. Ann Rheum Dis. 2020;79(10):1290–7.

Cytomegalovirus and Other Herpesviruses

20

Fuensanta Gavilán Guirao and Julian Torre Cisneros

Introduction

Members of the family *Herpesviridae* are encapsulated, double-stranded DNA viruses that are widely distributed in the animal kingdom. Although nearly 100 virus species are known, only eight are human pathogens. These species are grouped into three subfamilies according to their genomic and biological characteristics (Table 20.1): *Alfaherpesvirinae* (herpes simplex virus type 1 [HSV-1], herpes simplex virus type 2 [HSV-2], and varicella-zoster virus [VZV]), *Betaherpesvirinae* (cytomegalovirus [CMV], human herpesvirus type 6 [HHV-6] and human herpesvirus type 7 [HHV-7]), and *Gammaherpesvirinae* (Epstein-Barr virus [EBV] and human herpesvirus type 8 [HHV-8] associated with Kaposi's sarcoma). One of the

Table 20.1 Classification of human herpesviruses

Common name	Other denomination	Subfamily
Human viruses		
Herpes simplex virus type 1	Human herpesvirus type 1	Alpha
Herpes simplex virus type 2	Human herpesvirus type 2	Alpha
Varicella-zoster virus	Human herpesvirus type 3	Gamma
Epstein-Barr virus	Human herpesvirus type 4	Beta
Cytomegalovirus	Human herpesvirus type 5	Beta
Human herpesvirus type 6	–	Beta
Human herpesvirus type 7	–	Gamma
Human herpesvirus type 8	Kaposi's sarcoma herpesvirus	
Simian virus	Cercopithecine herpesvirus type 1	Alpha

F. G. Guirao · J. Torre Cisneros (✉)
Infectious Disease Service, Hospital Universitario Reina Sofia-Instituto Maimónides de Investigación Biomédica de Córdoba (IMIBIC). CIBERINFEC, Instituto de Salud Carlos III., Córdoba, Spain
e-mail: fuensantam.gavilan.sspa@juntadeandalucia.es; julian.torre.sspa@juntadeansalucia.es

C. Cervera, J. M. Aguado (eds.), *Infectious Complications in Biologic and Targeted Therapies*, https://doi.org/10.1007/978-3-031-11363-5_20

most relevant clinical characteristics of these viruses is their ability to remain in a state of latency in the host's infected cells for long periods of time with periodic reactivations. In order to remain in a state of latency, viruses have developed very complex mechanisms to evade and reach a state of equilibrium with the host immune system. The mechanisms that establish latency are under continuous investigation.

In immunocompromised patients, the reactivation of these viruses, especially CMV, is a cause of significant morbidity and mortality. In this chapter we review the available evidence of the association between biologic agents and herpesvirus reactivation. Special attention will be paid to CMV infection due to its potential severity and possible prevention and treatment.

Biologic therapies act by modulating or suppressing some mechanism of the immune system. Depending on the immunological pathway in which they exert their action, some drugs are more likely to cause herpes infections than others, either by reactivating a latent infection or through the acquisition of the infection for the first time.

Numerous biologic agents are authorized for clinical use and it is not the purpose of this chapter to describe all of them. We will review only those drugs for which there is evidence of a higher risk of herpes infection or reactivation and, depending on the case, establish whether antiviral prophylaxis is indicated or not.

Cytomegalovirus and Immune Control of Infection

Cytomegalovirus (CMV) is the largest virus of the family *Herpesviridae*. CMV consists of a double-stranded DNA, four classes of mRNA, a protein capsid, and a lipoprotein coating. Like other herpesviruses, it replicates in the cell nucleus and can produce a symptomatic lytic infection or a latent infection. In immunocompetent older children and adults, CMV causes a wide variety of disorders ranging from asymptomatic subclinical infection to mononucleosis syndrome, while it can cause disseminated disease with high morbidity and mortality in immunosuppressed patients.

Once infected, the individual is likely to carry the virus for life. Although the infection can remain in a latent state, reactivation may occur if T cell-mediated immunity is impaired.

Immune Control of Infection

Knowledge of the immune mechanism involved in the control of CMV reactivation helps to understand why this infection is more frequent in certain biologic therapies than others.

CMV enters human cells by direct fusion with the plasma membrane or by endocytosis through the interaction of viral glycoproteins (gB and gH) with specific plasma membrane receptors. The viral nucleocapsids are transported from the cytoplasm to the nucleus where they release the viral DNA which activates the "early" expression of IE1/IE2 genes that initiate viral replication. The replicated viral DNA is encapsulated in capsids, transported back to the cytoplasm—where it finishes assembling its envelope—and released by exocytosis.

In healthy patients, primary CMV infection usually begins in the epithelial mucosa and spreads to the myeloid-monocytic cells, including monocytes and CD34+ cells, where it establishes latency. This state implies the existence of mechanisms that restrict the expression of viral genes, thus limiting immune recognition by effector cells. The mechanisms that control latency are not yet well known. However, the ability of CMV to elude the destruction of infected cells by the immune system through downregulation of cell surface markers such as the major histocompatibility complex class I (HLA-I) may contribute to the ability of the virus to remain undetected [1].

The differentiation of infected monocytes into macrophages can trigger replication. The viral particles can be processed by antigen-presenting cells (APCs) and stimulate antigen-specific T lymphocytes. These APCs, which are activated by toll-like receptors (TLRs), can secrete cytokines and chemokines that activate innate immunity (natural killer [NK] cells). The activated T lymphocytes and NK cells can directly lyse CMV-infected cells or block virus replication by secreting cytokines such as interferon gamma (IFN-γ) and/or tumor necrosis factor (TNF). APCs also activate B lymphocytes that produce specific antibodies capable of neutralizing extracellular viruses.

When patients are immunosuppressed either due to other infectious processes or the administration of immunosuppressive therapy, CMV can reactivate and replicate until high titers are reached, resulting in life-threatening disseminated or organ disease.

Biologic Drugs and Risk of Herpes Infection

The main biologic drugs associated with a higher risk of producing herpes infections and specific indications for prophylaxis are listed in Table 20.2. In this section we will describe the available clinical evidence.

Table 20.2 Biologic drugs, main indications, risk of herpesvirus infection, and prophylaxis recommendations

Biologic drug	Clinical indications	Risk of HSV, VZV, CMV, and EBV infection	Prophylaxis recommendation
TNF-α inhibitors			
Adalimumab Certolizumab Etanercept Golimumab Infliximab	RA, Crohn's disease, UC, PP, and JIA	Yes, mainly due to herpes zoster. Risk is associated with the concomitant use of corticosteroids	None. CMV reactivation monitoring is not recommended either

(continued)

Table 20.2 (continued)

Biologic drug	Clinical indications	Risk of HSV, VZV, CMV, and EBV infection	Prophylaxis recommendation
B-cell-targeted drugs			
Anti-CD20 Obinutuzumab Ocrelizumab Ofatumumab Rituximab Y-ibritumomab tiuxetan	RA, CLL, NHL	Yes, VZV infections predominate	Consider prophylaxis depending on the existence of concomitant immunosuppression No recommendation for routine CMV reactivation monitoring
Anti-CD30 Brentuximab vedotin	HL, NHL	Yes, especially CMV replication	Consider antiviral prophylaxis. CMV-positive patients should be monitored by PCR to rule out reactivation/infection
Anti-CD38 Daratumumab	MM, NHL	Yes	Herpes zoster prophylaxis is recommended
PI3K inhibitors			
Idelalisib Buparlisib Rigosertib Duvelisib	Breast cancer, CLL, FL, CML, SLL	Yes	Consider acyclovir prophylaxis. CMV-positive patients should be monitored by PCR to rule out reactivation/infection
Biologic drug	Clinical indications	Risk of HSV, VZV, CMV, and EBV infection	Prophylaxis recommendation
T-cell-targeted drugs			
CTL-4IgG:CD28-CD80/86 Blockade Abatacept Belatacept	Melanoma, non-small cell lung cancer, renal cancer, head and neck squamous cell carcinoma	Possible increased risk	Systematic antiviral prophylaxis and CMV reactivation monitoring are not recommended
Direct T-cell inhibitors and agents targeting T-cell migration and chemotaxis			
Anti-CD52 Alemtuzumab	CLL, cutaneous T-cell lymphoma, cellular NHL, MS	Yes	Antiviral prophylaxis against HSV and VZV is recommended. CMV-positive patients should be monitored by PCR
IL-4, IL-5, IL-6 inhibitors			
IL-4 inhibitor Dupilumab	AD, AA, CRSwNP	Possible increased risk of herpes zoster infection	Routine antiviral prophylaxis is not recommended
IL-5 inhibitors Benralizumab Mepolizumab Reslizumab	AA	Possible increased risk of herpes zoster infection	Routine antiviral prophylaxis is not recommended

Table 20.2 (continued)

Biologic drug	Clinical indications	Risk of HSV, VZV, CMV, and EBV infection	Prophylaxis recommendation
IL-6 inhibitors Sarilumab Tocilizumab	RA, JIA, Castleman's disease, neuromyelitis optica	Increased risk of herpes zoster infection	Routine antiviral prophylaxis is not recommended
Biologic drug	Clinical indications	Risk of HSV, VZV, CMV, and EBV infection	Prophylaxis recommendation
Checkpoint inhibitors			
Atezolizumab Avelumab Cemiplimab Durvalumab Ipilimumab Nivolumab Pembrolizumab	Melanoma Renal cancer, non-small cell lung cancer, head and neck squamous cell carcinoma	No, but the treatment used for immune-mediated complications increases the risk of herpesvirus reactivation	
Tyrosine kinase inhibitors for hematologic malignancies			
Bafetinib Bosutinib Dasatinib Imatinib Nilotinib Ponatinib	CML, ALL, MDS, mastocytosis, hypereosinophilic syndrome	Yes	Routine antiviral prophylaxis and CMV reactivation monitoring are not recommended
Janus kinase inhibitors			
Baricitinib Ruxolitinib Tofacitinib	RA, MF	Increased risk of herpes zoster infection	Prophylaxis for HSV and VZV and monitoring of CMV reactivation/infection in CMV-positive patients is recommended
Others			
Proteasome inhibitors Bortezomib Carfilzomib Ixazomib	MM	Increased risk of herpes zoster infection	Antiviral prophylaxis should be considered
S1P receptor modulator Fingolimod	MS	Increased risk of herpes zoster infection	Routine antiviral prophylaxis is not recommended, but should be considered if corticosteroids are used concomitantly
Anti-CCR4 Mogamulizumab	CLL, cutaneous T-cell lymphoma, T-cell NHL	Yes	Antiviral prophylaxis is recommended. CMV-positive patients should be closely monitored

ALL acute lymphoblastic leukemia, *AA* allergic asthma, *AD* atopic dermatitis, *CLL* chronic lymphocytic leukemia, *CML* chronic myelogenous leukemia, *CRSwNP* chronic rhinosinusitis with nasal polyps, *FL* follicular lymphoma, *HL* Hodgkin's lymphoma, *JIA* juvenile idiopathic arthritis, *MDS* myelodysplastic syndrome, *MF* myelofibrosis, *MM* multiple myeloma, *MS* multiple sclerosis, *NHL* non-Hodgkin's lymphoma, *PA* psoriatic arthritis, *PP* plaque psoriasis, *RA* rheumatoid arthritis, *SLL* small-cell lymphocytic lymphoma, *UC* ulcerative colitis

Tumor Necrosis Factor Alpha (TNF-α) Inhibitor Drugs: Adalimumab, Certolizumab, Etanercept, Golimumab, and Infliximab

Although severe HSV and VZV infections, including hepatitis, encephalitis, and disseminated VZV infection, have been reported in patients treated with TNF-α inhibitors [2–4], it is not fully demonstrated that treatment with these drugs is significantly associated with an increased risk of VZV infection. Several European studies have suggested this association [5–7]. However, in a long-term multicenter study in the USA that compared a cohort of 33,324 patients with rheumatoid arthritis treated with anti-TNF-α to a cohort of 25,742 patients treated with disease-modifying antirheumatic drugs (DMARDs), no significant differences were found in rates of VZV infection [8]. These observed differences may be due to the more frequent use of corticosteroids for the treatment of these diseases in Europe.

Regarding CMV infection, cases of acute disseminated infection, retinitis, colitis, and hepatitis have been described in patients on infliximab therapy [9, 10].

Although CMV infections are usually of greater clinical significance, prophylaxis is not routinely recommended for CMV seropositive patients. However, the increased risk of these infections should be considered and patients undergoing anti-TNF-α treatment should be closely monitored.

Drugs Targeting Specific B-Cell Receptors

Anti-CD20: Obinutuzumab, Ocrelizumab, Ofatumumab, Rituximab, and Y-Ibritumomab Tiuxetan

Rituximab and obinutuzumab are the drugs that have been shown to have the greatest incidence of herpesvirus infections.

Rituximab was the first biologic drug authorized for clinical use. A recent review after 20 years of clinical experience, including several randomized studies, has shown that approximately 4% of patients treated with this drug in monotherapy had severe HSV, VZV, and CMV infections, with CMV infection being the least frequent [11–14].

In a phase III randomized clinical trial in which obinutuzumab was compared to rituximab as a first-line treatment for patients with follicular lymphoma, a higher incidence of infection was found in the obinutuzumab-treated group (20%, $n = 595$) than in the rituximab-treated group (16%, $n = 575$) [15]. Approximately 1% of patients in the obinutuzumab group and 1.3% in the rituximab group developed shingles, but no cases of CMV disease were reported.

There is little information about the association between other anti-CD20 drugs and the risk of herpes infections. In a phase III clinical trial, ocrelizumab was administered for the treatment of multiple sclerosis and showed a higher incidence of oral HSV reactivation compared to the placebo group [16]. Ofatumumab has been used to treat the reactivation of chronic lymphocytic leukemia and did not show an increased incidence of CMV infection [17]. Regarding Y-ibritumomab, no cases of herpes infections have been reported when the drug was administered for the treatment of advanced stages of follicular lymphoma [18].

Currently, there are no recommendations for routine antiviral prophylaxis.

Anti-CD30: Brentuximab Vedotin

A pivotal phase III randomized clinical trial studying brentuximab vedotin as consolidation therapy in autologous hematopoietic stem cell transplantation (HSCT) patients with Hodgkin's lymphoma did not demonstrate an increase in the reactivation of herpesvirus infections [19]. However, a subsequent safety analysis showed a higher number of herpes infections in the brentuximab vedotin arm (HSV 4%, HZV 7%) than in the placebo arm (HSV 1%, HZV 3%), despite the fact that patients received antiviral prophylaxis following clinical protocol [20].

In a real-life retrospective study involving 39 patients on brentuximab vedotin treatment, six patients with CMV reactivation and one case of severe retinitis were reported [21].

In conclusion, brentuximab vedotin seems to be associated with an increased risk of reactivation of herpesvirus infections. The indication of antiviral prophylaxis could be considered [22].

Anti-CD38: Daratumumab

Daratumumab is a biologic drug approved for the treatment of multiple myeloma and non-Hodgkin's lymphoma. The available studies on the risk of viral infections have pointed to a higher VZV reactivation rate, although it should be noted that patients in these studies were also receiving other immunomodulatory drugs, including proteasome inhibitors and corticosteroids [22]. This drug has been associated with cases of HSV encephalitis, mononucleosis syndrome, and CMV retinitis and encephalitis despite acyclovir prophylaxis [23–25].

Although prophylaxis against VZV reactivation is not universally recommended, it was used in most clinical trials conducted with this drug. Prophylaxis should be initiated in the first week of treatment and maintained for 3 months [26].

Phosphatidylinositol 3-Kinase (PI3K) Inhibitors: Idelalisib, Buparlisib, Rigosertib, and Duvelisib

The clinical use of PI3K inhibitors is accepted for the treatment of breast cancer, chronic lymphocytic leukemia, follicular lymphoma, small-cell lymphocytic lymphoma, and chronic myeloid leukemia. These inhibitors block intracellular signaling mechanisms and favor the destruction of tumor cells. Idelalisib was one of the first drugs to be authorized and, therefore, the one with more available clinical experience.

In a pivotal phase III randomized clinical trial [27] that studied idelalisib in combination with ofatumumab for the treatment of relapsed chronic lymphocytic leukemia, severe infections in the idelalisib group included three cases of CMV reactivation (2%), one case of disseminated HSV infection, and one case of oral herpes. Cases of CMV reactivation and disease have also been reported in other research studies [28, 29].

The available literature on the new PI3K inhibitors and their association with herpes infections is scarce. In therapies with buparlisib, which is authorized for the treatment of HR-positive/HER2-negative metastatic breast cancer, an increased risk of reactivation of herpesvirus infections has not been identified. However, it should be kept in mind that patients with chronic lymphocytic leukemia have a higher underlying risk of opportunistic infections than those with solid tumors. Duvelisib, like idelalisib, has been associated with CMV reactivation in 1% of cases [30]. Given that prophylaxis against HSV and VZV (and also *Pneumocystis jirovecii*) was indicated in the clinical trials carried out with this drug, the actual incidence of CMV reactivation may be higher [31, 32].

It is recommended that patients with hematologic malignancies who are going to receive treatment with these drugs undergo a serological study to determine or rule out the presence of anti-CMV antibodies. Patients who prove to be seropositive (IgG positive) should be monitored periodically to rule out CMV reactivation and consequent disease [30, 33]. Although systematic CMV prophylaxis is recommended when duvelisib is administered, this is not usually given in clinical practice, as valganciclovir prophylaxis is potentially myelotoxic and the prophylactic doses of acyclovir or valacyclovir for HSV and VZV are probably insufficient to prevent CMV reactivation.

Drugs Targeting T-Cell Activation

IgG Against Cytotoxic T-Lymphocyte-Associated Protein 4: Blockade of CD28-CD80/86 Interaction by Abatacept and Belatacept

Abatacept and belatacept are indicated for the treatment of some rheumatic diseases, urological cancer, and as immunosuppressive agents in solid organ transplantation. In rheumatoid arthritis, treatment with abatacept has been associated with a higher rate of severe infections [34] and a risk of VZV reactivation similar to that of anti-TNF-α therapy [35]. A phase II/III randomized clinical trial studying abatacept in lupus nephritis showed a higher incidence of VZV infection in the abatacept-treated compared to the placebo group [36].

In kidney transplant recipients, a phase III randomized clinical trial with belatacept initially showed no risk of herpesvirus infection [37]. However, more recent studies have shown that belatacept increases the risk of reactivation of herpesvirus infections, although the prevalence is low. A study evaluating safety and efficacy outcomes at 3 years in kidney transplant recipients treated with calcineurin inhibitors or belatacept showed a rate of viral infections in the belatacept group of 14.6% compared to 11% in the anti-calcineurin group. The described viral infections were herpesvirus infection (1.71% vs. 0.84%), CMV viremia (1.71% vs. 0), and VZV (1.29% vs. 0.85%) [38]. Another phase III randomized clinical trial evaluating long-term outcomes in kidney transplant patients treated with belatacept versus cyclosporine showed a slightly higher incidence of CMV and VZV infection in the belatacept arm [39]. In addition, two cases of CMV retinitis [40] and one fatal case of disseminated VZV infection [41] have been reported.

Although the risk of herpesvirus reactivation is slightly higher using these agents, systematic use of prophylaxis is not recommended.

Direct T-Cell Inhibitors

Anti-CD52 Drugs: Alemtuzumab

Alemtuzumab is a monoclonal antibody approved by the FDA for the treatment of B-cell chronic lymphocytic leukemia and relapsing-remitting forms of multiple sclerosis. However, it has also been widely studied for other uses, including treatment of other hematologic malignancies and graft-versus-host disease after hematopoietic progenitor cell transplantation, as well as immunosuppressive induction therapy in solid organ transplantation.

Regarding hematologic malignancies treated with alemtuzumab, one study showed that 15–66% treated patients developed CMV reactivation [42]. In another study, CMV reactivation after treatment with alemtuzumab was prospectively monitored. All patients had CMV reactivation, including cases of pneumonitis and hepatitis [43]. Randomized clinical trials have shown a significant increase in asymptomatic CMV reactivation in patients treated with alemtuzumab compared to the comparator [44, 45]. Therefore, CMV reactivation should be monitored during treatment with alemtuzumab in order to initiate early treatment and to prevent the development of severe infections.

In relation to the use of alemtuzumab for the treatment of multiple sclerosis, disease for which the doses are generally lower, several studies have shown an increased risk of HSV and VZV infections associated with this drug. A phase III randomized clinical trial comparing interferon β-1a to alemtuzumab showed that 16% of patients (62 out of 376) treated with alemtuzumab had herpesvirus reactivation (12 cases of VZV and 50 cases of HSV) versus 2% of patients (three out of 187) treated with interferon β-1a, all of which were HSV [46]. This higher incidence of herpesvirus reactivation occurred even when acyclovir prophylaxis was administered [47]. With respect to CMV reactivation, several randomized clinical trials have shown no increased risk, but isolated cases of reactivation with associated organ disease have been reported [48–50].

Finally, in solid organ recipients who receive alemtuzumab as induction therapy, the risk of herpesvirus reactivation is difficult to establish, since patients usually receive protocolized antiviral prophylaxis.

In conclusion, given the significant risk of HSV and VZV infection in patients treated with alemtuzumab, it is recommended to have prophylactic treatment with acyclovir from the start of treatment and continued for up to 2 months after the end of treatment or until the CD4 cell count reaches 200 c/μL or higher. CMV-positive patients should be closely monitored for symptoms of CMV infection or reactivation.

Interleukin-4, Interleukin-5, and Interleukin-6 Inhibitors

Interleukin-4 Inhibitors: Dupilumab

Dupilumab is indicated for the treatment of moderate-to-severe atopic dermatitis. The available data on the risk of infection with this drug is based on a systematic review of seven randomized clinical trials involving adult patients with moderate-to-severe atopic dermatitis [51]. The dupilumab-treated group demonstrated greater risk of herpesvirus reactivation than the placebo group, but in most cases this consisted of oral herpes. In this systematic review, no herpesvirus infections of clinical relevance such as eczema herpeticum or herpes zoster disease were evident [51]. However, isolated cases of HSV uveitis and VZV meningitis have been reported [52].

Given that the incidence of herpesvirus reactivation in these patients is not high, prophylaxis is not indicated.

Interleukin-5 Inhibitors: Benralizumab, Mepolizumab, and Reslizumab

Benralizumab, mepolizumab, and reslizumab are authorized for the treatment of allergic asthma. Although isolated cases of VZV reactivation have been reported [53], these drugs are not associated with a significant increase in the risk of herpesvirus infections [54, 55].

Interleukin-6 Inhibitors: Tocilizumab, Sarilumab, and Siltuximab

Tocilizumab, sarilumab, and siltuximab are clinically indicated for the treatment of some immunological diseases, including rheumatoid arthritis, juvenile idiopathic arthritis, neuromyelitis optica, and Castleman's disease.

In general, these drugs have been associated with an increased risk of infectious complications including those caused by herpesvirus. Tocilizumab is the most widely used and scientifically studied interleukin-6 inhibitor.

In a postmarketing study carried out in Japan that followed 7901 patients with rheumatoid arthritis treated with tocilizumab, 86 cases of herpes zoster were detected, representing an incidence of 1.09% and incidence rate of 2.24 episodes per 100 patient-years [56]. According to data provided by Medicare, the incidence rate of herpes zoster infection in the elderly population with rheumatoid arthritis treated with tocilizumab was 2.15 cases per 100 patient-years [57]. Cases of severe CMV disease associated with this drug have also been described [58, 59].

Regarding sarilumab, clinical trials have shown no major increase in herpesvirus infections [60–62]. There is not enough available information on the risk of herpesvirus infections associated to siltuximab.

Checkpoint Inhibitors

Agents Targeting Cytotoxic T-Lymphocyte-Associated Protein 4 (Ipilimumab and Tremelimumab) and Programmed Cell Death Protein-1 and Ligand-1 (Nivolumab, Pembrolizumab, and Atezolizumab)

These drugs have been shown to be useful for the treatment of melanoma, non-small cell lung cancer, head and neck squamous cell carcinoma, urothelial carcinoma, and solid organ transplant rejection. Their use has not been associated with increased reactivation of herpesvirus infections, but they are responsible for adverse effects that mimic infectious syndromes. In many cases, the therapeutic management of the adverse reactions caused by these drugs requires the use of corticosteroids or other immunosuppressive drugs such as TNF-α inhibitors that are associated with reactivation of herpesvirus infections. For example, patients requiring corticosteroids and/or infliximab for the treatment of immune-mediated colitis may develop CMV enterocolitis [63, 64]. In a retrospective review of 740 melanoma patients who were treated with ipilimumab and nivolumab, 54 patients (7.3%) presented serious infectious complications, including three cases of disseminated/facial herpes zoster and one case of CMV enterocolitis [65]. The main risk factor for the development of infectious complications was the prior use of corticosteroids and/or infliximab, but it is not known if patients who presented herpesvirus infections had received other types of immunosuppressants.

According to the above, these drugs probably do not directly increase the risk of herpesvirus reactivation. However, in patients who present signs or symptoms compatible with infection during treatment of immune-related adverse events, herpesvirus reactivation should be considered.

Tyrosine Kinase Inhibitors Used in Hematologic Malignancies

BCR-ABL Tyrosine Kinase Inhibitor: Bosutinib, Dasatinib, Imatinib, Nilotinib, and Ponatinib

The clinical utility of these drugs has been demonstrated in the following hematologic malignancies: chronic myeloid leukemia, acute lymphoblastic leukemia, myelodysplastic syndrome, gastrointestinal stromal tumor (GIST), mastocytosis, and hypereosinophilic syndrome. These drugs exert their mechanism of action by interfering with T-cell activation and suppressing CMV-specific CD8+ T-cell responses [66, 67]. Interestingly, in vitro studies have shown that tyrosine kinase inhibitors exert direct antiviral action against CMV by binding to the platelet-derived growth factor receptor-α. This receptor is essential for the virus to enter the cell [68]. A phase II study using nilotinib for CMV infection prophylaxis after allogeneic hematopoietic progenitor cell transplantation showed that this drug may be safe, and a randomized clinical trial is being conducted with this objective [69].

Despite the described potential mechanistic inhibition, the anti-CMV effect of tyrosine kinase inhibitors has yet to be demonstrated in clinical practice. Dasatinib has been associated with cases of CMV reactivation and disease, including hepatitis, colitis, and pneumonitis [70–73]. Sporadic cases of oral herpes or herpes zoster have also been described for this drug. In a retrospective study of 771 patients treated with imatinib for chronic myeloid leukemia, 16 presented VZV infection or reactivation, resulting in 5.25 cases per 100 patient-years [74]. Although the incidence of herpesvirus reactivation appears to increase with these drugs, prophylaxis is not generally recommended.

Janus Kinase Inhibitors

Ruxolitinib, Tofacitinib, and Baricitinib

These drugs alter intracellular signaling by inhibiting Janus kinase (JAK) and are indicated for the treatment of rheumatoid arthritis and myeloproliferative disorders. As several studies have demonstrated, the use of these drugs is associated with an increased risk of infectious complications, especially by VZV. In a phase III clinical trial comparing ruxolitinib versus standard of care for the treatment of polycythemia vera, VZV infection occurred in 6% of patients treated with ruxotinib compared to 0% of the control group [75]. In another postmarketing study involving 1144 patients, VZV infection was the most frequent infectious complication with an incidence of 8%. Finally, a recent meta-analysis has shown a significantly higher risk of VZV infection with ruxolitinib (odds ratio of 7.39 compared to controls) [76]. The use of tofacitinib for the treatment of psoriasis, rheumatoid arthritis, and inflammatory bowel disease has also been shown to increase the risk of VZV reactivation [77–82]. In a study on the incidence of VZV infection in a cohort of 3623 psoriatic patients, 130 (3.6%) presented some form of infection. Of these, nine patients (7%) required hospitalization and eight (6%) had multimetameric disease [83]. Baricitinib has been studied for the treatment of rheumatoid arthritis, and clinical trials have shown an increased risk of VZV infections with the use of this drug [84].

JAK inhibitors do not appear to significantly increase the risk of CMV reactivation. In a study involving 5671 patients with rheumatoid arthritis treated with tofacitinib and long follow-up, only six cases of disease, including hepatitis, retinitis, and gastritis, were detected [85]. Tofacitinib was compared to cyclosporine A as an immunosuppressive therapy in kidney transplant recipients and showed a higher incidence of CMV viremia and disease than cyclosporine. This higher incidence was reduced by one-third when CMV prophylaxis was indicated [86].

In summary, JAK inhibitors significantly increase the risk of infectious complications, including VZV infection. Therefore, antiviral prophylaxis is recommended. VZV vaccination can be considered if it is administered at least 4 weeks before starting immunosuppressive therapy, but the efficacy of VZV vaccination in this setting has not been studied [87]. CMV reactivation is uncommon but should be considered, particularly in transplant patients.

mTOR Inhibitors

Everolimus, Sirolimus, and Temsirolimus

These drugs are primarily used as immunosuppressants to prevent solid organ transplantation rejection. In kidney transplant recipients treated with these inhibitors, a low risk of EBV reactivation and associated lymphoproliferative disorders has been observed compared to the use of calcineurin inhibitors [88, 89]. These agents have not been associated with an increased risk of infection by other herpesviruses.

Other Biologic Drugs Associated with the Risk of Herpesvirus Infections

Sphingosine 1-Phosphate Receptor Modulator: Fingolimod

Fingolimod is indicated for the treatment of multiple sclerosis. This drug acts by preventing the release of lymphocytes from the lymph nodes and causes a marked reduction in CD3 T cells. Patients treated with fingolimod have a reduced antiviral T-cell response [90] and VZV reactivation is more frequent [90, 91].

Clinical studies carried out with fingolimod for the treatment of relapsing-remitting multiple sclerosis have shown that the incidence of VZV infection is low (7–11 per 1000 patient-years) but higher than in the placebo group [92]. Severe cases were also rare. Experts recommend determining VZV serological status before initiating treatment with fingolimod and evaluating the immunization of patients susceptible to primary infection (negative IgG and IgM against VZV). Systematic prophylaxis is not necessary in most cases, but the risk/benefit ratio should be assessed in the event that the patient is to receive concomitant pulse corticosteroid therapy [92].

Proteasome Inhibitors: Bortezomib, Carfilzomib, and Ixazomib

These drugs are mainly indicated for the treatment of multiple myeloma and as an immunosuppressant in hematopoietic transplantation.

Bortezomib significantly reduces cell-mediated immunity to VZV, and several clinical studies have shown a higher incidence of VZV disease with its use [93–95]. For this reason, antiviral prophylaxis during treatment with this drug is indicated [94]. Patients undergoing autologous hematopoietic progenitor cell transplantation have also shown a higher risk of CMV and HHV-6 reactivation [96, 97].

There is little data in the literature on the use of ixazomib and carfilzomib.

CCR4 Inhibitors: Mogamulizumab

Mogamulizumab is the most commonly used drug for the treatment of cutaneous T-cell lymphoma, chronic lymphocytic leukemia, and non-Hodgkin's T-cell lymphoma.

The use of mogamulizumab has been associated with a higher incidence of herpesvirus diseases, especially CMV. In a postmarketing surveillance study, CMV reactivation was the most frequent adverse infectious effect. Forty cases of CMV disease were recorded, including chorioretinitis, enterocolitis, and pneumonia, and 484 patients (8.3%) presented viremia [98]. Fatal cases of CMV disease have also been reported [99, 100].

Antiviral Prophylaxis Against Herpesvirus Infection

Throughout this review we have described the risks of herpesvirus reactivation associated with the administration of biologic treatments or targeted therapy (Table 20.2). As we have shown, not all drugs have the same risk of reactivating latent herpesviruses and not all herpesviruses produce diseases of equal severity. In situations where the risk of reactivation and severe disease is high, specific prophylaxis is indicated (Table 20.2). In this section we will discuss the main therapeutic strategies available for preventing herpesvirus reactivation. Infections caused by Epstein-Barr virus, HHV-6, HHV-7, and HHV-8 are not mentioned because no drugs are currently approved for prophylaxis or treatment.

Prophylaxis Against Herpes Simplex Virus and Varicella-Zoster Virus

The antivirals used for prophylaxis and treatment of HSV and VZV infection are acyclovir/valacyclovir and famciclovir. All these antivirals act by inhibiting the viral DNA polymerase and preventing the replication of the virus. Other drugs that are also active but less used due to their toxicity are ganciclovir (and the ganciclovir ester, valganciclovir), foscarnet, and cidofovir. Foscarnet and cidofovir are the drugs of choice when HSV and VZV are resistant to acyclovir or for CMV when it is resistant to ganciclovir.

Acyclovir prophylaxis to prevent VZV reactivation has been widely studied in the context of hematopoietic progenitor cell transplantation. The prescribed dosage varies significantly and can range from daily doses of 200 mg to 2400 mg. It should be noted that low doses (200 or 400 mg daily) are effective for the prevention of VZV reactivation. The most frequently used drugs and doses for the prevention of HSV and VZV reactivation are 1) acyclovir 400 mg twice daily or 800 mg twice daily, 2) valacyclovir 500 mg once or twice daily, and 3) famciclovir 250 mg twice daily.

A new class of antivirals active against HSV and VZV is currently being developed. These new antivirals have a novel mechanism of action that could be useful for the treatment of these infections when they are resistant to acyclovir or famciclovir. Of these agents, pritelivir has been studied in a randomized clinical trial for the treatment of genital herpes caused by HSV-2 [101, 102], and amenamevir has been evaluated for the treatment of herpes zoster [103].

Another efficacious prevention method is vaccination. Currently, there are no vaccines against HSV, but several vaccines have been available for years to prevent VZV infection. Attenuated live virus vaccine (Zostavax®) is contraindicated in severely immunosuppressed patients but can be administered at least 4 weeks before initiating immunosuppressive therapy. In October 2017, the FDA approved the use of an inactivated recombinant vaccine (Shingrix®) for the prevention of VZV infection in patients 50 years and older. This vaccine has been shown to be highly effective and provide long-lasting protection. It has been studied in immunocompromised patients including autologous hematopoietic cell transplant patients [104], HIV-infected patients [105], and kidney transplant recipients [106], proving to be immunogenic and safe [107]. Although it has not been specifically evaluated in populations undergoing treatment with biologics, it is reasonable to think that it could also be associated with a decrease in VZV infections.

Cytomegalovirus

Valganciclovir or ganciclovir prophylaxis against cytomegalovirus is usually given to solid organ transplant patients. In hematopoietic progenitor cell transplantation are usually avoided due to the high risk of myelotoxicity [108]. Letermovir, a new drug with activity against CMV, has recently been approved for the prophylaxis of CMV infection in allogeneic hematopoietic progenitor cell transplant recipients [109]. At present, several clinical trials are underway to assess the usefulness of this drug for the prophylaxis and treatment of CMV infection in solid organ transplantation. Maribavir is also an antiviral which is currently under development and has been shown to be active against CMV by preventing the release of viral capsids from the infected cell through inhibition of the UL97. Several clinical trials have evaluated the safety and efficacy of maribavir for the treatment and prophylaxis of CMV infection [110–112]. Foscarnet and cidofovir, although useful for the treatment of infection, are not appropriate for prophylaxis due to their intravenous formulation and nephrotoxicity. Brincidofovir (also called CMX001), an oral prodrug of cidofovir, was evaluated for the prophylaxis of CMV infection in hematopoietic progenitor cell transplantation patients but failed to show a reduction in clinically significant CMV infections at 24 weeks and increased the rates of diarrhea and graft-versus-host disease [113] so its use was never approved by the FDA. Studies are currently being conducted to treat other DNA viruses with this drug [114].

As we have seen, some biologic therapies favor replication and CMV disease. Anti-CMV prophylaxis in patients undergoing these therapies is not generally indicated. In the context of hematopoietic progenitor transplant recipients at risk of CMV reactivation, CMV viral load should be periodically monitored by PCR, and specific treatment should be initiated as soon as viremia is detected. This preemptive therapy is not accepted in most patients treated with biologics, who are closely followed for signs and symptoms of disease. Although CMV PCR is useful to detect peripheral replication of the virus, CMV can cause specific organ disease that is not always accompanied by viremia. Therefore, it is necessary to perform diagnostic tests targeted at the organ with clinical suspicion of infection, such as bronchoscopies, endoscopies, or biopsies.

Although several vaccines are currently being tested, they have not yet been approved for clinical use.

References

1. Collins-Mc Millan D, Buehler J, Peppenelli M, et al. Molecular determinants and the regulation of human cytomegalovirus latency and reactivation. Viruses. 2018;10(8):E444.
2. Manzano V, Ruiz P, Torres M, et al. Severe pneumonia by aciclovir-resistant varicella-zoster virus during etanercept therapy. Rheumatology (Oxford). 2010;49(9):1791–3.
3. Skuhala T, Atelj A, Prepolec J, et al. A case report of severe recurrent varicella in an ankylosing spondylitis patient treated with adalimumab—a new side effect after 15 years of usage. BMC Infect Dis. 2019;19(1):127.

4. Ma C, Walters B, Fedorak RN. Varicella zoster meningitis complicating combined anti-tumor necrosis factor and corticosteroid therapy in Crohn's disease. World J Gastroenterol. 2013;19(21):3347–51.
5. Galloway JB, Mercer LK, Moseley A, et al. Risk of skin and soft tissue infections(including shingles) in patients exposed to anti-tumour necrosis factor therapy: results from the British Society for Rheumatology Biologics Register. Ann Rheum Dis. 2013;72(2):229–34.
6. Garcia-Doval I, Perez-Zafrilla B, Descalzo MA, et al. Incidence and risk of hospitalisation due to shingles and chickenpox in patients with rheumatic diseases treated with TNF antagonists. Ann Rheum Dis. 2010;69(10):1751–5.
7. Serac G, Tubach F, Mariette X, et al. Risk of herpes zoster in patients receiving anti-TNF-alpha in the prospective French RATIO registry. J Invest Dermatol. 2012;132(3 Pt 1):726–9.
8. Winthrop KL, Baddley JW, Chen L, et al. Association between the initiation of anti-tumor necrosis factor therapy and the risk of herpes zoster. JAMA. 2013;309(9):887–95.
9. Mizuta M, Schuster MG. Cytomegalovirus hepatitis associated with use of antitumor necrosis factor-alpha antibody. Clin Infect Dis. 2005;40(7):1071–2.
10. Helbling D, Breitbach TH, Krause M. Disseminated cytomegalovirus infection in Crohn's disease following anti-tumour necrosis factor therapy. Eur J Gastroenterol Hepatol. 2002;14(12):1393–5.
11. Salles G, Barrett M, Foa R, et al. Rituximab in B-cell hematologic malignancies: a review of 20 years of clinical experience. Adv Ther. 2017;34(10):2232–73.
12. Okamoto A, Abe A, Okamoto M, et al. Severe hepatitis associated with varicela zoster virus infection in a patient with diffuse large B cell lymphoma treated with rituximab-CHOP chemotherapy. Int J Hematol. 2012;96(4):516–20.
13. Okamoto A, Abe A, Okamoto M, et al. A varicella outbreak in B-cell lymphoma patients receiving rituximab-containing chemotherapy. J Infect Chemother. 2014;20(12):774–7.
14. Aksoy S, Harputluoglu H, Kilickap S, et al. Rituximab-related viral infections in lymphoma patients. Leuk Lymphoma. 2007;48(7):1307–12.
15. Marcus R, Davies A, Ando K, et al. Obinutuzumab for the first-line treatment of follicular lymphoma. N Engl J Med. 2017;377(14):1331–44.
16. Montalban X, Hauser SL, Kappos L, et al. Ocrelizumab versus placebo in primary progressive multiple sclerosis. N Engl J Med. 2017;376(3):209–20.
17. van Oers MH, Kuliczkowski K, Smolej L, et al. Ofatumumab maintenance versus observation in relapsed chronic lymphocytic leukaemia (PROLONG): an openlabel, multicentre, randomised phase 3 study. Lancet Oncol. 2015;16(13):1370–9.
18. Morschhauser F, Radford J, Van Hoof A, et al. Phase III trial of consolidation therapy with yttrium-90-ibritumomab tiuxetan compared with no additional therapy after first remission in advanced follicular lymphoma. J Clin Oncol. 2008;26(32):5156–64.
19. Moskowitz CH, Nademanee A, Masszi T, et al. Brentuximab vedotin as consolidation therapy after autologous stem-cell transplantation in patients with Hodgkin's lymphoma at risk of relapse or progression (AETHERA): a randomised, double-blind, placebo-controlled, phase 3 trial. Lancet. 2015;385(9980):1853–62.
20. Nademanee A, Sureda A, Stiff P, et al. Safety analysis of brentuximab vedotin from the phase III AETHERA trial in hodgkin lymphoma in the post-transplant consolidation setting. Biol Blood Marrow Transplant. 2018;24(11):2354–9.
21. Clarivet B, Vincent L, Vergely L, et al. Adverse reactions related to brentuximab vedotin use: a real-life retrospective study. Therapie. 2019;74(3):343–6.
22. Drgona L, Gudiol C, Lanini S, et al. ESCMID study Group for Infections in compromised hosts (ESGICH) consensus document on the safety of targeted and biological therapies: an infectious diseases perspective (agents targeting lymphoid or myeloid cells surface antigens [II]: CD22, CD30, CD33, CD38, CD40, SLAMF-7 and CCR4). Clin Microbiol Infect. 2018;24(Suppl 2):S83–94.
23. Frerichs KA, Bosman PWC, Nijhof IS, et al. Cytomegalovirus reactivation in a patient with extensively pretreated multiple myeloma during daratumumab treatment. Clin Lymphoma Myeloma Leuk. 2019;19(1):e9–11.

24. Lavi N, Okasha D, Sabo E, et al. Severe cytomegalovirus enterocolitis developing following daratumumab exposure in three patients with multiple myeloma. Eur J Haematol. 2018. https://doi.org/10.1111/ejh.13164.
25. Nahi H, Chrobok M, Gran C, et al. Infectious complications and NK cell depletion following daratumumab treatment of multiple myeloma. PLoS One. 2019;14(2):e0211927.
26. https://www.accessdata.fda.gov/drugsatfda_docs/label/2016/761036s004lbl.pdf.
27. Jones JA, Robak T, Brown JR, et al. Efficacy and safety of idelalisib in combination with ofatumumab for previously treated chronic lymphocytic leukaemia: an open-label, randomised phase 3 trial. Lancet Haematol. 2017;4(3):e114–26.
28. Goldring L, Kumar B, Gan TE, et al. Idelalisib induced CMV gastrointestinal disease: the need for vigilance with novel therapies. Pathology. 2017;49(5):555–7.
29. Lampson BL, Kasar SN, Matos TR, et al. Idelalisib given front-line for treatment of chronic lymphocytic leukemia causes frequent immune-mediated hepatotoxicity. Blood. 2016;128(2):195–203.
30. https://www.accessdata.fda.gov/drugsatfda_docs/label/2018/211155s000lbl.pdf.
31. Flinn IW, Hillmen P, Montillo M, et al. The phase 3 DUO trial: duvelisib vs ofatumumab in relapsed and refractory CLL/SLL. Blood. 2018;132(23):2446–55.
32. Flinn IW, Miller CB, Ardeshna KM, et al. DYNAMO: a phase II study of duvelisib (IPI-145) in patients with refractory indolent non-Hodgkin lymphoma. J Clin Oncol. 2019;37(11):912–22.
33. Reinwald M, Silva JT, Mueller NJ, et al. ESCMID study Group for Infections in compromised hosts (ESGICH) consensus document on the safety of targeted and biological therapies: an infectious diseases perspective (intracellular signaling pathways: tyrosine kinase and mTOR inhibitors). Clin Microbiol Infect. 2018;24(Suppl 2):S53–70.
34. Blair HA, Deeks ED. Abatacept: a review in rheumatoid arthritis. Drugs. 2017;77(11):1221–33.
35. Furie R, Nicholls K, Cheng TT, et al. Efficacy and safety of abatacept in lupus nephritis: a twelve-month, randomized, double-blind study. Arthritis Rheumatol. 2014;66(2):379–89.
36. Chen SK, Liao KP, Liu J, et al. Risk of hospitalized infection and initiation of abatacept versus TNF inhibitors among patients with rheumatoid arthritis: a propensity score-matched cohort study. Arthritis Care Res (Hoboken). 2020;72(1):9–17.
37. Vincenti F, Rostaing L, Grinyo J, et al. Belatacept and long-term outcomes in kidney transplantation. N Engl J Med. 2016;374(4):333–43.
38. Grinyo JM, Del Carmen RM, Alberu J, et al. Safety and efficacy outcomes 3 years after switching to belatacept from a calcineurin inhibitor in kidney transplant recipients: results from a phase 2 randomized trial. Am J Kidney Dis. 2017;69(5):587–94.
39. Durrbach A, Pestana JM, Florman S, et al. Long-term outcomes in belatacept versus cyclosporine-treated recipients of extended criteria donor kidneys: final results from BENEFIT-EXT, a phase III randomized study. Am J Transplant. 2016;16(11):3192–201.
40. Helou E, Grant M, Landry M, et al. Fatal case of cutaneous-sparing orolaryngeal zoster in a renal transplant recipient. Transpl Infect Dis. 2017;19(4). https://doi.org/10.1111/tid.12704.
41. Fan J, Gong D, Truong C, et al. Cytomegalovirus retinitis with belatacept immunosuppression. Retin Cases Brief Rep. 2019;16:199. https://doi.org/10.1097/ICB.0000000000000928.
42. Thursky KA, Worth LJ, Seymour JF, et al. Spectrum of infection, risk and recommendations for prophylaxis and screening among patients with lymphoproliferative disorders treated with alemtuzumab. Br J Haematol. 2006;132(1):3–12.
43. Cheung WW, Tse E, Leung AY, et al. Regular virologic surveillance showed very frequent cytomegalovirus reactivation in patients treated with alemtuzumab. Am J Hematol. 2007;82(2):108–11.
44. Mikulska M, Lanini S, Gudiol C, et al. ESCMID study Group for Infections in compromised hosts (ESGICH) consensus document on the safety of targeted and biological therapies: an infectious diseases perspective (agents targeting lymphoid cells surface antigens [I]: CD19, CD20 and CD52). Clin Microbiol Infect. 2018;24(Suppl 2):S71–82.
45. Skoetz N, Bauer K, Elter T, et al. Alemtuzumab for patients with chronic lymphocytic leukaemia. Cochrane Database Syst Rev. 2012;(2):CD008078.

46. Cohen JA, Coles AJ, Arnold DL, et al. Alemtuzumab versus interferon beta 1a as first-line treatment for patients with relapsing-remitting multiple sclerosis: a randomised controlled phase 3 trial. Lancet. 2012;380(9856):1819–28.
47. Coles AJ, Twyman CL, Arnold DL, et al. Alemtuzumab for patients with relapsing multiple sclerosis after disease-modifying therapy: a randomised controlled phase 3 trial. Lancet. 2012;380(9856):1829–39.
48. Clerico M, De Mercanti S, Artusi CA, et al. Active CMV infection in two patients with multiple sclerosis treated with alemtuzumab. Mult Scler. 2017;23(6):874–6.
49. Barone S, Scannapieco S, Torti C, et al. Hepatic microabscesses during CMV reactivation in a multiple sclerosis patient after alemtuzumab treatment. Mult Scler Relat Disord. 2018;20:68.
50. Buonomo AR, Sacca F, Zappulo E, et al. Bacterial and CMV pneumonia in a patient treated with alemtuzumab for multiple sclerosis. Mult Scler Relat Disord. 2019;27:44–5.
51. Eichenfield LF, Bieber T, Beck LA, et al. Infections in dupilumab clinical trials in atopic dermatitis: a comprehensive pooled analysis. Am J Clin Dermatol. 2019;20(3):443–56.
52. Ivert LU, Wahlgren CF, Ivert L, et al. Eye complications during dupilumab treatment for severe atopic dermatitis. Acta Derm Venereol. 2019;99(4):375–8.
53. Haldar P, Brightling CE, Hargadon B, et al. Mepolizumab and exacerbations of refractory eosinophilic asthma. N Engl J Med. 2009;360(10):973–84.
54. Bjermer L, Lemiere C, Maspero J, et al. Reslizumab for inadequately controlled asthma with elevated blood eosinophil levels: a randomized phase 3 study. Chest. 2016;150(4):789–98.
55. Castro M, Zangrilli J, Wechsler ME, et al. Reslizumab for inadequately controlled asthma with elevated blood eosinophil counts: results from two multicentre, parallel, double-blind, randomised, placebo-controlled, phase 3 trials. Lancet Respir Med. 2015;3(5):355–66.
56. Koike T, Harigai M, Inokuma S, et al. Effectiveness and safety of tocilizumab: postmarketing surveillance of 7901 patients with rheumatoid arthritis in Japan. J Rheumatol. 2014;41(1):15–23.
57. Yun H, Xie F, Delzell E, et al. Risks of herpes zoster in patients with rheumatoid arthritis according to biologic disease-modifying therapy. Arthritis Care Res (Hoboken). 2015;67(5):731–6.
58. Fromhold-Treu S, Erbersdobler A, Turan M, et al. CMV associated acute liver failure in a patient receiving tocilizumab for systemic lupus erythematosus. Z Gastroenterol. 2017;55(5):467–72. [in German]
59. Komura T, Ohta H, Nakai R, et al. Cytomegalovirus reactivation induced acute hepatitis and gastric erosions in a patient with rheumatoid arthritis under treatment with an anti-il-6 receptor antibody, tocilizumab. Intern Med. 2016;55(14):1923–7.
60. Genovese MC, van Adelsberg J, Fan C, et al. Two years of sarilumab in patients with rheumatoid arthritis and an inadequate response to MTX: safety, efficacy and radiographic outcomes. Rheumatology (Oxford). 2018;57(8):1423–31.
61. Burmester GR, Lin Y, Patel R, et al. Efficacy and safety of sarilumab monotherapy versus adalimumab monotherapy for the treatment of patients with active rheumatoid arthritis (MONARCH): a randomised, double-blind, parallel-group phase III trial. Ann Rheum Dis. 2017;76(5):840–7.
62. Fleischmann R, Genovese MC, Lin Y, et al. Long-term safety of sarilumab in rheumatoid arthritis: an integrated analysis with up to 7 years' follow-up. Rheumatology. 2020;59(2):292–302.
63. Franklin C, Rooms I, Fiedler M, et al. Cytomegalovirus reactivation in patients with refractory checkpoint inhibitor-induced colitis. Eur J Cancer. 2017;86:248–56.
64. Uslu U, Agaimy A, Hundorfean G, et al. Autoimmune colitis and subsequent CMV-induced hepatitis after treatment with ipilimumab. J Immunother. 2015;38(5):212–5.
65. Del Castillo M, Romero FA, Arguello E, et al. The spectrum of serious infections among patients receiving immune checkpoint blockade for the treatment of melanoma. Clin Infect Dis. 2016;63(11):1490–3.
66. Seggewiss R, Lore K, Greiner E, et al. Imatinib inhibits T-cell receptor-mediated T-cell proliferation and activation in a dose-dependent manner. Blood. 2005;105(6):2473–9.

67. Fei F, Yu Y, Schmitt A, et al. Dasatinib exerts an immunosuppressive effect on CD81 T cells specific for viral and leukemia antigens. Exp Hematol. 2008;36(10):1297–308.
68. Soroceanu L, Akhavan A, Cobbs CS. Platelet-derived growth factor-alpha receptor activation is required for human cytomegalovirus infection. Nature. 2008;455(7211):391–5.
69. Lin CT, Hsueh PR, Wu SJ, et al. Repurposing nilotinib for cytomegalovirus infection prophylaxis after allogeneic hematopoietic stem cell transplantation: a single-arm, phase II trial. Biol Blood Marrow Transplant. 2018;24(11):2310–5.
70. Davalos F, Chaucer B, Zafar W, et al. Dasatinib-induced CMV hepatitis in an immunocompetent patient: a rare complication of a common drug. Transl Oncol. 2016;9(3):248–50.
71. Yassin MA, Nashwan AJ, Soliman AT, et al. Cytomegalovirus-induced hemorrhagic colitis in a patient with chronic myeloid leukemia (chronic phase) on dasatinib as an upfront therapy. Clin Med Insights Case Rep. 2015;8:77–81.
72. Aldoss I, Gaal K, Al Malki MM, et al. Dasatinib-induced colitis after allogeneic stem cell transplantation for Philadelphia chromosome-positive acute lymphoblastic leukemia. Biol Blood Marrow Transplant. 2016;22(10):1900–3.
73. Knoll BM, Seiter K. Infections in patients on BCR-ABL tyrosine kinase inhibitor therapy: cases and review of the literature. Infection. 2018;46(3):409–18.
74. Mattiuzzi GN, Cortes JE, Talpaz M, et al. Development of varicella-zoster virus infection in patients with chronic myelogenous leukemia treated with imatinib mesylate. Clin Cancer Res. 2003;9(3):976–80.
75. Vannucchi AM, Kiladjian JJ, Griesshammer M, et al. Ruxolitinib versus standard therapy for the treatment of polycythemia vera. N Engl J Med. 2015;372(5):426–35.
76. Lussana F, Cattaneo M, Rambaldi A, et al. Ruxolitinib-associated infections: a systematic review and meta-analysis. Am J Hematol. 2018;93(3):339–47.
77. Asahina A, Etoh T, Igarashi A, et al. Oral tofacitinib efficacy, safety and tolerability in Japanese patients with moderate to severe plaque psoriasis and psoriatic arthritis: a randomized, double-blind, phase 3 study. J Dermatol. 2016;43(8):869–80.
78. Cohen SB, Tanaka Y, Mariette X, et al. Long-term safety of tofacitinib for the treatment of rheumatoid arthritis up to 8.5 years: integrated analysis of data from the global clinical trials. Ann Rheum Dis. 2017;76(7):1253–62.
79. Gladman D, Rigby W, Azevedo VF, et al. Tofacitinib for psoriatic arthritis in patients with an inadequate response to TNF inhibitors. N Engl J Med. 2017;377(16):1525–36.
80. Mease P, Hall S, FitzGerald O, et al. Tofacitinib or adalimumab versus placebo for psoriatic arthritis. N Engl J Med. 2017;377(16):1537–50.
81. Winthrop KL, Melmed GY, Vermeire S, et al. Herpes zoster infection in patients with ulcerative colitis receiving tofacitinib. Inflamm Bowel Dis. 2018;24(10):2258–65.
82. Caldera F, Hayney MS, Cross RK. Using number needed to harm to put the risk of herpes zoster from tofacitinib in perspective. Inflamm Bowel Dis. 2019;25(6):955–7.
83. Winthrop KL, Lebwohl M, Cohen AD, et al. Herpes zoster in psoriasis patients treated with tofacitinib. J Am Acad Dermatol. 2017;77(2):302–9.
84. Genovese MC, Kremer J, Zamani O, et al. Baricitinib in patients with refractory rheumatoid arthritis. N Engl J Med. 2016;374(13):1243–52.
85. Winthrop KL, Park SH, Gul A, et al. Tuberculosis and other opportunistic infections in tofacitinib-treated patients with rheumatoid arthritis. Ann Rheum Dis. 2016;75(6):1133–8.
86. Vincenti F, Tedesco Silva H, Busque S, et al. Randomized phase 2b trial of tofacitinib (CP-690,550) in de novo kidney transplant patients: efficacy, renal function and safety at 1 year. Am J Transplant. 2012;12(9):2446–56.
87. Fleischmann R, Mysler E, Hall S, et al. Efficacy and safety of tofacitinib monotherapy, tofacitinib with methotrexate, and adalimumab with methotrexate in patients with rheumatoid arthritis (ORAL strategy): a phase 3b/4, double-blind, head-to-head, randomised controlled trial. Lancet. 2017;390(10093):457–68.
88. Pascual J, Royuela A, Fernández AM, et al. Role of mTOR inhibitors for the control of viral infection in solid organ transplant recipients. Transpl Infect Dis. 2016;18:819–31.

89. Hymes LC, Warshaw BL. Five-year experience using sicrolimus based, calcineurin inhibitor-free inmunosuppression in pediatric renal transplantation. Pediatr Transplant. 2011;15:437–44.
90. Ricklin ME, Lorscheider J, Waschbisch A, et al. T-cell response against varicella-zoster virus in fingolimod-treated MS patients. Neurology. 2013;81(2):174–81.
91. Aramideh Khouy R, Karampoor S, Keyvani H, et al. The frequency of varicella zoster virus infection in patients with multiple sclerosis receiving fingolimod. J Neuroimmunol. 2019;328:94–7.
92. Arvin AM, Wolinsky JS, Kappos L, et al. Varicella-zoster virus infections in patients treated with fingolimod: risk assessment and consensus recommendations for management. JAMA Neurol. 2015;72(1):31–9.
93. Kim JW, Min CK, Mun YC, et al. Varicella-zoster virus-specific cell-mediated immunity and herpes zoster development in multiple myeloma patients receiving bortezomib- or thalidomide-based chemotherapy. J Clin Virol. 2015;73:64–9.
94. Richardson PG, Sonneveld P, Schuster MW, et al. Bortezomib or high-dose dexamethasone for relapsed multiple myeloma. N Engl J Med. 2005;352(24):2487–98.
95. San Miguel JF, Schlag R, Khuageva NK, et al. Bortezomib plus melphalan and prednisone for initial treatment of multiple myeloma. N Engl J Med. 2008;359(9):906–17.
96. Marchesi F, Mengarelli A, Giannotti F, et al. High incidence of post-transplant cytomegalovirus reactivations in myeloma patients undergoing autologous stem cell transplantation after treatment with bortezomib-based regimens: a survey from the Rome transplant network. Transpl Infect Dis. 2014;16(1):158–64.
97. Horowitz N, Oren I, Lavi N, et al. New rising infection: human herpesvirus 6 is frequent in myeloma patients undergoing autologous stem cell transplantation after induction therapy with bortezomib. Bone Marrow Res. 2012;2012:409765.
98. Ishitsuka K, Yurimoto S, Kawamura K, et al. Safety and efficacy of mogamulizumab in patients with adult T-cell leukemia-lymphoma in Japan: interim results of postmarketing all case surveillance. Int J Hematol. 2017;106(4):522–32.
99. Ishii Y, Itabashi M, Numata A, et al. Cytomegalovirus pneumonia after anti-CC chemokine receptor 4 monoclonal antibody (mogamulizumab) therapy in an angioimmunoblastic T-cell lymphoma patient. Intern Med. 2016;55(6):673–5.
100. Ohyama Y, Kumode T, Eguchi G, et al. Induction of molecular remission by using anti-CC-chemokine receptor 4 (anti-CCR4) antibodies for adult T cell leukemia: a risk of opportunistic infection after treatment with anti-CCR4 antibodies. Ann Hematol. 2014;93(1):169–71.
101. Wald A, Corey L, Timmler B, et al. Helicase-primase inhibitor pritelivir for HSV-2 infection. N Engl J Med. 2014;370(3):201–10.
102. Wald A, Timmler B, Magaret A, et al. Effect of pritelivir compared with valacyclovir on genital HSV-2 shedding in patients with frequent recurrences: a randomized clinical trial. JAMA. 2016;316(23):2495–503.
103. Kawashima M, Nemoto O, Honda M, et al. Amenamevir, a novel helicase primase inhibitor, for treatment of herpes zoster: a randomized, double-blind, valaciclovir-controlled phase 3 study. J Dermatol. 2017;44(11):1219–27.
104. Stadtmauer EA, Sullivan KM, Marty FM, et al. A phase 1/2 study of an adjuvanted varicella-zoster virus subunit vaccine in autologous hematopoietic cell transplant recipients. Blood. 2014;124(19):2921–9.
105. Berkowitz EM, Moyle G, Stellbrink HJ, et al. Safety and immunogenicity of an adjuvanted herpes zoster subunit candidate vaccine in HIV-infected adults: a phase 1/2a randomized, placebo-controlled study. J Infect Dis. 2015;211(8):1279–87.
106. https://idsa.confex.com/idsa/2017/webprogram/Paper65338.html.
107. James SF, Chahine EB, Sucher AJ, et al. Shingrix: the new adjuvanted recombinant herpes zoster vaccine. Ann Pharmacother. 2018;52(7):673–80.
108. Zaia JA. Cytomegalovirus infection. In: Forman SJ, Negrin RS, Antin JH, et al., editors. Thomas' hematopoietic cell transplantation, vol. 2. West Sussex: Wiley; 2016. p. 1069–77.

109. Razonable RR. Role of Letermovir for prevention of cytomegalovirus infection after allogeneic haematopoietic stem cell transplantation. Curr Opin Infect Dis. 2018;31(4):286–91.
110. Maertens J, Cordonnier C, Jaksch P, et al. Maribavir for preemptive treatment of cytomegalovirus reactivation. N Engl J Med. 2019;381(12):1136–47.
111. Marty FM, Ljungman P, Papanicolaou GA, et al. Maribavir prophylaxis for prevention of cytomegalovirus disease in recipients of allogeneic stem-cell transplants: a phase 3, double-blind, placebo-controlled, randomised trial. Lancet Infect Dis. 2011;11(4):284–92.
112. Winston DJ, Saliba F, Blumberg E, et al. Efficacy and safety of maribavir dosed at 100 mg orally twice daily for the prevention of cytomegalovirus disease in liver transplant recipients: a randomized, double-blind, multicenter controlled trial. Am J Transplant. 2012;12(11):3021–30.
113. Marty FM, Winston DJ, Rowley SD, et al. CMX001 to prevent cytomegalovirus disease in hematopoietic-cell transplantation. N Engl J Med. 2013;369(13):1227–36.
114. Hiwarkar P, Amrolia P, Sivaprakasam P, et al. Brincidofovir is highly efficacious in controlling adenoviremia in pediatric recipients hematopoietic cell transplant. Blood. 2017;129(14):2033–7.

Invasive Fungal Disease 21

Emma Paige, Scott J. Abbinga, and Monica A. Slavin

Introduction

Invasive fungal disease (IFD) is a commonly encountered problem in immunocompromised patients, and traditionally has been associated with neutropenia and the use of corticosteroids and other high-grade immunosuppressants. Over recent years, however, the advent of biologic and targeted therapies has introduced new risk groups for IFD. It is critical that medical professionals caring for these patients and prescribing biologic and targeted agents are aware of the potential for IFD, where this exists.

Overall, IFD risk is relatively low in patients receiving biologic and targeted therapies. A limited number of agents, however, have been associated with significant IFD risk; infrequent cases of IFD have also been reported in patients receiving a broader range of biologic and targeted agents. It is important to take into account the specific agent being used, in addition to the IFD risk associated with the underlying disease being treated, the presence of neutropenia and the current or recent use of other immunosuppressants.

Routine antifungal prophylaxis is not required in most patients receiving biologic and targeted therapies, although prophylaxis against *Pneumocystis jirovecii* is indicated in some specific patient groups. It is, however, important to recognise that

E. Paige · S. J. Abbinga
Department of Infectious Diseases, Alfred Health, Melbourne, VIC, Australia
e-mail: abbingascott@gmail.com

M. A. Slavin (✉)
Department of Infectious Diseases, Peter MacCallum Cancer Centre, Melbourne, VIC, Australia
e-mail: monica.slavin@petermac.org

C. Cervera, J. M. Aguado (eds.), *Infectious Complications in Biologic and Targeted Therapies*, https://doi.org/10.1007/978-3-031-11363-5_21

IFD risk is in flux for many of these agents, particularly those with limited clinical experience to date, and any clinical symptoms or signs of IFD should be investigated promptly. Morbidity and mortality associated with IFD in the setting of the use of biologic or targeted therapies can be significant.

Selected categories of biologic and targeted agents associated with IFD, with examples of specific agents in each category and common indications for their use, are listed in Table 21.1.

Table 21.1 Selected biologic and targeted therapies associated with invasive fungal disease

Biologic category	Examples of specific agents	Common indications for use
TNF-α inhibitors	Infliximab Etanercept Adalimumab Certolizumab Golimumab	Rheumatoid arthritis Other inflammatory arthritides Inflammatory bowel disease
Anti-IL-17 agents	Secukinumab Ixekizumab Brodalumab	Plaque psoriasis Psoriatic arthritis Ankylosing spondylitis
Anti-T-lymphocyte agents	Basiliximab Abatacept Belatacept	Immunosuppression induction prior to solid organ transplantation Inflammatory arthritides
CD52-targeted agents	Alemtuzumab	Immunosuppression induction prior to solid organ transplantation Lymphoproliferative disorders Multiple sclerosis
IL-6 inhibitors	Tocilizumab	Rheumatoid arthritis
JAK inhibitors	Tofacitinib Baricitinib Ruxolitinib	Rheumatoid arthritis Psoriatic arthritis Myelofibrosis Polycythaemia rubra vera
BTK inhibitors	Ibrutinib Acalabrutinib	Lymphoproliferative disorders Graft-versus-host disease
BCR-Abl inhibitors	Imatinib Dasatinib Nilotinib Ponatinib	Myeloproliferative and lymphoproliferative disorders Gastrointestinal stromal tumour
PI3K inhibitors	Idelalisib Copanlisib Duvelisib Alpelisib	Lymphoproliferative disorders Breast cancer
Anti-CD20 agents	Rituximab	Inflammatory arthritides Lymphoproliferative disorders

TNF-α tumour necrosis factor-alpha, *JAK* Janus associated kinases, *BTK* Bruton's tyrosine kinase, *PI3K* phosphatidylinositol 3-kinase

Invasive Candidiasis

Clinical Presentation of Invasive Candidiasis

Changes have recently been made to the classification and nomenclature of several fungal species, including some of those previously known as *Candida* species [1]. For simplicity, the generic terms *Candida* and 'candidiasis' in this chapter refer to those species currently and recently known as *Candida* species.

Invasive candidiasis can manifest as candidaemia, deep-seated *Candida* infection or as a combination of both. Candidaemia may present as sepsis or septic shock or more subtly with low-grade fever and other non-specific symptoms. Potential distant sites of infection in the setting of candidaemia can include the eyes (e.g. endophthalmitis), heart valves (e.g. infective endocarditis) and other organs including the kidneys, bone, joints or brain. Oropharyngeal and oesophageal candidiasis, although not strictly invasive in nature, can also occur in isolation or in association with candidaemia.

The sensitivity of blood cultures for the diagnosis of invasive candidiasis is relatively low, in the realm of 50% [2], and therefore empiric antifungal treatment may be required in cases in which there is a high degree of suspicion.

Biologics and Targeted Therapies Associated with Increased Risk of Invasive Candidiasis

Invasive candidiasis is a relatively infrequent complication of the use of biologics and targeted therapies. However, the use of biologics in combination with other immunosuppressants, including corticosteroids, can result in invasive candidiasis in settings where the risk associated with single-agent biologic or targeted therapy is low.

TNF-α Inhibitors (E.G. Infliximab, Etanercept, Adalimumab, Certolizumab, Golimumab)

Tumour necrosis factor alpha (TNF-α) is involved in the immune response to fungal pathogens, including *Candida* species [3], and the risk of IFD is increased in association with the use of anti-TNF-α agents, particularly in the setting of combination immunosuppression [4].

Infrequent cases of candidaemia and oesophageal candidiasis have been reported in association with the use of TNF-α inhibitors for IBD and inflammatory arthritis in both children [5] and adults [6], although these have often occurred in patients with other risk factors for invasive candidiasis, including central venous access lines and corticosteroid use. There is some evidence of infliximab conferring a higher risk for invasive candidiasis than etanercept [7]. Certolizumab and golimumab, also, have been responsible for occasional cases of oesophageal candidiasis [8, 9].

A 2008 review of IFD reported with the use of the TNF-α inhibitors available at the time (infliximab, etanercept and adalimumab) found that candidiasis represented 23% of published cases of IFD in this setting [10]. These reports however included cases of oropharyngeal and oesophageal candidiasis, and the majority of patients were receiving TNF-α inhibitors for graft-versus-host disease and therefore likely had other immunodeficiencies that may have contributed to their risk of invasive candidiasis. The overall frequency of invasive candidiasis in patients taking TNF-α inhibitors is low; a 2013 meta-analysis of more than 4000 patients receiving these agents found only six cases of oral or oesophageal candidiasis and no further cases of invasive candidiasis [11].

Anti-IL-17 Agents (Secukinumab, Ixekizumab, Brodalumab)

An increased risk of mucocutaneous, but not invasive, candidiasis is seen in association with the use of anti-IL-17 agents. It has been previously noted that individuals with functional deficiencies in or antibodies against IL-17 are at risk of developing chronic mucocutaneous candidiasis [12], suggesting that this pathway plays an important role in the defence against candidal infection. A 2017 review of published clinical trials of patients with psoriasis or psoriatic arthritis receiving IL-17 inhibitors reported *Candida* infections in 4.0% of patients on brodalumab, 3.3% of patients on ixekizumab and 1.7% of patients on secukinumab [13]. The majority of these infections were mild or moderate in severity and did not require discontinuation of treatment. Most could be managed with topical therapy. Long-term data suggest similar findings, with an increased frequency of mucocutaneous candidiasis but no cases of invasive candidiasis in more than 96,000 patient-years of exposure to secukinumab [14].

Other Agents with Reported Associations with Invasive Candidiasis

Occasional cases of invasive candidiasis have been reported in association with the use of a number of other biologic and targeted agents, including anti-T-lymphocyte therapies, anti-CD52 agents, IL-6-targeted agents, Janus associated kinase (JAK) inhibitors and Bruton's tyrosine kinase (BTK) inhibitors. Whether these agents are directly responsible for the development of invasive candidiasis has not been elucidated.

Basiliximab and abatacept are anti-T-lymphocyte biologics. Although cases of invasive candidiasis have been reported in patients receiving basiliximab, a study comparing basiliximab to placebo in renal transplant recipients prescribed three other immunosuppressants found no difference in the rate of fungal infections, of which candidiasis was the most common, in the 6 months following basiliximab administration [15]. Invasive candidiasis has also been reported in paediatric patients receiving basiliximab for immunosuppression induction in the setting of small bowel transplantation [16], although these patients have multiple other risk factors for invasive candidiasis. Abatacept has been associated with infrequent cases of invasive candidiasis; in an integrated safety analysis of abatacept use in over 4000 patients with rheumatoid arthritis, cases of systemic candidiasis occurred at a rate of 0.01 events/100 patient-years [17].

Alemtuzumab, a CD52-targeted agent, has also been associated with cases of invasive candidiasis [18]. In a retrospective cohort of 85 solid organ transplant patients receiving alemtuzumab, 10% developed fungal infections, most of which were due to *Candida* species. In 68% of these cases, fungal infection was disseminated [19].

Occasional cases of invasive candidiasis have been reported in patients receiving tocilizumab, an IL-6 inhibitor. Cumulative safety data examining over 8000 patient-years of exposure however demonstrated only six cases of invasive candidiasis [20]. Case reports of oesophageal candidiasis have been reported in association with the use of tofacitinib, a JAK inhibitor [21, 22]. Candidaemia has also been infrequently seen during the use of ibrutinib, a BTK inhibitor, although non-*Candida* IFD is much more common in this setting [23].

Impact of Biologics and Targeted Therapies on Investigation, Treatment and Prophylaxis of Invasive Candidiasis

The small increased risk of invasive candidiasis in patients taking TNF-α inhibitors does not warrant anti-*Candida* prophylaxis. TNF-α inhibitors should be withheld in the setting of serious infection, including invasive candidiasis, and recommenced only when the infection has been adequately treated and a clinical response observed [24]. Mucocutaneous candidiasis can be treated using usual treatment protocols without discontinuation of the TNF-α inhibitor.

Patients planned for IL-17 inhibitors should be screened with history and examination for evidence of mucocutaneous candidiasis, which should be treated prior to commencement. These patients should also be monitored during treatment for symptoms and signs of candidiasis, with prompt treatment instituted if necessary. In most cases, topical antifungal therapy and continuation of IL-17 inhibitor treatment are appropriate, but culture and susceptibility testing, in addition to systemic antifungal treatment, should be considered in refractory cases [13]. Antifungal prophylaxis is not required.

In most cases, other biologic or targeted therapies should be temporarily withheld in patients who develop invasive candidiasis. These agents can be recommenced when the infection has been treated and the patient has begun to clinically recover.

Cryptococcosis

Clinical Presentation of Cryptococcosis

Cryptococcosis is an invasive fungal infection caused by *Cryptococcus neoformans* or *Cryptococcus gattii*, environmental basidiomycetous encapsulated yeasts. *Cryptococcus* spp. typically cause meningoencephalitis or pneumonia but have a wide range of clinical manifestations including cryptococcoma formation, skin disease, ophthalmitis, osteomyelitis and disseminated disease, which may initially present as fever or undifferentiated sepsis. There is a high incidence of acute respiratory distress syndrome, severe neurologic complications and death [25]. Cryptococcosis should be strongly considered in any patient with risk factors who presents with fevers, headache, encephalopathy, respiratory symptoms or suspicious skin lesions.

Cryptococcus neoformans typically infects immunocompromised patients, with the majority of cases worldwide occurring in patients with advanced HIV or other immunocompromising conditions that impair cell-mediated immunity, such as haematologic malignancy and solid organ transplants. *Cryptococcus gattii* represents 5–40% of cryptococcosis worldwide with higher incidence in the tropics and Australasia [26]. Both *C. neoformans* and *C. gattii* have similar predisposing risk factors; however unlike *C. neoformans* the majority of *C. gattii* cases occur in immunocompetent hosts. *C. gattii* has a similar spectrum of clinical presentation with a stronger predilection for pulmonary disease and large cryptococcoma formation [27].

Biologics and Targeted Therapies Associated with Increased Risk of Cryptococcosis

Cryptococcosis has been reported with the use of biologics including TNF-α inhibitors, BTK inhibitors and many others. Agents which impair either CD4+ T cells or macrophages are particularly high risk. The precise risk attributable to each biologic therapy is unclear given that many patients are also receiving cytotoxic chemotherapy or steroids, many are immunosuppressed due to malignancy and because cryptococcosis also occurs in immunocompetent hosts.

TNF-α Inhibitors

TNF-α is a proinflammatory cytokine produced by macrophages and T lymphocytes and is essential for many elements of the antifungal immune response including phagocyte activation and chemotaxis, neutrophil activation and oxidative bursts and granuloma formation and integrity [28].

There are case reports of cryptococcosis associated with the use of infliximab [29, 30], adalimumab [31], etanercept [32], golimumab [33] and certolizumab [34]. A 2014 meta-analysis of biologic therapies demonstrated an increased risk of opportunistic infections in the subgroup taking TNF-α inhibitors (OR 2.10, 95% CI 1.27–3.45), but there were only nine cases of IFD in all studies analysed, eight in the biologic treatment group (five aspergillosis, two histoplasmosis and one coccidioidomycosis) and one in the control group (cryptococcosis) [35]. Therefore, the association is uncertain.

Infliximab may confer the highest risk for cryptococcosis among TNF-α inhibitors, and this has been attributed to its antagonism of both membrane-bound and soluble receptors [28].

Ibrutinib and Other Tyrosine Kinase Inhibitors

Ibrutinib has been linked to increased incidence of IFD, including cryptococcosis [36, 37]. Ibrutinib is thought to increase susceptibility to cryptococcosis through direct inhibition of B cells, impaired monocyte and macrophage function, decreased levels of anti-cryptococcal IgM and off-target kinase inhibition, which inhibits CD4+ T cell-mediated phagocytosis [36, 38]. In the largest study thus far of patients with CLL receiving ibrutinib (n = 841), in which patients with prior HSCT were excluded, overall IFD incidence was 2.5% and cryptococcosis incidence was 0.6% [39]. In one review of published cases of cryptococcosis in patients receiving ibrutinib, 66% developed within the first 6 months of ibrutinib therapy [40]. There are no specific recommendations for cryptococcal prophylaxis in patients receiving ibrutinib.

Acalabrutinib, a BTK inhibitor closely related to ibrutinib, has also been linked to cases of cryptococcosis [41, 42].

Ruxolitinib has been linked to IFD, including cases of cryptococcosis [43, 44]. It is thought to increase susceptibility to fungal infections by inhibition of JAK-STAT signalling which impairs T-cell-macrophage crosstalk, affecting macrophage and effector cell functions. One 2017 study of infections associated with ruxolitinib in patients with myelofibrosis found cryptococcosis represented 9% of all reported infections [45]. Another 2017 multicentre study of patients with myelofibrosis treated with ruxolitinib however reported a lower total IFD incidence of 0.8/100 person-years [46].

Cryptococcal infections have been occasionally reported with many other small molecule kinase inhibitors including BCR-Abl inhibitors such as imatinib [47], phosphatidylinositol 3-kinase (PI3K) inhibitors such as idelalisib [48] and copanlisib [49], JAK-STAT inhibitors such as tofacitinib [21, 50] and multitargeted kinase inhibitors such as crizotinib [51].

Other Biologic and Targeted Therapies with Reported Associations with Cryptococcosis

Alemtuzumab targets CD52, which is present on lymphocytes, monocytes and natural killer cells. It causes profound lymphocyte depletion lasting up to 18 months and has been linked to cryptococcosis.

One study of 121 patients with pancreas transplants receiving alemtuzumab induction therapy in addition to other immunosuppressants reported 6.6% incidence of IFD, including three cases (0.24%) of cryptococcosis [52]. Another study of 542 solid organ transplant recipients receiving alemtuzumab induction therapy reported 3.3% IFD incidence, with two cases (0.37%) of cryptococcosis [53].

Cryptococcosis risk due to alemtuzumab may be dose-dependent. In a cohort of 1561 solid organ transplant recipients, incidence of cryptococcosis was 0.26% in those who received neither alemtuzumab nor anti-thymocyte globulin, 0.3% in those who received one dose and 2.24% in those who received two doses or more [54].

Cryptococcosis has been reported with the use of checkpoint inhibitors such as nivolumab, pembrolizumab and ipilimumab; however this risk is probably conferred by concurrent steroid use and lymphopenia [55]. Anti-PD1 therapy has been used to treat cryptococcosis with success in murine trials [56].

Other agents with case reports of cryptococcal infection during therapy include rituximab [57], tocilizumab [20, 58], natalizumab [59], fingolimod [60] and bortezomib [61].

Impact of Biologics and Targeted Therapies on Investigation, Treatment and Prophylaxis of Cryptococcosis

Treatment of non-HIV cryptococcosis is largely extrapolated from the HIV literature. Cryptococcosis treatment includes antifungal therapy, immune modulation (if possible) and intracranial hypertension management. Antifungal therapy in patients receiving biologic or targeted therapies is generally in keeping with standard treatment guidelines.

If possible, immunosuppression should be reduced in a sequential manner to reduce the chance of immune reconstitution inflammatory syndrome (IRIS) and other risks such as allograft loss in transplant patients [62]. Steroid therapy should generally be reduced first given its significant contribution to cryptococcosis risk [62, 63]. High-risk agents such as infliximab should be ceased during treatment of any serious infection, including cryptococcosis [64]. All patients should be monitored for clinical relapse and for IRIS, which develops in 5–11% of solid organ transplant recipients after initiation of antifungal therapy for cryptococcosis and requires adjuvant steroid treatment [62]. Patients with intensive immunosuppression regimens may require consolidation therapy with fluconazole beyond 12 months.

Common drug interactions in cohorts with cryptococcosis include those involving fluconazole, which inhibits CYP3A4 metabolism and increases serum concentrations of calcineurin inhibitors, mTOR inhibitors and ibrutinib.

Invasive Mould Disease

Clinical Presentation of Invasive Mould Disease

Aspergillosis is the most common cause of invasive mould disease (IMD) and most often manifests as pulmonary disease. Invasive pulmonary aspergillosis often presents with subacute respiratory symptoms, fevers unresponsive to antibacterial therapy or pulmonary changes on imaging with or without clinical symptoms and signs. Bronchoscopic samples and molecular and serological testing are often required for diagnosis. Less common forms of invasive aspergillosis can include tracheobronchitis, rhinosinusitis, central nervous system (CNS) infection, endophthalmitis, endocarditis and cutaneous or gastrointestinal infection. Disseminated disease is a particular concern in immunocompromised hosts, and an increased incidence of CNS aspergillosis has been observed in some patients receiving ibrutinib therapy

[37, 65], Infections involving other atypical sites, including the eye, have also been reported in patients receiving ibrutinib [65].

Other potential causes of IMD include *Fusarium* species, mucormycosis, *Scedosporium* and *Lomentospora* species and occasionally other rare moulds. Invasive fusariosis often presents with fungaemia in the immunocompromised, but can also involve the upper and lower respiratory tracts, including the sinuses, and the skin. Central line-associated infections have also occurred. *Scedosporium* and *Lomentospora* species can infect the respiratory tract or manifest in the eye, CNS, skin and bone. Disseminated infections can occur in significantly immunocompromised hosts. Mucormycosis can be associated with potentially aggressive invasive rhinocerebral disease or pulmonary, cutaneous, gastrointestinal, CNS or disseminated disease.

Biologics and Targeted Therapies Associated with Increased Risk of Invasive Mould Disease

IMD is an uncommon complication of biologic and targeted therapies in most settings. Patients with haematological malignancies, however, and particularly those who have received multiple previous lines of treatment and have relapsed or refractory disease, appear to be at increased risk. This may be at least partially related to immune deficits associated with the underlying condition, as is the case with chronic lymphocytic leukaemia (CLL). The concomitant use of other immunosuppressive agents, such as corticosteroids or conventional chemotherapy, in addition to disease- or therapy-related neutropenia, also significantly increases the risk of IMD.

BTK Inhibitors

Ibrutinib and acalabrutinib are BTK inhibitors; BTK mediates B-cell receptor signalling and may also play a role in T-cell-mediated immunity and macrophage function [66].

BTK inhibition has been clearly associated with an increased risk of invasive mould infections, particularly aspergillosis, although this is partially confounded by the underlying immune deficits seen in patients with CLL, which affect the complement system, cell-mediated immunity and humoural immunity [67]. Although IMD was not identified in initial clinical trials of ibrutinib as a significant adverse effect, post-marketing clinical experience has clearly demonstrated an association. Early reports of IMD complicating ibrutinib therapy were published in 2017 and included patients who developed invasive aspergillosis, including CNS aspergillosis, whilst receiving single-agent ibrutinib [68]. IMD incidence in some of these early studies was extremely high, up to 39% [68] in patients with CNS lymphoma receiving ibrutinib in combination with other chemotherapeutic agents, but subsequent studies have generally reported lower rates. Several retrospective reviews including patients with CLL or other lymphoproliferative disorders receiving ibrutinib have subsequently reported IMD incidence ranging from 1.7% to 12% [23, 39, 65, 69].

The most common manifestation of IMD in patients on ibrutinib appears to be invasive aspergillosis [70], and a greater than expected incidence of CNS invasive aspergillosis has also been reported in this patient cohort. Up to 60% of patients receiving ibrutinib who develop invasive aspergillosis have CNS involvement, often without pulmonary or sinus disease [38]. This risk of CNS disease appears to be particularly high in patients receiving ibrutinib for the treatment of CNS lymphoma, possibly due to the concomitant use of other immunosuppressants, including corticosteroids [68, 71]. IMD tends to occur relatively early in the course of ibrutinib therapy, with a median duration of ibrutinib therapy of 3 months prior to IMD onset [72, 73]. Patients with refractory or relapsed disease, or those who have been heavily pre-treated, appear to be at higher risk of developing IMD whilst taking ibrutinib [74].

Non-*Aspergillus* IMD has also been reported with the use of BTK inhibitors. Cases of mucormycosis [73, 75–77], fusariosis [78, 79] and *Lomentospora prolificans* [65] infection highlight the broad spectrum of IMD potentially associated with ibrutinib.

Other Agents with Reported Associations with Invasive Mould Disease

Cases of IMD have been reported during the use of multiple other biologic and targeted therapies, although at a lower frequency than in patients receiving ibrutinib. Infrequent cases of IMD have been documented in patients receiving TNF-α inhibitors [7, 80, 81], anti-B-cell agents including ofatumumab [82], the multikinase inhibitor sorafenib [83], the JAK inhibitor ruxolitinib [84], anti-CD52 agent alemtuzumab [85] and the PI3K inhibitors idelalisib [86] and copanlisib [87]. Factors increasing the risk of IMD in these patients include neutropenia and concomitant corticosteroid use [36]. The underlying disease for which the biologic is being administered is also often a contributing factor, particularly in the case of CLL and other haematological malignancies, which may be associated with broad immune system effects.

A 2008 literature review of fungal infections associated with the use of TNF-α inhibitors found 64 reported cases of invasive aspergillosis, 75% of which occurred in patients receiving infliximab for graft-versus-host disease and who were also receiving other immunosuppressants [10]. IMD associated with the use of TNF-α inhibitors alone appears to be rare.

Impact of Biologics and Targeted Therapies on Investigation, Treatment and Prophylaxis of Invasive Mould Disease

Although the risk of IMD associated with ibrutinib therapy is moderate (<10% in most published studies), a high degree of suspicion should be maintained, particularly during the first 6 months of therapy when IMD risk is highest. Any concerning clinical features of possible IMD, particularly those suggesting CNS involvement, should be promptly investigated as the potential for significant morbidity and mortality is high. Routine anti-mould prophylaxis is not recommended [71], but prophylaxis can be considered in patients with other risk factors for IMD, such as a history of relapsed or refractory underlying haematological malignancy [74]. Ibrutinib should be withheld in patients with IMD until the infection has been appropriately treated [88]. Secondary propylaxis should be considered.

There is the potential for significant drug interactions between both ibrutinib and idelalisib and CYP3A4 inhibitors, such as azoles. Exposure to ibrutinib increases significantly when it is given with azoles, and ibrutinib dose reduction is recommended in this setting [89]. Close monitoring for signs of ibrutinib toxicity is required [89, 90]. No dose adjustment is required for idelalisib when this agent is used with azoles but close monitoring for idelalisib toxicity is recommended [89].

IMD should be considered in the differential diagnosis of respiratory, sinus or other unexplained symptoms in patients receiving other biologic and targeted therapies, particularly if other immunosuppressants are also being used or the patient is neutropenic. In general, biologic and targeted therapies should be withheld in patients being treated for IMD and only reinstituted once clinical recovery has occurred.

Pneumocystis jirovecii Pneumonia

Clinical Presentation of *Pneumocystis jirovecii* Pneumonia

Pneumocystis jirovecii (previously *Pneumocystis carinii*) is a unicellular fungus which is a common and life-threatening cause of pneumonia in immunocompromised patients [91]. *Pneumocystis jirovecii* pneumonia (PJP) classically presents with a fever, dry cough and hypoxia. The clinical course of PJP may be more fulminant or atypical in immunocompromised patients without HIV, who can progress rapidly to hypoxic respiratory failure and death [92]. Almost all patients are hypoxic at rest or on minimal exertion. Pneumothoraces are common complications, whilst extrapulmonary disease is very rare. Diagnosis can be confirmed with an induced sputum or bronchoalveolar lavage with dye-based staining, fluorescent antibody staining or polymerase chain reaction assay confirming the presence of *Pneumocystis jirovecii.*

PJP prophylaxis with trimethoprim-sulfamethoxazole (TMP-SMX) in high-risk groups reduces infections and mortality. In a Cochrane systematic review, TMP-SMX prophylaxis reduced PJP incidence by 85% (relative risk [RR] 0.15, 95% confidence interval [CI] 0.04–0.62) and PJP-related mortality by 83% in non-HIV immunocompromised patients (RR 0.17, 95% CI 0.03–0.95) [93].

Biologics and Targeted Therapies Associated with Increased Risk of *Pneumocystis jirovecii* Pneumonia

It is difficult to precisely attribute risk of PJP to many biologics due to coexisting risk factors such as malignancy, transplants or steroid use, the impact of prophylaxis and the novelty of many agents [93]. This review will discuss the biologics with the strongest evidence of risk for PJP.

Anti-CD52 Therapy

Alemtuzumab has been linked to increased incidence of many bacterial, viral and fungal infections, including PJP, although precise risk estimates are lacking. Universal PJP prophylaxis is recommended for alemtuzumab recipients [94].

In a Center for International Blood and Marrow Transplant Research database analysis of allogeneic and autologous haematopoietic stem cell transplant (HSCT) recipients, overall PJP incidence was 0.63% and 0.28%, respectively [95]. Eighty-five percent of all patients received PJP prophylaxis and those receiving alemtuzumab had a higher relative risk of PJP compared to those receiving traditional graft-versus-host disease prophylaxis with methotrexate and a calcineurin inhibitor (RR = 5, $P < 0.022$, prevalence 4.6%).

A 2018 study of 6270 kidney or combined kidney-pancreas transplant recipients receiving universal PJP prophylaxis reported a 0.45% incidence of PJP with a non-significant trend towards increased risk of PJP in patients who received alemtuzumab (19/28 PJP cases, OR 4.4, $P > 0.05$) [96].

PI3K Inhibitors

Phosphatidylinositol 3-kinase (PI3K) is a lipid kinase downstream to the B-cell receptor which is key in B-cell proliferation, survival and motility and is pathologically activated in several B-cell malignancies [28].

Idelalisib significantly increases the risk of PJP and prophylaxis is universally recommended, although precise risk estimates are lacking [28]. Incidence of PJP in clinical trials ranged from 2 to 5%, including trials where it was often co-administered with other treatments that increase PJP risk such as bendamustine, rituximab and ofatumumab [86, 97]. In a post-marketing cohort of 2198 patients receiving idelalisib, with or without rituximab ± bendamustine, reported PJP incidence was 2.5% in patients receiving idelalisib and 0.2% in patients receiving only rituximab ± bendamustine [98]. PJP prophylaxis appears to reduce the incidence of PJP infection in patients receiving idelalisib; in one large phase III trial, despite an overall PJP incidence of 2%, only one case of PJP occurred in the 66% of patients prescribed with PJP prophylaxis [86]. A 2020 retrospective review, however, reported a lower rate of PJP (1%) in 900 patients with lymphoid malignancies, despite low PJP prophylaxis coverage of 25–37% [99].

Cases of PJP have also been reported in association with copanlisib and duvelisib. Some authors, and the drug manufacturer, suggest universal PJP prophylaxis for patients receiving copanlisib, as for idelalisib, whilst other authors recommend prophylaxis only in high-risk patients [100]. A 2019 review of copanlisib in non-Hodgkin's lymphoma reported a PJP incidence of 0.6% and recommended considering prophylaxis for high-risk patients but not universally [101].

A phase I/II study of 32 patients with refractory CLL receiving duvelisib reported three cases of PJP despite the use of prophylaxis in all three cases [102]. The US Food and Drug Administration (FDA) data in respect to patients receiving duvelisib suggested an overall PJP incidence of 1% and recommends universal prophylaxis until treatment cessation and CD4 cell counts are >200 cells per microlitre [103].

No cases of PJP have been reported to date in association with the use of alpelisib, an oral inhibitor of PI3K alpha [104].

TNF-α Inhibitors

TNF-α is a proinflammatory cytokine produced by macrophages and T lymphocytes with many downstream effects including macrophage and neutrophil activation (including neutrophil-mediated oxidative bursts for fungal disease), promotion of phagocytic function, chemotaxis and granuloma formation and integrity [28]. Anti-TNF-α agents have a risk gradient of infection, with the highest risk associated with infliximab followed by adalimumab and the lowest risk associated with etanercept, which is thought to reflect the lack of membrane-bound receptor antagonism in etanercept [28].

Studies and post-marketing surveillance in patients on TNF-α inhibitors have reported PJP incidences from 0.1% to 0.4% [35, 105, 106]. A Japanese study of 702 patients with rheumatoid arthritis receiving TNF-α inhibitors or tocilizumab showed a significant increase in PJP incidence in those with age ≥ 65 (relative risk [RR] 4.37), coexisting pulmonary disease (RR 8.13) and glucocorticoid use (RR 11.4) [105]. A second-stage protocol of administering PJP prophylaxis to all patients with ≥2 of these three risk factors reduced overall incidence from 0.93 per 100 person-years to zero, with a number needed to treat of 19.9 and no severe adverse effects from prophylaxis [105].

There are no authorities which recommend universal PJP prophylaxis in patients receiving TNF-α inhibitors; however prophylaxis should be considered in the presence of coexisting risk factors [105].

BTK Inhibitors

BTK inhibitors (ibrutinib and acalabrutinib) inhibit BTK, a protein which is present in B cells, myeloid cells, mast cells and platelets, in order to downregulate their immune activity.

Many serious infections have been linked to BTK inhibitors, including PJP [37]. In a multicentre cohort examining IFD in CLL patients receiving ibrutinib, invasive aspergillosis was the most common form of IFD, representing 82% of IFD, followed by PJP at 12% [73]. It has been postulated that increased fungal susceptibility is the result of off-target effects of ibrutinib on other kinases, such as IL-2-inducible T-cell kinases, which weakens the immune response of T helper cells [74].

A 2020 study of 217 patients with CLL receiving ibrutinib or acalabrutinib alone or in combination with umbralisib or chemotherapy, in which 41% of patients were prescribed PJP prophylaxis, reported a 3.4% incidence of PJP in those without prophylaxis and no cases among patients who received prophylaxis [107]. Other studies involving patients with lymphoid malignancies taking ibrutinib have found incidences from 0.8–3%, including many PJP cases in patients without concurrent immunosuppression or lymphopenia [23, 108].

Ibrutinib used alone is not considered a sufficient indication for routine PJP prophylaxis; however it may be considered in the presence of other risk factors such as haematopoietic stem cell transplant, chemotherapy, neutropenia or prolonged steroid use [109].

Acalabrutinib is a more selective oral irreversible BTK inhibitor than ibrutinib. Acalabrutinib safety data are limited although it has been linked to cases of serious and opportunistic infections, including PJP [42]. A phase III trial comparing it to ibrutinib for relapsed CLL is ongoing (NCT02477696—completion due March 2021).

Other Agents with Reported Associations with PJP

Many other new biologic agents have been linked to cases of PJP, although the attributable risk of biologic therapy is often difficult to distinguish among other risk factors among the immunocompromised cohort receiving it.

Rituximab use has been linked to increased risk of PJP infection, and mortality rates of 30% have been reported in this setting [110]. In a 2015 systematic review of PJP in rituximab-treated lymphoma patients, rituximab was associated with an increased risk of PJP (2.9% vs. 0.5%; $p = 0.001$) [111]. Prescribing prophylaxis to such patients significantly reduced the risk of infection (0% vs. 2.6%; $p = 0.04$). Another study of CLL patients treated with idelalisib compared to idelalisib and rituximab found no statistical difference in PJP incidence between groups with a 3% total overall incidence [112]. PJP incidence is lower in patients with inflammatory arthritides receiving rituximab than in those with haematological malignancies receiving the agent [113]. Currently, the FDA recommends PJP prophylaxis in patients with lymphoma, granulomatosis with polyangiitis and microscopic polyangiitis treated with rituximab but not in patients with inflammatory arthritides [114].

Cases of PJP have been reported in patients with solid organ cancers and lymphoma receiving checkpoint inhibitors such as PD-1 inhibitors (e.g. nivolumab, pembrolizumab) and CTLA-4 inhibitors (e.g. ipilimumab) [115, 116]. These therapies frequently cause immune toxicities requiring high-dose corticosteroid and other immunosuppressive treatments, which are thought to drive the increased infection risk observed [117].

JAK inhibitors inhibit lymphocyte proliferation and also affect dendritic cells and cytokine production. They confer a small increased risk of serious infections, and PJP has also been reported [28, 118]. A Japanese post-marketing surveillance study of patients on tofacitinib for rheumatoid arthritis reported PJP incidence of 0.4% [119]. PJP prophylaxis is not indicated without coexisting risk factors.

Belatacept binds to CD80 and CD86, inhibiting a CD28-mediated interaction between antigen-presenting cells and T cells, reducing cytokine production and T-lymphocyte proliferation. A retrospective case-control study of renal transplant patients treated with belatacept demonstrated increased risk of PJP in this subgroup (4.3%); however this may have been caused by older age, more baseline lymphopenia and lower eGFR in this cohort [120].

Abatacept also blocks CD86 and CD28, albeit less completely than belatacept. Post-marketing surveillance has shown a PJP incidence of 0.1% [106], and there are no recommendations for PJP prophylaxis.

Many other biologics have occasionally been associated with PJP in the literature: IL-1 antagonists (e.g. anakinra), IL-2 antagonists (basiliximab), α-4 integrin inhibitors (natalizumab), CD3 receptor inhibitors (muromonab), proteasome inhibitors (bortezomib) [121] and BCR-Abl inhibitors (e.g. imatinib, ponatinib, dasatinib). These agents do not require prophylaxis without coexisting indications.

Impact of Biologics and Targeted Therapies on Investigation, Treatment and Prophylaxis of *Pneumocystis jirovecii* Pneumonia

PJP may lead to more fulminant respiratory failure in patients without HIV, including those on biologics, than in patients with HIV. When PJP is suspected, the biologic therapy should be withheld. In confirmed PJP, any agents that confer a significant risk of PJP should be discontinued, including alemtuzumab, idelalisib, copanlisib, duvelisib, rituximab and infliximab. PJP should otherwise be treated according to normal protocols including antibiotics, steroids and respiratory support where indicated. Secondary prophylaxis may be considered.

Table 21.2 displays commonly used biologics and whether PJP prophylaxis is recommended in the absence of coexisting indications such as corticosteroids, prolonged lymphopenia, solid organ or haematopoietic stem cell transplantation, certain malignancies or chemotherapies. Biologics for which universal PJP prophylaxis is recommended include alemtuzumab, idelalisib and copanlisib, whilst many other agents are linked to PJP but only require prophylaxis in the setting of additional risk factors.

Table 21.2 Common biologic therapies and whether PJP prophylaxis is indicated [24, 28, 122–126]

Drug	PJP prophylaxis indicated?	Duration	Incidence without prophylaxis	Indication summary
Alemtuzumab (anti-CD52)	Universally indicated	6–12 months after cessation	0.5–4.5% [95, 96]	Most guidelines recommend PJP prophylaxis after alemtuzumab for whichever is greater of 6–12 months or until CD4 counts are >200 cells/μL [18, 94, 95, 127]
Idelalisib (PI3K inhibitor)	Universally indicated	2–6 months post cessation	1–5% [86, 97, 128]	Universal PJP prophylaxis recommended [28, 71, 129]
Duvelisib (PI3K inhibitor)	Universally indicated	Until CD4 ≥ 200	Data lacking 1–9%	FDA recommendation for universal prophylaxis [103]

(continued)

Table 21.2 (continued)

Drug	PJP prophylaxis indicated?	Duration	Incidence without prophylaxis	Indication summary
Copanlisib (PI3K inhibitor)	Universally or sometimes indicated according to source	No consensus	Data lacking, 0.6% in one study of non-Hodgkin's lymphoma	Some authors and the manufacturer recommended universal prophylaxis, the FDA only for high-risk patients [100, 101, 130]
Rituximab and ocrelizumab (anti-CD20 agents)	Indicated in high-risk patients	Up to 12 months (FDA)	Varies depending on indication	FDA recommends prophylaxis in CLL, GPA, MPA, solid organ transplant or with other risk factors[a] [111]
Ibrutinib (BTK inhibitors)	Indicated in high-risk patients	Unknown	0.7–3% in lymphoid malignancy	Not recommended unless concurrent indication [109]
Infliximab, etanercept, adalimumab (TNF inhibitors)	Indicated in high-risk patients (no consensus)	Unknown	0.1–0.3% in RA	Some authors suggest prophylaxis indicated if ≥2 of age > 65, comorbid lung disease and steroid usage [105]. Infliximab is highest risk
Belatacept, abatacept (anti-T-cell agents)	Not usually indicated[a]	–	Rare	
Nivolumab, pembrolizumab (checkpoint inhibitors)	Not usually indicated[a]	–	Rare	Indicated if immune complications treated with high-dose steroids[b]
Imatinib, ponatinib, dasatinib (BCR-Abl inhibitors)	Not usually indicated[a]	–	Rare [129]	
Anakinra (IL-1 antagonist)	Not usually indicated[a]		Rare	
Natalizumab (a4 integrin inhibitors)	Not usually indicated[a]		Rare	

[a] Common coexisting risk factors which may indicate PJP prophylaxis include allogeneic stem cell transplant, solid organ transplant, corticosteroid dose ≥20 mg prednisolone daily for ≥4 weeks, acute lymphocytic leukaemia, non-Hodgkin's lymphoma or Hodgkin's lymphoma with high-intensity chemotherapy (e.g. R-CHOP, fludarabine, gemcitabine, high-dose methotrexate, temozolomide), T-cell-depleting therapy

[b] Corticosteroids equivalent of ≥20 mg prednisolone daily for ≥4 weeks

Other Invasive Fungal Diseases Including Endemic Mycoses

Clinical Presentation of Endemic Mycoses

Endemic mycoses include, most commonly, histoplasmosis, coccidioidomycosis, paracoccidioidomycosis, blastomycosis and talaromycosis.

Histoplasmosis is the most prevalent endemic mycosis in the United States, although cases have occurred worldwide. It most often causes pulmonary or asymptomatic disease, although immunocompromised patients may present with disseminated disease manifested by pancytopenia, hepatosplenomegaly and multiorgan involvement. Histoplasmosis can present soon after an exposure or reactivate many years later, particularly in the context of immunosuppression.

Blastomycosis and coccidioidomycosis are also most commonly found in the United States and cause primarily pulmonary disease, although multiple body sites can be involved and disseminated disease can occur in immunocompromised hosts. Clinical reactivation can occur in the context of immunosuppression after previous exposure. Paracoccidioidomycosis occurs in Central and South America and again can cause pulmonary or disseminated disease. Talaromycosis occurs in Asia and causes disseminated infection in immunocompromised hosts.

Biologics and Targeted Therapies Associated with Increased Risk of Endemic Mycoses

TNF-α Inhibitors (Infliximab, Etanercept, Adalimumab, Golimumab, Certolizumab)

TNF-α appears to be the most important endogenous cytokine involved in the immune response to *Histoplasma capsulatum* infection [131], and the use of TNF-α inhibitors has been associated with a significantly increased risk of histoplasmosis and other endemic mycoses. The role of TNF-α in the T-cell and macrophage response to infection and in maintenance of granulomas is thought to be responsible for the increased risk of histoplasmosis seen in patients receiving TNF-α inhibitors [10]. Histoplasmosis was identified as the most common manifestation of invasive fungal disease (IFD) in patients taking TNF-α inhibitors in a 2008 review of published cases [10].

Infliximab is associated with the highest frequency of histoplasmosis of all the TNF-α inhibitors [132]. A 2004 review of granulomatous infections associated with the use of TNF-α inhibitors in the United States reported histoplasmosis incidence of 16.7 cases per 100,000 patients treated with infliximab and 2.7 cases per 100,000 patients treated with etanercept [132]. A 2015 multicentre retrospective review of patients receiving TNF-α inhibitors who developed histoplasmosis identified concomitant corticosteroid use as an independent predictor of disease severity; 75.5% of patients had disseminated disease [133].

Occasional cases of other endemic mycoses have been reported with the use of TNF-α inhibitors, including coccidioidomycosis [134], paracoccidioidomycosis [135] and talaromycosis [136]. Infliximab seems to be the TNF-α inhibitor associated with the greatest degree of risk for coccidioidomycosis [132, 134].

Other Agents with Reported Associations with Endemic Mycoses
Infrequent cases of histoplasmosis have been reported in association with the use of the BTK inhibitor ibrutinib [137, 138] the JAK inhibitor ruxolitinib [139] and the anti-T-cell agent abatacept [140]. Cases of blastomycosis have been reported in patients on ibrutinib [138] and abatacept [17], and talaromycosis has occurred in patients receiving ruxolitinib and the multikinase inhibitor sorafenib [141].

It should be noted that clinical trials have rarely been conducted in many regions where endemic fungi exist, and therefore the true incidence of these infections in patients receiving biologic therapies is unknown in many geographic areas.

Impact of Biologics and Targeted Therapies on Investigation, Treatment and Prophylaxis of Endemic Mycoses

In general, TNF-α inhibitors should be withheld in patients diagnosed with invasive endemic mycoses. Treatment of histoplasmosis and reduction of immunosuppression may be associated with immune reconstitution inflammatory syndrome (IRIS) in immunocompromised patients; in one multicentre retrospective review, median time to IRIS onset was 6 weeks after cessation of the TNF-α inhibitor [133]. Timing and safety of TNF-α inhibitor recommencement should be considered on a case-by-case basis.

It has been suggested that patients living in or with previous exposure to endemic areas, and who are planned for TNF-α inhibitor therapy, should have serological testing for *Histoplasma capsulatum*, *Blastomyces dermatitidis* and *Coccidioides immitis* prior to commencement of the TNF-α inhibitor [7, 142]. There is, however, no clear consensus on the optimal management of asymptomatic patients with serological evidence of histoplasmosis or coccidioidomycosis receiving, or about to commence, TNF-α inhibitors or whether these patients should receive antifungal prophylaxis [143–145]. Some authors also recommend a screening chest X-ray prior to commencement of TNF-α inhibitors in patients living in, or with exposure to, areas endemic for histoplasmosis [146].

Patients taking TNF-α inhibitors who live in endemic areas should also be counselled to avoid risk activities, such as caving and cleaning chicken coops or bird roosts [7, 146].

Conclusion

Although the overall incidence of IFD in patients receiving biologic or targeted therapies is low, awareness of these potentially serious complications of therapy is essential. Recognition of the increased IFD risk associated with specific agents, such as IMD in patients receiving BTK inhibitors, PJP in patients receiving PI3K inhibitors or endemic mycoses in patients receiving TNF-α inhibitors, is particularly important. In some instances, pre-treatment screening or prophylaxis is recommended.

The additive effect of biologic or targeted therapies to baseline IFD risk associated with the underlying disease process or other immunosuppressive agents being used should also be taken into account. The concomitant use of corticosteroids or other immunosuppressants may significantly increase the risk for IFD in patients receiving biologic and targeted therapies.

Evidence for the risk of IFD associated with biologic and targeted therapies is constantly changing as a result of growing clinical experience with these agents and with the release of new novel agents.

References

1. Borman AM, Johnson EM. Name changes for fungi of medical importance, 2018–2019. J Clin Microbiol. 2021;59:e01811.
2. Clancy CJ, Nguyen MH. Diagnosing invasive candidiasis. J Clin Microbiol. 2018;56(5):e01909.
3. Ferrante A. Tumor necrosis factor alpha potentiates neutrophil antimicrobial activity: increased fungicidal activity against Torulopsis glabrata and Candida albicans and associated increases in oxygen radical production and lysosomal enzyme release. Infect Immun. 1989;57(7):2115–22.
4. McConachie SM, Wilhelm SM, Bhargava A, Kale-Pradhan PB. Biologic-induced infections in inflammatory bowel disease: the TNF-α antagonists. Ann Pharmacother. 2018;52(6):571–9.
5. Toussi SS, Pan N, Walters HM, Walsh TJ. Infections in children and adolescents with juvenile idiopathic arthritis and inflammatory bowel disease treated with tumor necrosis factor–α inhibitors: systematic review of the literature. Clin Infect Dis. 2013;57(9):1318–30.
6. Lichtenstein GR, Feagan BG, Cohen RD, Salzberg BA, Diamond RH, Price S, et al. Serious infection and mortality in patients with Crohn's disease: more than 5 years of follow-up in the TREAT™ registry. Am J Gastroenterol. 2012;107(9):1409–22.
7. Tragiannidis A, Kyriakidis I, Zündorf I, Groll AH. Invasive fungal infections in pediatric patients treated with tumor necrosis alpha (TNF-α) inhibitors. Mycoses. 2017;60(4):222–9.
8. Bykerk VP, Cush J, Winthrop K, Calabrese L, Lortholary O, de Longueville M, et al. Update on the safety profile of certolizumab pegol in rheumatoid arthritis: an integrated analysis from clinical trials. Ann Rheum Dis. 2015;74(1):96–103.
9. Vallabhaneni S, Chiller TM. Fungal infections and new biologic therapies. Curr Rheumatol Rep. 2016;18(5):29.
10. Tsiodras S, Samonis G, Boumpas DT, Kontoyiannis DP. Fungal infections complicating tumor necrosis factor alpha blockade therapy. Mayo Clin Proc. 2008;83(2):181–94.
11. Ford AC, Peyrin-Biroulet L. Opportunistic infections with anti-tumor necrosis factor-α therapy in inflammatory bowel disease: meta-analysis of randomized controlled trials. Am J Gastroenterol. 2013;108(8):1268–76.
12. Puel A, Döffinger R, Natividad A, Chrabieh M, Barcenas-Morales G, Picard C, et al. Autoantibodies against IL-17A, IL-17F, and IL-22 in patients with chronic mucocutaneous candidiasis and autoimmune polyendocrine syndrome type I. J Exp Med. 2010;207(2):291–7.
13. Saunte DM, Mrowietz U, Puig L, Zachariae C. Candida infections in patients with psoriasis and psoriatic arthritis treated with interleukin-17 inhibitors and their practical management. Br J Dermatol. 2017;177(1):47–62.

14. Deodhar A, Mease PJ, McInnes IB, Baraliakos X, Reich K, Blauvelt A, et al. Long-term safety of secukinumab in patients with moderate-to-severe plaque psoriasis, psoriatic arthritis, and ankylosing spondylitis: integrated pooled clinical trial and post-marketing surveillance data. Arthritis Res Ther. 2019;21(1):111.
15. Ponticelli C, Yussim A, Cambi V, Legendre C, Rizzo G, Salvadori M, et al. A randomized, double-blind trial of basiliximab immunoprophylaxis plus triple therapy in kidney transplant recipients. Transplantation. 2001;72(7):1261–7.
16. Florescu DF, Islam KM, Grant W, Mercer DF, Langnas A, Botha J, et al. Incidence and outcome of fungal infections in pediatric small bowel transplant recipients. Transpl Infect Dis. 2010;12(6):497–504.
17. Schiff M. Abatacept treatment for rheumatoid arthritis. Rheumatology. 2010;50(3):437–49.
18. Thursky KA, Worth LJ, Seymour JF, Miles Prince H, Slavin MA. Spectrum of infection, risk and recommendations for prophylaxis and screening among patients with lymphoproliferative disorders treated with alemtuzumab*. Br J Haematol. 2006;132(1):3–12.
19. Safdar N, Smith J, Knasinski V, Sherkow C, Herrforth C, Knechtle S, et al. Infections after the use of alemtuzumab in solid organ transplant recipients: a comparative study. Diagn Microbiol Infect Dis. 2010;66(1):7–15.
20. Schiff MH, Kremer JM, Jahreis A, Vernon E, Isaacs JD, van Vollenhoven RF. Integrated safety in tocilizumab clinical trials. Arthritis Res Ther. 2011;13(5):R141.
21. Winthrop KL, Park SH, Gul A, Cardiel MH, Gomez-Reino JJ, Tanaka Y, et al. Tuberculosis and other opportunistic infections in tofacitinib-treated patients with rheumatoid arthritis. Ann Rheum Dis. 2016;75(6):1133–8.
22. Cohen S, Curtis JR, DeMasi R, Chen Y, Fan H, Soonasra A, et al. Worldwide, 3-year, post-marketing surveillance experience with tofacitinib in rheumatoid arthritis. Rheumatol Ther. 2018;5(1):283–91.
23. Varughese T, Taur Y, Cohen N, Palomba ML, Seo SK, Hohl TM, et al. Serious infections in patients receiving Ibrutinib for treatment of lymphoid cancer. Clin Infect Dis. 2018;67(5):687–92.
24. Baddley JW, Cantini F, Goletti D, Gómez-Reino JJ, Mylonakis E, San-Juan R, et al. ESCMID Study Group for Infections in Compromised Hosts (ESGICH) Consensus Document on the safety of targeted and biological therapies: an infectious diseases perspective (Soluble immune effector molecules [I]: anti-tumor necrosis factor-α agents). Clin Microbiol Infect. 2018;24(Suppl 2):S10–s20.
25. Kiertiburanakul S, Wirojtananugoon S, Pracharktam R, Sungkanuparph S. Cryptococcosis in human immunodeficiency virus-negative patients. Int J Infect Dis. 2006;10(1):72–8.
26. Cogliati M. Global molecular epidemiology of Cryptococcus neoformans and Cryptococcus gattii: an atlas of the molecular types. Scientifica (Cairo). 2013;2013:675213.
27. Sun H-Y, Wagener MM, Singh N. Cryptococcosis in solid-organ, hematopoietic stem cell, and tissue transplant recipients: evidence-based evolving trends. Clin Infect Dis. 2009;48(11):1566–76.
28. Davis JS, Ferreira D, Paige E, Gedye C, Boyle M. Infectious complications of biological and small molecule targeted immunomodulatory therapies. Clin Microbiol Rev. 2020;33(3):e00035–19.
29. Takazono T, Sawai T, Tashiro M, Saijo T, Yamamoto K, Imamura Y, et al. Relapsed pulmonary cryptococcosis during tumor necrosis factor α inhibitor treatment. Intern Med. 2016;55(19):2877–80.
30. Yamada S, Kajihara I, Johno T, Fukushima S, Jinnin M, Masunaga A, et al. Symptomless pulmonary cryptococcosis in a psoriatic arthritis patient during Infliximab therapy. Ann Dermatol. 2016;28(2):269–70.
31. Liao TL, Chen YM, Chen DY. Risk factors for cryptococcal infection among patients with rheumatoid arthritis receiving different immunosuppressive medications. Clin Microbiol Infect. 2016;22(9):815.e1–3.
32. Chávez-López M, Márquez-Díaz F, Aguayo-Leytte G. Meningitis criptocócica tras tratamiento con etanercept. Enferm Infecc Microbiol Clin. 2006;24(4):288.

33. Tesser J, Kafka S, DeHoratius RJ, Xu S, Hsia EC, Turkiewicz A. Efficacy and safety of intravenous golimumab plus methotrexate in patients with rheumatoid arthritis aged <65 years and those ≥65 years of age. Arthritis Res Ther. 2019;21(1):190.
34. Wysocki JD, Said SM, Papadakis KA. An uncommon cause of abdominal pain and fever in a patient with Crohn's disease. Gastroenterology. 2015;148(5):e12–3.
35. Kourbeti IS, Ziakas PD, Mylonakis E. Biologic therapies in rheumatoid arthritis and the risk of opportunistic infections: a meta-analysis. Clin Infect Dis. 2014;58(12):1649–57.
36. Zarakas MA, Desai JV, Chamilos G, Lionakis MS. Fungal infections with Ibrutinib and other small-molecule kinase inhibitors. Curr Fungal Infect Rep. 2019;13(3):86–98.
37. Chamilos G, Lionakis MS, Kontoyiannis DP. Call for action: invasive fungal infections associated with ibrutinib and other small molecule kinase inhibitors targeting immune signaling pathways. Clin Infect Dis. 2018;66(1):140–8.
38. Reynolds G, Slavin M, Teh BW. Ibrutinib and invasive fungal infections: the known, the unknown and the known unknowns. Leuk Lymphoma. 2020;61(10):2292–4.
39. Frei M, Aitken SL, Jain N, Thompson P, Wierda W, Kontoyiannis DP, et al. Incidence and characterization of fungal infections in chronic lymphocytic leukemia patients receiving ibrutinib. Leuk Lymphoma. 2020;61(10):2488–91.
40. Brochard J, Morio F, Mahe J, Le Pape P, Guimard T, Mahe B, et al. Ibrutinib, a Bruton's tyrosine kinase inhibitor, a new risk factor for cryptococcosis. Med Mal Infect. 2020;50:742–5.
41. Wilson PA, Melville K. Disseminated cryptococcal infection in a patient receiving Acalabrutinib for chronic lymphocytic leukemia. Infect Dis Clin Pract. 2019;27(3):160–2.
42. Byrd JC, Owen R, O'Brien SM, Brown JR, Hillmen P, Bitman B, et al. Pooled analysis of safety data from clinical trials evaluating Acalabrutinib monotherapy in hematologic malignancies. Blood. 2017;130(Supplement 1):4326.
43. Wysham NG, Sullivan DR, Allada G. An opportunistic infection associated with ruxolitinib, a novel janus kinase 1,2 inhibitor. Chest. 2013;143(5):1478–9.
44. Chen CC, Chen YY, Huang CE. Cryptococcal meningoencephalitis associated with the long-term use of Ruxolitinib. Ann Hematol. 2016;95(2):361–2.
45. Dioverti MV, Abu Saleh OM, Tande AJ. Infectious complications in patients on treatment with Ruxolitinib: case report and review of the literature. Infect Dis (Lond). 2018;50(5):381–7.
46. Verstovsek S, Mesa RA, Gotlib J, Gupta V, DiPersio JF, Catalano JV, et al. Long-term treatment with Ruxolitinib for patients with myelofibrosis: 5-year update from the randomized, double-blind, placebo-controlled, phase 3 COMFORT-I trial. J Hematol Oncol. 2017;10(1):55.
47. Anthony N, Shanks J, Terebelo H. Occurrences of opportunistic infections in chronic myelogenous leukemia patients treated with imatinib mesylate. Leuk Res. 2010;34(9):1250–1.
48. Hengeveld PJ, de Jongh E, Westerweel PE, Levin M-D. Disseminated cryptococcal disease during treatment with idelalisib and corticosteroids for follicular lymphoma. BMJ Case Rep. 2020;13(7):e235216.
49. Dreyling M, Morschhauser F, Bouabdallah K, Bron D, Cunningham D, Assouline SE, et al. Phase II study of copanlisib, a PI3K inhibitor, in relapsed or refractory, indolent or aggressive lymphoma. Ann Oncol. 2017;28(9):2169–78.
50. Seminario-Vidal L, Cantrell W, Elewski BE. Pulmonary cryptococcosis in the setting of tofacitinib therapy for psoriasis. J Drugs Dermatol. 2015;14(8):901–2.
51. Su C, Ren S, Li X, Hou L, Zhou C. Pseudo-progression in a patient with lung adenocarcinoma and ALK fusion who responded to crizotinib. Int J Clin Exp Med. 2016;9(6):12290–3.
52. Nath DS, Kandaswamy R, Gruessner R, Sutherland DE, Dunn DL, Humar A. Fungal infections in transplant recipients receiving alemtuzumab. Transplant Proc. 2005;37(2):934–6.
53. Peleg AY, Husain S, Kwak EJ, Silveira FP, Ndirangu M, Tran J, et al. Opportunistic infections in 547 organ transplant recipients receiving alemtuzumab, a humanized monoclonal CD-52 antibody. Clin Infect Dis. 2007;44(2):204–12.
54. Silveira FP, Husain S, Kwak EJ, Linden PK, Marcos A, Shapiro R, et al. Cryptococcosis in liver and kidney transplant recipients receiving anti-thymocyte globulin or alemtuzumab. Transpl Infect Dis. 2007;9(1):22–7.

55. Li X, Lau SKP, Woo PCY. Fungal infection risks associated with the use of cytokine antagonists and immune checkpoint inhibitors. Exp Biol Med. 2020;245(13):1104–14.
56. Roussey JA, Viglianti SP, Teitz-Tennenbaum S, Olszewski MA, Osterholzer JJ. Anti-PD-1 antibody treatment promotes clearance of persistent cryptococcal lung infection in mice. J Immunol. 2017;199(10):3535–46.
57. Wingfield T, Jani M, Krutikov M, Mayer J, Uriel A, Marks J, et al. Cryptococcal meningitis in an HIV-negative patient with rheumatoid arthritis treated with rituximab. Rheumatology. 2011;50(9):1725–7.
58. Nishioka H, Takegawa H, Kamei H. Disseminated cryptococcosis in a patient taking tocilizumab for Castleman's disease. J Infect Chemother. 2018;24(2):138–41.
59. Valenzuela RM, Pula JH, Garwacki D, Cotter J, Kattah JC. Cryptococcal meningitis in a multiple sclerosis patient taking natalizumab. J Neurol Sci. 2014;340(1–2):109–11.
60. Chong I, Wang KY, Lincoln CM. Cryptococcal meningitis in a multiple sclerosis patient treated with Fingolimod: a case report and review of imaging findings. Clin Imaging. 2019;54:53–6.
61. Marr KA, Sun Y, Spec A, Lu N, Panackal A, Bennett J, et al. A multicenter, longitudinal cohort study of cryptococcosis in human immunodeficiency virus-negative people in the United States. Clin Infect Dis. 2020;70(2):252–61.
62. Gupta AO, Singh N. Immune reconstitution syndrome and fungal infections. Curr Opin Infect Dis. 2011;24(6):527–33.
63. Henao-Martínez AF, Chastain DB, Franco-Paredes C. Treatment of cryptococcosis in non-HIV immunocompromised patients. Curr Opin Infect Dis. 2018;31(4):278–85.
64. Remicade (infliximab) [package insert]. U.S. Food and Drug Administration website. 2020. https://www.accessdata.fda.gov/drugsatfda_docs/label/2020/103772s5389s5391s5394lbl.pdf. Accessed 18 Nov 2020.
65. Teh BW, Chui W, Handunnetti S, Tam C, Worth LJ, Thursky KA, et al. High rates of proven invasive fungal disease with the use of ibrutinib monotherapy for relapsed or refractory chronic lymphocytic leukemia. Leuk Lymphoma. 2019;60(6):1572–5.
66. Fiorcari S, Maffei R, Vallerini D, Scarfò L, Barozzi P, Maccaferri M, et al. BTK inhibition impairs the innate response against fungal infection in patients with chronic lymphocytic leukemia. Front Immunol. 2020;11:2158.
67. Hilal T, Gea-Banacloche JC, Leis JF. Chronic lymphocytic leukemia and infection risk in the era of targeted therapies: linking mechanisms with infections. Blood Rev. 2018;32(5):387–99.
68. Lionakis MS, Dunleavy K, Roschewski M, Widemann BC, Butman JA, Schmitz R, et al. Inhibition of B cell receptor signaling by Ibrutinib in primary CNS lymphoma. Cancer Cell. 2017;31(6):833–43.e5.
69. Lewis KL, Chin CK, Manos K, Casey J, Hamad N, Crawford J, et al. Ibrutinib for central nervous system lymphoma: the Australasian Lymphoma Alliance/MD Anderson Cancer Center experience. Br J Haematol. 2020;192:1049–53.
70. Tillman BF, Pauff JM, Satyanarayana G, Talbott M, Warner JL. Systematic review of infectious events with the Bruton tyrosine kinase inhibitor ibrutinib in the treatment of hematologic malignancies. Eur J Haematol. 2018;100(4):325–34.
71. Maschmeyer G, De Greef J, Mellinghoff SC, Nosari A, Thiebaut-Bertrand A, Bergeron A, et al. Infections associated with immunotherapeutic and molecular targeted agents in hematology and oncology. A position paper by the European Conference on Infections in Leukemia (ECIL). Leukemia. 2019;33(4):844–62.
72. Ruchlemer R, Ben-Ami R, Bar-Meir M, Brown JR, Malphettes M, Mous R, et al. Ibrutinib-associated invasive fungal diseases in patients with chronic lymphocytic leukaemia and non-Hodgkin lymphoma: An observational study. Mycoses. 2019;62(12):1140–7.
73. Ghez D, Calleja A, Protin C, Baron M, Ledoux MP, Damaj G, et al. Early-onset invasive aspergillosis and other fungal infections in patients treated with ibrutinib. Blood. 2018;131(17):1955–9.
74. Teh BW, Tam CS, Handunnetti S, Worth LJ, Slavin MA. Infections in patients with chronic lymphocytic leukaemia: mitigating risk in the era of targeted therapies. Blood Rev. 2018;32(6):499–507.

75. Rogers KA, Luay M, Zhao Q, Wiczer T, Levine L, Zeinab EB, et al. Incidence and type of opportunistic infections during ibrutinib treatment at a single academic center. Blood. 2017;130(Supplement 1):830.
76. Grossi O, Pineau S, Sadot-Lebouvier S, Hay B, Delaunay J, Miailhe AF, et al. Disseminated mucormycosis due to Lichtheimia corymbifera during ibrutinib treatment for relapsed chronic lymphocytic leukaemia: a case report. Clin Microbiol Infect. 2019;25(2):261–3.
77. Mascarella MA, Schweitzer L, Alreefi M, Silver J, Caglar D, Loo VG, et al. The infectious thyroid nodule: a case report of mucormycosis associated with ibrutinib therapy. J Otolaryngol Head Neck Surg. 2019;48(1):49.
78. Chan TS, Au-Yeung R, Chim CS, Wong SC, Kwong YL. Disseminated fusarium infection after ibrutinib therapy in chronic lymphocytic leukaemia. Ann Hematol. 2017;96(5):871–2.
79. Anastasopoulou A, DiPippo AJ, Kontoyiannis DP. Non-Aspergillus invasive mould infections in patients treated with ibrutinib. Mycoses. 2020;63(8):787–93.
80. Marty FM, Lee SJ, Fahey MM, Alyea EP, Soiffer RJ, Antin JH, et al. Infliximab use in patients with severe graft-versus-host disease and other emerging risk factors of non-Candida invasive fungal infections in allogeneic hematopoietic stem cell transplant recipients: a cohort study. Blood. 2003;102(8):2768–76.
81. Camargo JF, Yakoub D, Cho-Vega JH. Successful treatment of primary cutaneous mucormycosis complicating anti-TNF therapy with a combination of surgical debridement and oral posaconazole. Mycopathologia. 2015;180(3):187–92.
82. Wierda WG, Kipps TJ, Mayer J, Stilgenbauer S, Williams CD, Hellmann A, et al. Ofatumumab as single-agent CD20 immunotherapy in fludarabine-refractory chronic lymphocytic leukemia. J Clin Oncol. 2010;28(10):1749–55.
83. Bazaz R, Denning DW. Subacute invasive aspergillosis associated with sorafenib therapy for hepatocellular carcinoma. Clin Infect Dis. 2018;67(1):156–7.
84. Moruno-Rodríguez A, Sánchez-Vicente JL, Rueda-Rueda T, Lechón-Caballero B, Muñoz-Morales A, López-Herrero F. Invasive aspergillosis manifesting as retinal necrosis in a patient treated with ruxolitinib. Arch Soc Esp Oftalmol. 2019;94(5):237–41.
85. Russo CV, Saccà F, Paternoster M, Buonomo AR, Gentile I, Scotto R, et al. Post-mortem diagnosis of invasive pulmonary aspergillosis after alemtuzumab treatment for multiple sclerosis. Mult Scler. 2020;26(1):123–6.
86. Zelenetz AD, Barrientos JC, Brown JR, Coiffier B, Delgado J, Egyed M, et al. Idelalisib or placebo in combination with bendamustine and rituximab in patients with relapsed or refractory chronic lymphocytic leukaemia: interim results from a phase 3, randomised, double-blind, placebo-controlled trial. Lancet Oncol. 2017;18(3):297–311.
87. Dreyling M, Santoro A, Mollica L, Leppä S, Follows GA, Lenz G, et al. Phosphatidylinositol 3-kinase inhibition by Copanlisib in relapsed or refractory indolent lymphoma. J Clin Oncol. 2017;35(35):3898–905.
88. Gribben JG, Bosch F, Cymbalista F, Geisler CH, Ghia P, Hillmen P, et al. Optimising outcomes for patients with chronic lymphocytic leukaemia on ibrutinib therapy: European recommendations for clinical practice. Br J Haematol. 2018;180(5):666–79.
89. Lindsay J, Teh BW, Micklethwaite K, Slavin M. Azole antifungals and new targeted therapies for hematological malignancy. Curr Opin Infect Dis. 2019;32(6):538–45.
90. de Zwart L, Snoeys J, De Jong J, Sukbuntherng J, Mannaert E, Monshouwer M. Ibrutinib dosing strategies based on interaction potential of CYP3A4 perpetrators using physiologically based pharmacokinetic modeling. Clin Pharmacol Ther. 2016;100(5):548–57.
91. Sokulska M, Kicia M, Wesołowska M, Hendrich AB. Pneumocystis jirovecii—from a commensal to pathogen: clinical and diagnostic review. Parasitol Res. 2015;114(10):3577–85.
92. Roux A, Gonzalez F, Roux M, Mehrad M, Menotti J, Zahar JR, et al. Update on pulmonary pneumocystis jirovecii infection in non-HIV patients. Med Mal Infect. 2014;44(5):185–98.
93. Stern A, Green H, Paul M, Vidal L, Leibovici L. Prophylaxis for pneumocystis pneumonia (PCP) in non-HIV immunocompromised patients. Cochrane Database Syst Rev. 2014;2014(10):Cd005590.
94. Mikulska M, Lanini S, Gudiol C, Drgona L, Ippolito G, Fernández-Ruiz M, et al. ESCMID Study Group for Infections in Compromised Hosts (ESGICH) Consensus Document on the

safety of targeted and biological therapies: an infectious diseases perspective (Agents targeting lymphoid cells surface antigens [I]: CD19, CD20 and CD52). Clin Microbiol Infect. 2018;24(Suppl 2):S71–s82.

95. Williams KM, Ahn KW, Chen M, Aljurf MD, Agwu AL, Chen AR, et al. The incidence, mortality and timing of Pneumocystis jirovecii pneumonia after hematopoietic cell transplantation: a CIBMTR analysis. Bone Marrow Transplant. 2016;51(4):573–80.
96. Garg N, Jorgenson M, Descourouez J, Saddler CM, Parajuli S, Astor BC, et al. Pneumocystis jirovecii pneumonia in kidney and simultaneous pancreas kidney transplant recipients in the present era of routine post-transplant prophylaxis: risk factors and outcomes. BMC Nephrol. 2018;19(1):332.
97. Jones JA, Robak T, Brown JR, Awan FT, Badoux X, Coutre S, et al. Efficacy and safety of idelalisib in combination with ofatumumab for previously treated chronic lymphocytic leukaemia: an open-label, randomised phase 3 trial. Lancet Haematol. 2017;4(3):e114–e26.
98. Sehn LH, Hallek M, Jurczak W, Brown JR, Barr PM, Catalano J, et al. A retrospective analysis of *Pneumocystis jirovecii* pneumonia infection in patients receiving Idelalisib in clinical trials. Blood. 2016;128(22):3705.
99. Bird ST, Tian F, Flowers N, Przepiorka D, Wang R, Jung T-H, et al. Idelalisib for treatment of relapsed follicular lymphoma and chronic lymphocytic leukemia: a comparison of treatment outcomes in clinical trial participants vs medicare beneficiaries. JAMA Oncol. 2020;6(2):248–54.
100. Mensah FA, Blaize JP, Bryan LJ. Spotlight on copanlisib and its potential in the treatment of relapsed/refractory follicular lymphoma: evidence to date. Onco Targets Ther. 2018;11:4817–27.
101. Cheson BD, O'Brien S, Ewer MS, Goncalves MD, Farooki A, Lenz G, et al. Optimal management of adverse events from copanlisib in the treatment of patients with non-Hodgkin lymphomas. Clin Lymphoma Myeloma Leuk. 2019;19(3):135–41.
102. Davids MS, Fisher DC, Tyekucheva S, McDonough M, Hanna J, Lee B, et al. A phase 1b/2 study of duvelisib in combination with FCR (DFCR) for frontline therapy for younger CLL patients. Leukemia. 2020;35:1064–72.
103. Copiktra (duvelisib) [package insert]. U.S. Food and Drug Administration website. 2019. https://www.accessdata.fda.gov/drugsatfda_docs/label/2019/211155s001lbl.pdf. Accessed 14 Nov 2020.
104. Piqray (alpelisib) [package insert]. U.S. Food and Drug Administration website. 2019. https://www.accessdata.fda.gov/drugsatfda_docs/label/2019/212526s000lbl.pdf. Accessed 14 Nov 2020.
105. Katsuyama T, Saito K, Kubo S, Nawata M, Tanaka Y. Prophylaxis for Pneumocystis pneumonia in patients with rheumatoid arthritis treated with biologics, based on risk factors found in a retrospective study. Arthritis Res Ther. 2014;16(1):R43.
106. Mori S, Sugimoto M. Pneumocystis jirovecii infection: an emerging threat to patients with rheumatoid arthritis. Rheumatology (Oxford). 2012;51(12):2120–30.
107. Ryan CE, Cheng MP, Issa NC, Brown JR, Davids MS. Pneumocystis jirovecii pneumonia and institutional prophylaxis practices in CLL patients treated with BTK inhibitors. Blood Adv. 2020;4(7):1458–63.
108. Ahn IE, Jerussi T, Farooqui M, Tian X, Wiestner A, Gea-Banacloche J. Atypical Pneumocystis jirovecii pneumonia in previously untreated patients with CLL on single-agent ibrutinib. Blood. 2016;128(15):1940–3.
109. Imbruvica (Ibrutinib) [package insert]. U.S. Food and Drug Administration website. 2018. https://www.accessdata.fda.gov/drugsatfda_docs/label/2018/210563s000lbl.pdf. Accessed 14 Nov 2020.
110. Martin-Garrido I, Carmona EM, Specks U, Limper AH. Pneumocystis pneumonia in patients treated with rituximab. Chest. 2013;144(1):258–65.
111. Jiang X, Mei X, Feng D, Wang X. Prophylaxis and treatment of Pneumocystis jirovecii pneumonia in lymphoma patients subjected to rituximab-contained therapy: a systemic review and meta-analysis. PLoS One. 2015;10(4):e0122171.

112. Furman RR, Sharman JP, Coutre SE, Cheson BD, Pagel JM, Hillmen P, et al. Idelalisib and rituximab in relapsed chronic lymphocytic leukemia. N Engl J Med. 2014;370(11):997–1007.
113. Zalmanovich A, Ben-Ami R, Rahav G, Alon D, Moses A, Olshtain-Pops K, et al. Rituximab identified as an independent risk factor for severe PJP: A case-control study. PLoS One. 2020;15(9):e0239042.
114. Truxima (rituximab-abbs) [package insert]. U.S. Food and Drug Administration website. 2018. https://www.accessdata.fda.gov/drugsatfda_docs/label/2018/761088s000lbl.pdf. Accessed 31 Dec 2020.
115. Schwarz M, Kocher F, Niedersuess-Beke D, Rudzki J, Hochmair M, Widmann G, et al. Immunosuppression for immune checkpoint-related toxicity can cause Pneumocystis jirovecii Pneumonia (PJP) in non-small-cell lung cancer (NSCLC): a report of 2 cases. Clin Lung Cancer. 2019;20(3):e247–e50.
116. Si S, Erickson K, Evageliou N, Silverman M, Kersun L. An usual presentation of Pneumocystis jirovecii Pneumonia in a woman treated with immune checkpoint inhibitor. J Pediatr Hematol Oncol. 2021;43(2):e163.
117. Redelman-Sidi G, Michielin O, Cervera C, Ribi C, Aguado JM, Fernández-Ruiz M, et al. ESCMID Study Group for Infections in Compromised Hosts (ESGICH) Consensus Document on the safety of targeted and biological therapies: an infectious diseases perspective (Immune checkpoint inhibitors, cell adhesion inhibitors, sphingosine-1-phosphate receptor modulators and proteasome inhibitors). Clin Microbiol Infect. 2018;24(Suppl 2):S95–S107.
118. Grigoropoulos I, Thomas K, Christoforou P, Fanidi I, Papavdi M, Kyriakou F, et al. Pneumocystis jirovecii pneumonia after initiation of Tofacitinib therapy in rheumatoid arthritis: case-based review. Mediterr J Rheumatol. 2019;30(3):167–70.
119. Mimori T, Harigai M, Atsumi T, Kuwana M, Takei S, Tamura N, et al. AB0431 post-marketing surveillance of tofacitinib in Japanese patients with rheumatoid arthritis: an interim report of safety data. Ann Rheum Dis. 2017;76(Suppl 2):1200.
120. Brakemeier S, Dürr M, Bachmann F, Schmidt D, Gaedeke J, Budde K. Risk evaluation and outcome of Pneumocystis jirovecii pneumonia in kidney transplant patients. Transplant Proc. 2016;48(9):2924–30.
121. Swan CD, Reid AB. Three cases of presumed pneumocystis pneumonia in patients receiving bortezomib therapy for multiple myeloma. IDCases. 2014;1(3):32–5.
122. Cooley L, Dendle C, Wolf J, Teh BW, Chen SC, Boutlis C, et al. Consensus guidelines for diagnosis, prophylaxis and management of Pneumocystis jirovecii pneumonia in patients with haematological and solid malignancies, 2014. Intern Med J. 2014;44(12b):1350–63.
123. Maertens J, Cesaro S, Maschmeyer G, Einsele H, Donnelly JP, Alanio A, et al. ECIL guidelines for preventing Pneumocystis jirovecii pneumonia in patients with haematological malignancies and stem cell transplant recipients. J Antimicrob Chemother. 2016;71(9):2397–404.
124. Green H, Paul M, Vidal L, Leibovici L. Prophylaxis of Pneumocystis pneumonia in immunocompromised non-HIV-infected patients: systematic review and meta-analysis of randomized controlled trials. Mayo Clin Proc. 2007;82(9):1052–9.
125. Avino LJ, Naylor SM, Roecker AM. Pneumocystis jirovecii Pneumonia in the non-HIV-infected population. Ann Pharmacother. 2016;50(8):673–9.
126. Drgona L, Gudiol C, Lanini S, Salzberger B, Ippolito G, Mikulska M. ESCMID Study Group for Infections in Compromised Hosts (ESGICH) Consensus Document on the safety of targeted and biological therapies: an infectious diseases perspective (Agents targeting lymphoid or myeloid cells surface antigens [II]: CD22, CD30, CD33, CD38, CD40, SLAMF-7 and CCR4). Clin Microbiol Infect. 2018;24(Suppl 2):S83–94.
127. Winthrop KL, Mariette X, Silva JT, Benamu E, Calabrese LH, Dumusc A, et al. ESCMID Study Group for Infections in Compromised Hosts (ESGICH) Consensus Document on the safety of targeted and biological therapies: an infectious diseases perspective (Soluble immune effector molecules [II]: agents targeting interleukins, immunoglobulins and complement factors). Clin Microbiol Infect. 2018;24(Suppl 2):S21–40.
128. Zydelig (idelalisib) [package insert]. U.S. Food and Drug Administration website. 2014. https://www.accessdata.fda.gov/drugsatfda_docs/label/2014/205858lbl.pdf. Accessed 14 Nov 2020.

129. Reinwald M, Silva JT, Mueller NJ, Fortún J, Garzoni C, de Fijter JW, et al. ESCMID Study Group for Infections in Compromised Hosts (ESGICH) Consensus Document on the safety of targeted and biological therapies: an infectious diseases perspective (Intracellular signaling pathways: tyrosine kinase and mTOR inhibitors). Clin Microbiol Infect. 2018;24(Suppl 2):S53–s70.
130. Aliqopa (copanlisib) [package insert]. U.S. Food and Drug Administration website. 2017. https://www.accessdata.fda.gov/drugsatfda_docs/label/2017/209936s000lbl.pdf. Accessed 14 Nov 2020.
131. Deepe GS Jr. Modulation of infection with Histoplasma capsulatum by inhibition of tumor necrosis factor-alpha activity. Clin Infect Dis. 2005;41(Suppl 3):S204–7.
132. Wallis RS, Broder MS, Wong JY, Hanson ME, Beenhouwer DO. Granulomatous infectious diseases associated with tumor necrosis factor antagonists. Clin Infect Dis. 2004;38(9):1261–5.
133. Vergidis P, Avery RK, Wheat LJ, Dotson JL, Assi MA, Antoun SA, et al. Histoplasmosis complicating tumor necrosis factor–α blocker therapy: a retrospective analysis of 98 cases. Clin Infect Dis. 2015;61(3):409–17.
134. Bergstrom L, Yocum DE, Ampel NM, Villanueva I, Lisse J, Gluck O, et al. Increased risk of coccidioidomycosis in patients treated with tumor necrosis factor alpha antagonists. Arthritis Rheum. 2004;50(6):1959–66.
135. Covre LCP, Hombre PM, Falqueto A, Peçanha PM, Valim V. Pulmonary paracoccidioidomycosis: a case report of reactivation in a patient receiving biological therapy. Rev Soc Bras Med Trop. 2018;51(2):249–52.
136. Yoshinari H, Saito K, Nakano K, Fukuyo S, Miyagawa I, Tanaka Y. A case of rheumatoid arthritis treated with infliximab who developed disseminated Penicillium marneffei infection after visit to Thailand. Mod Rheumatol Case Rep. 2017;1(2):43–8.
137. Wang ML, Blum KA, Martin P, Goy A, Auer R, Kahl BS, et al. Long-term follow-up of MCL patients treated with single-agent ibrutinib: updated safety and efficacy results. Blood. 2015;126(6):739–45.
138. Rogers KA, Mousa L, Zhao Q, Bhat SA, Byrd JC, El Boghdadly Z, et al. Incidence of opportunistic infections during ibrutinib treatment for B-cell malignancies. Leukemia. 2019;33(10):2527–30.
139. Prakash K, Richman D. A case report of disseminated histoplasmosis and concurrent cryptococcal meningitis in a patient treated with ruxolitinib. BMC Infect Dis. 2019;19(1):287.
140. Jain N, Doyon JB, Lazarus JE, Schaefer IM, Johncilla ME, Agoston AT, et al. A case of disseminated histoplasmosis in a patient with rheumatoid arthritis on Abatacept. J Gen Intern Med. 2018;33(5):769–72.
141. Chan JF, Chan TS, Gill H, Lam FY, Trendell-Smith NJ, Sridhar S, et al. Disseminated infections with Talaromyces marneffei in non-AIDS patients given monoclonal antibodies against CD20 and kinase inhibitors. Emerg Infect Dis. 2015;21(7):1101–6.
142. Galgiani JN, Ampel NM, Blair JE, Catanzaro A, Geertsma F, Hoover SE, et al. 2016 Infectious Diseases Society of America (IDSA) Clinical Practice Guideline for the treatment of Coccidioidomycosis. Clin Infect Dis. 2016;63(6):e112–e46.
143. Garrett AL, Cha SS, Wack E, Blair JE. Divergence in the approach to tumor necrosis factor α-inhibitor recipients with coccidioidomycosis. Infection. 2017;45(4):539–43.
144. Bilal J, Kollampare S, Bode B, Lisse JR, Hoover SE, Sudano D, et al. Management of asymptomatic coccidioidomycosis in patients with rheumatic diseases. Rheumatol Int. 2019;39(7):1257–62.
145. Wheat LJ, Freifeld AG, Kleiman MB, Baddley JW, McKinsey DS, Loyd JE, et al. Clinical Practice Guidelines for the management of patients with histoplasmosis: 2007 update by the Infectious Diseases Society of America. Clin Infect Dis. 2007;45(7):807–25.
146. Hage CA, Bowyer S, Tarvin SE, Helper D, Kleiman MB, Wheat LJ. Recognition, diagnosis, and treatment of histoplasmosis complicating tumor necrosis factor blocker therapy. Clin Infect Dis. 2010;50(1):85–92.

Progressive Multifocal Leukoencephalopathy

22

Rafael San-Juan and Mario Fernández-Ruiz

Introduction

The John Cunningham virus (JCV) is a neurotropic DNA virus belonging to the polyomavirus family that binds to N-linked glycoproteins and serotonergic 5-HT receptors presented on the surface of many human cells including kidney epithelial cells, B-cells, platelets, glial cells, and neurons [1].

JCV infection is common, with seroprevalence rates increasing with age from 10% in children to more than 80% in adulthood [2]. Primary infection is usually asymptomatic, and JCV usually remains quiescent in the kidneys, bone marrow, and lymphoid tissues. Through intermittent episodes of viremia, JCV may reach the brain [1]. Nevertheless, adequate humoral and, more importantly, cellular immunity are capable of controlling viral replication in glial tissue and therefore avoid tissue damage [3].

Progressive multifocal leukoencephalopathy (PML) is a rare disease related to JCV infection-derived pathogenic lesions on oligodendrocytes, and, to a lesser extent, astrocytes, that trigger the development of areas of demyelination sparing spinal cord and optical nerves, clinically expressed by muscle weakness, sensory

R. San-Juan (✉)
Unit of Infectious Diseases, Hospital Universitario "12 de Octubre", Instituto de Investigación Sanitaria Hospital "12 de Octubre" (imas12), Madrid, Spain

Spanish Network for Research in Infectious Diseases (REIPI RD16/0016/0002), Instituto de Salud Carlos III, Madrid, Spain

School of Medicine, Universidad Complutense, Madrid, Spain

M. Fernández-Ruiz
Unit of Infectious Diseases, Hospital Universitario "12 de Octubre", Instituto de Investigación Sanitaria Hospital "12 de Octubre" (imas12), Madrid, Spain

Spanish Network for Research in Infectious Diseases (REIPI RD16/0016/0002), Instituto de Salud Carlos III, Madrid, Spain

C. Cervera, J. M. Aguado (eds.), *Infectious Complications in Biologic and Targeted Therapies*, https://doi.org/10.1007/978-3-031-11363-5_22

deficit, cognitive dysfunction, confusion, aphasia, coordination, or gait difficulties [1]. Replication and cytopathic effects of JCV in myelin-producing cells occur in situations of failure of immunological control by CD4+ and CD8+ T-cells, which hampers clearance of the virus from the cerebrospinal fluid [4]. Therefore, PML had been reported as a rare disease restricted to immunosuppressed hosts with hematological malignancies, organ transplant recipients, and with chronic inflammatory disorders. Since the emergence of the human immunodeficiency virus (HIV) epidemic, the prevalence of PML substantially increased so that more than 80% of cases of PML reported in the USA between 1998 and 2005 were AIDS-related [5].

More recently, PML has been increasingly reported as a rare, serious adverse event related with some new targeted and biological therapies. The first monoclonal antibodies (mAbs) approved for the treatment of cancer or autoimmune diseases that have been reported to incur an increased risk of PML included natalizumab, efalizumab, rituximab, and alemtuzumab [6]. Nevertheless, novel therapies approved for B-cell hematologic malignancies and autoimmune diseases as brentuximab vedotin, alemtuzumab, ofatumumab, ibrutinib, obinutuzumab, belimumab, and idelalisib had also been reported as potentially of risk in view of data from passive FDA pharmacovigilance surveillance program in the USA (Table 22.1).

With exception of α4-integrin-targeting agents natalizumab and efalizumab, in which the underlying mechanisms behind the development of PML have been clearly demonstrated, drug-related cases of PML are mostly based on statistical relationship and confusion by other potential risk factors are usually difficult to discard.

In the present chapter, we will revise currently available data on PML in patients receiving targeted and biological therapy, focusing on the underlying mechanisms and potential preventive management of natalizumab-related PML. Nevertheless, we will also discuss current information regarding drug-related PML by other targeted biological drugs with the most established statistical relationships and as is the case of alemtuzumab, anti-CD20 mAbs, brentuximab, and novel intracellular signaling pathway inhibitors.

Table 22.1 Cases of PML associated with the use of immune-targeted therapies (2009–2016) with significant signal detection results included in the FDA adverse event reporting system (FAERS)

Drug	PML cases	Drug courses	% PML	PRR (CI 95%)
Brentuximab vedotin[a]	15	1017	1.47	24.49 (14.79–40.56)
Ofatumumab[a]	14	1478	0.95	16.26 (9.64–27.42)
Alemtuzumab[a]	15	3038	0.49	9.87 (5.95–6.38)
Obinutuzumab[a]	3	655	0.46	7.36 (2.38–22.8)
Ibrutinib[a]	10	2860	0.35	5.63 (3.02–10.49)
Belimumab[a]	8	2985	0.27	4.5 (2.25–9)
Idelalisib	3	1089	0.46	4.05 (1.31–12.58)

Adapted from [7]

Only drugs with more than two PML cases and PRR (proportional reporting ratios with respect to other drugs) greater than 2.0 are included

PML progressive multifocal leukoencephalopathy, *FAERS* FDA Adverse Event Reporting System

[a] PML risk included in labeling

PML Related with α4-Integrin-Targeted Agents

Natalizumab (Tysabri®, Elan Pharmaceuticals and Biogen Idec) is a humanized IgG4 mAb targeting the α4 integrin subunit that constituted the first anti-integrin agent approved for clinical use. The α4 chain forms two different integrins, α4β1 (also known as very late antigen [VLA]-4]) and α4β7, respectively [8]. VLA-4 is expressed on practically all leukocytes (except mature granulocytes) and mediates binding to endothelial cell layers, including the blood-brain barrier (BBB), via vascular cell adhesion molecule (VCAM)-1. The VLA-4/VCAM-1 interaction is required for immune cell trafficking into the central nervous system (CNS). Through blockade of α4β1 integrin (VLA-4), natalizumab inhibits T-cell migration across the BBB, thereby reducing CNS inflammation [9, 10]. This drug received FDA regulatory approval to treat relapsing-remitting multiple sclerosis (MS) in 2004 [11] and for moderate-to-severe Crohn's disease (CD) in 2008 [12].

Efalizumab (Raptiva®, Genentech) is also a recombinant humanized mAb targeted against CD11a, one of the two subunits of the αLβ2 integrin (also known as leukocyte function antigen-1 [LFA-1]) and prevents binding of T-cells to the intercellular adhesion molecule-1 (ICAM-1), found on antigen-presenting cells (endothelial cells and keratinocytes), interfering with inflammatory mechanisms involved in the formation of the psoriatic plaque. After approval for the treatment of adult patients with moderate-to-severe chronic plaque psoriasis, the high number of cases of PML under this treatment led to drug withdrawn from the market, so it is no longer available [10]. Vedolizumab (Entyvio®, Millennium Pharmaceuticals) is the other currently approved α-integrin-targeted drug that selectively targets the α4β7 integrin, which binds to mucosal addressin cell adhesion molecule-1 (MAdCAM-1) mediating T-cell migration to the lamina propria of the small intestine [10]. This drug has been approved for the treatment of moderately to severely active ulcerative colitis and Crohn's disease in adults who have failed at least one conventional therapy. Unlike natalizumab or efalizumab, vedolizumab does not affect CNS immune modulation as α4β7 integrin acts exclusively on intestinal lymphocytes and no cases of vedolizumab-induced PML have been reported to date [13–15]. We therefore will focus the present section on natalizumab-related PML.

Underlying Mechanisms of Natalizumab-Related PML

PML is the result of the infection (and subsequent degeneration) of oligodendrocytes in the white matter due to the JCV [16]. The archetypal form of JCV is the cause for primary infection and latency. In patients receiving natalizumab, several subtypes of mononuclear cells (central memory T-cells, effector memory T-cells, and activated monocytes) that express α4β1 and α4β7 on their surface are affected, and inhibition of their migration into the CNS is described [8]. This leads to a decrease in the CD4+/CD8+ T-cell ratio and B-cell and CD138+ plasma cell counts in the cerebrospinal fluid (CSF) [17, 18] and in the number of dendritic cells and CD4+ T-cells in cerebral perivascular spaces [19] allowing asymptomatic reactivation of JCV in plasma and urine in parallel with a decrease in JCV-specific cellular immune responses [20]. Natalizumab treatment also induces rearrangements in the noncoding control region (NCCR) of the JCV genome [21] promoting replication of the so-called prototypical form (or PML-type) of the virus capable of promoting replication and pathogenic effect of JCV in oligodendrocytes.

Epidemiology and Risk Factors for Natalizumab-Related PML

Natalizumab initially seemed to be well tolerated in phase 3 randomized clinical trials (RCTs) leading to approval. However, the first cases of PML in natalizumab-treated patients recruited in pivotal trials were early reported through extended follow-up [12, 22, 23]. This circumstance led to a voluntary suspension of marketing in February 2005. Natalizumab was reintroduced in the US market in 2006 with a black box warning for PML and under a restricted distribution program (Tysabri® Outreach: Unified Commitment to Health [TOUCH]) [24]. The European Medicines Agency (EMA) furtherly approved natalizumab as monotherapy only for patients with highly active or rapidly evolving forms of relapsing-remitting MS despite an adequate course with at least one disease-modifying agent. On the basis of more than 150,000 patients treated with natalizumab worldwide, the overall current incidence of PML has been currently estimated in 4.22 cases per 1000 patients [24].

Three major clinical risk factors have been identified to stratify the risk of PML in patients receiving natalizumab [25]:

- *Treatment duration.* The annualized seroconversion rate among JCV-seronegative patients exposed to natalizumab has been estimated in 7.1% [26], reaching an incidence of two cases per 1000 treated patients beyond 48 months of therapy. However, although the incidence increases abruptly after 72 months, more information is needed to delineate the risk of PML after prolonged treatment courses [27, 28].
- *Exposure to JCV* (as assessed by a positive status for anti-JCV IgG antibodies). The risk of early natalizumab-induced PML seems to be negligible if pretreatment JCV-specific IgG antibodies are negative. The incidence among JCV-seropositive patients was estimated at 3.87 cases per 1000 natalizumab-treated patients, as compared to zero cases per 1000 in seronegative individuals [27]. Among JCV-seropositive subjects, those with an IgG index ≤1.5 have a lower incidence of PML compared to the remaining population of anti-JCV antibody-positive patients [29].
- *Previous or even remote history of immunosuppressive therapy* (including relatively mild agents such as methotrexate) double the incidence of PML among natalizumab-exposed patients [27], an observation likely explained by the higher risk of having latent infection due to the prototype form of JCV at therapy initiation.

By combining these variables into a risk stratification algorithm, different categories may be established, with expected PML incidences ranging from less than 0.09 cases per 1000 patients in the lowest-risk subgroup to 11.1 cases per 1000 patients in the highest-risk category [27]. The quantification of anti-JCV IgG titers by enzyme-linked immunosorbent assay (ELISA) has been proven to provide further refinement in risk prediction. The anti-JCV antibody index is the normalized ratio between the signal (in optical densities) obtained from the patient's serum and that from a cutoff calibrator prepared with pooled sera collected from JCV-seropositive healthy volunteers. Patients not previously treated with immunosuppressive agents with an index value ≤0.9 carried a risk of 0.1 cases per 1000 during the first 24 months of therapy, which gradually increased up to 0.4 per 1000 with 49 to 72 months of exposure. In contrast, the expected incidence during the first 24 months among patients with an index >1.5 was of 1.0 cases per 1000, reaching 10.12 per 1000 between months 49 and 72 [30]. An FDA-cleared second-generation ELISA test (STRATIFY JCV™, Focus Diagnostics) is now commercially available [31]. Other biomarkers that are being evaluated to stratify the risk of PML include decreased CD4+ T-cell expression of L-selectin CD62L [32] and lipid-specific immunoglobulin M bands in CSF [33].

Clinical Features and Management

The prognosis of natalizumab-associated PML critically depends on early recognition [24]. Typical clinical and radiological characteristics are detailed in Table 22.2. The clinical presentation of natalizumab-induced PML includes motor weakness, cognitive deficits, dysarthria, and ataxia [34]. Cranial magnetic resonance imaging

Table 22.2 Main clinical and radiological features of PML in patients treated with natalizumab (modified from McGuigan et al.) [29]

Clinical presentation
• Subacute (weeks) onset and progressive course
• Aphasia, behavioral, and neuropsychological alterations, visual deficits, hemiparesis, and seizures
MRI features
• Large (>3 cm) lesions with unifocal, multifocal, or widespread distribution
• Subcortical location rather than periventricular
• Frequent involvement of cortical gray matter (50% of cases), posterior fossa less commonly affected
• No mass effect even in large lesions
• T2-weighted sequences: Diffuse hyperintensity (often with punctate microcystic appearance) within the lesions
• T1-weighted sequences: Lightly hypointensity at onset, with signal intensity decreasing over time
• Paramagnetic contrast enhancement in <50% of cases at the time of presentation (often patchy or punctate appearance)
• Diffusion-weighted imaging: Hyperintense appearance of acute lesions

MRI magnetic resonance imaging

(MRI) typically shows T2-weighted hyperintense lesions in subcortical white matter without gadolinium enhancement [35]. The detection of viral DNA in the CSF or brain biopsy is required for the definitive diagnosis [35]. JCV PCR on CSF has a high sensitivity and even higher specificity, but a negative result does not rule out the diagnosis of PML, and testing should be repeated in case of high clinical suspicion. Early discontinuation of natalizumab is the first step in the management of PML [4], whereas antiviral therapy has not shown clear benefit. Early removal of natalizumab from the bloodstream via plasma exchange or immunoadsorption is also indicated [35, 36], although such approach has been associated with the subsequent development of immune reconstitution inflammatory syndrome [37, 38].

Preventive Algorithms

In order to minimize the risk of PML under natalizumab treatment, different preventive algorithms have been developed based on pre-treatment serological risk stratification of patients and active clinical and virological surveillance in high-risk patients [38, 39] which is represented in Fig. 22.1:

- **Test for anti-JCV IgG antibodies** is recommended before starting treatment in natalizumab-*naïve* MS patients [29, 38]. An index cutoff value of >1.5 constitutes a reasonable threshold to guide the clinical decision process. Patients with an index >1.5 are to be already considered at high risk and no further testing is required. JCV-seronegative patients and those with IgG antibody index ≤1.5 should be retested every 6 months after the first year of treatment.

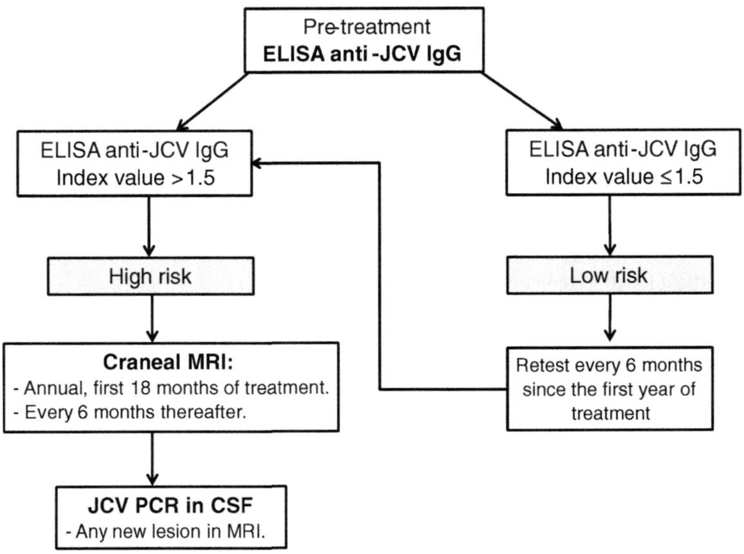

Fig. 22.1 Natalizumab-related PML risk stratification algorithm

- **Cerebral MRI** with diffusion-weighted imaging (DWI) and fluid-attenuated inversion recovery (FLAIR) should be performed at baseline and repeated at scheduled intervals in seropositive patients:
  - Annual MRI scans during the first 18 months of therapy.
  - After the first 18 months of treatment at least 6-month intervals for patients with an index ≤1.5 and 3- to 4-month intervals for those with index >1.5.
- **PCR testing on cerebrospinal fluid specimens**. Should be performed whenever any new lesion on subsequent MRI [29].

A recent study from France found an annual reduction of 23.0% in the crude incidence of natalizumab-associated PML since 2013 (in contrast to the steady increase observed before that year), supporting the efficacy of this risk minimization strategy [40]. The decision of discontinuing therapy with natalizumab in patients at high risk of PML (positive anti-JCV serology with an IgG antibody index >1.5 and therapy duration of 48 months or more) is difficult and should be shared by the MS specialist and the patient [38].

PML Related to Monoclonal Antibodies Against Lymphoma and Leukemia Surface Antigens

Anti-CD20 Monoclonal Antibodies

In 1997, rituximab was the first anti-cancer mAb approved for clinical use. Since June 2017, there are six different anti-CD20 mAbs authorized for clinical use. In the European Union, a PML warning was added to the prescribing information of rituximab in 2007 based on pharmacovigilance signaling. In 2009, the Research on Adverse Drug Events and Reports (RADAR) group published the first case series of rituximab-related PML [41]. Although PML is still nowadays considered as a "very rare" complication of rituximab therapy, with current incidence rates estimation ranging from 0.2 to 2.56 per 10,000 exposed patients [42, 43], most experts take into consideration the risk of this serious complication in patients receiving anti-CD20 mAbs [44–46]. In spite of isolated cases of PML reported with other anti-CD20 antibodies as obinutuzumab [47] or ofatumumab [48], the possibility that PML could be a class effect of all anti-CD20 antibodies is currently debated as no conclusive evidence is yet available. However, as for cautionary approach, obinutuzumab, ofatumumab, and ocrelizumab labels included PML among potential adverse reactions since the first day of marketing and probably deserve similar precaution and surveillance than with rituximab [45].

About 65% of PML cases are diagnosed within the first 2 years after the first rituximab dose, and more than 70% of cases were reported during remission induction therapy for non-Hodgkin's lymphoma [46]. In contrast to what has been established with natalizumab-related PML, no cumulative dose-effect relationship has been demonstrated for rituximab, and concurrent drug analysis in PML cases has suggested potential confusion or synergies with other drugs which inhibit cellular immunity as fludarabine or bendamustine [46]. Indeed, in a recent global post-marketing safety and clinical trial, all rituximab-related cases of PML had at least one additional potential risk factor [49].

The mechanisms underlying the increased risk of PML in patients receiving anti-CD20 mAbs are incompletely understood. Whereas rituximab has shown quantitative impact on other cell lines apart from CD20+ B-cells clinically expressed as neutropenia and thrombocytopenia, the impact on T-cell immunity has been more difficult to ascertain. A drop in CD4+ T-cell counts intensified through repeated treatment cycles has been reported in some series including rheumatoid arthritis patients treated with rituximab [43, 50, 51]. Nevertheless, available databases of post-marketing surveillance argue against the role of rituximab at causing severe CD4+ T-cell lymphopenia (with most of the cases providing alternative explanation, mainly concurrent use of bendamustine) and no definite conclusion whether rituximab induces a clinically relevant deleterious effect on the cell-mediated immunity in patients with normal T-cell counts at baseline can be made [46].

Regarding potential functional effect on T-cells, whereas animal models could not demonstrate that B-cells affect secondary T-cell responses against viral pathogens, B-cell depletion before or during primary viral infection significantly impairs cytokine production and generation of new memory CD4+ T-cells, thus increasing the risk of systemic primary infections [52]. In addition to B-cell-dependent mechanism, direct effect on T-cells of CD20-targeted agents could be suggested in view of efficacy data for graft rejection treatment after solid organ transplantation and graft versus host disease following allogenic hematopoietic stem cell transplantation. Finally, there is a population of 3%–5% of T-cells represented in different cell compartments, including the CNS, that express CD20 (CD3+ CD20+ T-cells) and are selectively depleted by CD20-targeted agents [53]. Although the natural function of this T-cell subset is currently unclear, their depletion seems to be crucial in the efficacy of anti-CD20 mAbs in the treatment of multiple sclerosis [53].

Unfortunately, there is no validated risk stratification strategy directed to the prevention of potential PML cases in patients under anti-CD20 treatments. CD4+ T-cell counts appear to be a reasonable marker for the risk of PML and possibly more cost-effective than using JCV detection techniques in contrast to what occurs with drugs with a higher and more clearly established risk such as natalizumab.

Antibodies Against Lymphoma and Leukemia Cell Surface Antigens

Alemtuzumab

Alemtuzumab is a humanized IgG1 mAb that binds to CD52 and leads to the lysis of targeted cells by means of complement-dependent cytotoxicity. CD52 is expressed on most mature lymphocytes, monocytes, and macrophages, thereby inducing severe depletion of peripheral blood lymphocytes (both T- and B-cells, especially CD4+), an effect that is more profound and long-lasting with repeated infusions. Even with the lower doses of alemtuzumab used in multiple sclerosis, decreased CD4+ T-cell counts (<200 cells/μL) have been reported to persist months after the completion of therapy [54]. Lymphodepletion is evident by 2–4 weeks from the first dose with the lowest values typically found after 1 month [55] and remains below 25% from baseline levels beyond 9 months [56]. Recovery to the normal range can take 8 months for B-cells and up to 3 years for CD4+ and CD8+ T-cells, although lymphocyte counts rarely return to baseline values [54]. In view of the notable impact on the CD4+ T-cell subset, the expected infection risk is similar to the spectrum observed in advanced HIV infection, with increased incidence of classic opportunistic infections, including scattered cases of PML, that have been reported mostly in patients with hematological malignancy treated with this drug [57–59]. In spite of the potential risk of this complication under this treatment, no specific preventive recommendations are currently available [45].

Brentuximab

Brentuximab vedotin (Adcetris®, Takeda) is an antibody-drug conjugate composed of a human/murine chimeric anti-CD30 IgG1 mAb approved in 2011 by the FDA and in 2012 by EMA for the treatment of relapsed/refractory Hodgkin's lymphoma (HL) and anaplastic large T-cell lymphoma. CD30 is expressed in various cellular types, including T-cells, B-cells, monocytes, and activated natural killer cells. Taking into account that CD30 has been implied in the regulation of the balance between Th1 and Th2 responses and in the generation of memory and effector T-cells [60, 61], CD30-targeted agents may affect antibody-dependent cell-mediated cytotoxicity and exert a deleterious impact on humoral immunity.

PML has been described in patients receiving brentuximab vedotin, although the concomitant use of other cytostatic and immunosuppressive agents administered in affected patients makes it difficult to establish causality [62–65]. Time from initiation of therapy to symptom onset (second or third dose) has been reported as much shorter than PML cases related with anti-CD20 mAbs or natalizumab, and the case fatality rate among reported cases was 80% [62–65]. These clinical observations prompted the FDA to launch a Risk Evaluation and Mitigation Strategy (REMS) program including appropriate label warning [7, 65].

Clinical monitoring of neurological symptoms of new onset among brentuximab-treated patients in order to achieve prompt suspicion of PML and early drug discontinuation with appropriate diagnostic work-up is currently recommended [45].

Drugs Targeted to Intracellular Signaling Pathways

Several cases of fatal PML have been reported following the use of Bruton's tyrosine kinase inhibitor ibrutinib, although in the context of multiple prior treatment lines, including rituximab [7, 66–68]. In the same line, Janus kinase inhibitor ruxolitinib has also been recently associated with PML even in the absence of lymphopenia [69].

As cases of PML derived from these targeted therapies are currently emerging, there is still scant epidemiological data and little information on the underlying pathophysiological mechanisms causing increased risk. Therefore, preventive algorithms have not yet been developed. As discussed for other targeted biological drugs potentially associated to PML, specific clinical surveillance of new onset of neurological symptoms in patients treated with ibrutinib or ruxolitinib seems to be advisable [70].

References

1. Tan CS, Koralnik IJ. Progressive multifocal leukoencephalopathy and other disorders caused by JC virus: clinical features and pathogenesis. Lancet Neurol. 2010;9(4):425–37. https://doi.org/10.1016/S1474-4422(10)70040-5.
2. Knowles WA, Pipkin P, Andrews N, Vyse A, Minor P, Brown DW, et al. Population-based study of antibody to the human polyomaviruses BKV and JCV and the simian polyomavirus SV40. J Med Virol. 2003;71(1):115–23. https://doi.org/10.1002/jmv.10450.
3. Berger JR, Houff SA, Major EO. Monoclonal antibodies and progressive multifocal leukoencephalopathy. MAbs. 2009;1(6):583–9. https://doi.org/10.4161/mabs.1.6.9884.
4. Warnke C, Menge T, Hartung HP, Racke MK, Cravens PD, Bennett JL, et al. Natalizumab and progressive multifocal leukoencephalopathy: what are the causal factors and can it be avoided? Arch Neurol. 2010;67(8):923–30. https://doi.org/10.1001/archneurol.2010.161.
5. Molloy ES, Calabrese LH. Progressive multifocal leukoencephalopathy: a national estimate of frequency in systemic lupus erythematosus and other rheumatic diseases. Arthritis Rheum. 2009;60(12):3761–5. https://doi.org/10.1002/art.24966.
6. Toussirot E, Bereau M. The risk of progressive multifocal leukoencephalopathy under biological agents used in the treatment of chronic inflammatory diseases. Inflamm Allergy Drug Targets. 2014;13(2):121–7. https://doi.org/10.2174/1871528113666140224103712.
7. Raisch DW, Rafi JA, Chen C, Bennett CL. Detection of cases of progressive multifocal leukoencephalopathy associated with new biologicals and targeted cancer therapies from the FDA's adverse event reporting system. Expert Opin Drug Saf. 2016;15(8):1003–11. https://doi.org/10.1080/14740338.2016.1198775.
8. Ransohoff RM. Natalizumab for multiple sclerosis. N Engl J Med. 2007;356(25):2622–9. https://doi.org/10.1056/NEJMct071462.
9. Yednock TA, Cannon C, Fritz LC, Sanchez-Madrid F, Steinman L, Karin N. Prevention of experimental autoimmune encephalomyelitis by antibodies against alpha 4 beta 1 integrin. Nature. 1992;356(6364):63–6. https://doi.org/10.1038/356063a0.
10. Ley K, Rivera-Nieves J, Sandborn WJ, Shattil S. Integrin-based therapeutics: biological basis, clinical use and new drugs. Nat Rev Drug Discov. 2016;15(3):173–83. https://doi.org/10.1038/nrd.2015.10.
11. Natalizumab: AN 100226, anti-4alpha integrin monoclonal antibody. Drugs R D. 2004;5(2):102–7. https://doi.org/10.2165/00126839-200405020-00007.
12. Van Assche G, Van Ranst M, Sciot R, Dubois B, Vermeire S, Noman M, et al. Progressive multifocal leukoencephalopathy after natalizumab therapy for Crohn's disease. N Engl J Med. 2005;353(4):362–8. https://doi.org/10.1056/NEJMoa051586.
13. Haanstra KG, Hofman SO, Lopes Estevao DM, Blezer EL, Bauer J, Yang LL, et al. Antagonizing the alpha4beta1 integrin, but not alpha4beta7, inhibits leukocytic infiltration of the central nervous system in rhesus monkey experimental autoimmune encephalomyelitis. J Immunol. 2013;190(5):1961–73. https://doi.org/10.4049/jimmunol.1202490.
14. Wyant T, Fedyk E, Abhyankar B. An overview of the mechanism of action of the monoclonal antibody Vedolizumab. J Crohns Colitis. 2016;10(12):1437–44. https://doi.org/10.1093/ecco-jcc/jjw092.

15. Parikh A, Stephens K, Major E, Fox I, Milch C, Sankoh S, et al. A Programme for risk assessment and minimisation of progressive multifocal leukoencephalopathy developed for Vedolizumab clinical trials. Drug Saf. 2018;41(8):807–16. https://doi.org/10.1007/s40264-018-0669-8.
16. Ferenczy MW, Marshall LJ, Nelson CD, Atwood WJ, Nath A, Khalili K, et al. Molecular biology, epidemiology, and pathogenesis of progressive multifocal leukoencephalopathy, the JC virus-induced demyelinating disease of the human brain. Clin Microbiol Rev. 2012;25(3):471–506. https://doi.org/10.1128/CMR.05031-11.
17. Stuve O, Marra CM, Bar-Or A, Niino M, Cravens PD, Cepok S, et al. Altered CD4+/CD8+ T-cell ratios in cerebrospinal fluid of natalizumab-treated patients with multiple sclerosis. Arch Neurol. 2006;63(10):1383–7. https://doi.org/10.1001/archneur.63.10.1383.
18. Stuve O, Marra CM, Jerome KR, Cook L, Cravens PD, Cepok S, et al. Immune surveillance in multiple sclerosis patients treated with natalizumab. Ann Neurol. 2006;59(5):743–7. https://doi.org/10.1002/ana.20858.
19. del Pilar MM, Cravens PD, Winger R, Frohman EM, Racke MK, Eagar TN, et al. Decrease in the numbers of dendritic cells and CD4+ T cells in cerebral perivascular spaces due to natalizumab. Arch Neurol. 2008;65(12):1596–603. https://doi.org/10.1001/archneur.65.12.noc80051.
20. Chen Y, Bord E, Tompkins T, Miller J, Tan CS, Kinkel RP, et al. Asymptomatic reactivation of JC virus in patients treated with natalizumab. N Engl J Med. 2009;361(11):1067–74. https://doi.org/10.1056/NEJMoa0904267.
21. Reid CE, Li H, Sur G, Carmillo P, Bushnell S, Tizard R, et al. Sequencing and analysis of JC virus DNA from natalizumab-treated PML patients. J Infect Dis. 2011;204(2):237–44. https://doi.org/10.1093/infdis/jir256.
22. Langer-Gould A, Atlas SW, Green AJ, Bollen AW, Pelletier D. Progressive multifocal leukoencephalopathy in a patient treated with natalizumab. N Engl J Med. 2005;353(4):375–81. https://doi.org/10.1056/NEJMoa051847.
23. Kleinschmidt-DeMasters BK, Tyler KL. Progressive multifocal leukoencephalopathy complicating treatment with natalizumab and interferon beta-1a for multiple sclerosis. N Engl J Med. 2005;353(4):369–74. https://doi.org/10.1056/NEJMoa051782.
24. McGinley MP, Moss BP, Cohen JA. Safety of monoclonal antibodies for the treatment of multiple sclerosis. Expert Opin Drug Saf. 2017;16(1):89–100. https://doi.org/10.1080/14740338.2017.1250881.
25. Ho PR, Koendgen H, Campbell N, Haddock B, Richman S, Chang I. Risk of natalizumab-associated progressive multifocal leukoencephalopathy in patients with multiple sclerosis: a retrospective analysis of data from four clinical studies. Lancet Neurol. 2017;16(11):925–33. https://doi.org/10.1016/s1474-4422(17)30282-x.
26. Vennegoor A, van Rossum JA, Leurs C, Wattjes MP, Rispens T, Murk JL, et al. High cumulative JC virus seroconversion rate during long-term use of natalizumab. Eur J Neurol. 2016;23(6):1079–85. https://doi.org/10.1111/ene.12988.
27. Bloomgren G, Richman S, Hotermans C, Subramanyam M, Goelz S, Natarajan A, et al. Risk of natalizumab-associated progressive multifocal leukoencephalopathy. N Engl J Med. 2012;366(20):1870–80. https://doi.org/10.1056/NEJMoa1107829.
28. Cervera C. Natalizumab-associated progressive multifocal leukoencephalopathy. N Engl J Med. 2012;367(9):871; author reply 2. https://doi.org/10.1056/NEJMc1207116.
29. McGuigan C, Craner M, Guadagno J, Kapoor R, Mazibrada G, Molyneux P, et al. Stratification and monitoring of natalizumab-associated progressive multifocal leukoencephalopathy risk: recommendations from an expert group. J Neurol Neurosurg Psychiatry. 2016;87(2):117–25. https://doi.org/10.1136/jnnp-2015-311100.
30. Plavina T, Subramanyam M, Bloomgren G, Richman S, Pace A, Lee S, et al. Anti-JC virus antibody levels in serum or plasma further define risk of natalizumab-associated progressive multifocal leukoencephalopathy. Ann Neurol. 2014;76(6):802–12. https://doi.org/10.1002/ana.24286.

31. Lee P, Plavina T, Castro A, Berman M, Jaiswal D, Rivas S, et al. A second-generation ELISA (STRATIFY JCV DxSelect) for detection of JC virus antibodies in human serum and plasma to support progressive multifocal leukoencephalopathy risk stratification. J Clin Virol. 2013;57(2):141–6. https://doi.org/10.1016/j.jcv.2013.02.002.
32. Schwab N, Schneider-Hohendorf T, Melzer N, Cutter G, Wiendl H. Natalizumab-associated PML: Challenges with incidence, resulting risk, and risk stratification. Neurology. 2017;88(12):1197–205. https://doi.org/10.1212/WNL.0000000000003739.
33. Toboso I, Tejeda-Velarde A, Alvarez-Lafuente R, Arroyo R, Hegen H, Deisenhammer F, et al. New algorithms improving PML risk stratification in MS patients treated with Natalizumab. Front Neurol. 2020;11:579438. https://doi.org/10.3389/fneur.2020.579438.
34. Maas RP, Muller-Hansma AH, Esselink RA, Murk JL, Warnke C, Killestein J, et al. Drug-associated progressive multifocal leukoencephalopathy: a clinical, radiological, and cerebrospinal fluid analysis of 326 cases. J Neurol. 2016;263(10):2004–21. https://doi.org/10.1007/s00415-016-8217-x.
35. Hellwig K, Gold R. Progressive multifocal leukoencephalopathy and natalizumab. J Neurol. 2011;258(11):1920–8. https://doi.org/10.1007/s00415-011-6116-8.
36. Khatri BO, Man S, Giovannoni G, Koo AP, Lee JC, Tucky B, et al. Effect of plasma exchange in accelerating natalizumab clearance and restoring leukocyte function. Neurology. 2009;72(5):402–9. https://doi.org/10.1212/01.wnl.0000341766.59028.9d.
37. Clifford DB, De Luca A, Simpson DM, Arendt G, Giovannoni G, Nath A. Natalizumab-associated progressive multifocal leukoencephalopathy in patients with multiple sclerosis: lessons from 28 cases. Lancet Neurol. 2010;9(4):438–46. https://doi.org/10.1016/S1474-4422(10)70028-4.
38. Redelman-Sidi G, Michielin O, Cervera C, Ribi C, Aguado JM, Fernandez-Ruiz M, et al. ESCMID study Group for Infections in compromised hosts (ESGICH) consensus document on the safety of targeted and biological therapies: an infectious diseases perspective (immune checkpoint inhibitors, cell adhesion inhibitors, sphingosine-1-phosphate receptor modulators and proteasome inhibitors). Clin Microbiol Infect. 2018;24(Suppl 2):S95–S107. https://doi.org/10.1016/j.cmi.2018.01.030.
39. Fernandez-Ruiz M, Aguado JM. Direct T-cell inhibition and agents targeting T-cell migration and chemotaxis. Infect Dis Clin North Am. 2020;34(2):191–210. https://doi.org/10.1016/j.idc.2020.02.002.
40. Vukusic S, Rollot F, Casey R, Pique J, Marignier R, Mathey G, et al. Progressive multifocal leukoencephalopathy incidence and risk stratification among Natalizumab users in France. JAMA Neurol. 2020;77(1):94–102. https://doi.org/10.1001/jamaneurol.2019.2670.
41. Carson KR, Evens AM, Richey EA, Habermann TM, Focosi D, Seymour JF, et al. Progressive multifocal leukoencephalopathy after rituximab therapy in HIV-negative patients: a report of 57 cases from the research on adverse drug events and reports project. Blood. 2009;113(20):4834–40. https://doi.org/10.1182/blood-2008-10-186999.
42. Lanini S, Molloy AC, Fine PE, Prentice AG, Ippolito G, Kibbler CC. Risk of infection in patients with lymphoma receiving rituximab: systematic review and meta-analysis. BMC Med. 2011;9:36. https://doi.org/10.1186/1741-7015-9-36.
43. Piantoni S, Scarsi M, Tincani A, Airo P. Circulating CD4+ T-cell number decreases in rheumatoid patients with clinical response to rituximab. Rheumatol Int. 2015;35(9):1571–3. https://doi.org/10.1007/s00296-015-3295-0.
44. Wick W, Hertenstein A, Platten M. Neurological sequelae of cancer immunotherapies and targeted therapies. Lancet Oncol. 2016;17(12):e529–e41. https://doi.org/10.1016/S1470-2045(16)30571-X.
45. Mikulska M, Lanini S, Gudiol C, Drgona L, Ippolito G, Fernandez-Ruiz M, et al. ESCMID study Group for Infections in compromised hosts (ESGICH) consensus document on the safety of targeted and biological therapies: an infectious diseases perspective (agents targeting lymphoid cells surface antigens [I]: CD19, CD20 and CD52). Clin Microbiol Infect. 2018;24(Suppl 2):S71–82. https://doi.org/10.1016/j.cmi.2018.02.003.

46. Focosi D, Tuccori M, Maggi F. Progressive multifocal leukoencephalopathy and anti-CD20 monoclonal antibodies: what do we know after 20 years of rituximab. Rev Med Virol. 2019;29(6):e2077. https://doi.org/10.1002/rmv.2077.
47. Turine G, London F. Obinutuzumab use complicated by progressive multifocal leukoencephalopathy in a patient with chronic lymphocytic leukemia: a case report. Acta Neurol Belg. 2020;121:781. https://doi.org/10.1007/s13760-020-01520-1.
48. Moreno C, Montillo M, Panayiotidis P, Dimou M, Bloor A, Dupuis J, et al. Ofatumumab in poor-prognosis chronic lymphocytic leukemia: a phase IV, non-interventional, observational study from the European research initiative on chronic lymphocytic leukemia. Haematologica. 2015;100(4):511–6. https://doi.org/10.3324/haematol.2014.118158.
49. Berger JR, Malik V, Lacey S, Brunetta P, Lehane PB. Progressive multifocal leukoencephalopathy in rituximab-treated rheumatic diseases: a rare event. J Neurovirol. 2018;24(3):323–31. https://doi.org/10.1007/s13365-018-0615-7.
50. Melet J, Mulleman D, Goupille P, Ribourtout B, Watier H, Thibault G. Rituximab-induced T cell depletion in patients with rheumatoid arthritis: association with clinical response. Arthritis Rheum. 2013;65(11):2783–90. https://doi.org/10.1002/art.38107.
51. Lavielle M, Mulleman D, Goupille P, Bahuaud C, Sung HC, Watier H, et al. Repeated decrease of CD4+ T-cell counts in patients with rheumatoid arthritis over multiple cycles of rituximab treatment. Arthritis Res Ther. 2016;18(1):253. https://doi.org/10.1186/s13075-016-1152-5.
52. Misumi I, Whitmire JK. B cell depletion curtails CD4+ T cell memory and reduces protection against disseminating virus infection. J Immunol. 2014;192(4):1597–608. https://doi.org/10.4049/jimmunol.1302661.
53. Schuh E, Berer K, Mulazzani M, Feil K, Meinl I, Lahm H, et al. Features of human CD3+CD20+ T cells. J Immunol. 2016;197(4):1111–7. https://doi.org/10.4049/jimmunol.1600089.
54. Hill-Cawthorne GA, Button T, Tuohy O, Jones JL, May K, Somerfield J, et al. Long term lymphocyte reconstitution after alemtuzumab treatment of multiple sclerosis. J Neurol Neurosurg Psychiatry. 2012;83(3):298–304. https://doi.org/10.1136/jnnp-2011-300826.
55. Li Z, Richards S, Surks HK, Jacobs A, Panzara MA. Clinical pharmacology of alemtuzumab, an anti-CD52 immunomodulator, in multiple sclerosis. Clin Exp Immunol. 2018;194(3):295–314. https://doi.org/10.1111/cei.13208.
56. Lundin J, Porwit-MacDonald A, Rossmann ED, Karlsson C, Edman P, Rezvany MR, et al. Cellular immune reconstitution after subcutaneous alemtuzumab (anti-CD52 monoclonal antibody, CAMPATH-1H) treatment as first-line therapy for B-cell chronic lymphocytic leukaemia. Leukemia. 2004;18(3):484–90. https://doi.org/10.1038/sj.leu.2403258.
57. Gerevini S, Capra R, Bertoli D, Sottini A, Imberti L. Immune profiling of a patient with alemtuzumab-associated progressive multifocal leukoencephalopathy. Mult Scler. 2019;25(8):1196–201. https://doi.org/10.1177/1352458519832259.
58. Thursky KA, Worth LJ, Seymour JF, Miles Prince H, Slavin MA. Spectrum of infection, risk and recommendations for prophylaxis and screening among patients with lymphoproliferative disorders treated with alemtuzumab*. Br J Haematol. 2006;132(1):3–12. https://doi.org/10.1111/j.1365-2141.2005.05789.x.
59. Malek SK, Obmann MA, Gotoff RA, Foltzer MA, Hartle JE, Potdar S. Campath-1H induction and the incidence of infectious complications in adult renal transplantation. Transplantation. 2006;81(1):17–20. https://doi.org/10.1097/01.tp.0000189713.14993.db.
60. Romagnani S, Del Prete G, Maggi E, Chilosi M, Caligaris-Cappio F, Pizzolo G. CD30 and type 2 T helper (Th2) responses. J Leukoc Biol. 1995;57(5):726–30. https://doi.org/10.1002/jlb.57.5.726.
61. Stanciu LA, Roberts K, Lau LC, Coyle AJ, Johnston SL. Induction of type 2 activity in adult human CD8(+) T cells by repeated stimulation and IL-4. Int Immunol. 2001;13(3):341–8. https://doi.org/10.1093/intimm/13.3.341.
62. Wagner-Johnston ND, Bartlett NL, Cashen A, Berger JR. Progressive multifocal leukoencephalopathy in a patient with Hodgkin lymphoma treated with brentuximab vedotin. Leuk Lymphoma. 2012;53(11):2283–6. https://doi.org/10.3109/10428194.2012.676170.

63. Jalan P, Mahajan A, Pandav V, Bekker S, Koirala J. Brentuximab associated progressive multifocal leukoencephalopathy. Clin Neurol Neurosurg. 2012;114(10):1335–7. https://doi.org/10.1016/j.clineuro.2012.03.019.
64. von Geldern G, Pardo CA, Calabresi PA, Newsome SD. PML-IRIS in a patient treated with brentuximab. Neurology. 2012;79(20):2075–7. https://doi.org/10.1212/WNL.0b013e3182749f17.
65. Carson KR, Newsome SD, Kim EJ, Wagner-Johnston ND, von Geldern G, Moskowitz CH, et al. Progressive multifocal leukoencephalopathy associated with brentuximab vedotin therapy: a report of 5 cases from the Southern Network on Adverse Reactions (SONAR) project. Cancer. 2014;120(16):2464–71. https://doi.org/10.1002/cncr.28712.
66. Lutz M, Schulze AB, Rebber E, Wiebe S, Zoubi T, Grauer OM, et al. Progressive multifocal leukoencephalopathy after Ibrutinib therapy for chronic lymphocytic leukemia. Cancer Res Treat. 2017;49(2):548–52. https://doi.org/10.4143/crt.2016.110.
67. Hsiehchen D, Arasaratnam R, Raj K, Froehlich T, Anderson L. Ibrutinib use complicated by progressive multifocal leukoencephalopathy. Oncology. 2018;95(5):319–22. https://doi.org/10.1159/000490617.
68. Teixeira LLC, Nunes VRH, Perini GF, Feres CCP, Ovigli D, Hamerschlak N. Progressive multifocal leukoencephalopathy in a patient with relapsed chronic lymphocytic leukemia treated with Ibrutinib. Hematol Transfus Cell Ther. 2020. https://doi.org/10.1016/j.htct.2020.11.006.
69. Wathes R, Moule S, Milojkovic D. Progressive multifocal leukoencephalopathy associated with Ruxolitinib. N Engl J Med. 2013;369(2):197–8. https://doi.org/10.1056/NEJMc1302135.
70. Reinwald M, Silva JT, Mueller NJ, Fortun J, Garzoni C, de Fijter JW, et al. ESCMID study Group for Infections in compromised hosts (ESGICH) consensus document on the safety of targeted and biological therapies: an infectious diseases perspective (intracellular signaling pathways: tyrosine kinase and mTOR inhibitors). Clin Microbiol Infect. 2018;24(Suppl 2):S53–70. https://doi.org/10.1016/j.cmi.2018.02.009.

Hepatitis Viruses

23

Mark Robbins and Karen Doucette

Introduction

The viral hepatidities include hepatitis A, B, C, D, and E viruses, with the latter four having the ability to lead to chronic infection. In the context of immunomodulatory therapy, chronic viral hepatitis requires careful attention. Reactivation may occur with variable risk depending on both host and viral factors as well as features of the underlying immunosuppressive regimen, with the possibility of fulminant liver failure or death as possible outcomes in the most severe cases. An understanding of the relative risk of these complications based on the planned biologic therapy allows appropriate monitoring and/or prophylactic antiviral therapy. Here we will focus on the impact of targeted biologic therapies in those with hepatitis B or C.

Hepatitis B

Hepatitis B is a small, partially double-stranded DNA virus in the *Hepadnaviridae* family. There are an estimated 257 million people chronically infected with hepatitis B virus (HBV) worldwide with the highest prevalence rates noted in the Western Pacific (6.2%) and African regions (6.1%) with rates <0.5% in North America and Western Europe [1].

Following acute infection, the likelihood of progressing to chronic infection is inversely proportional to age at the time of acquisition, occurring in more than 80–90% of infants, 10–25% of young children, and less than 5% of adults. Chronic hepatitis B (CHB) is defined by the presence of hepatitis B surface antigen (HBsAg) for more than 6 months. Based on the underlying serologic pattern, it is further

M. Robbins · K. Doucette (✉)
Division of Infectious Diseases, Department of Medicine, University of Alberta, Edmonton, AB, Canada
e-mail: mrobbin1@ualberta.ca; karen.doucette@ualberta.ca

C. Cervera, J. M. Aguado (eds.), *Infectious Complications in Biologic and Targeted Therapies*, https://doi.org/10.1007/978-3-031-11363-5_23

Table 23.1 Phases of CHB infection

	Phase 1: HBeAg+ chronic infection	Phase 2: HBeAg+ chronic hepatitis	Phase 3: HBeAg− chronic infection	Phase 4: HBeAg− chronic hepatitis	Phase 5: Resolved hepatitis B infection
HBsAg	Positive	Positive	Positive	Positive	Negative
Anti-HBs	Negative	Negative	Negative	Negative	Positive or negative
HBeAg	Positive	Positive	Negative	Negative	Negative
Anti-HBc	Positive	Positive	Positive	Positive	Positive
HBV DNA (IU/mL)	Often $>10^7$	10^4–10^7	Often <2000	10^3–10^7	Negative or trace levels
ALT	Normal	Elevated or fluctuating	Normal	Often fluctuating	Normal

Modified from Coffin et al. [2]

classified into five distinct phases as follows: (1) hepatitis B e antigen positive (HBeAg+) chronic infection, (2) HBeAg+ chronic hepatitis, (3) HBeAg negative (HBeAg−) chronic infection, (4) HBeAg− chronic hepatitis, and (5) resolved HBV infection (see Table 23.1). Both patients seropositive for HBsAg (phase 1–4) and those with resolved infection (positive for antibody to HBV core [anti-HBc] in the absence of HBsAg (phase 5)) are at risk of HBV reactivation with certain biologic therapies.

Following exposure, which globally is predominantly mother to child, percutaneous or through sexual exposure, viral entry occurs through the binding of the HBV pre-surface 1 region to the sodium taurocholate cotransporter polypeptide. Following this, genetic material is converted into covalently closed circular DNA (cccDNA) which can persist in hepatocytes despite apparent immune control and HBsAg loss. This phase of infection is identified by reactive anti-HBc serology and is noteworthy as HBV reactivation in this setting is well described with various immunomodulatory therapies. Worldwide it is also five to tenfold more prevalent than the background rate of chronic HBV infection in the corresponding population.

Although the complete mechanism of immune control of CHB is not fully elucidated, it is well established that both the cell-mediated and humoral arms of the immune system play vital roles. Cell-mediated immunity targets HBV eradication from infected cells, and the humoral immune system serves to clear circulating virus and prevent further spread. When considering the likely risks of HBV reactivation of various classes of immunomodulatory therapies, remembering these broad functions provides a useful framework.

In terms of cell-mediated immunity, the CD4+ T-cell response against HBV is predominantly Th1-driven, resulting in IFN-γ, TNF-α, and IL-2 production. The CD8+ T-cell response plays a prominent role in the immune control of HBV through both direct cytolytic and non-cytolytic mechanisms, with the later predominating. The non-cytolytic mechanism involves, in part, IFN-γ and TNF-α-related effects with IFN-γ decreasing intracellular cccDNA and repressing cccDNA transcriptional activity through epigenetic modification [3–5]. The action of TNF-α has an established role in disrupting cccDNA integrity and targeting post-transcriptional events [6, 7]. However, cell-mediated immunity is unable to eradicate HBV infection in a subset of the population, and, in the setting of CHB, functionally exhausted CD8+ T cells predominate which are characterized, in part, by increased expression of co-inhibitory receptors PD-1 and CTLA-4 [8, 9]. Regulatory T (Treg) cells, with a classic cytokine profile of IL-10, IL-35, and TGF-β, are generally overexpressed in CHB and appear to contribute to CD8+ T-cell exhaustion [10]. Th17 cells, with a classic cytokine profile of IL-17A, IL-17F, and IL-22, also seem to be overexpressed in CHB and contribute to immune-mediated damage and progression to cirrhosis [11]. The importance of humoral immunity in CHB, through production of antibodies against HBsAg and HBcAg, which function to clear circulating virus and prevent further spread and infection of additional hepatocytes, is evidenced indirectly through studies showing exceptionally high rates of CHB reactivation with B-cell-depleting agents such as rituximab and anti-CD20 antibody [12].

Waning adaptive immunity can lead to HBV reactivation in those with CHB (HBsAg+) and anti-HBc + patients. HBV reactivation in HBsAg+ patients is defined by any of the following criteria: (1) ≥2 log increase in HBV DNA as compared to baseline, (2) ≥3 log increase if baseline HBV DNA was undetectable, or (3) ≥4 log absolute HBV DNA level if no baseline is available [13]. Alternatively, for anti-HBc + patients HBV reactivation is defined by either of the following: (1) HBV DNA is detectable at any level or (2) sero-reversion from HBsAg− to HBsAg+ serostatus [13]. HBV reactivation, as previously defined, can then progress to hepatitis flares, which are defined as elevation in ALT ≥3 times the patient baseline value and ≥100 U/L. The period during which HBV reactivation can occur in those receiving immunomodulatory therapy is quite variable with HBV reactivations occurring as early as a few days following initiation of therapy and can occur as late as months to years following cessation of therapy. While not all patients who experience HBV reactivation go on to develop hepatitis flares, should this occur it typically develops within days to weeks of viral reactivation [14].

Given the possibility of HBV reactivation in the context of immunomodulatory therapy, it is recommended that patients be screened with HBsAg, anti-HBc, and anti-HBs prior to therapy. A comprehensive approach considering serologic results, host factors, and the planned therapeutic regimen should then be undertaken as the risk of CHB reactivation depends on these three factors. Established serologic risk factors that increase risk of HBV reactivation include HBsAg+ status which carries a higher risk than HBsAg−/anti-HBc + status, presence of HBeAg, higher baseline HBV viral loads, and absence of anti-HBs in those HBsAg negative/anti-HBc+ [15–17]. Established host factors that predispose to hepatitis B reactivation include older age and male sex [16, 18]. Current knowledge on specific risks of HBV reactivation associated with various biologic agents is summarized in following sections while a general approach to the management of patients with CHB receiving biologic therapy can be found in Fig. 23.1.

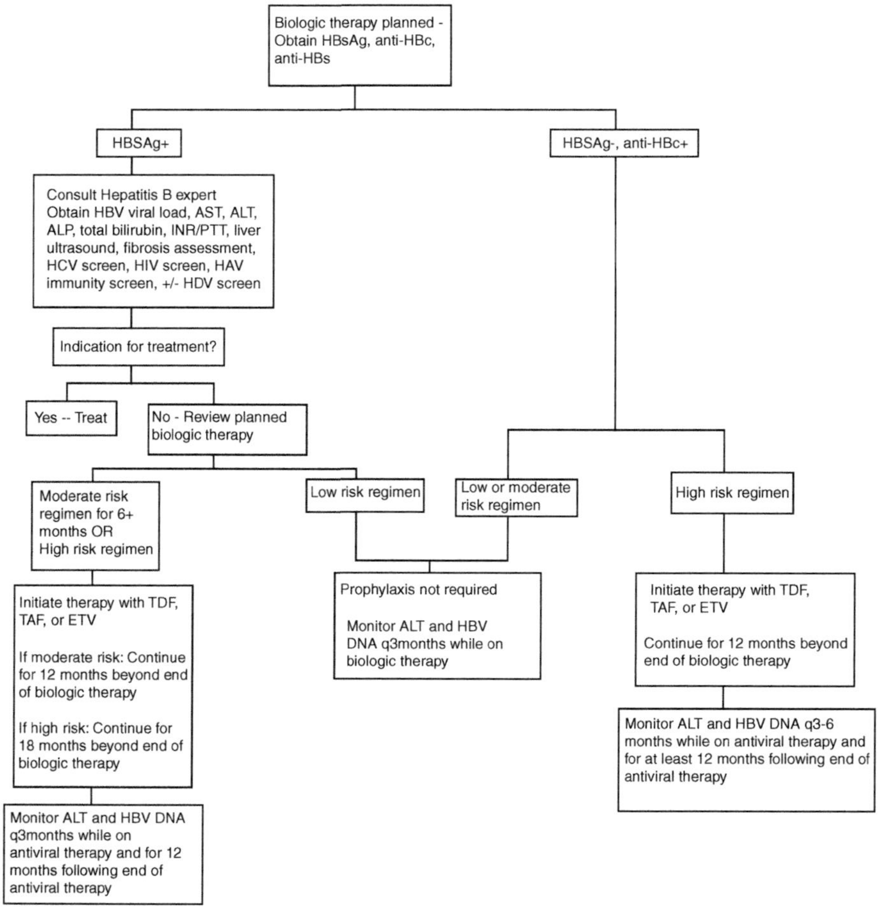

Fig. 23.1 Algorithm for management of CHB in patients receiving biologic therapy. (Adapted from Coffin et al. [2])

Patients who are HBsAg positive should be linked to specialist care and, if indicated based on guidelines in the general population, be initiated on antiviral therapy on that basis. For HBsAg+ patients, for whom therapy is not otherwise indicated, but who are receiving a regimen associated with a moderate risk (1–10%) of HBV reactivation for ≥6 months or receiving a therapy of high risk (≥10% risk of HBV reactivation), they should initiate antiviral prophylaxis and continue this for at least 12 months beyond the end of therapy. HBV DNA and ALT measurement every 3 to 6 months while on antiviral therapy and for 12 months following cessation of antiviral therapy is recommended. Alternatively, for those receiving low-risk biologics, prophylaxis is not required, and preemptive monitoring with HBV DNA and ALT every 3 months while on therapy is suggested [2, 13]. A discussion of this in the context of specific classes of biologics follows.

For anti-HBc + patients receiving a high-risk regimen, it is suggested that patients initiate antiviral prophylaxis throughout their course of immunosuppression and for at least 12 months beyond the end of therapy. These patients should also undergo HBV DNA and ALT measurements every 3 to 6 months while on antiviral therapy and for 12 months following cessation. Alternatively, for those receiving moderate- or low (≤1% risk of HBV reactivation)-risk regimens, prophylaxis is not required and preemptive monitoring with clinical follow-up and ALT measurements every 3 months while on therapy is suggested [2, 13].

Should HBV reactivation or HBV hepatitis flare occur in patients receiving biologic therapy, prompt initiation of antiviral therapy under the guidance of an experienced practitioner is advised.

With respect to whether biologic agents or classes are best classified as low, moderate, or high risk for triggering HBV reactivation, this is fairly well established for older and more commonly used agents, such as TNF-α inhibitors. Data is more limited however for newer biologic therapies, and evidence on associated risks is summarized in following sections.

Hepatitis C

Hepatitis C is an enveloped, positive-sense, single-stranded RNA virus in the *Flaviviridae* family. There are currently eight identified genotypes and 86 subtypes with genotype 1 predominating globally [19, 20] . There are an estimated 71.1 million people chronically infected worldwide with prevalence rates highest in the Eastern Mediterranean region (2.3%) and European regions (1.5%) with most of the rest of the world ranging from 0.5 to 1% [21]. Hepatitis C virus (HCV) infection follows a bimodal age distribution with higher rates in those aged 20–40, predominantly related to transmission through injection drug use, and in those aged >50 years, particularly those in the birth cohort of 1945–1975 in North America. The primary route of transmission in developing regions is related to unsafe medical practices while, in developed regions, transmission through percutaneous exposure in the form of intravenous drug use predominates.

Following acute infection, approximately 20–25% of patients spontaneously clear HCV infection while 75–80% of patients progress to chronic HCV infection, which is characterized by the presence of HCV RNA for more than 6 months.

Following exposure, HCV virion-associated apoE interacts with cell-surface LDL receptors and glycosaminoglycans, and with further interactions with a number of additional cell-surface molecules, viral entry and subsequent replication in hepatocytes can occur. Initial innate immune responses to infection occur and for the subset of patients who go on to develop chronic HCV infection. As with CHB, mechanisms of immune control of chronic HCV infection have not been fully elucidated, although contributions from T-cell-mediated cytolytic and non-cytolytic mechanisms and humoral immunity have been established, and this provides useful information when considering the likely risks of various immunosuppressive and immunomodulatory therapies. In terms of cell-mediated immunity, the CD4+ T-cell response against HCV is predominantly Th1-driven, resulting in IFN-γ, TNF-α, and IL-2 production while the CD8+ T-cell response plays a prominent role in the immune control of HCV through both direct cytolytic effects, mediated through perforin-granzymes as well as cell-surface death receptors such as FAS/FASL. This results in hepatocyte apoptosis and, through non-cytolytic effects, mediated through a number of cytokines including IFN-γ and TNF-α, inhibition of HCV replication. However, cell-mediated immunity is unable to eradicate HCV infection in a subset of the population, and in the setting of chronic HCV infection, functionally exhausted CD8+ T cells predominate which are characterized, in part, by increased expression of co-inhibitory receptors PD-1 and CTLA-4 [22]. Regulatory T (Treg) cells, with a classic cytokine profile of IL-10, IL-35, and TGF-β, are generally found to be overexpressed in chronic HCV infection and appear to contribute to CD8+ T cell exhaustion [23]. The importance of humoral immunity in the immune control of chronic HCV infection appears to play a less significant role than cell-mediated immunity, although neutralizing antibodies against envelope glycoproteins E1 and E2 have been postulated to play a role in partial protection against reinfection and, therefore, may limit further hepatocyte damage during HCV reactivation, although this remains largely speculative.

In the context of immunomodulation, impaired adaptive immunity can lead to HCV reactivation and hepatitis flare in those with chronic hepatitis C with HCV reactivation being defined as an increase in HCV RNA of ≥1 log as compared to baseline and with HCV hepatitis flare being defined as HCV reactivation with concomitant elevation in ALT ≥3 times the patient baseline value and ≥100 U/L [24].

For those with chronic HCV receiving biologic therapy, international guidelines for the treatment of psoriasis, rheumatoid arthritis, and other medical conditions for which biologic therapy is often used suggest pre-treatment HCV screening [25, 26]. For those in whom chronic HCV infection has been identified, the following three approaches to management can be considered: (1) sequential therapy with biologic therapy administration preceding HCV treatment, (2) concomitant therapy with HCV treatment and biologic therapy being given simultaneously, or (3) inverted sequential therapy with HCV treatment preceding biologic therapy administration.

Advantages of the sequential approach include earlier treatment and control of the underlying disease requiring biologic therapy while disadvantages include the potential for HCV reactivation and hepatitis flare with reduced immune control of chronic HCV related to immunomodulatory therapy. This approach has derived support from a number of studies showing relatively low risk of HCV reactivation and hepatitis flare with the majority in biologic therapies (see following sections for agent-specific summary). Advantages of the concomitant approach include earlier treatment of chronic HCV and potential avoidance of HCV reactivation and hepatitis flare while disadvantages are similar as for the sequential approach. This approach has similarly derived support from the relatively low risk of HCV reactivation or hepatitis flares associated with the majority of biologic therapies. Advantages of the inverse sequential approach include having the lowest risk of HCV reactivation, hepatitis flare, and drug-drug interactions while disadvantages include delays in achieving underlying disease control while awaiting direct-acting antiviral therapy completion.

For patients who have not yet received treatment for chronic HCV in the setting of biologic therapy, unlike for CHB infection, the role for routine viral load or transaminase monitoring is not well established. However, should clinical or laboratory suspicion for HCV reactivation or hepatitis flare occur while on biologic therapy, prompt review by an experienced practitioner is advisable with consideration for initiation of HCV therapy.

B-Cell-Depleting Antibodies

The B-cell-depleting antibody family of medications includes rituximab, ofatumumab, ocrelizumab, veltuzumab, ublituximab, ocaratuzumab, and 90Y-ibritumomab tiuxetan. These agents are variably approved for the treatment of diffuse large B-cell lymphoma, follicular lymphoma, chronic lymphocytic leukemia, rheumatoid arthritis, granulomatosis with polyangiitis, microscopic polyangiitis, and relapsed or progressive multiple sclerosis, although these agents are often used for a variety of off-label indications.

Their immunosuppressive effect is mediated through their effects on B cells between the pre-B phase and the mature B-cell phase, although they do not affect mature plasma cells, with subsequent impaired antibody production in response to antigen stimulation, possible induction of hypogammaglobulinemia, and, perhaps more importantly, indirect impairments of cell-mediated immunity [27].

With respect to HBV, the impact of rituximab therapy on reactivation is complex and impacted by a number of factors including patient serologic status, indication for therapy, and both dose and number of treatments. The highest risk generally involves combination chemotherapy for hematological malignancies. A recent systematic review of 42 trials, which included patients undergoing cytotoxic chemotherapy or hematopoietic stem cell transplantation for hematological malignancies, demonstrated HBV reactivation in the absence of prophylaxis in 24.4–85% of HBsAg+ patients and in 4.1–41.5% of anti-HBc + patients [28]. The risk of HBV reactivation varies somewhat in those administered rituximab for rheumatologic conditions, with a recent observational study demonstrating HBV reactivation in 5/20 (25%) of anti-HBc+/anti-HBs- patients and 4/83 (4.8%) of anti-HBc+/anti-HBs + patients [29].

With respect to HCV, a multicenter retrospective analysis comparing 131 HCV+ patients and 422 HCV- patients undergoing combined chemotherapy with rituximab therapy for diffuse large B-cell lymphoma found that HCV RNA levels increased significantly during chemotherapy for the HCV+ group, and the rate of severe, grade 3–4, hepatic toxicity was significantly higher in the HCV+ group (27% vs. 3%) [30]. The literature on the risk of HCV reactivation during rituximab therapy for rheumatologic indications is less robust. A recent prospective study evaluating the safety of TNF-α inhibitors as compared to rituximab in HCV+ rheumatoid arthritis patients found that, while 6/6 patients receiving rituximab had a median twofold increase in HCV viral load, there was no associated hepatotoxicity or ALT elevation in any patient [31].

National guidelines and consensus statements suggest antiviral prophylaxis be given to both HBsAg+ and anti-HBc + patients both during and following rituximab therapy [2, 32]. HCV should generally be treated at the first available opportunity, although biologic therapy need not be withheld until direct-acting antiviral therapy has been administered and sustained virologic response demonstrated.

Anti-TNF-α

The anti-TNF-α antibody family of medications includes etanercept, adalimumab, infliximab, certolizumab, and golimumab. While infliximab, adalimumab, and golimumab are monoclonal antibodies against TNF-α, etanercept is a decoy soluble TNF-α receptor and certolizumab is a pegylated agent. These agents are variably approved for inflammatory bowel disease, rheumatoid arthritis, psoriatic arthritis, seronegative spondyloarthropathies, and uveitis.

Their immunosuppressive effect is mediated through inhibition of the pleotropic effects of TNF-α, which include (1) induction of various proinflammatory cytokines, (2) induction of acute-phase reactants, (3) activation of cellular adhesion processes, (4) chemoattraction, (5) macrophage activation, and (6) phagosome development [33].

In one retrospective study including patients with HBsAg+ or anti-HBc+ status undergoing anti-TNF-α therapy for a variety of autoimmune conditions, HBV reactivation was observed in 9/23 (39%) of HBsAg+ patients with no cases of HBV reactivation among 178 anti-HBc+ patients [34]. This finding was supported in a systematic review including 49 studies and 312 patients that demonstrated HBV reactivation in 8/40 (20%) HBsAg+ patients and 2/175 (1.1%) anti-HBc+ patients [35].

There is much less evidence on the safety of anti-TNF-α agents in the setting of chronic hepatitis C virus infection, especially with newer agents such as certolizumab and golimumab. Brunasso et al. performed a meta-analysis including 37 publications with 153 patients with chronic hepatitis C virus infection undergoing treatment with anti-TNF-α agents, predominately for rheumatoid arthritis. They found two cases of confirmed or probable worsening of HCV liver disease out of 153 evaluable patients [35]. In addition, Pompili et al. performed a comprehensive literature review on the topic and found reports of 216 patients with HCV receiving anti-TNF-α therapy for a median period of 1.2 years with only three cases of drug withdrawal due to suspected worsening of HCV liver disease [36].

For those undergoing TNF-α therapy, national guidelines and consensus statements suggest antiviral prophylaxis be given to HBsAg+ patients while anti-HBc+ patients can be safely managed with laboratory monitoring [2, 32]. While HCV should generally be treated at the first available opportunity, TNF-α therapy generally need not be withheld until direct-acting antiviral therapy has been administered and sustained virologic response demonstrated.

Anti-IL-1R Antagonists

Agents targeting the function of IL-1 include the anti-IL-1Ra antibody anakinra, which is approved for rheumatoid arthritis, juvenile idiopathic arthritis, and neonatal-onset multisystem inflammatory disease, as well as the anti-IL-1b antibody canakinumab, which is approved for the treatment of cryopyrin-associated periodic fever syndromes.

Their immunomodulatory effect is mediated through the pleiotropic effects of IL-1, which include promotion of inflammatory cytokine release, inflammasome formation, and production of IL-2 with subsequent proliferative and differentiation of T cells [37].

To date there have been no published reports of HBV or HCV reactivation in the setting of anakinra use, although reports of safe use in HBsAg+, anti-HBc+, or HCV+ patients are also lacking. Data are limited to a small cohort of three anti-HBc+ patients who received anakinra for underlying rheumatologic conditions, none of whom showed evidence of HBV reactivation [38]. Along these lines, there is no warning regarding either HBV or HCV on the product monograph, and the manufacturer has reported no cases of reactivated viral hepatitis with anakinra use [39].

Given the paucity of data related to the risk of HBV reactivation during anakinra use, national guidelines and consensus statements remain silent on any specific recommendations related to either antiviral prophylaxis or monitoring approaches. However, in the absence of compelling evidence of significantly elevated risk of HBV reactivation, monitoring of HBV DNA every 3 months in HBsAg+ patients seems reasonable.

Anti-IL-6/Anti-IL-6R

Agents targeting the function of IL-6 include the anti-IL-6 antibody siltuximab, which is approved for multicentric Castleman's disease, as well as the anti-IL-6R antibodies tocilizumab and sarilumab, which are variably approved for rheumatoid arthritis, juvenile idiopathic arthritis, and giant cell arteritis.

Their immunosuppressive effect is mediated through the effects of IL-6 as a proinflammatory cytokine, thereby activating peripheral blood mononuclear cells and promoting B-cell differentiation. In addition, as outlined above, IL-6 plays a role in HBV immune control through entry into hepatocytes, epigenetic control of cccDNA, and transcription of HBV RNA [40].

With respect to HBV, Chen et al. prospectively followed seven HBsAg+ and 41 anti-HBc+ patients with rheumatoid arthritis who received tocilizumab without antiviral prophylaxis and found 3/7 (43%) of HBsAg+ patients and 0/41 anti-HBc+ patients developed HBV reactivation [41]. Similarly, Ahn et al. prospectively followed 15 anti-HBc+ patients receiving tocilizumab for rheumatoid arthritis and found no evidence of HBV reactivation in their relatively small cohort [42].

With respect to HCV, a number of case reports have shown no significant increase in HCV viral loads or transaminase levels during tocilizumab therapy for rheumatoid arthritis [43, 44]. More recently, Chen et al. performed a prospective study that included eight HCV viremic patients treated with tocilizumab for rheumatoid arthritis and showed no changes in HCV viral load before therapy and 1 year after therapy with tocilizumab [45].

Consensus statements suggest, given similar overall infection rates with anti-IL-6 and anti-IL-6R antibodies as compared to TNF-a inhibitors, that a similar approach be applied to management of HBsAg+ and anti-HBc+ patients, with administration of prophylactic antivirals to HBsAg+ patients while anti-HBc+ patients can be safely managed with laboratory monitoring [2, 32]. HCV should be treated at the first available opportunity, and biologic therapy need not be withheld until direct-acting antiviral therapy has been completed.

Anti-IL-12/23

The anti-IL-12/23 antibody family of medications includes ustekinumab, which is approved for psoriasis, psoriatic arthritis, and Crohn's disease, and the anti-IL-23 antibody family of medications (guselkumab, tildrakizumab, risankizumab) which are approved for psoriasis and, in the case of guselkumab, for psoriatic arthritis as well.

Their immunosuppressive effect is mediated through the effects of IL-12 as an IFN-γ-inducing signal, though Th1 biasing, and through Th17 cell and NK cell activation while the immunosuppressive effect of IL-23 stems, in part, from its ability to promote differentiation of Th17 cells and consequent B-cell function [46].

With respect to HBV, a recent prospective study of eight HBsAg+ and 44 anti-HBc+ patients treated with ustekinumab for plaque psoriasis, none of whom received antiviral prophylaxis, showed reactivation rates of 25% (2/8) in HBsAg+ and 2.3% (1/44) in anti-HBc+ patients [47]. Similarly, a second recent prospective study included 11 HBsAg+, four of whom received antiviral prophylaxis and seven of whom did not, who were treated with ustekinumab for plaque psoriasis. They observed HBV reactivation in none of the cohort of HBsAg+ patients receiving prophylaxis and 2/7 (28.5%) in the cohort of HBsAg+ patients not receiving prophylaxis [48].

With respect to HCV, Chiu et al. performed a prospective study that included four patients with chronic HCV infection who were treated with ustekinumab for psoriasis and found HCV reactivation occurred in 1/4 (25%) patients although no significant differences in transaminase levels were observed among the group [48]. Similar results were seen in a retrospective study by Navarro et al. that included three HCV+ patients treated with ustekinumab for psoriasis, none of whom had elevations in hepatic transaminases or of baseline HCV viral load with therapy [49].

Thus, similar overall reactivation rates are seen with use of anti-IL-12/23 antibody family as are seen with anti-TNF-α agents, and thus it seems prudent to follow a similar management strategy for this class of drugs with antiviral prophylaxis being given to HBsAg+ patients and monitoring of anti-HBc+ patients. HCV should be treated at the first available opportunity, without the need to delay biologic therapy until its completion.

Anti-IL-17

The anti-IL-17 antibody family of medications includes secukinumab, ixekizumab, and brodalumab that are approved for use in psoriasis, psoriatic arthritis, and ankylosing spondylitis.

Their immunosuppressive effect is mediated through the effects of IL-17 in promoting proinflammatory cytokine production, chemokine production, proinflammatory cytokine, induction of innate host antimicrobial peptides, and phagocyte activation [50].

With respect to HBV, Chiu et al. performed a multicenter prospective cohort study including 25 HBsAg+ and 24 anti-HBc+ patients receiving secukinumab for psoriasis. They found HBV reactivation occurred in 6/25 (24%) of HBsAg+ patients, despite very high rates of antiviral prophylaxis, and 1/24 (4.2%) of anti-HBc+ patients, again with almost universal antiviral prophylaxis administration [51]. Otherwise, literature on the safety of secukinumab therapy in HBV+ patients is limited to case series and case reports which generally support the safety of secukinumab although definitive conclusions are difficult in the setting of variable antiviral prophylaxis administration, variable reporting of HBsAg+ as opposed to anti-HBc+ patients, and a small evidence base overall [52].

With respect to HCV, the previously mentioned prospective cohort study by Chiu et al. also included 14 HCV+ patients receiving secukinumab for psoriasis and found HCV reactivation occurred in 1/14 (7.1%) cases [51]. As for HBV, literature on the topic of risk of reactivation with secukinumab in HCV+ patients is otherwise limited to case reports which generally seem to support the safety of secukinumab use in patients with HCV infection [53].

Thus, although data are more limited, similar overall reactivation rates are seen with use of the anti-IL-17 antibody family as are seen with anti-IL-12/23 agents and with anti-TNF-α agents. Therefore, it seems prudent to follow a similar management strategy for this class of drugs with antiviral prophylaxis being given to HBsAg+ patients. For anti-HBc+ patients, regular (at least every 3 months) laboratory monitoring is suggested pending further data. HCV should be treated at the first available opportunity, without the need to delay biologic therapy pending its completion.

Integrin Inhibitors

The integrin inhibitor family of medications includes natalizumab (α4), which is approved for the treatment of multiple sclerosis, and vedolizumab (α4/β7) which is approved for ulcerative colitis and Crohn's disease.

Their immunosuppressive effect is mediated through impaired leukocyte adhesion and trafficking. In the case of natalizumab, this results in prevention of monocyte and memory T-cell trafficking into the central nervous system while, in the case of vedolizumab, this results in prevention of lymphocyte trafficking into gut-associated lymphoid tissue [54].

Information regarding the risk of HBV or HCV reactivation with natalizumab and vedolizumab are quite limited at this time with a single case report of fulminant

HBV infection reported, although whether this represented acute infection or reactivation is unclear [55]. Ng et al. utilized the Global Safety Database to identify 14 HBV+ patients, three of whom were HBsAg+ and the remainder of whom had unreported baseline serologic status, and 15 HCV+ patients treated with vedolizumab for inflammatory bowel disease. Only two liver-related adverse events were noted, neither of which were related to HBV or HCV reactivation or transaminase elevation [56].

Despite the paucity of evidence, consensus statements recommend antiviral prophylaxis administration to HBsAg+ patients and either antiviral prophylaxis or preemptive monitoring for anti-HBc+ patients treated with integrin inhibitors [32, 57].

JAK/STAT

The JAK/STAT family of medications includes tofacitinib, baricitinib, and ruxolitinib which are variably approved for rheumatoid arthritis, psoriatic arthritis, ulcerative colitis, myelofibrosis, and polycythemia rubra vera.

The immunosuppressive effects of tofacitinib and baricitinib, in particular, are mediated through impaired Th1, Th2, and Th17 cell differentiation as well as through impaired dendritic cell maturation [58].

With respect to HBV, Chen et al. performed a retrospective cohort study including six HBsAg+ and 75 anti-HBc+ patients treated with tofacitinib. They found HBV reactivation occurred in 2/4 (50%) HBsAg+ patients not receiving antiviral prophylaxis and 0/2 (0%) HBsAg+ patients receiving antiviral prophylaxis. Among anti-HBc+ patients, no cases of HBV reactivation were observed among their cohort of 75 patients, with no patient receiving antiviral prophylaxis [59]. Similarly, Serling-Boyd et al. performed a retrospective study including eight anti-HBc+ patients treated with tofacitinib, two of whom received antiviral prophylaxis, and found no episodes of HBV reactivation over 3 years of therapy [60].

With respect to HCV, Chen et al. recently performed a prospective study that included nine HCV viremic patients treated with tofacitinib for rheumatoid arthritis and showed no changes in HCV viral load before therapy compared to 1 year on therapy with tofacitinib [45].

National guidelines and consensus statements suggest antiviral prophylaxis be given to HBsAg+ patients receiving tofacitinib while anti-HBc+ patients can be monitored [2, 32]. Those with chronic HCV should be treated at the first available opportunity, without delay of biologic therapy pending completion.

CTLA-4 Fusion Proteins

The CTLA-4 fusion protein family of medications, namely, abatacept, is approved for use in rheumatoid arthritis, psoriatic arthritis, and juvenile idiopathic arthritis.

The immunosuppressive effects of abatacept are mediated through costimulatory CD28 interactions with CD80/86, thereby preventing T-cell activation [61].

With respect to HBV, Padovan et al. performed an observational retrospective study that included 51 HBsAg+ patients, 13 of whom received antiviral prophylaxis, and 21 anti-HBc+ patients, four of whom received antiviral prophylaxis, who were being treated with abatacept for rheumatoid arthritis [62]. Results demonstrated no cases of HBV reactivation in the cohort, including patients not receiving antiviral prophylaxis. This conflicts with a retrospective study by Kim et al. that included eight HBsAg+ patients receiving abatacept for rheumatoid arthritis where HBV reactivations were observed in 4/8 (50%) of patients, with reactivation rates of 100% (4/4) in those not receiving antiviral prophylaxis and 0% (0/4) in those receiving antiviral prophylaxis [63].

With respect to HCV, Chen et al. recently performed a prospective study that included 15 HCV+ patients treated with abatacept for rheumatoid arthritis and showed a statistically significant decrease in HCV viral load following 1 year of abatacept therapy when compared to pretreatment levels [45].

National guidelines and consensus statements suggest antiviral prophylaxis be given to HBsAg+ patients receiving abatacept while anti-HBc+ patients can be monitored [2, 32]. Those with chronic HCV infection should be treated at the first available opportunity without delay of biologic therapy pending its completion.

CTLA-4 Inhibitors

The CTLA-4 inhibitor family of medications includes ipilimumab and tremelimumab, which are currently approved for use in melanoma and renal cell carcinoma.

Their immunosuppressive effect is thought to be minimal, as CTLA-4 has an inhibitory signaling function, thereby negatively regulating T-cell priming by antigen-presenting cells. This function is abrogated by CTLA-4 inhibitors, thereby enhancing T-cell priming [61]. As a result of subsequent immune stimulation, however, medication-induced immune-mediated hepatitis may occur and be confused with reactivation of viral hepatitis.

With respect to both HBV and HCV, Ravi et al. conducted a retrospective case series of three HBsAg+ patients, two anti-HBc+ patients, and four chronic HCV patients receiving ipilimumab [64]. There were no cases of HBV reactivation in HBsAg+ patients and one of two anti-HBc+ patients receiving antiviral prophylaxis. Two of the four HCV+ patients experienced HCV reactivation while the other two patients had significant declines in viral load while on ipilimumab. In contrast, a small prospective study by Hosry et al. that included three chronic HCV patients treated with ipilimumab demonstrated elevated transaminase levels in each patient without associated HCV reactivation [65].

Due to a paucity of published evidence and limited clinical experience with the risk of HBV and HCV reactivation or hepatitis flare with CTLA-4 inhibitors, there are no firm recommendations on the management of CHB and chronic HCV infection with their use at this time.

PD-1/PD-L1 Inhibitors

The PD-1/PD-L1 inhibitor family of medications includes nivolumab, pembrolizumab, cemiplimab, atezolizumab, avelumab, and durvalumab, which are variably approved for melanoma, non-small cell lung cancer, urothelial and bladder carcinoma, metastatic renal cell carcinoma, Hodgkin's lymphoma, Merkel cell carcinoma, and head and neck squamous cell carcinoma.

Their immunomodulatory effect is mediated through the key role of PD-1, which is predominately expressed on CD4+ and CD8+ T cells, upon activation by PD-L1 or, to a lesser extent, PD-L2, inhibiting CD8+ T-cell effector function [66]. As with CTLA-4 inhibitors, given their underlying mechanism generally involves immune activation, it has been postulated that loss of immune control of chronic viral hepatitis may be unlikely, and in fact such agents may be useful in the treatment of chronic viral hepatitis while immune-mediated hepatitis may occur and be confused with reactivation of viral hepatitis.

With respect to HBV, a retrospective cohort study by Zhang et al. included 114 HBsAg+ patients undergoing anti-PD-1/PD-L1 therapy demonstrated HBV reactivation in 6/114 (5.3%) patients [67]. Of the six cases of HBV reactivation, only one patient had received antiviral prophylaxis. Similarly, a recent retrospective pharmacovigilance study and literature review by Muhsen identified 15 cases of HBV reactivation using the FDA Adverse Event Reporting System, along with seven additional published reports [68]. While interpretation is limited given unclear baseline HBV serologic information on participants, the authors presented an overall reporting odds ratio of 1.2 (95% CI 0.72–1.99) with only pembrolizumab having a statistically significant association with HBV reactivation with a reporting odds ratio of 2.93 (95% CI 1.57–5.46). Finally, the most comprehensive evidence comes from a systematic review by Pu et al. which included 188 patients in total, 137 of which were treated with PD-1 inhibitor monotherapy, with 89 patients being HBV-infected and 98 patients being HCV-infected [69]. Among these cohorts, HBV reactivation was observed in only 2/89 (2.25%) and HCV reactivation in only 1/98 (1.02%) of individuals. However, lack of granular data on the distribution of HBsAg+ versus anti-HBc+ serostatus and on the distribution of antiviral prophylaxis between groups, firm conclusions from the data remain difficult.

With respect to HCV, in addition to previously mentioned data published by Pu et al. suggesting low rates of HCV reactivation with PD-1/L1 inhibitor therapy, Tsimafeyeu et al. conducted a matched cohort study that included 44 matched patients receiving nivolumab. Of the 14/22 evaluable patients with baseline HCV infection, they found no significant impact of nivolumab therapy on HCV concentration with a mean change of 210 IU/mL ($p = 0.82$) [70].

As with the CTLA-4 inhibitor family of checkpoint inhibitors, due to a paucity of published evidence and limited clinical experience with the risk of HBV and HCV reactivation or hepatitis flare with the PD-1/PD-L1 inhibitor family of inhibitor agents, there are no firm recommendations on the management of CHB and chronic HCV infection with their use at this time.

Anti-CD52

The anti-CD52 inhibitor family of medications includes alemtuzumab which is approved for use in relapsing-remitting multiple sclerosis and B-cell chronic lymphocytic leukemia.

Their immunosuppressive effect is mediated through binding of CD52, which is expressed on B cells, T cells, NK cells, and macrophages, with resultant profound and persistent lymphocyte depletion [71].

With respect to HBV, a retrospective study by Kim et al. included 182 patients receiving alemtuzumab for a variety of hematologic malignancies with 15 patients identified as HBsAg+, seven of whom received antiviral prophylaxis. In follow-up, they identified four patients with HBV reactivation, one of whom was HBsAg+ but discontinued prophylaxis (1/15, 7%) and three of whom were anti-HBc+ but were not receiving prophylaxis, although the denominator for this group is not reported [72]. These results contrast somewhat with the presumed high theoretical risk of HBV reactivation given profound T-cell depletion with alemtuzumab, and recommendations generally suggest that antiviral prophylaxis be administered to HBsAg+ patients and either a prophylactic or preemptive strategy be used in anti-HBc+ patients receiving alemtuzumab [73].

With respect to HCV, while case reports of HCV reactivation with associated hepatitis have been sparsely published [74], more evidence on the safety of alemtuzumab administration in HCV-infected individuals, presuming direct-acting antiviral therapy will be administered, comes from studies using alemtuzumab induction immunosuppression in the setting of organ transplantation in HCV+ recipients [75, 76].

Anti-CCR4

The anti-CCR4 inhibitor family of medications includes mogamulizumab which is approved for use in adult T-cell leukemia/lymphoma, peripheral T-cell lymphoma, and cutaneous T-cell lymphoma.

Their immunosuppressive effect is mediated through blocking the activity of chemokines CCL2, CCL4, CCL5, CCL17, and CCL22 at the CCR4 receptor, which is expressed broadly including on Th2 cells, CD4+ memory cells, and regulatory T cells [77].

With respect to HBV, Totani et al. performed a retrospective review of 24 anti-HBc+ patients with adult T-cell leukemia who had received systemic chemotherapy, 11 of whom received mogamulizumab, and identified HBV reactivation in 2/11 (18%). None had received antiviral prophylaxis [78]. In addition, a recent report by Wang et al. using the Food and Drug Administration Adverse Event Reporting System and identified 338 total adverse cases during the study period of 2011–2019, with eight cases of HBV reactivation resulting in five patient deaths for a reporting odds ratio of 143.67 (95% CI 71.17–290.04) [79]. These results have informed recommendations that antiviral prophylaxis be administered to HBsAg+ patients receiving mogamulizumab while either preemptive monitoring or antiviral prophylaxis is suggested in anti-HBc+ patients.

Relevant evidence regarding the impact of mogamulizumab on chronic hepatitis C infection is lacking, and thus definitive recommendations cannot be made at this time.

Summary

The prevention of viral hepatitis reactivation and hepatitis flare in HBsAg+, anti-HBc+, and chronic HCV patients receiving biological and small molecule targeted immunomodulatory therapy is complex and depends on underlying host risk factors, serologic status, and therapy-specific considerations. For HBV, the risk of reactivation is generally much higher in those HBsAg+ than those anti-HBc+, and Table 23.2 summarizes the risk by serologic status and class of biologic agent. For

Table 23.2 Risk of HBV reactivation among HBsAg+/anti-HBc + patients receiving immunomodulatory therapy

Drug class	Examples	Hepatitis B serology	Risk class(high risk >10%, moderate risk 1–10%, low risk <1%)
B-cell-depleting agents	Rituximab, ofatumumab, ocrelizumab, veltuzumab, ublituximab, ocaratuzumab, ^{90}Y-ibritumomab tiuxetan	HBsAg+ Anti-HBc+	High High
Anti-TNF-α	Etanercept, adalimumab, infliximab, certolizumab, golimumab	HBsAg+ Anti-HBc+	High Moderate
Anti-IL1Ra	Anakinra	HBsAg+ Anti-HBc+	Low/moderate Low
Anti-IL-6/ anti-IL-6R	Tocilizumab, sarilumab	HBsAg+ Anti-HBc+	High Low/moderate
Anti-IL-12/23 and anti-IL-23	Ustekinumab, guselkumab, tildrakizumab, risankizumab	HBsAg+ Anti-HBc+	High Moderate
Anti-IL-17	Secukinumab, ixekizumab, brodalumab	HBsAg+ Anti-HBc+	High Moderate
Integrin inhibitors	Natalizumab, vedolizumab	HBsAg+ Anti-HBc+	Moderate Moderate
CTLA-4 fusion proteins	Abatacept	HBsAg+ Anti-HBc+	Moderate Low
CTLA-4 inhibitors	Ipilimumab, tremelimumab	HBsAg+ Anti-HBc+	Moderate Moderate
PD-1/PD-L1 inhibitors	Nivolumab, pembrolizumab, cemiplimab, atezolizumab, avelumab, durvalumab	HBsAg+ Anti-HBc+	Moderate Moderate
JAK/STAT	Tofacitinib, baricitinib, ruxolitinib	HBsAg+ Anti-HBc+	Moderate/high Low
Anti-CD52	Alemtuzumab	HBsAg+ Anti-HBc+	High High
Anti-CCR4	Mogamulizumab	HBSAg+ Anti-HBc+	High Moderate/high

traditional immunosuppressive therapies and non-biologic disease-modifying antirheumatic drugs, extensive clinical experience allows for more definitive recommendations on patient management, decisions regarding prophylaxis or preemptive therapy for HBV+ patients, and sequential versus concomitant versus inverse sequential therapy for HCV+ patients. For many small molecule targeted immunomodulatory therapies, however, data are limited by the typical exclusion of such patients from large registration trials and an evidence base that relies predominantly on small retrospective studies as well as case reports and case series. Additionally, the armamentarium of biological and small molecule targeted immunomodulatory therapies continues to expand at a rapid pace, leaving the clinical infection prevention and management of such patients a vexing challenge for practitioners.

References

1. Papastergiou V, Lombardi R, MacDonald D. Global epidemiology of hepatitis B virus (HBV) infection. Curr Hepatol Rep. 2015;14:171–8.
2. Coffin CS, et al. Management of chronic hepatitis B: Canadian Association for the Study of the liver consensus guidelines. Can J Gastroenterol. 2012;26(12):917–38.
3. Chuaypen N, et al. Kinetics of serum HBsAg and intrahepatic cccDNA during pegylated interferon therapy in patients with HBeAg-positive and HBeAg-negative chronic hepatitis B. J Med Virol. 2017;89(1):130–8.
4. Mu D, et al. Baseline value of intrahepatic HBV DNA over cccDNA predicts patient's response to interferon therapy. Sci Rep. 2017;7(1):5937.
5. Belloni L, et al. IFN-alpha inhibits HBV transcription and replication in cell culture and in humanized mice by targeting the epigenetic regulation of the nuclear cccDNA minichromosome. J Clin Invest. 2012;122(2):529–37.
6. Xia Y, et al. Interferon-gamma and tumor necrosis factor-alpha produced by T cells reduce the HBV persistence form, cccDNA, without cytolysis. Gastroenterology. 2016;150(1):194–205.
7. Biermer M, Puro R, Schneider RJ. Tumor necrosis factor alpha inhibition of hepatitis B virus replication involves disruption of capsid integrity through activation of NF-kappaB. J Virol. 2003;77(7):4033–42.
8. Blackburn SD, et al. Coregulation of CD8+ T cell exhaustion by multiple inhibitory receptors during chronic viral infection. Nat Immunol. 2009;10(1):29–37.
9. Chen L, Flies DB. Molecular mechanisms of T cell co-stimulation and co-inhibition. Nat Rev Immunol. 2013;13(4):227–42.
10. Yang G, et al. Association of CD4+CD25+Foxp3+ regulatory T cells with chronic activity and viral clearance in patients with hepatitis B. Int Immunol. 2007;19(2):133–40.
11. Sun HQ, et al. Increased Th17 cells contribute to disease progression in patients with HBV-associated liver cirrhosis. J Viral Hepat. 2012;19(6):396–403.
12. Chen KL, et al. Hepatitis B virus reactivation and hepatitis in diffuse large B-cell lymphoma patients with resolved hepatitis B receiving rituximab-containing chemotherapy: risk factors and survival. Chin J Cancer. 2015;34(5):225–34.
13. Terrault NA, et al. Update on prevention, diagnosis, and treatment of chronic hepatitis B: AASLD 2018 hepatitis B guidance. Hepatology. 2018;67(4):1560–99.
14. Yeo W, et al. Hepatitis B virus reactivation during cytotoxic chemotherapy-enhanced viral replication precedes overt hepatitis. J Med Virol. 2001;65(3):473–7.
15. Lau GK, et al. High hepatitis B virus (HBV) DNA viral load as the most important risk factor for HBV reactivation in patients positive for HBV surface antigen undergoing autologous hematopoietic cell transplantation. Blood. 2002;99(7):2324–30.

16. Lok AS, et al. Reactivation of hepatitis B virus replication in patients receiving cytotoxic therapy. Report of a prospective study. Gastroenterology. 1991;100(1):182–8.
17. Paul S, et al. Role of surface antibody in hepatitis B reactivation in patients with resolved infection and hematologic malignancy: a meta-analysis. Hepatology. 2017;66(2):379–88.
18. Yeo W, et al. Frequency of hepatitis B virus reactivation in cancer patients undergoing cytotoxic chemotherapy: a prospective study of 626 patients with identification of risk factors. J Med Virol. 2000;62(3):299–307.
19. Messina JP, et al. Global distribution and prevalence of hepatitis C virus genotypes. Hepatology. 2015;61(1):77–87.
20. Robaeys G, et al. Global genotype distribution of hepatitis C viral infection among people who inject drugs. J Hepatol. 2016;65(6):1094–103.
21. Shepard CW, Finelli L, Alter MJ. Global epidemiology of hepatitis C virus infection. Lancet Infect Dis. 2005;5(9):558–67.
22. Golden-Mason L, et al. Upregulation of PD-1 expression on circulating and intrahepatic hepatitis C virus-specific CD8+ T cells associated with reversible immune dysfunction. J Virol. 2007;81(17):9249–58.
23. Hall CH, et al. HCV+ hepatocytes induce human regulatory CD4+ T cells through the production of TGF-beta. PLoS One. 2010;5(8):e12154.
24. Torres HA, et al. Hepatitis C virus reactivation in patients receiving cancer treatment: a prospective observational study. Hepatology. 2018;67(1):36–47.
25. Menter A, et al. Joint AAD-NPF guidelines of care for the management and treatment of psoriasis with biologics. J Am Acad Dermatol. 2019;80(4):1029–72.
26. Bykerk VP, et al. Canadian rheumatology association recommendations for pharmacological management of rheumatoid arthritis with traditional and biologic disease-modifying antirheumatic drugs. J Rheumatol. 2012;39(8):1559–82.
27. Pescovitz MD. Rituximab, an anti-cd20 monoclonal antibody: history and mechanism of action. Am J Transplant. 2006;6(5 Pt 1):859–66.
28. Gentile G, et al. Screening, monitoring, prevention, prophylaxis and therapy for hepatitis B virus reactivation in patients with haematologic malignancies and patients who underwent haematologic stem cell transplantation: a systematic review. Clin Microbiol Infect. 2017;23(12):916–23.
29. Chen YM, et al. Reactivation of hepatitis B virus infection following rituximab treatment in HBsAg-negative, HBcAb-positive rheumatoid arthritis patients: a long-term, real-world observation. Int J Rheum Dis. 2019;22(6):1145–51.
30. Ennishi D, et al. Hepatic toxicity and prognosis in hepatitis C virus-infected patients with diffuse large B-cell lymphoma treated with rituximab-containing chemotherapy regimens: a Japanese multicenter analysis. Blood. 2010;116(24):5119–25.
31. Chen YM, et al. A comparison of safety profiles of tumour necrosis factor alpha inhibitors and rituximab therapy in patients with rheumatoid arthritis and chronic hepatitis C. Ann Rheum Dis. 2015;74(3):626–7.
32. Reddy KR, et al. American Gastroenterological Association Institute guideline on the prevention and treatment of hepatitis B virus reactivation during immunosuppressive drug therapy. Gastroenterology. 2015;148(1):215–9; quiz e16–7.
33. Cessak G, et al. TNF inhibitors - mechanisms of action, approved and off-label indications. Pharmacol Rep. 2014;66(5):836–44.
34. Pauly MP, et al. Incidence of hepatitis B virus reactivation and hepatotoxicity in patients receiving long-term treatment with tumor necrosis factor antagonists. Clin Gastroenterol Hepatol. 2018;16(12):1964–1973 e1.
35. Snast I, et al. Risk for hepatitis B and C virus reactivation in patients with psoriasis on biologic therapies: a retrospective cohort study and systematic review of the literature. J Am Acad Dermatol. 2017;77(1):88–97 e5.
36. Pompili M, et al. Tumor necrosis factor-alpha inhibitors and chronic hepatitis C: a comprehensive literature review. World J Gastroenterol. 2013;19(44):7867–73.

37. Dinarello CA. Overview of the IL-1 family in innate inflammation and acquired immunity. Immunol Rev. 2018;281(1):8–27.
38. Barone M, et al. Safety of long-term biologic therapy in rheumatologic patients with a previously resolved hepatitis B viral infection. Hepatology. 2015;62(1):40–6.
39. Carroll MB. The impact of biologic response modifiers on hepatitis B virus infection. Expert Opin Biol Ther. 2011;11(4):533–44.
40. Lan T, et al. IL-6 plays a crucial role in HBV infection. J Clin Transl Hepatol. 2015;3(4):271–6.
41. Chen LF, et al. Short-course tocilizumab increases risk of hepatitis B virus reactivation in patients with rheumatoid arthritis: a prospective clinical observation. Int J Rheum Dis. 2017;20(7):859–69.
42. Ahn SS, et al. Safety of Tocilizumab in rheumatoid arthritis patients with resolved hepatitis B virus infection: data from real-world experience. Yonsei Med J. 2018;59(3):452–6.
43. Nagashima T, et al. Unchanged serum viral load and liver function during tocilizumab treatment in a patient with rheumatoid arthritis and hepatitis C virus infection. Rheumatol Int. 2012;32(7):2231–2.
44. Dragonas C, Ehrenstein B, Fleck M. Tocilizumab treatment in a patient suffering from rheumatoid arthritis and concomitant chronic hepatitis C infection. Rheumatology (Oxford). 2012;51(8):1520–1.
45. Chen YM, et al. Comparisons of hepatitis C viral replication in patients with rheumatoid arthritis receiving tocilizumab, abatacept and tofacitinib therapy. Ann Rheum Dis. 2019;78(6):849–50.
46. Aggeletopoulou I, et al. Interleukin 12/interleukin 23 pathway: biological basis and therapeutic effect in patients with Crohn's disease. World J Gastroenterol. 2018;24(36):4093–103.
47. Ting SW, Chen YC, Huang YH. Risk of hepatitis B reactivation in patients with psoriasis on Ustekinumab. Clin Drug Investig. 2018;38(9):873–80.
48. Chiu HY, et al. The safety profile of Ustekinumab in the treatment of patients with psoriasis and concurrent hepatitis B or C. Br J Dermatol. 2013;169(6):1295–303.
49. Navarro R, et al. Safety and effectiveness of Ustekinumab and antitumour necrosis factor therapy in patients with psoriasis and chronic viral hepatitis B or C: a retrospective, multicentre study in a clinical setting. Br J Dermatol. 2013;168(3):609–16.
50. Onishi RM, Gaffen SL. Interleukin-17 and its target genes: mechanisms of interleukin-17 function in disease. Immunology. 2010;129(3):311–21.
51. Chiu HY, et al. Safety pro fi le of Secukinumab in treatment of patients with psoriasis and concurrent hepatitis B or C: a multicentric prospective cohort study. Acta Derm Venereol. 2018;98(9):829–34.
52. Moneva-Leniz LM, et al. Risk of hepatitis B virus reactivation in patients on Secukinumab for psoriasis: a series of 4 cases. Actas Dermosifiliogr. 2020;111(7):613–4.
53. Siegel S, Winthrop K, Ehst BD, Ortega Loayza A. 191 Secukinumab treatment of individuals with psoriasis infected with hepatitis B and/or hepatitis C virus. J Investig Dermatol. 2017;137:S32.
54. Ley K, et al. Integrin-based therapeutics: biological basis, clinical use and new drugs. Nat Rev Drug Discov. 2016;15(3):173–83.
55. Hillen ME, et al. Fatal acute liver failure with hepatitis B virus infection during nataluzimab treatment in multiple sclerosis. Neurol Neuroimmunol Neuroinflamm. 2015;2(2):e72.
56. Ng SC, et al. Low frequency of opportunistic infections in patients receiving Vedolizumab in clinical trials and post-marketing setting. Inflamm Bowel Dis. 2018;24(11):2431–41.
57. Epstein DJ, Dunn J, Deresinski S. Infectious complications of multiple sclerosis therapies: implications for screening, prophylaxis, and management. Open Forum Infect Dis. 2018;5(8):174.
58. Hodge JA, et al. The mechanism of action of tofacitinib—an oral Janus kinase inhibitor for the treatment of rheumatoid arthritis. Clin Exp Rheumatol. 2016;34(2):318–28.
59. Chen YM, et al. Reactivation of hepatitis B virus infection in patients with rheumatoid arthritis receiving tofacitinib: a real-world study. Ann Rheum Dis. 2018;77(5):780–2.

60. Serling-Boyd N, et al. The use of tocilizumab and tofacitinib in patients with resolved hepatitis B infection: a case series. Ann Rheum Dis. 2021;80(2):1–2.
61. Herrero-Beaumont G, Martinez Calatrava MJ, Castaneda S. Abatacept mechanism of action: concordance with its clinical profile. Reumatol Clin. 2012;8(2):78–83.
62. Padovan M, et al. Safety of Abatacept in rheumatoid arthritis with serologic evidence of past or present hepatitis B virus infection. Arthritis Care Res (Hoboken). 2016;68(6):738–43.
63. Kim PS, et al. Safety and efficacy of abatacept in eight rheumatoid arthritis patients with chronic hepatitis B. Arthritis Care Res (Hoboken). 2012;64(8):1265–8.
64. Ravi S, et al. Ipilimumab administration for advanced melanoma in patients with pre-existing hepatitis B or C infection: a multicenter, retrospective case series. J Immunother Cancer. 2014;2(1):33.
65. Hosry J, Naing A, Torres H. 2226. Immune checkpoint inhibitors in solid tumor patients with chronic hepatitis C virus infection: a prospective case-series. Open Forum Infect Dis. 2018;5:S658.
66. Wu Q, et al. Small molecule inhibitors targeting the PD-1/PD-L1 signaling pathway. Acta Pharmacol Sin. 2021;42(1):1–9.
67. Zhang X, et al. Hepatitis B virus reactivation in cancer patients with positive hepatitis B surface antigen undergoing PD-1 inhibition. J Immunother Cancer. 2019;7(1):322.
68. Burns EA, et al. Hepatitis B virus reactivation in cancer patients treated with immune checkpoint inhibitors. J Immunother. 2021;44:132–9.
69. Pu D, et al. Safety and efficacy of immune checkpoint inhibitors in patients with HBV/HCV infection and advanced-stage cancer: a systematic review. Medicine (Baltimore). 2020;99(5):e19013.
70. Tsimafeyeu I, et al. Nivolumab in patients with metastatic renal cell carcinoma and chronic hepatitis C virus infection. Cancer Immunol Immunother. 2020;69(6):983–8.
71. Li Z, et al. Clinical pharmacology of alemtuzumab, an anti-CD52 immunomodulator, in multiple sclerosis. Clin Exp Immunol. 2018;194(3):295–314.
72. Kim SJ, et al. Non-bacterial infections in Asian patients treated with alemtuzumab: a retrospective study of the Asian lymphoma study group. Leuk Lymphoma. 2012;53(8):1515–24.
73. Mikulska M, et al. ESCMID study Group for Infections in compromised hosts (ESGICH) consensus document on the safety of targeted and biological therapies: an infectious diseases perspective (agents targeting lymphoid cells surface antigens [I]: CD19, CD20 and CD52). Clin Microbiol Infect. 2018;24(Suppl 2):S71–82.
74. Anoop P, Wotherspoon A, Matutes E. Severe liver dysfunction from hepatitis C virus reactivation following alemtuzumab treatment for chronic lymphocytic leukaemia. Br J Haematol. 2010;148(3):484–6.
75. Del Gaudio M, et al. Induction therapy with alemtuzumab (campath) in combined liver-kidney transplantation: University of Bologna experience. Transplant Proc. 2013;45(5):1969–70.
76. Vivanco M, et al. Campath induction in HCV and HCV/HIV-seropositive kidney transplant recipients. Transpl Int. 2013;26(10):1016–26.
77. Hagemann UB, et al. Fully human antagonistic antibodies against CCR4 potently inhibit cell signaling and chemotaxis. PLoS One. 2014;9(7):e103776.
78. Totani H, et al. Reactivation of hepatitis B virus (HBV) infection in adult T-cell leukemia-lymphoma patients with resolved HBV infection following systemic chemotherapy. Int J Hematol. 2015;101(4):398–404.
79. Wang S, et al. Risk of hepatitis B reactivation and cytomegalovirus related infections with Mogamulizumab: a retrospective study of international pharmacovigilance database. EClin Med. 2020;28:100601.

Immune-Targeted Therapies for COVID-19

24

Michele Bartoletti and Renato Pascale

Introduction

SARS-CoV-2 is a *Betacoronavirus* belonging to the family of *Coronaviridae*. Coronaviruses are large, enveloped, single-stranded RNA virus largely distributed in nature and in animals, which occasionally may infect human beings. SARS-CoV-2 targets mainly nasal and bronchial epithelial cells and pneumocytes through the SARS-CoV-2 spike glycoprotein (S) that binds the host cell surface via angiotensin-converting enzyme-2 (ACE2) receptor, allowing virus cell entry and replication. As the ACE2 receptor is widely distributed in several organs and tissues, a variety of organ involvement has been described due to tropism to central nervous system, kidneys, myocardium, and gut [1–5].

The pathological features of SARS-CoV-2 are similar to SARS-CoV and MERS-CoV infections. After infection, profound lymphopenia may occur as SARS-CoV-2 infects and kills T lymphocyte cells. Additionally, impaired lymphopoiesis and increased lymphocyte apoptosis may occur during the viral inflammatory response, with compromise in adaptive and innate immune responses [5].

It is believed that the delayed type I interferon (IFN) response plays a role in the process of SARS-CoV-2 infection. In the initial phase, the virus evades pattern recognition receptors and antagonizes the type I INF response in the airway and alveolar epithelial cells, which leads to rapid viral replication. However, plasmacytoid dendritic cell and macrophage response to SARS-CoV-2 leads to a strong but delayed type I IFN response as well as releasing other inflammatory cytokines. The

M. Bartoletti (✉) · R. Pascale
Division of Infectious Diseases, IRCCS Azienda Ospedaliero-Universitaria di Bologna, Bologna, Italy

Department of Medical and Surgical Sciences, Alma Mater Studiorum University of Bologna, Bologna, Italy
e-mail: m.bartoletti@unibo.it; renato.pascale@aosp.bo.it

C. Cervera, J. M. Aguado (eds.), *Infectious Complications in Biologic and Targeted Therapies*, https://doi.org/10.1007/978-3-031-11363-5_24

activation of type I IFN signaling cascades attracts neutrophils, inflammatory monocyte-macrophages, dendritic cells, and natural killer (NK) cells to the lung, and a cytokine-driven cycle occurs [5, 6].

The clinical spectrum of COVID-19 is broad with the majority of infected individuals experiencing only a mild or subclinical illness, especially in the early phase of disease [7]. However, between 14 and 30% of hospitalized patients diagnosed with COVID-19 develop a severe respiratory failure requiring intensive care [8–11].

As the median time from symptom onset to worsening is on average 7 days, it has been hypothesized that the main cause of illness progression is a cytokine storm characterized by dysregulated release of inflammatory products leading to organ failure and acute respiratory distress syndrome (ARDS). For this reason, it has been hypothesized that corticosteroids and other immunomodulators may have a role in reducing the inflammatory cascade [5]. Consistently, the use of corticosteroids was associated to lower mortality rate in randomized and non-randomized trials when compared with controls [12–14].

From a pathophysiological perspective, the inflammatory response of COVID-19 is characterized by the release of many different cytokines and inflammatory markers such as interleukins (IL-1, IL-6, IL-8, IL-120, and IL-12), tumor necrosis factor-α (TNF-α), IFN-λ and IFN-β, CXCL-10, monocyte chemoattractant protein-1 (MCP-1), and macrophage inflammatory protein-1α (MIP-1α). Cytokines and chemokines act as chemoattractants for neutrophils, CD4 helper T cells, and CD8 cytotoxic T cells, which are recruited in the lung tissue. If on the one hand this is necessary to fight against the virus, on the other these cells are responsible for inducing uncontrolled inflammation of the lung. The host cell undergoes apoptosis with the release of new viral particles, which then infect the adjacent type 2 alveolar epithelial cells in the same manner. Due to the persistent injury caused by the sequestered inflammatory cells and viral replication leading to loss of both type 1 and type 2 pneumocytes, there is diffuse alveolar damage eventually culminating ARDS [15–18].

Immunomodulatory Agents for the Treatment of COVID-19

SARS-CoV-2 triggers a strong immune response which may cause CRS. Thus, immunomodulatory agents that inhibit the excessive inflammatory response may be a potential adjunctive therapy for COVID-19.

Dexamethasone is a corticosteroid often used in a wide range of conditions to relieve inflammation through its anti-inflammatory and immunosuppressant effects. Results from RCTs showed that corticosteroid treatment was associated with reduced mortality and need for mechanical ventilation [19–26]. The largest experience come from the RECOVERY trial, which enrolled 2104 patients assigned to receive dexamethasone and 4321 to receive usual care [19]. In RECOVERY, dexamethasone reduced mortality by about one third in hospitalized patients with COVID-19 who received invasive mechanical ventilation (29.3% vs. 41.4%; RR, 0.64; 95% CI, 0.51 to 0.81) and by one fifth in patients receiving oxygen (23.3% vs.

26.2%; rate ratio, 0.82; 95% CI, 0.72 to 0.94). By contrast, no benefit was found in patients without respiratory support (17.8% vs. 14.0%; rate ratio, 1.19; 95% CI, 0.92 to 1.55). Furthermore, in patients who did not require oxygen, corticosteroids seem not to be associated with improved outcome but also increased mortality [19]. Worthy of mention, corticosteroid administration is not affected by severe adverse events and superinfections compared with other treatment [19, 20, 22].

Interleukin-6 Antagonists

Tocilizumab

Tocilizumab is a humanized IL-6 receptor antagonist. It is approved for the treatment rheumatoid arthritis, systemic juvenile idiopathic arthritis, juvenile idiopathic polyarthritis, and giant cell arteritis in adults [27–29]. More recently, tocilizumab was successfully used to treat CRS in patients receiving chimeric antigen receptor T (CAR-T) cells as treatment for refractory B-cell malignancies [17].

Tocilizumab was used early in the course of the pandemic for the treatment of severe COVID-19 patients based on several considerations. First the CRS is considered the main pathophysiological feature of the disease leading to ARDS. Second, the initial reports from China and Italy revealed that most patients with critical COVID-19 had higher levels of IL-6. Third, initial retrospective observational studies showed promising results for the use of tocilizumab in terms of reduction in mortality [30–32].

Tocilizumab efficacy was further assessed in seven large randomized clinical trials (RCTs) with conflicting results (Table 24.1). Most smaller trials did not show any mortality benefits [33–37]. Conversely the REMAP-CAP and the RECOVERY trial showed significant, though small, benefits [38, 39]. The REMAP-CAP study is an ongoing international, multifactorial, adaptive platform trial including ICU patients randomly assigned to receive tocilizumab, sarilumab, or standard of care. The primary outcome was respiratory and cardiovascular organ support-free days, on an ordinal scale combining in-hospital death and days free of organ support to day 21. Overall, the group treated with IL-6 receptor blocker had an in-hospital mortality of 27%, as compared with 36% in the control group, and those receiving the receptor blocker had a median of 10–11 organ support-free days, as compared with zero days for controls [39].

The RECOVERY trial is an ongoing large adaptive trial enrolling COVID-19 patient with different levels of disease severity which already led to important findings regarding the clinical benefits of corticosteroids. In the study assessing the efficacy of tocilizumab, patients were enrolled and assigned to the tocilizumab or standard of care group if they had oxygen saturation <92% on air or requiring oxygen therapy and evidence of systemic inflammation defined by a level of C-reactive protein CRP ≥75 mg/L. The primary outcome was all-cause 28-day mortality and was assessed in 4116 adults. Overall, 29% patients allocated tocilizumab and 33%

Table 24.1 Summary if available randomized controlled trial to assess efficacy of tocilizumab in COVID-19 patients

RCT	Design	Number of patients	Country, centers	Inclusion criteria	Tocilizumab	Primary outcome	Main results (based on primary endpoint)
RCT-TCZ-COVID-19 [33] NCT04346355	Open label	60 TCZ versus 66 controls	Italy, 24 centers	COVID-19 pneumonia + PaO_2/FIO_2 between 200 and 300 mmHg and an inflammatory phenotype defined by fever and elevated CRP	8 mg/kg up to a maximum of 800 mg, followed by a second dose after 12 h	Composite outcome: ICU admission for MV, death from all causes, or clinical aggravation documented by the finding of a PaO_2/FIO_2 ratio < 150 mmHg, whichever came first	17 of 60 (28.3%) in the TCZ arm vs. 17 of 63 (27.0%) in the standard care group (rate ratio, 1.05; 95% CI, 0.59–1.86)
CORIMUNO-19 [34] NCT04331808	Open label	64 TCZ versus 67 controls	France, nine centers	COVID-19 and moderate or severe pneumonia requiring at least 3 L/min of oxygen but without ventilation or admission to ICU	8 mg/kg on day 1 and on day 3 if clinically indicated	Scores >5 on the World Health Organization 10-point Clinical Progression Scale (WHO-CPS) on day 4 and survival without need of ventilation (including noninvasive ventilation) at day 14	In the TCZ group, 12 patients had a WHO-CPS score > 5 at day 4 vs. 19 in the UC group (median posterior absolute risk difference −9.0%; 90% credible interval, −21.0 to 3.1)
BACC Bay Tocilizumab Trial [36] NCT04356937	Double-blind, placebo-controlled trial	161 TCZ versus 81 controls	USA, seven centers	SARS-CoV-2 infection, hyperinflammatory states, and at least two of the following signs: fever (body temperature >38 °C), pulmonary infiltrates, or the need for supplemental oxygen in order to maintain an oxygen saturation >92%	Single dose of tocilizumab 8 mg/kg	Intubation or death	HR for intubation or death in the tocilizumab group as compared with the placebo group was 0.83 (95% CI, 0.38 to 1.81; $P = 0.64$), and the hazard ratio for disease worsening was 1.11 (95% CI, 0.59 to 2.10; $P = 0.73$)

COVACTA NCT04320615 [35]	Double-blind, placebo-controlled trial	294 TCZ versus 144 controls	Nine countries (Canada, Denmark, France, Germany, Italy, the Netherlands, Spain, UK, USA), 67 centers	Patients ≥18 years with severe COVID-19 pneumonia confirmed by PCR test in any body fluid and evidenced by bilateral chest infiltrates. Blood oxygen saturation ≤93% or partial pressure of oxygen/fraction of inspired oxygen <300 mm/Hg	8 mg/kg infusion, maximum 800 mg second infusion could be administered 8–24 h after the first	Clinical status on a 7-category ordinal scale at day 28 (1, discharged/ready for discharge; 7, death)	Median value for clinical status on the ordinal scale at day 28 was 1.0 (95% CI, 1.0 to 1.0) in the TCZ group and 2.0 (95% CI, 1.0 to 4.0) in the placebo group (between-group difference, −1.0; 95% CI, −2.5 to 0; $P = 0.31$) Mortality at day 28: 19.7% in the TCZ group and 19.4% in the placebo group ($P = 0.94$)
EMPACTA NCT04372186 [90]	Double-blind, placebo-controlled trial	194 TCZ versus 195 controls	Six countries (Brazil, Kenya, Mexico, Peru, South Africa, USA), 69 centers	COVID-19 pneumonia confirmed by PCR of any specimen and radiographic imaging SpO_2 <94% while on ambient air	8 mg/kg × 1, possible second dose	Death or MV by day 28	Primary endpoint: 12.0% (95% CI, 8.5 to 16.9) in the tocilizumab group and 19.3% (95% CI, 13.3 to 27.4) in the placebo group (HR for MV or death, 0.56; 95% CI, 0.33 to 0.97; $P = 0.04$ by the log-rank test)

(continued)

Table 24.1 (continued)

RCT	Design	Number of patients	Country, centers	Inclusion criteria	Tocilizumab	Primary outcome	Main results (based on primary endpoint)
RECOVERY (NCT04381936) [38]	Open label	2022 in the TCZ group 2094 in the usual care group	UK, 131 centers	Clinically suspected or laboratory confirmed SARS-CoV-2 infection	One dose (8 mg/kg max 800 mg) followed by a second dose 12–24 h later on clinical judgment basis	All-cause mortality at day 28	Primary endpoint 29% in tocilizumab group vs. 33% of in the usual care (rate ratio 0.86; 95% CI 0.77–0.96; $p = 0.007$
REMAP-CAP NCT02735707 [39]	International, multifactorial, adaptive platform trial	353 in the TCZ group 48 to sarilumab and 402 controls	Over 200 centers across 19 countries	Adult patients with Covid-19, within 24 h of commencing organ support in an ICU	Tocilizumab (8 mg/kg) or sarilumab (400 mg)	Ordinal scale combining in-hospital mortality (assigned −1) and days free of organ support to day 21	Median organ support-free days were 10 (interquartile range [IQR] −1, 16), 11 (IQR 0, 16) and 0 (IQR −1, 15) for tocilizumab, sarilumab and control, respectively
TOCIBRAS NCT04403685 [37]	Open label	65 in TCZ 64 standard of care	Brazil (six centers)	Adults with confirmed COVID-19 who were receiving supplemental oxygen or MV and had abnormal levels of at least two serum biomarkers (CRP, D-dimer, lactate dehydrogenase, or ferritin	Single intravenous infusion of 8 mg/kg	Composite of death or mechanical ventilation	TCZ: 18 of 65 (28%) patients in the tocilizumab group SOC 13 of 64 (20%) (OR 1.54, 95% CI 0.66 to 3.66; $P = 0.32$

CI confidence interval, *CRP* C-reactive protein, *ICU* intensive care unit, *IQR* interquartile range, *HR* hazard ratio, *MV* mechanical ventilation, *OR* odds ratio, *PCR* polymerase chain reaction, *TCZ* tocilizumab of patients allocated to usual care died within 28 days (rate ratio 0.86; 95% confidence interval [CI] 0.77–0.96; $p = 0.007$) [38].

To date, the clinical benefit of IL-6 receptor blocker remains unclear. However, it seems that there is an advantage at least under some circumstances. These may be the type of patients, type of inflammation, or timing between the clinical diagnosis and drug administrations. Although the combination of different drugs has not been explored, in the RECOVERY trial the subgroup of patients that received corticosteroids appeared to have higher benefit from tocilizumab [13, 38].

Tocilizumab use was not associated to an increase rate of adverse events in most clinical trials. However, in observational studies and case series, an association with bacterial infections and life-threatening reactivation of herpes simplex virus was found [40].

Siltuximab

Siltuximab is a monoclonal antibody that blocks IL-6 signaling by binding IL-6 itself and preventing it from activating immune effector cells. It is approved for the treatment of adults with multicentric Castleman's disease who are human immunodeficiency virus and human herpes virus-8 negative [41].

Additionally, it was used as salvage treatment for cytokine-releasing syndrome complicating patients undergoing chimeric antigen receptor (CAR) T cell therapy [29]. Compared with tocilizumab, siltuximab has a higher affinity for IL-6 than tocilizumab has for the IL-6 receptor making it an attractive drug in managing COVID-19 patients.

In a recent observational study of patients receiving ventilator support, the use of siltuximab was associated with lower mortality compared with patients receiving usual treatment even after adjustment for confounders and matching using propensity scores [42]. To date, siltuximab has not been evaluated in randomized trial. Therefore, its use in clinical practice is under debate.

JAK/STAT Pathway Inhibitor

Cytokines regulate different cellular and immune processes, and their activation is controlled by the Janus kinases and the signal transducers and activators of transcription (JAK/STAT, Janus kinase signal transducer and activator of transcription proteins) signaling pathway [43]. Different therapeutic strategies to overcome hyperinflammation in COVID-19 include the use of JAK/STAT pathway inhibitors [44].

The JAK/STAT pathway is one of the main regulatory cell signaling pathway. The JAK non-receptor tyrosine kinases receive different extracellular signals (growth factor, cytokine, and hormone) from host receptors and transfer these responses to the nucleus via the intracellular STATs. Depending on the physiological signal, the JAK/STAT pathway regulates critical cellular homeostasis processes including immune response, proliferation, differentiation, migration, and apoptosis [45]. The IL6/JAK/STAT3 signaling pathway represents a specific branch of the pathway that includes IL-6, one of the most highly expressed cytokines in COVID-19 as mentioned above [46, 47]. However, other cytokines stimulated by JAK/STAT pathway, such as IL-2, IL-7, IL-10, IFN-γ, G-CSF, and GM-CSF, are also elevated and may be equally or more important in the inflammatory response in patients with severe COVID-19 [46]. Moreover, SARS-CoV-2 enters the cells through receptor-mediated endocytosis. One of the known regulators of endocytosis is the AP2-associated protein kinase 1 (AAK1). Therefore, another potential target of anti-SARS-CoV-2 drug could be the inhibition of AAK1 interrupting the endocytosis of the virus into cells stopping the intracellular assembly of virus particles [48].

Ruxolitinib

Ruxolitinib is a JAK inhibitor that blocks JAK kinase activity and prevents STAT activation and nuclear translocation. Ruxolitinib was approved in the USA and European Union for the treatments of myelofibrosis, polycythemia vera, and acute graft-versus-host disease, diseases characterized by over-inflammation cytokine-driven [49]. In addition, ruxolitinib has begun to take its place in the treatment of autoimmune diseases such as rheumatoid arthritis, psoriasis, and lupus erythematosus, as well as other allergic and inflammatory diseases [50]. Ruxolitinib inhibits IL-6/JAK/STAT3 pathway, thus reducing circulating IL-6 levels [51, 52]. In all these syndromes, ruxolitinib shows to have reduction of the cytokine burden and levels of these pro-inflammatory biomarkers [51, 53, 54]. The effect of ruxolitinib in animal model showed a significant reduction in the inflammatory cytokines in circulation, but no differences were observed in the proportion of peripheral CD4+ or CD8+ T cells. These data suggest that ruxolitinib has immunomodulatory but not immunodepleting effects [55, 56].

Ruxolitinib is characterized by rapid oral absorption and a with an half-life of approximately 3 h, shorter than other JAK inhibitors [57, 58]. It has a concentration-dependent and reversible pharmacodynamic effect. A therapy cycle of 14 days with dose ranges of 5 to 15 mg BID could be effective enough in inhibition of cytokine signaling and minimize adverse events, especially risk of long-term infection or other complication. As regard adverse effects, thrombocytopenia and anemia are the most frequently observed during ruxolitinib treatment. A reversible cytopenia, elevated lipid parameters, and non-melanoma skin cancers are also reported [53, 59–61].

Suppression of the JAK/STAT pathway by ruxolitinib can also result in reactivation of different herpesvirus family members like varicella-zoster virus (VZV), Epstein-Barr virus, and cytomegalovirus (CMV) with several clinical manifestations ranging from gastric ulcer to meningoencephalitis and secondary lymphoproliferative disorders [60, 62–64]. Furthermore the development of polyomavirus JC virus-related fatal encephalopathy and meningitis has been reported [65, 66] as well as hepatitis B virus (HBV) reactivation [67]. Of note, opportunistic infections are reported during long-course therapy, and, currently, increased infectious adverse events are not yet reported during short-course treatment for COVID-19.

Few clinical experiences are available for treatment with ruxolitinib for COVID-19, mainly case reports or small case series [58–62, 68–71].

There are few relevant clinical trials. A prospective experience was reported by La Rosee et al. [72]. In this study the efficacy of ruxolitinib was demonstrated in 14 patients with severe COVID-19. Patients were stratified using an internal score to receive targeted inhibition of cytokine with ruxolitinib. In this study, the dose of ruxolitinib was 7.5 mg BID and then increased to a maximum of 15 mg BID, over 9 days median. Among patients who received ruxolitinib, 12 (86%) achieved significant reduction of hyperinflammation, and 11 (76%) had clinical improvement without developing toxicity.

The largest available experience comes from an Italian report of 34 patients with COVID-19 who received ruxolitinib via compassionate-use protocol [73]. All patients analyzed had severe pulmonary disease not requiring mechanical ventilation. Ruxolitinib was administered at a starting dose of 5 mg BID increasing until 25 mg daily in case of worsening. Median treatment duration was 13 days. Of note, patients also received any other available therapies for COVID-19 (antiviral drugs, hydroxychloroquine, antimicrobials, corticosteroids, and prophylactic doses of subcutaneous enoxaparin).

Of 34 patients analyzed, 29 (85.3%) were discharged home by the 28-day observation period; two patients died and three patients were hospitalized by day 28. Overall survival by day 28 was 94.1%. Cumulative incidence of significant clinical improvement in the ordinal scale was 82.4% (95% CI, 71–93). Improvement of inflammatory cytokine profile and activated lymphocyte subsets was observed at day 14. Adverse events or worsening of pre-existing laboratory abnormality developed in 82% of patients without leading to drug discontinuation. The most common adverse events were anemia, urinary tract infection, increase of creatinine and aminotransferases, and thrombocytopenia. All these abnormalities resulted largely restored after ruxolitinib discontinuation.

The efficacy of ruxolitinib in patients with advanced respiratory distress due to COVID-19 was also evaluated in the RESPIRE study [74], a multicenter retrospective study.

In this study ruxolitinib was used as off-label therapy in 18 patients with COVID-19-related ARDS with a dosage of 20 mg BID for the first 48 h and subsequent with a tapering strategy according to response achievement. A maximum total of 14 days of treatment was administered. Study analysis reported no progression from NIV to mechanical ventilation in a large majority of patients (16/18). After 7 days of ruxolitinib treatment, 11 patients showed fully recovered respiratory function. At day 14 of ruxolitinib treatment, 16/18 patients showed complete respiratory recovery. Compliance to ruxolitinib was good, and none of the patients discontinued the drug or needed a reduction of the dose. No relevant reductions in leukocyte count, erythrocytes, or platelets were observed.

Finally, the most promising trial is the RUXCOVID (NCT04362137), a phase III multicenter, randomized, double-blind, placebo-controlled, 29-day study. The trial is ongoing at time of writing and aims to evaluate the efficacy and safety of ruxolitinib plus standard of care therapy compared to placebo plus standard of care in patients aged ≥12 years hospitalized for COVID-19. Patients enrolled were not intubated or receiving ICU care prior to randomization. The study has enrolled 432 patients globally. Initial data available in December 2020 showed that there was no statistically significant reduction in the proportion of patients on ruxolitinib therapy who experienced severe complications, including death, respiratory failure, or admission to the intensive care unit, compared to standard of care alone. The trial also did not show clinically relevant benefit among secondary endpoints including mortality rate by day 29 and time to recovery. Of note, ruxolitinib was reported to be well tolerated, but analysis including safety data is ongoing at time of writing [75].

Baricitinib

Baricitinib is an inhibitor targeting Janus kinases, and it is approved by the FDA for the treatment of rheumatoid arthritis [76].

Using artificial intelligence algorithms, Richardson et al. [77] reviewed drugs inhibiting the AP2-associated protein kinase 1 (AAK1) pathway. The Janus kinase inhibitor baricitinib seemed to reduce both the viral entry and the inflammation in patients with COVID-19 without leading to serious side effects. Of note, there were some concerns about the use of baricitinib in SARS-CoV-2 patients due to the interference of drugs with endogenous interferon and immune response to virus and the risk of increasing thromboembolic events [68, 70, 76, 78].

One of the first small experiences using baricitinib for the treatment of COVID-19 comes from Italy [79]. In this open-label, non-randomized trial, patients treated with baricitinib plus lopinavir/ritonavir were compared with patients treated with standard of care therapy (lopinavir/ritonavir and hydroxychloroquine). Patients in the baricitinib group were treated for 2 weeks using a dosage of 4 mg/day. Twelve patients for baricitinib group were enrolled. Baricitinib treatment was well tolerated with no serious adverse events. No infections, thrombophlebitis, or hematologic toxicity were observed in the baricitinib group. The authors reported fever, respiratory parameters, and inflammatory markers improved at a statistically significant higher rate in the baricitinib-treated group compared with controls. In addition, ICU transfer was lower in the baricitinib group with also early discharge.

Another experience of baricitinib use for treatment of COVID-19 comes from a Spanish study [80]. In this retrospective observational study, a more homogeneous group of patients was studied. The authors compared 34 patients with COVID-19 treated with baricitinib (of them, 11 were treated also with tocilizumab) with patients treated with standard of care. Baricitinib was administered at an oral dose of 2 mg or 4 mg daily. Treatment with baricitinib was well tolerated and without serious side effects, but showing statistically significant improvement in ICU admission, mortality at 15 days, and duration of symptoms compared with control groups.

More interesting data come from the study of Rodriguez-Garcia and colleagues [81]. The authors presented an observational study enrolling patients with moderate to severe SARS-CoV-2 pneumonia receiving lopinavir/ritonavir and hydroxychloroquine therapy plus corticosteroids or corticosteroids and baricitinib. The baricitinib and corticosteroid group included 62 patients and the corticosteroid group 50 patients. Both groups received similar total doses of methylprednisolone and respiratory support. Baricitinib was administered under two regimens: a low-dose scheme with a loading dose of 4 mg the first day and then 2 mg daily (40 patients) or a high-dose scheme with 4 mg daily (22 patients). Patients older than 75 years received low-dose baricitinib. The length of therapy was 5–10 days in each group. The primary endpoint was the change in oxygen saturation (SpO_2/FiO_2) from hospitalization to discharge. A greater statistically significant improvement in SpO_2/FiO_2 from hospitalization to discharge was observed in the baricitinib group compared with the corticosteroid group ($P < 0.001$). Secondary endpoints included the proportion of patients requiring supplemental oxygen at discharge and 1 month later. Patients assigned to the baricitinib group had a lower proportion of patients requiring supplemental oxygen both at discharge (26% vs. 62%; $P < 0.001$) and 1 month later (12.9 vs. 28.0%; $P = 0.024$). Of note, there were no significant differences between the baricitinib group and the corticosteroid group regarding death and ICU admission. The authors also analyzed the low dose vs. high dose of baricitinib. In each group, the median time of therapy was 5 days. At admission to hospital, patients receiving high-dose baricitinib differed from low-dose patients in lower SpO_2/FiO_2 on ward and needed more intensive ventilatory support and a higher dose of methylprednisolone compared with patients on low-dose baricitinib. The proportion of patients requiring supplemental oxygen was similar at discharge and 1 month later. There were no differences in laboratory parameter changes between the high- and low-dose groups. This study showed a synergistic effect on respiratory function improvement of short-course baricitinib plus corticosteroid treatment in hospitalized patients, suggesting that baricitinib could improve both the host systemic inflammatory response to the virus and decrease the viral entry into the lung cells.

Another experience in patients treated with baricitinib comes from a small trial by Bronte and colleagues [82]. In this study 20 patients were treated with baricitinib (4 mg twice daily for 2 days, followed by 4 mg per day for the remaining 7 days) and compared with 56 patients who did not receive the drug. The patients enrolled in the baricitinib group did not develop deep vein thrombosis or pulmonary thromboembolism. Among the baricitinib-treated patients, the authors observed no significant difference in progression to ARDS or disease duration. Patients treated with baricitinib experienced a faster reduction in the need for oxygen ($P < 0.001$) and a more rapid increase in the P/F ratio compared to the control group ($P = 0.02$). Moreover, patients treated with baricitinib had a marked reduction in serum levels of inflammatory cytokines (IL-6, IL-1β, TNF-α), a faster recovery of circulating T and B cell, and increased antibody production against the SARS-CoV-2 spike protein.

The ACTT-2 [78], a randomized double-blind controlled trial, was designed to evaluate baricitinib plus remdesivir vs. remdesivir alone in hospitalized patients with COVID-19 pneumonia. All patients received standard supportive care. Of note, the use of glucocorticoids was not allowed and only permitted for standard indications (such as septic shock and acute respiratory distress syndrome). The study was conducted in 1033 patients, 515 assigned to the combination group and 518 to the control group. The baricitinib dose was 4 mg per day for 14 days. The primary outcome was the time to recovery within 29 days after randomization. The main secondary endpoint was clinical status on day 15. Overall, the baricitinib plus remdesivir combination regimen showed a 1-day shortening of recovery time (7 vs. 8 days, $P = 0.03$). The 28-day mortality rate was 5.1% in the baricitinib group vs. 7.8% in the control group (HR 0.65, CI 0.39–1.09). The effect size was greatest for those requiring noninvasive ventilation or high-flow oxygen and lowest for those who did not need oxygen, suggesting that stage and timing of treatment may be critical. The most commonly occurring adverse events were hyperglycemia, anemia, decreased lymphocyte count, and acute kidney injury. The incidence of these adverse events was similar in the two treatment groups. Of note, venous thromboembolism was similar in the combination group and the control group.

From this study, baricitinib plus remdesivir was superior to remdesivir alone in reducing recovery time and accelerating improvement in clinical status, especially among patients receiving high-flow oxygen or noninvasive mechanical ventilation.

At the time of writing this chapter, based on the results of the ACTT-2 trial, the combination of baricitinib with remdesivir has been granted emergency use authorization by the US Food and Drug Administration to treat COVID-19 in adults and pediatric patients [83].

Il-1 Antagonist

IL-1 includes two distinct cytokines, IL-1αand IL-1β, molecules that play important roles in the acute inflammatory response. IL-1 can be activated by a variety of triggers, such as infectious agents or endogenous signals generated by dying cells, like macrophages and monocytes. IL-1 inhibitors are approved for treating rheumatoid arthritis, systemic juvenile idiopathic arthritis, cryopyrin-associated periodic syndromes, and familial Mediterranean fever. There are also nonapproved indications in which IL-1 inhibitors seem to have a role, such as hemophagocytic lymphohistiocytosis and macrophage activation syndrome [77, 78]. All these diseases have many similar immunologic and clinical features to the inflammatory phase of COVID-19. Specifically, pulmonary macrophages are hyperactivated in COVID-19 either directly by the virus or indirectly by the products of damaged tissues [79].

Anakinra

Among the interleukin-1 inhibitors, anakinra has been used for the treatment of COVID-19. Compared with the doses used in approved indications, most studies conducted in patients with COVID-19 used higher doses of anakinra [80–82, 84–86].

Navarro-Millán et al. [84] reported a retrospective case series of 14 patients with severe COVID-19. In this case series, subcutaneous anakinra was administered in a dosage of 100 mg every 6 h for a maximum of 20 days. Primary endpoint was progression to mechanical ventilation. All patients receiving early treatment with anakinra did not require mechanical ventilation.

In another prospective observational study, the use of anakinra was evaluated in combination with methylprednisolone for severe COVID-19 pneumonia [85]. In this cohort 65 patients with severe COVID-19 pneumonia were treated with anakinra and methylprednisolone and compared to 55 patients from a historical cohort. Anakinra was administered subcutaneously at 200 mg TID for 3 days, then 100 mg TID up to day 14. Mortality was 13.9% in treated patients and 35.6% in controls ($p = 0.005$). On multivariable analysis, treatment with anakinra and methylprednisolone was found to be independently associated with survival (HR 0.18, 95%CI 0.07–0.50, $p = 0.001$). Treatment was well tolerated, and anakinra-treated patients had non-statistically significant higher gamma-glutamyl transferase and alanine transaminase increase and worse anemia and granulocytopenia than controls.

Another experience was the study of Cavalli et al. [87]. The authors conducted a retrospective cohort study including patients with COVID-19, moderate-to-severe ARDS, and hyperinflammation. They compared survival, mechanical ventilation-free survival, and changes in inflammation parameters in a cohort of 29 patients receiving anakinra (either 5 mg/kg twice a day intravenously or 100 mg twice a day subcutaneously) in addition to standard treatment to a retrospective cohort of 16 patients who did not receive anakinra. Survival was 90% in the anakinra group and 56% in the standard treatment group ($p = 0.009$). Mechanical ventilation-free survival was 72% in the anakinra group versus 50% in the standard treatment group ($p = 0.15$). Anakinra was well tolerated in all patients, with adverse events reported in seven (24%) patients (mainly increase in serum liver enzymes), but similar to those receiving standard treatment.

The largest experience of anakinra use came from a prospective, open-label, interventional study in adults hospitalized with severe COVID-19 pneumonia conducted by Balkhair et al. [88]. In this study patients received subcutaneous anakinra at dosage of 100 mg BID daily for 3 days followed by 100 mg daily for 7 days in addition to standard treatment. The authors compared 45 patients treated with anakinra with 24 historical controls. The outcomes were need for mechanical ventilation, in-hospital death, weaning from supplemental oxygen, and change in inflammatory biomarkers. Patients treated with anakinra were compared to historical controls who received standard treatment. The anakinra group was superior in all outcomes: need for mechanical ventilation (31% vs. 75%, $p < 0.001$), in-hospital mortality (29% vs. 46%, $p = 0.082$), and weaning from supplemental oxygen (63% vs. 27%, $p = 0.008$). In addition, patients who received anakinra compared with historical controls showed significant reduction in IL-6 ($p < 0.001$), C-reactive protein ($p = 0.001$), lactate dehydrogenase ($p = 0.011$), and D-dimer levels ($p = 0.001$).

Another prospective cohort of 52 patients with severe COVID-19 pneumonia treated with anakinra was compared with 44 patients from a historical control cohort with similar baseline characteristics [85]. Anakinra was used at 100 mg twice a day for 72 h, then 100 mg daily for 7 days. Patients in the historical group received standard treatments and supportive care. The need for invasive mechanical ventilation or death was 25% in the anakinra group vs. 73% in the historical cohort group (95% CI 0.10–0.49, $p = 0.0002$). An increase in liver aminotransferases occurred in seven (13%) patients in the anakinra group and four (9%) patients in the historical group.

Regarding laboratory abnormalities, anakinra can cause neutropenia, thrombocytopenia, and elevations of hepatic aminotransferases [86, 87]. The incidence of serious infection associated with IL-1 inhibitors is very low but not absent [87]. In a large observational study of anakinra for acute gout, no serious infectious complications were reported [89].

All these non-randomized studies seem promising for the use of anakinra in the treatment of severe COVID-19, but randomized, controlled trials are needed to confirm these results.

References

1. Hamming I, Timens W, Bulthuis ML, Lely AT, Navis G, van Goor H. Tissue distribution of ACE2 protein, the functional receptor for SARS coronavirus. A first step in understanding SARS pathogenesis. J Pathol. 2004;203:631–7.
2. Kang Y, Chen T, Mui D, Ferrari V, Jagasia D, Scherrer-Crosbie M, et al. Cardiovascular manifestations and treatment considerations in COVID-19. Heart. 2020;106:1132–41.
3. Su H, Yang M, Wan C, Yi LX, Tang F, Zhu HY, et al. Renal histopathological analysis of 26 postmortem findings of patients with COVID-19 in China. Kidney Int. 2020;98:219–27.
4. Pan L, Mu M, Yang P, Sun Y, Wang R, Yan J, et al. Clinical characteristics of COVID-19 patients with digestive symptoms in Hubei, China: a descriptive, cross-sectional, multicenter study. Am J Gastroenterol. 2020;115:766–73.
5. Hadjadj J, Yatim N, Barnabei L, Corneau A, Boussier J, Smith N, et al. Impaired type I interferon activity and inflammatory responses in severe COVID-19 patients. Science. 2020;369:718–24.
6. Lee JS, Shin EC. The type I interferon response in COVID-19: implications for treatment. Nat Rev Immunol. 2020;20:585–6.
7. Wu Z, McGoogan JM. Characteristics of and important lessons from the coronavirus disease 2019 (COVID-19) outbreak in China: summary of a report of 72314 cases from the Chinese Center for Disease Control and Prevention. JAMA. 2020;323:1239–42.
8. Richardson S, Hirsch JS, Narasimhan M, Crawford JM, McGinn T, Davidson KW, et al. Presenting characteristics, comorbidities, and outcomes among 5700 patients hospitalized with COVID-19 in the New York City Area. JAMA. 2020;323:2052–9.
9. Grasselli G, Pesenti A, Cecconi M. Critical care utilization for the COVID-19 outbreak in Lombardy, Italy: early experience and forecast during an emergency response. JAMA. 2020;323:1545–6.
10. Huang C, Wang Y, Li X, Ren L, Zhao J, Hu Y, et al. Clinical features of patients infected with 2019 novel coronavirus in Wuhan, China. Lancet. 2020;395:497–506.
11. Bartoletti M, Giannella M, Scudeller L, Tedeschi S, Rinaldi M, Bussini L, et al. Development and validation of a prediction model for severe respiratory failure in hospitalized patients with SARS-CoV-2 infection: a multicentre cohort study (PREDI-CO study). Clin Microbiol Infect. 2020;26:1545–53.
12. Horby P, Lim WS, Emberson JR, Mafham M, Bell JL, Linsell L, et al. Dexamethasone in hospitalized patients with Covid-19. N Engl J Med. 2021;384:693–704.

13. Bartoletti M, Azap O, Barac A, Bussini L, Ergonul O, Krause R, et al. ESCMID COVID-19 Living guidelines: drug treatment and clinical management. Clin Microbiol Infect. 2022;28:222–38.
14. Bartoletti M, Marconi L, Scudeller L, Pancaldi L, Tedeschi S, Giannella M, et al. Efficacy of corticosteroid treatment for hospitalized patients with severe COVID-19: a multicentre study. Clin Microbiol Infect. 2021;27:105–11.
15. Zhu Z, Cai T, Fan L, Lou K, Hua X, Huang Z, et al. Clinical value of immune-inflammatory parameters to assess the severity of coronavirus disease 2019. Int J Infect Dis. 2020;95:332–9.
16. Del Valle DM, Kim-Schulze S, Huang HH, Beckmann ND, Nirenberg S, Wang B, et al. An inflammatory cytokine signature predicts COVID-19 severity and survival. Nat Med. 2020;26:1636–43.
17. Mathew D, Giles JR, Baxter AE, Oldridge DA, Greenplate AR, Wu JE, et al. Deep immune profiling of COVID-19 patients reveals distinct immunotypes with therapeutic implications. Science. 2020;369:eabc8511.
18. Parasher A. COVID-19: current understanding of its pathophysiology, clinical presentation and treatment. Postgrad Med J. 2021;97:312–20.
19. Group RC, Horby P, Lim WS, Emberson JR, Mafham M, Bell JL, et al. Dexamethasone in hospitalized patients with Covid-19. N Engl J Med. 2021;384:693–704.
20. Dequin PF, Heming N, Meziani F, Plantefeve G, Voiriot G, Badie J, et al. Effect of hydrocortisone on 21-day mortality or respiratory support among critically ill patients with COVID-19: a randomized clinical trial. JAMA. 2020;324:1298–306.
21. Jeronimo CMP, Farias MEL, Val FFA, Sampaio VS, Alexandre MAA, Melo GC, et al. Methylprednisolone as adjunctive therapy for patients hospitalized with coronavirus disease 2019 (COVID-19; Metcovid): a randomized, double-blind, phase IIb, placebo-controlled trial. Clin Infect Dis. 2021;72:e373–e81.
22. Angus DC, Derde L, Al-Beidh F, Annane D, Arabi Y, Beane A, et al. Effect of hydrocortisone on mortality and organ support in patients with severe COVID-19: the REMAP-CAP COVID-19 corticosteroid domain randomized clinical trial. JAMA. 2020;324:1317–29.
23. Tomazini BM, Maia IS, Cavalcanti AB, Berwanger O, Rosa RG, Veiga VC, et al. Effect of dexamethasone on days alive and ventilator-free in patients with moderate or severe acute respiratory distress syndrome and COVID-19: the CoDEX randomized clinical trial. JAMA. 2020;324:1307–16.
24. Munch MW, Meyhoff TS, Helleberg M, Kjaer MN, Granholm A, Hjortso CJS, et al. Low-dose hydrocortisone in patients with COVID-19 and severe hypoxia: The COVID STEROID randomised, placebo-controlled trial. Acta Anaesthesiol Scand. 2021;65:1421–30.
25. Villar J, Ferrando C, Martinez D, Ambros A, Munoz T, Soler JA, et al. Dexamethasone treatment for the acute respiratory distress syndrome: a multicentre, randomised controlled trial. Lancet Respir Med. 2020;8:267–76.
26. Edalatifard M, Akhtari M, Salehi M, Naderi Z, Jamshidi A, Mostafaei S, et al. Intravenous methylprednisolone pulse as a treatment for hospitalised severe COVID-19 patients: results from a randomised controlled clinical trial. Eur Respir J. 2020;56.
27. Scott LJ. Correction to: Tocilizumab: a review in rheumatoid arthritis. Drugs. 2018;78:285.
28. Jones G, Ding C. Tocilizumab: a review of its safety and efficacy in rheumatoid arthritis. Clin Med Insights Arthritis Musculoskelet Disord. 2010;3:81–9.
29. Maude SL, Laetsch TW, Buechner J, Rives S, Boyer M, Bittencourt H, et al. Tisagenlecleucel in children and young adults with B-cell lymphoblastic leukemia. N Engl J Med. 2018;378:439–48.
30. Chilimuri S, Sun H, Alemam A, Kang KS, Lao P, Mantri N, et al. Tocilizumab use in patients with moderate to severe COVID-19: a retrospective cohort study. J Clin Pharm Ther. 2021;46:440–6.
31. Guaraldi G, Meschiari M, Cozzi-Lepri A, Milic J, Tonelli R, Menozzi M, et al. Tocilizumab in patients with severe COVID-19: a retrospective cohort study. Lancet Rheumatol. 2020;2:e474–e84.

32. Kewan T, Covut F, Al-Jaghbeer MJ, Rose L, Gopalakrishna KV, Akbik B. Tocilizumab for treatment of patients with severe COVID-19: a retrospective cohort study. EClin Med. 2020;24:100418.
33. Salvarani C, Dolci G, Massari M, Merlo DF, Cavuto S, Savoldi L, et al. Effect of tocilizumab vs standard care on clinical worsening in patients hospitalized with COVID-19 pneumonia: a randomized clinical trial. JAMA Intern Med. 2021;181:24–31.
34. Hermine O, Mariette X, Tharaux PL, Resche-Rigon M, Porcher R, Ravaud P. Effect of Tocilizumab vs usual care in adults hospitalized with COVID-19 and moderate or severe pneumonia: a randomized clinical trial. JAMA Intern Med. 2021;181:32–40.
35. Rosas IO, Brau N, Waters M, Go RC, Hunter BD, Bhagani S, et al. Tocilizumab in hospitalized patients with severe Covid-19 pneumonia. N Engl J Med. 2021;384:1503–16.
36. Stone JH, Frigault MJ, Serling-Boyd NJ, Fernandes AD, Harvey L, Foulkes AS, et al. Efficacy of Tocilizumab in patients hospitalized with Covid-19. N Engl J Med. 2020;383:2333–44.
37. Veiga VC, Prats J, Farias DLC, Rosa RG, Dourado LK, Zampieri FG, et al. Effect of tocilizumab on clinical outcomes at 15 days in patients with severe or critical coronavirus disease 2019: randomised controlled trial. BMJ. 2021;372:n84.
38. Horby P, Pessoa-Amorim G, Peto L, Brightling C, Sarkar R, Thomas K, et al. Tocilizumab in patients admitted to hospital with COVID-19 (RECOVERY): preliminary results of a randomised, controlled, open-label, platform trial, vol. 397; 2021. p. 1637–45.
39. Gordon AC, Mouncey PR, Al-Beidh F, Rowan KM, Nichol AD, Arabi YM, et al. Interleukin-6 receptor antagonists in critically ill patients with Covid-19. N Engl J Med. 2021;384:1491–502.
40. Busani S, Bedini A, Biagioni E, Serio L, Tonelli R, Meschiari M, et al. Two fatal cases of acute liver failure due to HSV-1 infection in COVID-19 patients following immunomodulatory therapies. Clin Infect Dis. 2020;73:e252–5.
41. van Rhee F, Wong RS, Munshi N, Rossi JF, Ke XY, Fossa A, et al. Siltuximab for multicentric Castleman's disease: a randomised, double-blind, placebo-controlled trial. Lancet Oncol. 2014;15:966–74.
42. Gritti G, Raimondi F, Bottazzi B, Ripamonti D, Riva I, Landi F, et al. Siltuximab downregulates interleukin-8 and pentraxin 3 to improve ventilatory status and survival in severe COVID-19. Leukemia. 2021;35(9):2734. https://doi.org/10.1038/s41375-021-01329-8.
43. Villarino AV, Kanno Y, Ferdinand JR, O'Shea JJ. Mechanisms of Jak/STAT signaling in immunity and disease. J Immunol. 2015;194:21–7.
44. Mehta RM, Bansal S, Bysani S, Kalpakam H. A shorter symptom onset to remdesivir treatment (SORT) interval is associated with a lower mortality in moderate-to-severe COVID-19: a real-world analysis. Int J Infect Dis. 2021;106:71–7.
45. Lee M, Rhee I. Cytokine signaling in tumor progression. Immune Netw. 2017;17:214–27.
46. Goker Bagca B, Biray AC. The potential of JAK/STAT pathway inhibition by ruxolitinib in the treatment of COVID-19. Cytokine Growth Factor Rev. 2020;54:51–62.
47. Mehta P, McAuley DF, Brown M, Sanchez E, Tattersall RS, Manson JJ. COVID-19: consider cytokine storm syndromes and immunosuppression. Lancet. 2020;395:1033–4.
48. Lu R, Zhao X, Li J, Niu P, Yang B, Wu H, et al. Genomic characterisation and epidemiology of 2019 novel coronavirus: implications for virus origins and receptor binding. Lancet. 2020;395:565–74.
49. Yeleswaram S, Smith P, Burn T, Covington M, Juvekar A, Li Y, et al. Inhibition of cytokine signaling by ruxolitinib and implications for COVID-19 treatment. Clin Immunol. 2020;218:108517.
50. Tasian SK, Casas JA, Posocco D, Gandre-Babbe S, Gagne AL, Liang G, et al. Mutation-specific signaling profiles and kinase inhibitor sensitivities of juvenile myelomonocytic leukemia revealed by induced pluripotent stem cells. Leukemia. 2019;33:181–90.
51. Caocci G, La Nasa G. Could ruxolitinib be effective in patients with COVID-19 infection at risk of acute respiratory distress syndrome (ARDS)? Ann Hematol. 2020;99:1675–6.
52. Kusoglu A, Bagca BG, Ay NPO, Saydam G, Avci CB. Ruxolitinib regulates the autophagy machinery in multiple myeloma cells. Anticancer Agents Med Chem. 2020;20:2316–23.

53. Harrison C, Kiladjian JJ, Al-Ali HK, Gisslinger H, Waltzman R, Stalbovskaya V, et al. JAK inhibition with ruxolitinib versus best available therapy for myelofibrosis. N Engl J Med. 2012;366:787–98.
54. Morimoto A, Nakazawa Y, Ishii E. Hemophagocytic lymphohistiocytosis: pathogenesis, diagnosis, and management. Pediatr Int. 2016;58:817–25.
55. Goldsmith SR, Saif Ur Rehman S, Shirai CL, Vij K, DiPersio JF. Resolution of secondary hemophagocytic lymphohistiocytosis after treatment with the JAK1/2 inhibitor ruxolitinib. Blood Adv. 2019;3:4131–5.
56. Choi J, Cooper ML, Alahmari B, Ritchey J, Collins L, Holt M, et al. Pharmacologic blockade of JAK1/JAK2 reduces GvHD and preserves the graft-versus-leukemia effect. PLoS One. 2014;9:e109799.
57. Zhang M, Xu CR, Shamiyeh E, Liu F, Yin JY, von Moltke LL, et al. A randomized, placebo-controlled study of the pharmacokinetics, pharmacodynamics, and tolerability of the oral JAK2 inhibitor fedratinib (SAR302503) in healthy volunteers. J Clin Pharmacol. 2014;54:415–21.
58. Shi JG, Chen X, McGee RF, Landman RR, Emm T, Lo Y, et al. The pharmacokinetics, pharmacodynamics, and safety of orally dosed INCB018424 phosphate in healthy volunteers. J Clin Pharmacol. 2011;51:1644–54.
59. Verstovsek S, Kantarjian H, Mesa RA, Pardanani AD, Cortes-Franco J, Thomas DA, et al. Safety and efficacy of INCB018424, a JAK1 and JAK2 inhibitor, in myelofibrosis. N Engl J Med. 2010;363:1117–27.
60. Vannucchi AM. Ruxolitinib versus standard therapy for the treatment of polycythemia vera. N Engl J Med. 2015;372:1670–1.
61. Zeiser R, von Bubnoff N, Butler J, Mohty M, Niederwieser D, Or R, et al. Ruxolitinib for glucocorticoid-refractory acute graft-versus-host disease. N Engl J Med. 2020;382:1800–10.
62. Kusano Y, Terui Y, Ueda K, Hatake K. Epstein-Barr virus gastric ulcer associated with ruxolitinib. Ann Hematol. 2016;95:1741–2.
63. Eyal O, Flaschner M, Ben Yehuda A, Rund D. Varicella-zoster virus meningoencephalitis in a patient treated with ruxolitinib. Am J Hematol. 2017;92:E74–E5.
64. Palmason R, Linden O, Richter J. Case-report: EBV driven lymphoproliferative disorder associated with Ruxolitinib. BMC Hematol. 2015;15:10.
65. Reoma LB, Trindade CJ, Monaco MC, Solis J, Montojo MG, Vu P, et al. Fatal encephalopathy with wild-type JC virus and Ruxolitinib therapy. Ann Neurol. 2019;86:878–84.
66. Ballesta B, Gonzalez H, Martin V, Ballesta JJ. Fatal Ruxolitinib-related JC virus meningitis. J Neurovirol. 2017;23:783–5.
67. Perricone G, Vinci M, Pungolino E. Occult hepatitis B infection reactivation after Ruxolitinib therapy. Dig Liver Dis. 2017;49:719.
68. Neubauer A, Wiesmann T, Vogelmeier CF, Mack E, Skevaki C, Gaik C, et al. Ruxolitinib for the treatment of SARS-CoV-2 induced acute respiratory distress syndrome (ARDS). Leukemia. 2020;34:2276–8.
69. Cao Y, Wei J, Zou L, Jiang T, Wang G, Chen L, et al. Ruxolitinib in treatment of severe coronavirus disease 2019 (COVID-19): a multicenter, single-blind, randomized controlled trial. J Allergy Clin Immunol. 2020;146(137–46):e3.
70. Innes AJ, Cook LB, Marks S, Bataillard E, Crossette-Thambiah C, Sivasubramaniam G, et al. Ruxolitinib for tocilizumab-refractory severe COVID-19 infection. Br J Haematol. 2020;190:e198–200.
71. Koschmieder S, Jost E, Cornelissen C, Muller T, Schulze-Hagen M, Bickenbach J, et al. Favorable COVID-19 course despite significant comorbidities in a ruxolitinib-treated patient with primary myelofibrosis. Eur J Haematol. 2020;105:655–8.
72. La Rosee F, Bremer HC, Gehrke I, Kehr A, Hochhaus A, Birndt S, et al. The Janus kinase 1/2 inhibitor ruxolitinib in COVID-19 with severe systemic hyperinflammation. Leukemia. 2020;34:1805–15.
73. Vannucchi AM, Sordi B, Morettini A, Nozzoli C, Poggesi L, Pieralli F, et al. Compassionate use of JAK1/2 inhibitor ruxolitinib for severe COVID-19: a prospective observational study. Leukemia. 2021;35:1121–33.

74. Capochiani E, Frediani B, Iervasi G, Paolicchi A, Sani S, Roncucci P, et al. Ruxolitinib rapidly reduces acute respiratory distress syndrome in COVID-19 disease. Analysis of data collection from RESPIRE protocol. Front Med. 2020;7:466.
75. Novartis. Novartis update on RUXCOVID study of ruxolitinib for hospitalized patients with COVID-19. 2021. https://www.novartis.com/news/media-releases/novartis-provides-update-ruxcovid-study-ruxolitinib-hospitalized-patients-covid-19. Accessed 28 Feb 2021.
76. Mayence A, Van den Eynde JJ. Baricitinib: a 2018 novel FDA-approved small molecule inhibiting janus kinases. Pharmaceuticals (Basel). 2019;12:37.
77. Richardson P, Griffin I, Tucker C, Smith D, Oechsle O, Phelan A, et al. Baricitinib as potential treatment for 2019-nCoV acute respiratory disease. Lancet. 2020;395:e30–e1.
78. Kalil AC, Patterson TF, Mehta AK, Tomashek KM, Wolfe CR, Ghazaryan V, et al. Baricitinib plus Remdesivir for hospitalized adults with Covid-19. N Engl J Med. 2021;384:795–807.
79. Cantini F, Niccoli L, Matarrese D, Nicastri E, Stobbione P, Goletti D. Baricitinib therapy in COVID-19: a pilot study on safety and clinical impact. J Infect. 2020;81:318–56.
80. Rosas J, Liano FP, Canto ML, Barea JMC, Beser AR, Rabasa JTA, et al. Experience with the use of Baricitinib and Tocilizumab monotherapy or combined, in patients with interstitial pneumonia secondary to coronavirus COVID19: a real-world study. Reumatol Clin. 2020;18:150–6.
81. Rodriguez-Garcia JL, Sanchez-Nievas G, Arevalo-Serrano J, Garcia-Gomez C, Jimenez-Vizuete JM, Martinez-Alfaro E. Baricitinib improves respiratory function in patients treated with corticosteroids for SARS-CoV-2 pneumonia: an observational cohort study. Rheumatology (Oxford). 2021;60:399–407.
82. Bronte V, Ugel S, Tinazzi E, Vella A, De Sanctis F, Cane S, et al. Baricitinib restrains the immune dysregulation in patients with severe COVID-19. J Clin Invest. 2020;130:6409–16.
83. (FDA) FaDA. Fact sheet for healthcare providers. Emergency use authorization (EUA) of baricitinib. US Food and Drug Administration. 2020. https://www.fda.gov/media/143823/download. Accessed 28 Feb 2021.
84. Navarro-Millan I, Sattui SE, Lakhanpal A, Zisa D, Siegel CH, Crow MK. Use of Anakinra to prevent mechanical ventilation in severe COVID-19: a case series. Arthritis Rheumatol. 2020;72:1990–7.
85. Bozzi G, Mangioni D, Minoia F, Aliberti S, Grasselli G, Barbetta L, et al. Anakinra combined with methylprednisolone in patients with severe COVID-19 pneumonia and hyperinflammation: an observational cohort study. J Allergy Clin Immunol. 2021;147:561–6e4.
86. Bresnihan B, Alvaro-Gracia JM, Cobby M, Doherty M, Domljan Z, Emery P, et al. Treatment of rheumatoid arthritis with recombinant human interleukin-1 receptor antagonist. Arthritis Rheum. 1998;41:2196–204.
87. Cavalli G, De Luca G, Campochiaro C, Della-Torre E, Ripa M, Canetti D, et al. Interleukin-1 blockade with high-dose anakinra in patients with COVID-19, acute respiratory distress syndrome, and hyperinflammation: a retrospective cohort study. Lancet Rheumatol. 2020;2:e325–e31.
88. Balkhair A, Al-Zakwani I, Al Busaidi M, Al-Khirbash A, Al Mubaihsi S, BaTaher H, et al. Anakinra in hospitalized patients with severe COVID-19 pneumonia requiring oxygen therapy: results of a prospective, open-label, interventional study. Int J Infect Dis. 2021;103:288–96.
89. Liew JW, Gardner GC. Use of Anakinra in hospitalized patients with crystal-associated arthritis. J Rheumatol. 2019;46:1345–9.
90. Salama C, Han J, Yau L, Reiss WG, Kramer B, Neidhart JD, et al. Tocilizumab in patients hospitalized with Covid-19 pneumonia. N Engl J Med. 2021;384:20–30.

Index

C. Cervera, J. M. Aguado (eds.), *Infectious Complications in Biologic and Targeted Therapies*, https://doi.org/10.1007/978-3-031-11363-5

GPSR Compliance

The European Union's (EU) General Product Safety Regulation (GPSR) is a set of rules that requires consumer products to be safe and our obligations to ensure this.

If you have any concerns about our products, you can contact us on ProductSafety@springernature.com

In case Publisher is established outside the EU, the EU authorized representative is:

Springer Nature Customer Service Center GmbH
Europaplatz 3
69115 Heidelberg, Germany

Batch number: 10732076

Printed by Printforce, the Netherlands